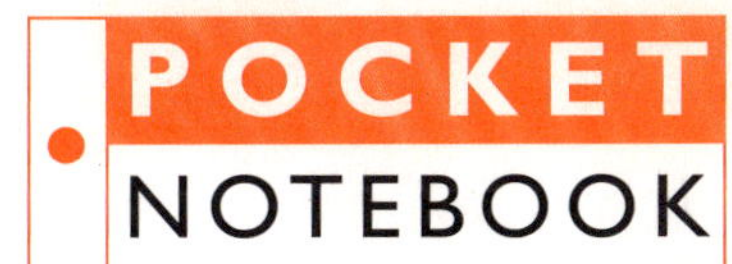

Pocket RADIATION ONCOLOGY

The MD Anderson Cancer Center Handbook of Radiation Oncology

Second Edition

Edited by

CHAD TANG, MD

AHSAN FAROOQI, MD, PhD

Advisors

ALBERT C. KOONG, MD, PhD

PRAJNAN DAS, MD, MPH

CHELSEA C. PINNIX, MD, PhD

THE UNIVERSITY OF TEXAS
MD Anderson Cancer Center
Making Cancer History®

Wolters Kluwer

Philadelphia • Baltimore • New York • London
Buenos Aires • Hong Kong • Sydney • Tokyo

Acquisitions Editor: Joe Cho
Development Editor: Cindy Yoo
Editorial Coordinator: Thirupura Sundari
Marketing Manager: Kirsten Watrud
Production Project Manager: Justin Wright
Design Coordinator: Stephen Druding
Manufacturing Coordinator: Lisa Bowling
Prepress Vendor: Straive
Second edition

10 9 8 7 6 5 4 3 2

Printed in Mexico

Cataloging-in-Publication Data available on request from the Publisher
ISBN: 978-1-9752-1894-2

---

shop.lww.com

QUADM0126

DEDICATION

We dedicate this book in memory of Dr. Cullen Taniguchi, MD, PhD, a true physician scientist and invaluable mentor, friend, and colleague to all.

CONTRIBUTORS

Chike Abana, MD, PhD
Resident Physician
Department of Radiation Oncology
The University of Texas MD Anderson Cancer Center
Houston, Texas

Lauren Andring, MD
Resident Physician
Department of Radiation Oncology
The University of Texas MD Anderson Cancer Center
Houston, Texas

Peter Balter, MD, PhD
Professor
Department of Radiation Physics
The University of Texas MD Anderson Cancer Center
Houston, Texas

Thomas Beckham, MD, PhD
Assistant Professor
Department of Radiation Oncology
The University of Texas MD Anderson Cancer Center
Houston, Texas

Vincent Bernard, MD, PhD
Resident
Department of Radiation Oncology
The University of Texas MD Anderson Cancer Center
Houston, Texas

Andrew Bishop, MD
Associate Professor
Department of Radiation Oncology
The University of Texas MD Anderson Cancer Center
Houston, Texas

Julianna Bronk, MD, PhD
Resident Physician
Department of Radiation Oncology
The University of Texas MD Anderson Cancer Center
Houston, Texas

Elaine Cha, MD
Resident Physician
Department of Radiation Oncology
The University of Texas MD Anderson Cancer Center
Houston, Texas

Joe Chang, MD, PhD
Professor
Department of Radiation Oncology
The University of Texas MD Anderson Cancer Center
Houston, Texas

Seungtaek Choi, MD
Professor
Department of Radiation Oncology
The University of Texas MD Anderson Cancer Center
Houston, Texas

Lauren Elizabeth Colbert, MD, MSCR
Assistant Professor
Department of Radiation Oncology
Division of Radiation Oncology
The University of Texas MD Anderson Cancer Center
Houston, Texas

Kelsey Corrigan, MD, MPH
Resident
Department of Radiation Oncology
The University of Texas MD Anderson Cancer Center
Houston, Texas

Bouthaina Dabaja, MD
Professor
Department of Radiation Oncology
Division of Radiation Oncology
The University of Texas MD Anderson Cancer Center
Houston, Texas

Prajnan Das, MD, MS, MPH
Professor
Department of Radiation Oncology
The University of Texas MD Anderson Cancer Center
Houston, Texas

Brian De, MD
Resident
Department of Radiation Oncology
The University of Texas MD Anderson Cancer Center
Houston, Texas

Kevin Diao, MD
Resident Physician
Department of Radiation Oncology
The University of Texas MD Anderson Cancer Center
Houston, Texas

Stephanie Dudzinski, MD, PhD
Resident Physician
Department of Radiation Oncology
The University of Texas MD Anderson Cancer Center
Houston, Texas

Penny Fang, MD, MBA
Assistant Professor
Department of Radiation Oncology
The University of Texas MD Anderson Cancer Center
Houston, Texas

Ahsan Farooqi, MD, PhD
Assistant Professor
Department of Radiation Oncology
The University of Texas MD Anderson Cancer Center
Houston, Texas

Steven J. Frank, MD
Deputy Division Head and Executive Director, Particle Therapy Institute
Department of Radiation Oncology
The University of Texas MD Anderson Cancer Center
Houston, Texas

Clifton David Fuller, MD, PhD
Professor
Department of Radiation Oncology
The University of Texas MD Anderson Cancer Center
Houston, Texas

Saumil Gandhi, MD, PhD
Assistant Professor
Department of Radiation Oncology
The University of Texas MD Anderson Cancer Center
Houston, Texas

Adam Garden, MD
Professor
Department of Radiation Oncology
The University of Texas MD Anderson Cancer Center
Houston, Texas

Amol Ghia, MD
Associate Professor
Department of Radiation Oncology
The University of Texas MD Anderson Cancer Center
Houston, Texas

Adam Grippin, MD, PhD
Resident
Department of Radiation Oncology
The University of Texas MD Anderson Cancer Center
Houston, Texas

Aaron Grossberg, MD, PhD
Assistant Professor
Department of Radiation Medicine
Oregon Health & Science University
Portland, Oregon

David Grosshans, MD, PhD
Professor
Department of Radiation Oncology
The University of Texas MD Anderson Cancer Center
Houston, Texas

Ashleigh Guadagnolo, MD, MPH
Professor
Department of Radiation Oncology
The University of Texas MD Anderson Cancer Center
Houston, Texas

Jillian Gunther, MD, PhD
Assistant Professor
Department of Radiation Oncology
The University of Texas MD Anderson Cancer Center
Houston, Texas

Karen E. Hoffman, MD, MHSc, MPH
Professor of Radiation Oncology
Department of Genitourinary Radiation Oncology
The University of Texas MD Anderson Cancer Center
Houston, Texas

Emma Holliday, MD
Associate Professor
Department of Gastrointestinal Radiation Oncology
The University of Texas MD Anderson Cancer Center
Houston, Texas

Anuja Jhingran, MD
Professor
Department of Radiation Oncology
The University of Texas MD Anderson Cancer Center
Houston, Texas

Ann Klopp, MD, PhD
Professor
Department of Radiation Oncology–Gynecology
The University of Texas MD Anderson Cancer Center
Houston, Texas

Eugene Koay, MD, PhD
Associate Professor
Department of Gastrointestinal Radiation Oncology
The University of Texas MD Anderson Cancer Center
Houston, Texas

Albert C. Koong, MD, PhD
Division Head and Chair
Department of Radiation Oncology
The University of Texas MD Anderson Cancer Center
Houston, Texas

Ramez Kouzy, MD
Resident Physician
Department of Radiation Oncology
The University of Texas MD Anderson Cancer Center
Houston, Texas

Jing Li, MD, PhD
Associate Professor
Department of Radiation Oncology
The University of Texas MD Anderson Cancer Center
Houston, Texas

Zhongxing Liao, MD
Professor
Department of Radiation Oncology
The University of Texas MD Anderson Cancer Center
Houston, Texas

Anna Likhacheva, MD, MPH
Staff Physician
Department of Radiation Oncology
Sutter Health
Sacramento, California

Lilie L. Lin, MD
Professor
Department of Radiation Oncology–Gynecology
The University of Texas MD Anderson Cancer Center
Houston, Texas

Steven Lin, MD, PhD
Professor
Department of Radiation Oncology
The University of Texas MD Anderson Cancer Center
Houston, Texas

Yufei Liu, MD, PhD
Resident Physician
Department of Radiation Oncology
The University of Texas MD Anderson Cancer Center
Houston, Texas

Ethan Ludmir, MD
Assistant Professor
Department of Gastrointestinal Radiation Oncology
The University of Texas MD Anderson Cancer Center
Houston, Texas

Gohar Manzar, MD, PhD
Resident Physician
Department of Radiation Oncology
The University of Texas MD Anderson Cancer Center
Houston, Texas

Kathryn Marqueen, MD
Resident Physician
Department of Radiation Oncology
The University of Texas MD Anderson Cancer Center
Houston, Texas

Mary McAleer, MD, PhD
Professor
Department of Radiation Oncology
The University of Texas MD Anderson Cancer Center
Houston, Texas

Wendy McGinnis, MD, MCR
Resident
Department of Radiation Oncology
The University of Texas MD Anderson Cancer Center
Houston, Texas

Susan L. McGovern, MD, PhD
Associate Professor
Department of Radiation Oncology
The University of Texas MD Anderson Cancer Center
Houston, Texas

Devarati Mitra, MD, PhD
Assistant Professor
Department of Radiation Oncology
The University of Texas MD Anderson Cancer Center
Houston, Texas

Amy Moreno, MD
Assistant Professor
Department of Radiation Oncology
The University of Texas MD Anderson Cancer Center
Houston, Texas

Quynh-Nhu Nguyen, MD, MHCM
Professor of Radiation Oncology
Department of Radiation Oncology
The University of Texas MD Anderson Cancer Center
Houston, Texas

Jared Ohrt, MS
Medical Physicist
Department of Radiation Physics
The University of Texas MD Anderson Cancer Center
Houston, Texas

Arnold Paulino, MD
Professor
Department of Radiation Oncology
The University of Texas MD Anderson Cancer Center
Houston, Texas

Subha Perni, MD
Assistant Professor
Department of Radiation Oncology
The University of Texas MD Anderson Cancer Center
Houston, Texas

Jack Phan, MD, PhD
Associate Professor
Department of Radiation Oncology
The University of Texas MD Anderson Cancer Center
Houston, Texas

Chelsea C. Pinnix, MD, PhD
Associate Professor
Department of Radiation Oncology
The University of Texas MD Anderson Cancer Center
Houston, Texas

Jay Reddy, MD, PhD
Assistant Professor
Department of Radiation Oncology
The University of Texas MD Anderson Cancer Center
Houston, Texas

Mike Rooney, MD
Resident
Department of Radiation Oncology
The University of Texas MD Anderson Cancer Center
Houston, Texas

Mohammad Salehpour, PhD
Professor and Director of Education
Department of Radiation Physics
The University of Texas MD Anderson Cancer Center
Houston, Texas

Ugur Selek, MD, FASTRO
Professor
Department of Radiation Oncology
Koc University
Istanbul, Turkey

Aaron Seo, MD, PhD
Resident Physician
Department of Radiation Oncology
The University of Texas MD Anderson Cancer Center
Houston, Texas

Shalin Shah, MD
Professor/Section Chief-Houston Area Locations
Department of Radiation Oncology
The University of Texas MD Anderson Cancer Center
Houston, Texas

Alex Sherry, MD
Resident
Department of Radiation Oncology
The University of Texas MD Anderson Cancer Center
Houston, Texas

Alan Sosa, MD
Resident Physician
Department of Radiation Oncology
The University of Texas MD Anderson Cancer Center
Houston, Texas

Shane Stecklein, MD, PhD
Assistant Professor
Department of Radiation Oncology
University of Kansas Cancer Center
Kansas City, Kansas

Chad Tang, MD
Associate Professor
Department of Radiation Oncology
The University of Texas MD Anderson Cancer Center
Houston, Texas

Cullen Taniguchi, MD, PhD
Associate Professor
Department of Gastrointestinal Radiation Oncology
The University of Texas MD Anderson Cancer Center
Houston, Texas

Martin Tom, MD
Assistant Professor
Department of Gastrointestinal Radiation Oncology
The University of Texas MD Anderson Cancer Center
Houston, Texas

Gary Walker, MD, MPH, MS
Adjunct Associate Professor
Department of Radiation Oncology
Banner MD Anderson Cancer Center
Gilbert, Arizona

Chenyang Wang, MD, PhD
Assistant Professor
Department of Radiation Oncology
The University of Texas MD Anderson Cancer Center
Houston, Texas

Wendy Woodward, MD, PhD
Professor and Chair
Department of Breast Radiation Oncology
The University of Texas MD Anderson Cancer Center
Houston, Texas

Susan Wu, MD
Assistant Professor
Department of Radiation Oncology
The University of Texas MD Anderson Cancer Center
Houston, Texas

Jinzhong Yang, PhD
Assistant Professor
Department of Radiation Physics
The University of Texas MD Anderson Cancer Center
Houston, Texas

D. Nana Yeboa, MD
Associate Professor
Department of Radiation Oncology
The University of Texas MD Anderson Cancer Center
Houston, Texas

Alison Yoder, MD, MPH
Resident Physician
Department of Radiation Oncology
The University of Texas MD Anderson Cancer Center
Houston, Texas

ACKNOWLEDGMENTS

The editors would like to acknowledge the contributors who worked on the first edition:

Mitchell S. Anscher, MD
Alexander Augustyn, MD, PhD
Zeina Ayoub, MD
Alexander F. Bagley, MD, PhD
Houda Bahig, MD
Michael Bernstein, MD
Eric D. Brooks, MD, MHS
Samantha M. Buszek, MD
Bhavana S. Vangara Chapman, MD
Kaitlin Christopherson, MD
Caroline Chung, MD, MSc
Brian J. Deegan, MD, PhD
Patricia J. Eifel, MD
Adnan Elhammali, MD, PhD
Daniel Gomez, MD
Stephen Grant, MD
Stephen Hahn, MD
Jennifer C. Ho, MD
Rachit Kumar, MD
Jennifer Logan, MD
Geoffrey V. Martin, MD
Shane Mesko, MD, MBA
Sarah Milgrom, MD
Bruce Minsky, MD
Shalini Moningi, MD
Hubert Young Pan, MD
Dario Pasalic, MD
Curtis A. Pettaway, MD
Courtney Pollard III, MD, PhD
Tommy Sheu, MD, MPH
Shervin 'Sean' Shirvani, MD, MPH
Lisa Singer, MD, PhD
Erik P. Sulman, MD, PhD
Nikhil G. Thaker, MD
Jeena Varghese, MD
Christopher Wilke, MD, PhD

FOREWORD

Rapid access to practical, up-to-date information is critical for the busy clinician juggling many demands. Given the multiple sources of information that is often just a mouse click away, it is near impossible to determine the most credible sources of medical information and to synthesize all of the data into actionable recommendations.

National guidelines regarding how to deliver radiation therapy for specific disease sites can be vague. Textbooks are either too broad or too lengthy for practitioners to interpret key concepts necessary to deliver care and become outdated rapidly. While we recognize that there are other pocket books available, we have intentionally narrowed our focus and scope of this pocket handbook to include the best practices that we have determined are necessary to deliver safe, multidisciplinary evidence-based care to our patients. This was accomplished by curating years of experience and expertise of senior radiation oncologists at MD Anderson, many of which created the cutting edge technologies discussed in this handbook. The MD Anderson residents and fellows both past and current played a major part in the creation of this pocket handbook and reviewed each of the chapters.

The goal of this pocket handbook is to provide an updated, practical set of radiation therapy guidelines that can be used to guide the active management and review of specific cases. This pocketbook is not intended to serve as a comprehensive resource; however, all of the fundamental principles are covered here to provide the practitioner with the necessary tools and information to dig deeper into specific cases as needed.

In this handbook, we have covered all of the major stages of commonly treated diseases and included treatment techniques for both common and rare malignancies. Unlike most pocket references, we have a section that is dedicated to treatment planning and dose constraints. This section also includes specific figures which are helpful in determining how treatment planning may be approached including normal tissue considerations for radiation therapy.

Recognizing the limited time that physicians and trainees have, we included only those references that drive the current clinical standards. We hope that this handbook will serve as a valuable resource for you and your peers as we endeavor to provide appropriate, safe, and quality care to our patients.

Albert C. Koong, MD, PhD
Professor and Department Chair, Radiation Oncology

PREFACE

We are delighted to introduce the second edition of *Pocket Radiation Oncology: The MD Anderson Cancer Center Handbook of Radiation Oncology*. While there are many excellent textbooks on radiation oncology, in an era of constantly evolving evidence and rapidly changing technology, there is a great need for an easily accessible handbook with clinically relevant and evidence-based information, presented in a concise and easily accessible format. We were very pleased by the response to the first edition, and we believe that the second edition will provide a timely update, while appealing to the learning styles of today's generation of adult learners.

We are grateful to all the current and past The University of Texas MD Anderson Cancer Center resident and faculty contributors who made Pocket Radiation Oncology possible. All chapters were created by resident and attending pairs, and all chapters were reviewed by a senior attending who specialized in that disease site. We are also grateful to the past and present faculty at The University of Texas MD Anderson Cancer Center, whose clinical experience and knowledge are reflected in this handbook.

Prajnan Das and Chelsea C. Pinnix, Advisors

CONTENTS

GASTROINTESTINAL

Section Editors: Brian De, Chike Abana and Prajnan Das

BREAST

Section Editors: Kelsey Corrigan and Wendy Woodward

GENITOURINARY

Section Editors: Kevin Diao and Seungtaek Choi

GYNECOLOGIC

Section Editors: Wendy McGinnis, Lauren Andring and Ann Klopp

SKIN/SARCOMA

Section Editors: Alison Yoder and Ashleigh Guadagnolo

LYMPHOMA

Section Editors: Gohar Manzar and Bouthaina Dabaja

METASTASES AND BENIGN DISEASE

Section Editors: Alex Sherry, Julianna Bronk and Amol Ghia

RADIATION BIOLOGY

STEPHANIE DUDZINSKI • AARON GROSSBERG •
CULLEN TANIGUCHI • SHANE STECKLEIN

4 Rs of Radiobiology

- **Repair**
  Lethal and sublethal ***damage repair*** *increases cell survival after fractionated radiation.*
- **Reoxygenation**
  Hypoxic cells *are radioresistant; hypoxic fraction ↑ with treatment.*
- **Redistribution**
  Lethality increases as cells redistribute to more radiosensitive stages of ***cell cycle****.*
- **Repopulation**
  Repopulation increases cell survival over a ***long treatment time****; accelerated in some cancers. Can be triggered by radiation.*

Molecular Signaling and Pathways

- **Oncogene:** Normal function is to positively regulate cellular growth, that is, *RAS, MYC, ABL, and ERBB2.*
- **Tumor suppressor gene:** Normal function is to negatively regulate cellular growth, that is, *TP53, RB, VHL, and PTEN.*
- **Cellular signaling pathways**
  - EGFR-MAPK: Prosurvival pathway involving the EGFR family of tyrosine kinases
    - EGFR (ErbB-1): Targeting by cetuximab
    - HER2/neu (ErbB-2): Targeted by trastuzumab
    - Her3 and Her4: Not as commonly mutated in cancer
  - Ras: G protein bound to cellular membrane that transmits signals from activated tyrosine kinases
    - K-RAS: Mutated in colon and lung cancer
    - N-RAS: Mutated in neuroblastoma
    - H-RAS: Bladder cancer
- VEGFR: Leads to angiogenesis, also involves tyrosine kinase pathways. Targeted by bevacizumab
- PI3K-Akt-mTOR pathway: PI3K is a membrane-bound protein that is negatively regulated by PTEN, and whose downstream targets include Akt and mTOR, which activate cellular survival, proliferation, and angiogenesis. Targeted by rapamycin, temsirolimus, and everolimus (immune-suppressive drugs), which can also inhibit various cancers that activate this pathway (ie, renal cell carcinoma)
- BCR-ABL: Tyrosine kinase pathway activated in chronic myelogenous leukemia (via classic 9:22 chromosomal translocation) that is targeted by imatinib
- ALK: Tyrosine kinase that is prosurvival and found mutated in NSCLC and hereditary neuroblastoma leading to constitutive activation. Targeted by ALK inhibitor crizotinib

Telomeres, Telomerase, and Cancer

- Due to the end replication problem, a cell loses between 50 and 200 bp per cell division.
- Telomeres are repetitive elements consisting of the (TTAGGG)n repeats found at the ends of our chromosomes that serve as a buffer to our coding DNA.
- After ~40-50 population doublings, most cell lines in culture reach critically short telomere lengths, which triggers senescence/apoptosis (Hayflick limit).
- Cancer cells counteract telomere shortening by activating telomere maintenance mechanisms.
  - Telomerase: Activated in ~85% of all cancers. Increased telomerase activity has been associated with mutations in the *TERT* promoter gene (which encodes the catalytic component of telomerase) seen in tumors of neural or mesenchymal origin (*Killela PNAS* 2013).
  - Alternative lengthening of telomeres: Activated in 10-15% of cancers. Poorly understood mechanism but thought to utilize homologous recombination machinery to maintain telomere length. Associated with mutations in *ATRX/DAXX/H3.3.*

DNA Damage and Repair

- **DNA damage:** Defined as any covalent modifications of the nucleotide backbone (exception being cytosine methylation)
    - Occurs at a high frequency from both endogenous and exogenous sources
- Approximately 1 Gy of ionizing radiation leads to ~40 double-strand breaks (DSBs), >1000 base damages, and ~1000 single-strand breaks (SSBs)
- DNA repair pathways
    - Base excision repair (*APE1, PCNA, FEN1, XRCC1*): Functions to repair base damage utilizing DNA glycosylase and endonucleases
    - Nucleotide excision repair: Can be initiated by either the global genomic pathway (*ERCC1, XPF, XPG*) or transcription coupled (stalled RNA polymerase complexes). Defects in this pathway lead to hereditary xeroderma pigmentosum.
    - Mismatch repair: *MLH1, MSH2, MSH4, MSH6*. Functions to excise the incorrect nucleotide and replace with the correct one. Mutations in genes involved in this pathway lead to microsatellite instability (MSI) and hereditary nonpolyposis colorectal cancer (HNPCC).
    - Nonhomologous end joining (NHEJ): Immediate response of a cell to correct a DNA double-strand break. Compared to homologous recombination, this process is rapid but is more prone to errors. First there is end recognition by binding of Ku proteins → recruitment of DNA-dependent protein kinases (DNA-PKcs) → end-processing, bridging, and ligation. Typically, active in the G1 phase of the cell cycle, where there is no sister chromatid, but occurs throughout the cell cycle.
    - Homologous recombination: High-fidelity mechanism compared to NHEJ for repair of DNA DSBs. Requires sequence homology to rejoin the broken DNA ends; hence this repair process is active in the S and G2 phases of the cell cycle. Following ATM-mediated DNA DSB recognition, the Mre11/Rad50/NBS1 complex is recruited for 3′ end resection. RAD51/RAD52 then mediate strand invasion of the homologous strand on the sister chromatid in conjunction with BRCA1 and BRCA2 proteins. Inactivation of HRR genes greatly increase radiosensitivity in in vitro models.

Mechanisms of Cell Death

- DNA is the target of radiation-induced cell lethality.
- Apoptosis: Programmed cell death mechanism that is common in embryonic development. Primary mode of cell death in hemopoietic and lymphoid cells following radiation. Importantly, this is a p53-mediated cellular death pathway (which is mutated in numerous cancers). BCL-2 counteracts the initiation of apoptosis. Can be initiated by the extrinsic pathway (via FAS-L and TRAILR) or intrinsic pathway (as a result of DNA damage, hypoxia, and metabolic stress). Both pathways lead to activation of caspases that disrupt mitochondrial outer membrane permeabilization leading to cytochrome c release and subsequent chromatin condensation → DNA fragmentation → cell death.
- Mitotic catastrophe: Results from aberrated mitosis due to radiation-induced lethal DNA DSBs. Primary mode of death following radiation in nonhematopoietic cells. Many tumors have deficient p53 and abrogated cell-cycle checkpoints that allow cells to progress into G2/M despite sustaining DNA DSBs as a result of radiation. **The three major lethal chromosomal aberrations induced from radiation are formation of dicentric chromosomes, rings, and anaphase bridges.**
- Radiation-induced senescence: Has been reported in in vitro models following extensive stress due to DNA damage induced from radiation. Classically, senescence (or permanent cellular arrest) occurs as a result of telomere shortening due to aging. However, DNA damage that results from low doses of radiation can induce accelerated senescence due to a persistently up-regulated DNA damage response proteins. There is some clinical evidence of radiation-induced senescence in slow growing tumors following radiation (ie, prostate cancer). Can stain for beta-galactosidase via immunohistochemistry to assess for senescence in vitro.

Acute Effects of Total Body Irradiation

Vomiting Onset	Est. Dose
<10 min	>8 Gy
10-30 min	6-8 Gy
30 min to 1 h	4-6 Gy
1-2 h	2-4 Gy
>2 h	<2 Gy

- **LD_{50}**
  - **3.25-4 Gy** (without treatment)
  - **~7 Gy** (with antibiotics, supportive care)
  - **~10 Gy** (with BMT)
  - *No survivors >10 Gy exposure*
- **Prodromal syndrome**
  - <50% lethal dose: Easy fatigability, anorexia, vomiting
  - Supralethal dose: Fever, hypotension, immediate diarrhea
- **REAC/TS triage based on vomiting onset time**
  - Vomit <4 hours → immediate hospital evaluation (median dose 3.6 Gy)
  - Vomit >4 hours → delayed (1-3 days) hospital evaluation (median dose 0.9 Gy)
- **Hematopoietic syndrome**
  - Dose: 2.5-5 Gy
  - Time: Death within 4-8 weeks
  - Symptoms: (1) Prodromal syndrome; (2) latent period; (3) ~3 weeks → chills, fatigue, petechial hemorrhages, loss of hair, infections (usually anemia not seen)
- **GI syndrome**
  - Dose: 5-12 Gy
  - Time: Death in 9-10 days, due to loss of intestinal lining
  - Symptoms: (1) Prodromal syndrome; (2) prolonged diarrhea (indicates *dose >10 Gy*)
- **Cerebrovascular syndrome**
  - Dose: >100 Gy
  - Time: Death in hours, due to capillary leakage in brain
  - Symptoms: (1) Nausea/vomiting *in minutes*; (2) disorientation, loss of coordination of muscular movement, respiratory distress, diarrhea, convulsive seizures, coma
- **Treatment**
  - <2 Gy: No treatment
  - 2-5 Gy: Expectant management (eg, antibiotics, transfusions)
  - 5-7 Gy: Prophylactic antibiotics, transfusions
  - 8-10 Gy: Bone marrow transplant
  - >10 Gy: GI death; supportive care
  - Colony-stimulating factors given for >2-3 Gy within 24-72 hours

Normal Tissue Toxicity

- **Early effects** <60 days; rapid cell turnover, due to acute cell killing; repaired within 2 months
  - High α/β; less sensitive to fraction size; toxicity based on total Gy and Gy/week
  - Prolonging radiation allows for repopulation (↓ acute effects)
  - **Latency period** = lifespan of functional cell
- **Late effects** >60 days; tissues without rapid turnover; **never completely repaired**
  - Low α/β; more sensitive to *fraction size*; toxicity based on *total Gy* and *Gy/fx*
  - *Fractionation decreases late effects, but not over a clinically relevant time.*
- **Serial organ:** Loss of function in one part causes whole organ dysfunction (CNS; GI tract).
  - No threshold volume; probability of damage proportional to volume irradiated
  - Risk dominated by D_{max}
- **Parallel organ:** Loss of function in one part only impacts that part (kidney, lung, liver).
  - Threshold volume effect
  - Risk dominated by **average dose** or **volume receiving threshold dose**
- **Skin tolerance:** ~60 Gy (depending on volume irradiated and fractionation)
  - Acute effects occur in epidermis: Erythema (rapid); desquamation (~14 days); epilation (~2-3 weeks, takes ~3 months to regrow)
  - Late effects occur in dermis: Telangiectasias and fibrosis

Oxygen Effects

- **Most potent modifying factor of cell kill by ionizing radiation**
- **Must be present within microseconds of IR**
  - **"Oxygen fixation"**: Formation of peroxyl radical permanently changes DNA structure.
  - Hydroxyl radical (·OH) most important radical for indirect damage to DNA
- **Oxygen enhancement ratio** $\frac{d_{hypoxic}}{d_{oxic}}$
  - OER range 2.5-3.0 (typically 2.8)
  - Requires very little O_2 (3 mmHg or ~0.5% O_2)
  - Higher LET reduces OER.
  - Optimal LET: 100 keV/μM (width of double helix)
- **Tumor hypoxia**
  - Hypoxic cells thought to be "treatment resistant"
  - Diffusional capacity of O_2 ~180 μM from capillary
  - Typical hypoxic fraction ~10-15% with standard fractionation
  - Hypoxic fraction ↑ as tumor size ↑
  - Hypoxic fraction ↑ as dose/fx ↑
- **Therapeutic approaches to hypoxia**
  - Raising tumor oxygenation: 100% O_2, hyperbaric, carbogen, transfusion, nicotinamide
  - Hypoxic cell sensitization
  - Nimorazole was tested as a hypoxic radiosensitizer in supraglottic laryngeal and pharyngeal cancer by the Danish HNC. It was found to improve LRC (49% vs 33%) and DSS (52% vs 41%) w/ minor side effects (*Overgaard et al. Radiother Oncol* 1998)
  - Hypoxic cell cytotoxins: Mitomycin C, doxorubicin, metronidazole, tirapazamine (no clear hypoxia-modulating clinical benefit shown)

Radioprotectors

Goal: Enhance therapeutic ratio

- Reoxygenation: Vasoconstriction or free radical scavenging
  - **Sulfhydryl compounds (amifostine)**, SOD, DMSO, CO, NaCN, epinephrine
- Repair: H donation to facilitate repair
  - **Sulfhydryl compounds (amifostine)**, glutathione, cysteine
- Reassortment: Induce senescence via p53; cell cycle arrest
- Repopulation: Enhance stem cell growth
  - For example, R-spondin for intestinal stem cells

Amifostine is the only FDA-approved radioprotector

- Administer 30 minutes prior to RT; reduces mucositis and xerostomia (head and neck ca); pneumonitis and esophagitis (lung ca); can also be renal protective in patients receiving cisplatin.
  - More effective if given in *morning*
- Selective for normal tissue because
  - Requires alk phos to activate (low in tumor tissue)
  - Hypovascularity and hypoxia of tumor limits amifostine penetration
  - Acidic environment of tumor prevents activation
- Side effects: Nausea and hypotension (~60% of pts; BP reverts w/in 15 minutes)

Carcinogenesis and Heritable Effects

Effective dose-Sievert (Sv) weighted for both radiation type and volume of tissue irradiated

$$\text{Effective dose }(\text{Sv}) = \text{dose }(\text{Gy}) \times \text{WF} \times \text{fraction of tissue irradiated}$$

- Photon/e^- *WF* = *1*; proton *WF* = *2*; neutron *WF up to 20*; heavy ion *WF* = *20*
- Can be calculated per *tissue* or per *whole body*

Average annual human exposure to ionizing radiation

- World: 3 mSv/y
- USA: 6 mSv/y
- **Deterministic:** Effect occurs after exceeding threshold dose and severity correlates with dose.
  - For example, skin erythema, epilation, sterility, cataracts, lethality, fetal abnormality

- **Stochastic:** Effect occurs randomly with probability proportional to dose (no safe threshold).
  - For example secondary malignancies and heritable effects

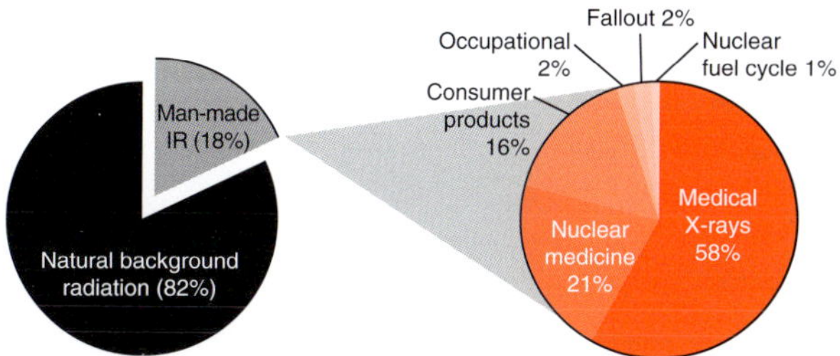

Data from the National Council on Radiation Protection and Measurements (NCRP). Report No. 93, Ionizing Radiation Exposure of the Population of the United States, 1987.

Radiation carcinogenesis

- **Solid tumors**
  - Within radiation field receiving >50 cGy
  - Latency ≥5 years
  - Usually different tumor type than original, most often a sarcoma
- **Leukemia**
  - Latency ≥5 years
  - Bone marrow >50 cGy
  - non-CLL
- Cancer induction: *Carcinogen dominant*
  - ↑ incidence of uncommon cancers assoc. w/ ↑ carcinogen exposure
  - Exposure stigmata (long-standing changes in affected tissues)
    - Radium-bone, aniline dye-bladder, uranium-lung, chimney sweep-scrotal, ALL
- Cancer enhancement: Predominant mechanism—*carcinogen participant*
  - ↑ incidence of common cancers assoc. w/ ↓ carcinogen exposure
  - Normal-appearing affected tissue
    - Thyroid (well-diff.), breast, skin (SCC/BCC ≫ sarcoma), ovary, lung, colon
    - RT for Hodgkin's ↑ breast ca risk (RR = 3.2 at 4 Gy; RR = 8 at 40 Gy)
    - RT for prostate ↑ secondary ca (rectal, bladder, sarcoma) RR = 1.34 at 10 years

Risk estimate for malignancy

- **10%/Sv** for entire population and high dose (>0.2 Gy) or dose rate (>0.1 Gy/h)
- **8%/Sv** for working population and high dose or dose rate
- **5%/Sv** for entire population and low dose or dose rate
- **4%/Sv** for working population and low dose or dose rate

Hereditary effects: Radiation effects that can be transferred from parent to progeny

- Radiation-caused changes in the genetic material of sex cells (germ-line mutations)
- Radiation does not produce new, unique mutations but *increases the incidence* of the same mutations that occur spontaneously.
- Doubling dose (increase spontaneous mutation rate twofold) = 1 Gy

Fertility effects

- **Male: >0.15 Gy** causes temporary infertility.
  - **3.5-6 Gy** causes permanent sterility.
  - 10-week delay for onset of infertility after exposure
  - Can take up to 6 months for fertility to return
- **Female: 2.6-6 Gy** causes permanent infertility
  - Sensitivity ↑ with age

ICRP risk estimate for hereditary effects (calculated using gonad dose)

0.41-0.64%/Sv/child of an irradiated individual
Total population **0.2%/Sv/individual;** working population **0.1%/Sv/individual**

Not more than 1-6% of spontaneous mutations ascribed to background radiation

Individual dose limits

- General public: 5 mSv total body, 15 mSv lens, 50 mSv other single organ
  - Continuous exposure: 1 mSv total body
- Radiation worker: 50 mSv total body, 150 mSv lens, 500 mSv other single organ
- Monthly limit of *declared pregnant woman* is **0.5 mSv/mo**

Area dose limits

- Uncontrolled area: ≤0.02 mSv/h and ≤0.1 mSv/wk
- Controlled area: ≤1 mSv/wk

Imaging	mSv	mrem	cGy
CXR	0.05	5	0.005
KUB	1	100	0.1
PET	4	400	0.4
Whole-body CT	~10	1000	1

Effects on the Embryo and Fetus

- **Sensitive period: 10 days to 26 weeks of gestation**
- **Preimplantation (0-9 days)**
  - Very low dose (0.05-0.15 Gy) leads to *prenatal death*; all or nothing effect
- **Organogenesis (10 days to 6 weeks)**
  - Structural malformation and IUGR most common; growth restriction resolves over time
  - Threshold dose >0.2 Gy
- **Fetal stage (>6 weeks)**
  - LD_{50} approaches that of adults (~3.5 Gy)
  - *Permanent* growth disturbances *without* malformation
- **Dose**
  - Microcephaly >10-19 cGy
  - Cognitive decline as low as 10 cGy; <5 cGy *probably* acceptable risk
  - Discussion of birth defects and possible actions at doses >0.1 cGy
  - Therapeutic abortion considered above 10 cGy to embryo during 10 days to 26 weeks
  - Max permissible dose to fetus is 5 mSv (0.5 rem); 0.5 mSv/mo (0.05 rem)
- **Teratogenesis**
  - Exposure of 1 cGy ↑ relative risk of cancer by 40%
  - Absolute excess risk is ~6%/Gy.

Equivalent Dose

- $$BED_{\alpha/\beta} = n \times d \times \left(1 + \frac{d}{\alpha/\beta}\right)$$
- $$EQD_{2Gy} = n \times d \times \left(\frac{\alpha/\beta + d}{\alpha/\beta + 2}\right)$$
- $$EQD_{\alpha/\beta} = n \times d_2 \times \left(\frac{\alpha/\beta + d_2}{\alpha/\beta + d_1}\right)$$

n = no. of fractions
d = dose/fraction

Linear Energy Transfer

Radiation	LET (keV/µm)
kV x-ray, γ	2-4
MV x-ray, γ, e^-	0.2-0.5
Fast protons	0.5

Radiation	LET (keV/μm)
Slow protons	~5
Fast neutrons	~100
α-Particles	~100
Heavy ions	200-1000
Optimal RBE	100

Alpha/Beta Ratios

Normal Tissue	Late Reaction	α/β
Spinal cord	Cervical	1.5-3.0
	Lumbar	2.3-4.9
Lung	Pneumonitis	4.0
	Fibrosis	3.1
Bladder	Frequency	5-10
Skin	Telangiectasia	2.6-2.8
	Fibrosis	1.7
Optic nerve	Neuropathy	1.6
Brachial plexus	Plexopathy	2-3.5
Small bowel		3.5-4.0
Supraglottic larynx		3.8
OC/OPX		0.8

Normal Tumor	α/β
Larynx	15-50
Nasopharynx	15-20
Oropharynx	13-19
Tonsil	7-10
Oral cavity	6.6
Skin	8.5
Esophagus	4-5
Breast	3-5
Rhabdomyosarcoma	2.8
Prostate	1-1.5
Melanoma	0.6
Liposarcoma	0.4

Normal Tissue	Early Reaction	α/β
Skin	Desquamation	9-12.5
Jejunum	Clones	6-10.7
Colon	Weight loss	13-19
	Clones	8-9
Testis	Clones	12-13
OC/OPX	Mucositis	8-15

RADIATION PHYSICS

AARON GROSSBERG • MOHAMMAD SALEHPOUR

PHOTON DOSIMETRY

Hand calcs *(make sure to include appropriate corrections for extended SSD/SAD)*

- **SAD**

$$MU = \frac{\text{Rx dose} \times \text{beam weight}}{OF \times \left(\frac{SCD}{SPD}\right)^2 \times S_c \times S_p \times TMR \times TF \times WF \times OAR}$$

Dose to a different depth (SAD)

$$Dose_B = Dose_A \times \frac{TMR_B}{TMR_A} \times \left(\frac{SPD_A}{SPD_B}\right)^2$$

- **SSD**

$$MU = \frac{\text{Rx dose} \times \text{beam weight}}{OF \times \left(\frac{SCD}{SSD + d_{max}}\right)^2 \times S_c \times S_p \times PDD \times TF \times WF \times OAR}$$

Mayneord *F* factor (at distance *d*)

$$F = \left[\frac{SSD + d_{max}}{100 + d_{max}} \times \frac{100 + d}{SSD + d}\right]^2$$

Dose to a different depth (SSD)

$$Dose_B = Dose_A \times \frac{PDD_B}{PDD_A}$$

OF = output factor calibrated at SCD
SCD = source to calibration distance
- Typically SCD = 100 cm for SAD and 100 cm + d_{max} for SSD

SPD = source to point distance
S_c = collimator scatter factor
S_p = phantom scatter factor
TMR = tissue maximum ratio
PDD = percent depth dose = dose at depth/d_{max}
- if SSD ≠ 100, then: **PDD_{new} = Mayneord *F* factor × $PDD_{(SSD = 100)}$**

Equivalent square: $ES = \frac{2WL}{W + L}$

Photon d_{max} (cm)	Photon Attenuation *in Tissue*	PDD
• ^{60}Co—0.5 • 4 MV—1.0 • 6 MV—1.5 • 10 MV—2.5 • 15 MV—3.0 • 18 MV—3.3 • 20 MV—3.5 • 25 MV—4.0	• ^{60}Co ~4.0%/cm • 6 MV ~3.3%/cm • 18 MV ~2.0%/cm 1 cm of air (eg, lung tissue) is equivalent to 0.3 cm of soft tissue/fluid	($SSD_{100\ cm}$, $ES_{10\ cm}$, d = 10 cm) • ^{60}Co—56% • 4 MV—61% • 6 MV—67% • 10 MV—73% • 20 MV—80% • 25 MV—83%

ELECTRON DOSIMETRY

Factors that affect PDD

- ↑ energy → ↑PDD
- ↑ field size → ↑ PDD
- ↑ SSD → ↑ PDD
- ↑ depth → ↓ PDD

Factors that affect skin dose

- ↑ energy → ↓ skin dose
- ↑ field size → ↑ skin dose
- ↑ SSD → ↓ skin dose
- ↑ obliquity → ↑ skin dose
- beam spoiler → ↑ skin dose
- bolus → ↑ skin dose
- underwedging → ↑ skin dose

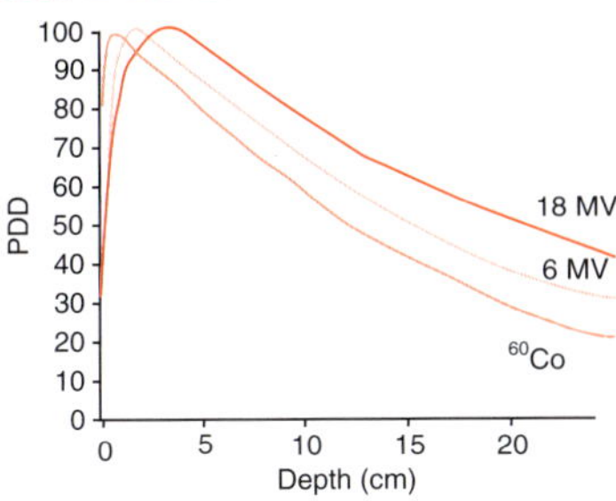

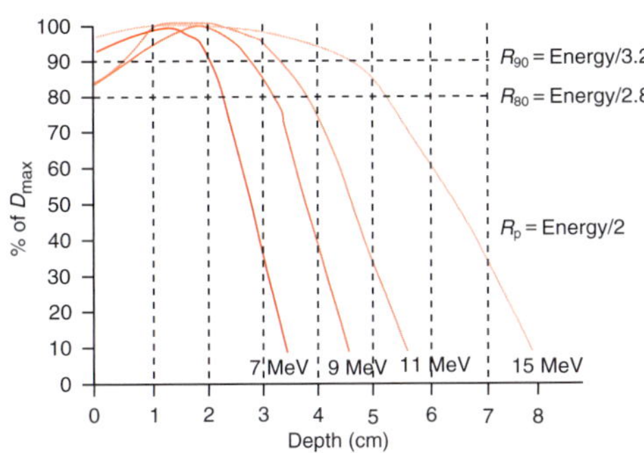

e⁻ Energy	R_{90}	R_{80}	R_p
7 MeV	2.1 cm	2.2 cm	3.5 cm
9 MeV	2.8 cm	3.2 cm	4.5 cm
11 MeV	3.4 cm	3.9 cm	5.5 cm
15 MeV	4.7 cm	5.4 cm	7.5 cm

Hand Calculations

$$\text{MU} = \frac{\text{Rx dose}}{\text{OF} \times \text{AF} \times \text{ISF} \times \text{Rx isodose}}$$

OF = output factor (typically 1 MU = 1 cGy for 10 × 10 applicator at d_{max}, 100 cm SSD)
AF = applicator factor

$$\text{ISF} = \left(\frac{\text{virtual SSD} + d_{max}}{\text{virtual SSD} + d_{max} + g}\right)^2; \quad g = \text{SSD} - 100$$

Electron shielding: Lead block thickness to attenuate 95% (mm)

Lead: t_{Pb} (mm) = (0.5 × e⁻ energy (MeV)) + 1
Cerrobend: t_{Cerr} (mm) = t_{Pb} (mm) × 1.2

Treatment Techniques

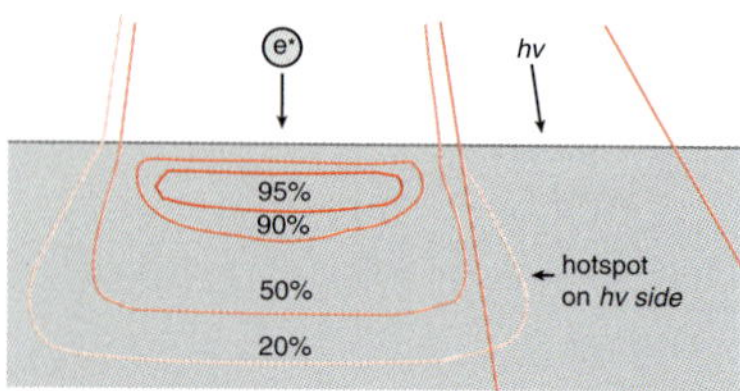

Matched photon/electron

- High electron isodose lines pull in
- Low electron isodose lines bow out
- Hotspot always on photon side
- Cold triangle on e⁻ side

Wedges

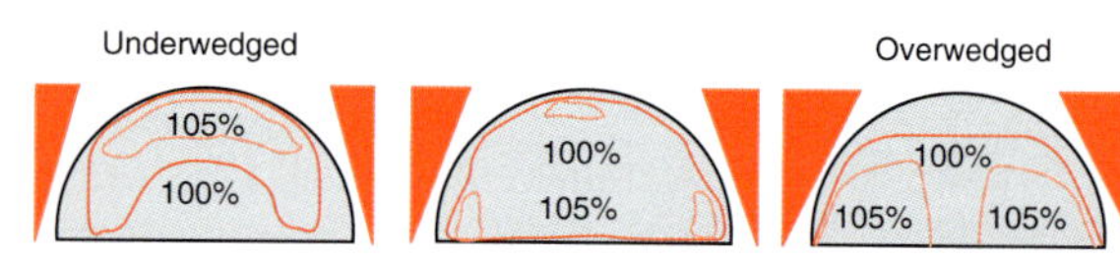

Wedge pair

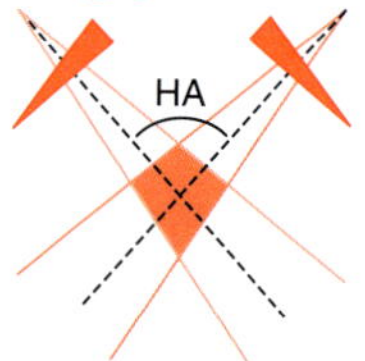

- Wedge angle (WA): Angle between wedged isodose line and a straight line at 10 cm depth
- Hinge angle (HA): Angle between central axes of incident beams
- **WA = 90 − HA/2**

Craniospinal irradiation

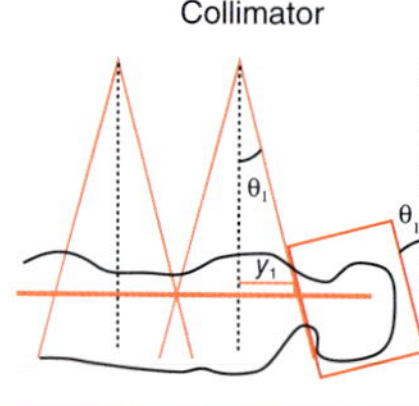

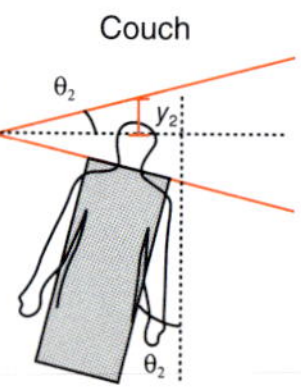

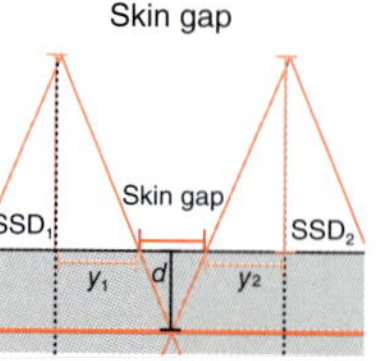

Collimator rot $\Theta_1 = \arctan\left(\frac{\text{spine } y_1}{\text{SAD}}\right)$	Skin gap $= d \times \frac{y_1}{\text{SSD}_1} + d \times \frac{y_2}{\text{SSD}_2}$
Couch kick $\Theta_2 = \arctan\left(\frac{\text{brain } y_2}{\text{SAD}}\right)$	

Brachytherapy

- 1 Becquerel (Bq) = 1 disintegration/second
- 1 curie (Ci) = 3.7×10^{10} Bq
- Source strength = air kerma rate at distance of 1 m. 1 U = 1 μGy/h/m²

Exponential decay: $A(t) = A_0\, e^{-\lambda t}$	Half-life: $t_{1/2} = \frac{\ln 2}{\lambda} = \frac{0.693}{\lambda}$
Mean life: $t_{avg} = 1.44 \times t_{1/2}$	Total dose $= \dot{D}_0 \times 1.44 \times t_{1/2}$ (permanent implant) $\dot{D}_0$ = initial dose rate
Effective half-life: $\frac{1}{t_{eff}} = \frac{1}{t_b} + \frac{1}{t_p}$ $\quad t_p$ = physical $t_{1/2}$; t_b = biological $t_{1/2}$	
Radium equivalent (mCi) = $\frac{\Gamma A \times \text{mgRaEq}}{8.25\text{R}/\text{cm}^2/\text{h}}$ for source of activity A and gamma constant Γ	

Hand calcs

$$\dot{D}(r,\Theta) = S_k \times \Lambda \times \frac{G(r,\Theta)}{D(1,\pi/2)} \times F(r,\Theta) \times g(r,\Theta)$$

- S_k: Air kerma rate
- Λ: Lambda (dose rate) constant. Converts kerma in air to dose in water
- $G(r,\Theta)$: Geometry Factor. Inverse square equation
  - Point source, $G(r) = 1/r^2$
  - Line source, $G(r,\Theta) = (\Theta_2 - \Theta_1)/Ly$
    - If $r \gg$ source length, $G(r,\Theta) \approx 1/r^2$
- $F(r,\Theta)$: Anisotropy factor
  - At perpendicular angles ($\Theta = \pi/2$), $F(r,\Theta) = 1$
  - Value changes as you move off axis
- $g(r)$: Radial dose function
  - High-energy γ sources (^{192}Ir), scatter $\approx$ attenuation ($r < 5$ cm)
    - $g(r) \approx 1$
  - Low-energy sources (^{125}I), attenuation $\gg$ scatter
    - $g(r) \ll 1$

Brachytherapy loading

- **Uniform loading:** More dose at center
- **Peripheral loading:** Uniform dose achieved by increasing source strength at ends

Brachytherapy systems

- **Fletcher-Suit:** Intracavitary tandem and ovoids; classically prescribed to *point A*
- **Patterson-Parker:** *Interstitial* crossed needles, peripheral loaded for uniform dose
- **Quimby:** *Interstitial* crossed needles, uniform loading, hot in center
- **Paris:** *Interstitial* parallel needles, hot in center
- **Modified peripheral loading**: Prostate interstitial implants

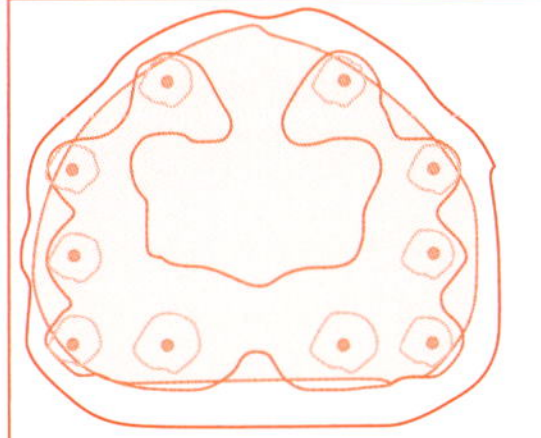	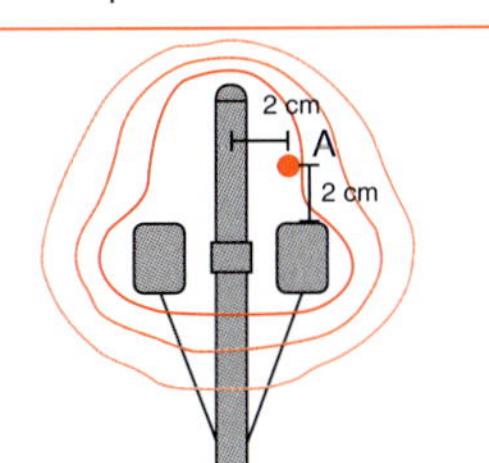
• Prostate interstitial brachytherapy using modified peripheral loading to achieve a gland coverage with a prescription dose while minimizing heterogeneity within the gland center.	• Fletcher-Suit applicator • Dose classically prescribed to point A • Start with 15/10/10 mgRaEq in tandem and 6-12 mgRaEq in each ovoid, and then optimize per GEC-ESTRO guidelines.

Common Radioisotopes

	$t_{1/2}$	Decay	Avg Energy	Use
^{60}Co	5.26 y	$\beta+ \rightarrow \gamma$ emis	1.25 MeV	EBRT, SRS
^{192}Ir	73.83 d	$\beta^- \rightarrow \gamma$ emis	0.38 MeV	brachy
^{125}I	60 d	e^- cap$\rightarrow\gamma$	28 keV	brachy
^{103}Pd	17 d	e^- cap	21 keV	brachy
^{131}Cs	9.7 d	e^- cap	30 keV	brachy
^{137}Cs	30.17 y	$\beta- \rightarrow \gamma$ emis	662 keV	brachy
^{223}Ra	11.4 d	α	5-7.5 MeV	bone mets
^{89}Sr	50 d	$\beta-$	1.46 MeV	bone mets
^{131}I	8 d	$\beta-$	190 keV	thyroid
^{32}P	14.3 d	$\beta-$	695 keV	craniopharyngeal
^{90}Y	64 h	$\beta-$	940 keV	liver
^{18}F	110 min	$\beta+$	640 keV	PET
^{99m}Tc	6 h	γ emis/IC	140 keV	Nuc med

Dose Specification

ICRU 50

- **GTV:** gross tumor volume—visually, palpably, or radiographically apparent disease
- **CTV:** clinical target volume—GTV + volume *suspected to harbor microscopic disease*
- **PTV:** planning target volume—CTV + margin for setup error and target motion
- **TV:** treated volume—volume receiving prescribed dose
- **IV:** irradiated volume—volume receiving dose appropriate for normal tissue toxicity
- **Dose reported to ICRU reference point** (PTV within 95-107% of Rx dose)
  - Relevant and representative of PTV dose
  - Easy to unambiguously define
  - Located where dose can be accurately calculated
  - Away from penumbra/steep dose gradients

ICRU 62

- **IM:** internal margin—physiologic variation in *shape* and *position*
- **ITV:** internal target volume—GTV + IM
- **SM:** setup margin—uncertainty in dose calc, machine alignment, and patient setup
- **PRV:** planning risk volume—organs at risk (OARs) + IM and SM
- **CI:** conformity index = TV/PTV
- *ICRU reference point not valid for IMRT*
  - Report DVHs for target volumes and OARs instead

Shielding

Half-value layer: HVL = ln 2/μ; **Tenth-value layer:** TVL = HVL × 3.3

μ = linear attenuation coefficient; dependent on material, energy, field size, and depth

Attenuation: $N = N_0 \times \left(\frac{1}{2}\right)^n$, where n is number of HVLs

Primary barrier: $P = \frac{WUT}{d^2} \times B$

Secondary barrier: $P = \frac{WUT}{d^2} \times B$

P = permissible dose-equivalent:
 Controlled area: 0.1 cGy/wk
 Uncontrolled area: 0.01 cGy/wk (infrequent exposure)

W = workload (# patients/wk × dose/patient = cGy/wk)

U = use factor (floor = 1, ceiling = ¼-½, walls = ¼, secondary barrier = 1)

T = occupancy factor (fraction of working day occupied; work areas/office/nurse station = 1, corridors/restrooms = ¼, waiting rooms/stairways/elevators = 1/16-1/8)

d = distance (m)

B = transmission factor (HVLs or TVLs)

Neutron shielding: Wax, concrete, or borated polyethylene

Basics of Radiation Physics

Radioactive decay

- *α-decay*: Releases a helium nucleus. Very heavy nuclei (Z > 52), monoenergetic, 2-8 MeV

$$ {}^{A}_{Z}X \rightarrow {}^{(A-4)}_{(Z-2)}Y + {}^{4}_{2}\alpha + E $$

- *β-decay*: Releases either b− (negatron) or b+ (positron). No change in *A*. Polyenergetic, energy shared between *β* and neutrino/antineutrino. Typical energy is 1/3 of maximum.

$$ \beta\text{-minus}: {}^{A}_{Z}X \rightarrow {}^{A}_{(Z+1)}Y + {}^{0}_{-1}\beta + \hat{v} + E $$

$$ \beta\text{-plus}: {}^{A}_{Z}X \rightarrow {}^{A}_{(Z-1)}Y + {}^{0}_{+1}\beta + v + E $$

- *Gamma emission*: Photon emitted by excited nucleus, typically after *α*- or *β*-decay
- *Electron capture*: Proton-rich nuclei; converts P→N and releases gamma ray/internal conversion electrons and characteristic x-rays or Auger e^-

Photon interactions

- *Rayleigh scatter*: Dominant <10 keV. Probability (*P*) *α* Z. Photon "bounces off" e^-. **No dose contribution**
- *Photoelectric effect*: Dominant at 10-26 keV. $P \alpha Z^3/E^3$. Photon ejects e^- and characteristic x-ray/Auger e^-. **Responsible for high-contrast imaging**
- *Compton scatter*: Dominant at 26 keV to 24 MeV. Photon hits e^- and sends it at angle ≤90 degrees. *P α* electron density (Z-independent). **Underlies radiotherapy dose delivery**. Poor for imaging
- *Pair production*: Dominant at >10 MeV. $P \alpha Z^2$ and dramatically increases with *E*. Photon splits energy of 1.02 MeV into electron and positron, which then release two additional photons (0.511 MeV each) via annihilation reaction. **Adds scatter** and widens margin around target

X-ray	Energy	Depth	Interaction	Uses
Diagnostic	20-150 kV	—	PE, Compton	Imaging
Superficial	50-200 kV	0-5 mm	Compton	Skin
Orthovoltage	200-500 kV	4-6 cm	Compton	Skin, ribs
Megavoltage	1-25 MV	1-30 cm	Compton, PP	Deep tissues

- Energy to produce an ion pair in gas: 33.97 eV
- Bremsstrahlung: Inelastic interaction between e^- and nucleus releases photon. Produces x-rays in x-ray tubes and linacs.

IMAGING AND RADIOLOGY

AARON GROSSBERG • CLIFTON DAVID FULLER

Imaging Radiation Basics

kVp: Peak x-ray energy (kV). Photons generated will have a range of energies with E_{max} = kVp.

mAs: E-current (milliamps) × time (seconds)

Quantity of x-rays produced in an exposure α *mAs* × *kV*^{2}

X-ray exposure that passes through patient to film α *mAs* × *kV*^{4}

- *Exposure of film/detector is very dependent on kV*

Imaging Examination	Approx. Effective Dose (mrem)	Lifetime Fatal Cancer Risk (per Million Persons)	Time for Equivalent Dose From Background Radiation
CXR	8	3	10 d
Lumbar spine film	127	51	155 d
Upper GI film	244	98	297 d
KUB	56	22	68 d

Imaging Examination	Approx. Effective Dose (mrem)	Lifetime Fatal Cancer Risk (per Million Persons)	Time for Equivalent Dose From Background Radiation
Pelvis	44	18	54 d
Barium enema	870	348	2.9 y
CT head	180	72	219 d
CT abdomen	760	304	2.53 y

Adapted from Dixon RL, Whitlow CT. In: Chen MYM, Pope TL, Ott DJ, eds. *Basic Radiology*. 2nd ed., 2011.

X-Ray Radiography

Production of two-dimensional images using (15-150 kV) low-energy x-rays

Use: Plain films (CXR, AXR, axial skeleton, extremities, etc.), mammography, kV IGRT

Physical interaction: Photoelectric (dominant) and Compton. Because interaction (P) α atomic number $(Z)^3$/photon energy $(E)^3$, interactions are more likely with higher Z material (bone, metal) and lower kVp x-ray.

X-ray generation: Bremsstrahlung (energy-dependent) and characteristic (anode material-dependent)

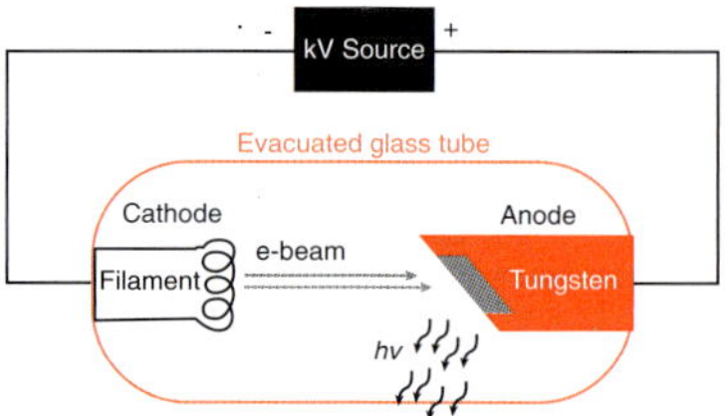

X-ray tube:

- ↑ kV: ↓ contrast, ↓ patient exposure (dose), ↓ exposure time (lower likelihood of interaction)
- ↑ mAs: ↓ exposure time
- ↑ size of focal spot (anode): ↑ penumbra, ↓ sharpness

Noise: Randomness of interactions within tissue. Compton interactions cause scatter electrons and increasing noise (energy independent in diagnostic range).

Mammography: To resolve glandular tissue or microcalcifications from fat, very low energy photons are needed. This is typically resolved by using an anode made from molybdenum (17.5 and 19.5 keV) or rhodium (20.2 and 22.7 keV), which emit characteristic x-rays of lower energy than tungsten (60-70 keV). Beryllium replaces glass as window of x-ray tube as it is lower Z and less attenuating.

Computed Tomography

Computer-processed combinations of multiple x-ray measures taken circumferentially around the patient to produce cross-sectional images (tomography). Because attenuation is closely related to tissue density and the probability of a Compton interaction is proportional to tissue density, CT number is used to calculate RT dose deposition.

Contrast: Dependent on differential attenuation, which reflects **physical density**. CT uses higher kVp and filtration (beam hardness), so interactions are mostly Compton scattering.

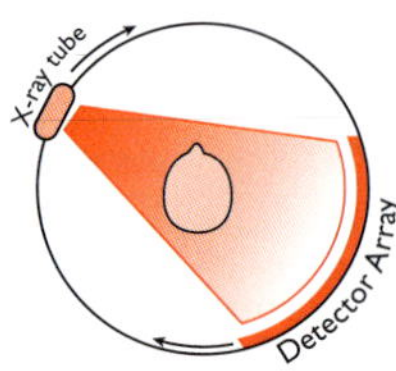

- **Hounsfield units (HU):** Linear CT contrast scale that normalizes the original linear attenuation coefficient measurement to the radio densities of water and air.

$$HU = 1000 \times \frac{\mu - \mu_{water}}{\mu_{water} - \mu_{air}}$$

- **Window (width) = range** of HU to be displayed
- **Level = midpoint** of the window

Substance	HU
Air	−1000
Water	0
Soft tissue	+100 to +300
Bone	+200 to +3000
Fat	−120 to −90
Blood	+13 to +50
Clotted blood	+50 to +75
Lung	−700 to −600
Liver	+55 to +65
Kidney	+20 to +45
Lymph nodes	+10 to +20
Muscle	+35 to +55
Gray matter	+37 to +45
White matter	+20 to +30
Gold, steel, brass	Up to 30 000

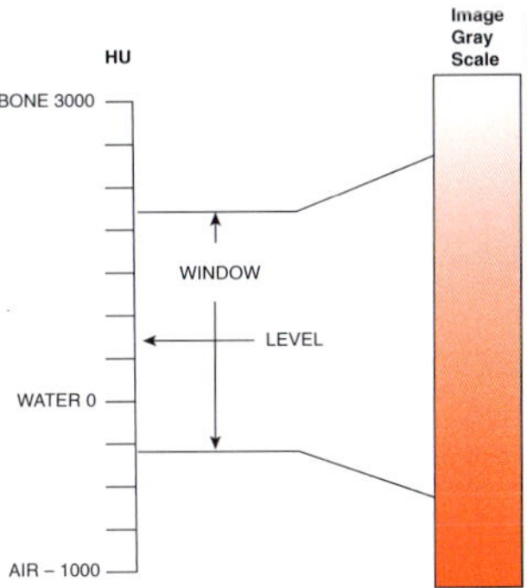

Image noise

Noise (graininess) is due to low number of x-rays contributing to each detector measurement.

- ↑ **mAs → ↑ number of x-rays → ↓ noise**; can be impacted by changing mA or scan time(s)
- ↑ **slice thickness → ↑ number of x-rays → ↓ noise** but decreased spatial resolution
- ↑ **kVp → ↑ number of x-rays → ↓ noise** but decreased contrast (slightly)
- ↑ **patient thickness → ↓ number of x-rays → ↑ noise**

Artifact: Any structure seen on an image that is not representative of actual anatomy

- **Shading artifact:** Lower than expected HU in regions downstream from high-density material—most commonly due to beam hardening that exceeds correction
- **Ring artifact:** Arise from errors, imbalances, or calibration drifts in part of the detector array. Errors are back projected along ray path to that detector, creating a ring.
- **Streak artifact:** Causes include bad detector measurement, motion, metal, insufficient x-ray intensity, partial volume effects, and tube arcing or system misalignment.

Additional limitations include bore size and field of view (FOV). Patient must be able to fit within the bore. FOV is always smaller than bore size. Contact with the CT bore or FOV limit can cause incomplete scanning and artifact that impact dose deposition calculations.

Special CT protocols

Head and neck: Thin-slice (<3 mm) IV contrast-enhanced with single phase collected ~70 seconds after contrast injection +/− upper and lower angles (in which case ½ the contrast is used for the angle scans)

Pancreatic (3-phase): Thin-slice (<3 mm) multidetector CT with triple-phase IV contrast and low-density/water oral contrast. Arterial phase (<30 seconds) shows arterial anatomy/involvement; parenchymal phase (45-50 seconds) shows parenchymal masses as hypointense lesions (PDAC) vs isodense (neuroendocrine); portal venous phase (75 seconds)—delineates venous structures and liver metastases.

Liver (3 phase): Includes late arterial phase (20-35 seconds after contrast administration), portal venous phase (60-90 seconds), and delayed phase (>3 minutes). Hypervascular tumors identified during arterial phase, hypovascular tumors during portal venous phase, washout evaluated during delayed phase.

4DCT: Continuous CT scan collected during breathing cycle. Tumor and normal tissue can be identified throughout breathing cycle, and the degree of movement can be represented on their simulation planning scan. Requires some level of respiratory management to ensure even, full breathing cycle during scan. The pitch of the scan is adjusted per the patient's respiratory rate.

Magnetic Resonance Imaging

Measures magnetic resonance: Frequency of energy released by protons as they "relax" from an energy pulse in a different direction from bore of the magnet (B_0). The local environment of each proton after excitation influences its return to alignment with B_0, yielding contrast. By changing the magnetic sequences and measured parameters, one can image different tissue characteristics.

T1: (spin-lattice relaxation) Time taken for spinning protons to realign with B_0 after 90 degrees pulse. "Longitudinal relaxation time." Dependent upon energy exchange with surrounding material

- Fat is bright; fluid (CSF) is dark.
- White matter is lighter than gray matter.
- Gadolinium increases brightness of blood/fluid by improving energy exchange (T1 + C = T1 with contrast).

T2: The component of T2* (transverse relaxation time) that is due to proton-proton interactions and thus tissue dependent. "Spin-spin relaxation"

- Fat is intermediate-bright, fluid (CSF) is bright.
- White matter is darker than gray matter.
- Gadolinium shortens T2 relaxation time → hypointense signal of blood/fluid.

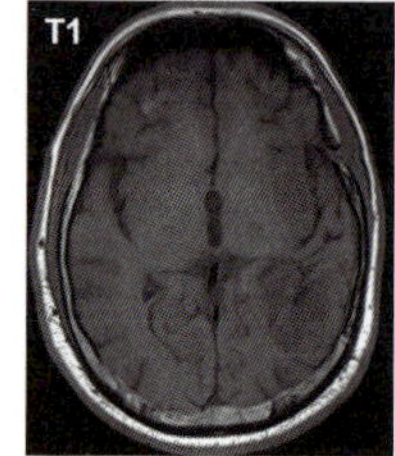

A

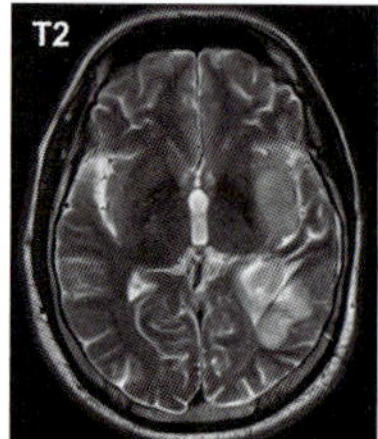

B

Special MRI sequences

- **STIR:** Short T1 inversion recovery. Used for fat suppression in T2-weighted images. Lower signal, poorer signal-to-noise, therefore often run at poorer spatial resolution to compensate
- **FLAIR:** Fluid-attenuation inversion recovery. Usually used in T2-weighted brain images to suppress CSF signal and improve sensitivity to pathology
  - Fat is dark; fluid (CSF) is dark.
  - White matter is darker than gray matter.
- **Diffusion-weighted imaging: detects random movements of water** protons by adding sequential diffusion gradients in opposing directions to T2-weighted sequences. Diffusion weighting depends on:
  1. Gradient amplitude
  2. Gradient pulse application time
  3. Interval between gradients
- **Apparent diffusion coefficient (ADC):** Calculated by comparing multiple diffusion-weighted scans with different *b*-values (a measure of the strength and duration of applied gradients). Areas of low diffusion lose the least signal on high *b*-value images (small ADC). Areas of fast diffusion appear bright (lose more signal on high *b*-value images).

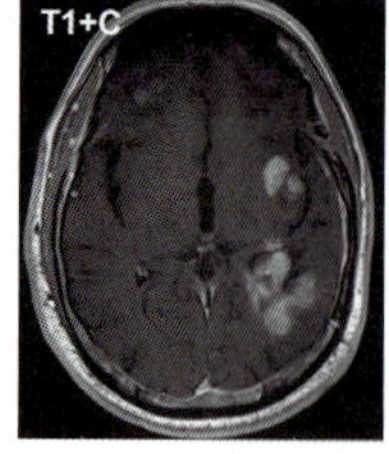

C

Positron Emission Tomography

Allows imaging of biological uptake of radiolabeled tracer that emits positrons. Positron annihilation results in pairs of 511 keV photons at 180 degrees, which are detected by coincidence detection allowing for back calculation of location in 2D space in each slice.

- **Coincidence detection:** Photons released by positron annihilation detected at same time by detectors at 180 degrees from each other. Detection within 6-12 ns considered "in coincidence." Majority (~99%) of photons are thus excluded from results.

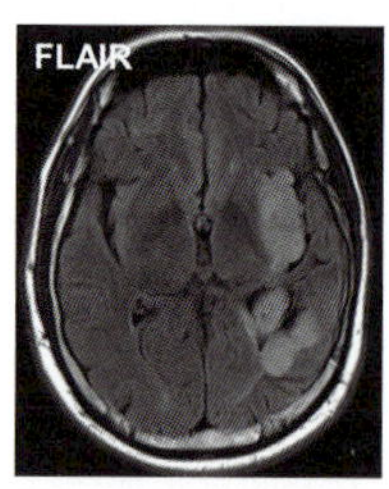

D

- ↑ **accumulated tracer** → ↑ **signal ^{18}FDG-PET images glucose uptake** (nonmetabolized glucose analog builds up in metabolically active cells). Most common use for PET imaging
- **SUV:** Standardized uptake value. FDG uptake in a region/tumor/tissue normalized to the injected radiotracer and patient's weight
  - SUV more accurate if normalized to patient's lean body mass or body surface area, but this is not standard practice
  - Normal tissues: SUV 0.5-2.5, tumor—SUV > 2.5 (usually)

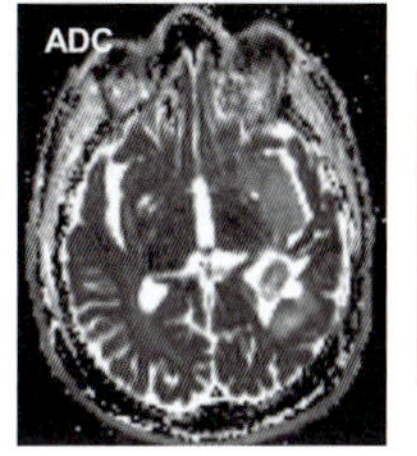

E

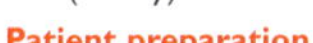

Patient preparation

- NPO 4-6 hours: FDG-PET to enhance FDG uptake by tumors. No caffeine/alcohol either. Blood glucose at time of injection <150 mg/dL
- No strenuous activity prior to imaging
- Typical dose of FDG **10 mCi**. Imaging initiated **60 minutes** after tracer injection
- Position: For HN, arms down; if below neck, arms above the head (decrease beam hardening during CT). Patient must be comfortable enough to lie for 45 minutes and instructed not to move.
  - PET can be done in treatment position (with immobilization) for better treatment planning image fusion. This is particularly important for INRT in lymphoma management.
- Duration: PET scanning typically takes 30-45 minutes.

Other PET tracers

- **Na^{18}F:** Images blastic and lytic bone lesions (alternative to traditional ^{99m}Tc bone scan)
- **^{11}C acetate:** Ketone body uptake. Related to enhanced lipid synthesis in prostate cancer tumor cells. Not cancer specific—also accumulates in BPH. 71% accuracy (*Jambor J Nucl Med* 2010)
- **^{11}C or ^{18}F choline:** Choline is used in cell membrane synthesis, which is increased in cancer cells. Highly sensitive for lymph node involvement or metastasis. High levels of uptake in liver, spleen, kidneys, pancreas, and salivary glands. Inflammation can confound interpretation of increased uptake.
- **^{18}F fluciclovine (Axumin):** Analogue of L-leucine. Uptake increased in prostate cancer. No physiologic accumulation in urinary tract or brain allowing for sensitive detection of localized and metastatic disease. Used for metastatic or recurrent disease, proven by rising PSA
- **^{11}C metomidate:** 11β-hydroxylase inhibitor, key enzyme in biosynthesis of cortisol and aldosterone. Used for detection of adrenocortical tumors
- **^{68}Ga or ^{18}F PSMA:** Refer to several small molecules or antibodies attached to PET tracers that target prostate-specific membrane antigen (PSMA). PSMA is highly expressed in most prostate cancer.
- **^{68}Ga or ^{64}Cu DOTA-TATE:** DOTA-TATE is an 8 amino acid long peptide, which binds to somatastatin receptors (SSR). SSRs are overexpressed in neuroendocrine tumors.

Other Nuclear Medicine Imaging

- **Bone scan:** ^{99m}Tc with methylene diphosphonate (MDP). MDP adsorbs to bone hydroxyapatite, which is present at sites of bone growth/increased turnover. Patient is typically injected with 740 MBq of tracer and scanned with a gamma camera (planar images).
- **Myocardial perfusion:** ^{99m}Tc tracers include teboroxime and sestamibi. Evaluates areas of infarction, ischemia, or reduced blood flow.
- **Renal scan:** aka renogram or MAG3 scan. May use ^{99m}Tc-conjugated mercaptoacetyltriglycine (MAG3) or diethylenetriaminepentaacetate (DTPA) injected intravenously. Progress through renal system tracked with gamma camera. Measures effective renal plasma flow. 40-50% of MAG3 (20% of DTPA) is removed by the proximal tubules during each pass.
- **V/Q scan:** Evaluates circulation of air and blood within patients' lungs. Used for pre-op/pre-RT estimate of lung function patients with lung ca. or mesothelioma. For the ventilation scan, aerosolized radionuclides are inhaled by the patient through nonrebreathing mask. Perfusion scan is ^{99m}Tc microaggregated albumin.

- **MIBG:** Metaiodobenzylguanidine labeled with ^{123}I or ^{131}I. Localized to adrenergic tissue and can be used to identify pheochromocytomas and neuroblastomas. Use of ^{131}I allows for treatment as well as imaging. Must undertake thyroid precautions by pretreating with potassium iodide
- **Sentinel node identification:** Injection of ^{99m}Tc-labelled sulfur colloid or albumin colloid injected 2-24 hours prior to operation. Preoperative lymphoscintigram is obtained to map axillary drainage pattern from tumor. Intraoperatively, a gamma counter is used to find the area of highest radioactivity.
- **^{123}I iodine scan:** Supplied as $Na^{131}I$ and administered orally vs IV Iodine is taken up by the thyroid and images obtained by gamma camera.
- **^{131}I iodine scan:** Like ^{123}I, it is taken up by the thyroid. 90% of decay is by β-decay, allowing for short-range therapeutic effects, with the remaining 10% via gamma decay, allowing for detection using gamma camera. Dose ranges from 2220 to 7400 MBq. Patients cannot be discharged until activity falls below 1100 MBq. Patients advised to collect urine, wear clothes and socks, and to regularly clean toilets, sinks, etc. Patients who undergo treatment may trigger airport radiation detectors up to 95 days after tx.

Image-Guided Radiation Therapy (IGRT)

Goal of IGRT is to minimize geometric uncertainty during treatment.

Sources of geometric uncertainties

- **Intrafraction**
  - Seconds: Cardiac cycle, breathing
  - Minutes: Patient movement, setup variation
- **Interfraction**
  - Hours: Patient movement, setup variation
  - Days to months: Anatomic changes, tumor response, normal tissue response

Corrections

Remember that you are moving the patient, not the imager. Often corrections involve moving patient in *opposite* direction to apparent misalignment.

- Isocenter too superior (target too inferior on daily imaging): Move patient *in*
- Isocenter too inferior (target too superior on daily imaging): Move patient *out*
- Isocenter too far on patient's left (target too far on patient's *right* on daily imaging): Move patient *left*
- Isocenter too far on patient's right (target too far on patient's *left* on daily imaging): Move patient *right*

IGRT approaches

- **Surface markers:** Use surface anatomy to infer internal anatomy. Usually in conjunction with immobilization devices. Establish position of multiple surface markers at simulation and in treatment room (relative to isocenter or ODI). *Not a good approach for mobile internal targets*
- **Stereotaxy:** 3D localization of structures using mechanical frame and precise coordinate system. Allows for reduction in PTV. Concepts have been adapted using 4DCT simulation and full-body immobilization to apply stereotaxy to extracranial sites, including lung cancer (~5 mm PTV).
- **MV electronic portal imaging devices (EPIDs):** Creating of radiographic images using RT x-ray beam. Advantage is that imaging represents actual treatment field. Disadvantage is that MV imaging exhibits negligible photoelectric effect, limiting contrast to detect only bony anatomy. Very difficult to align to soft tissue
- **Single exposure:** Only images treatment field
- **Double exposure:** Treatment field and open field both imaged for better anatomy
- **Localization film:** A few cGy for imaging verification of setup
- **Verification film:** Full fraction (~2 Gy) of exposure
- **kV imaging:** Most new radiation therapy machines have built in x-ray tube and EPID orthogonal to treatment ray. *Advantage* is that it offers increased contrast compared to MV. Can incorporate fluoroscopy for real-time monitoring. Due to increased contrast detection due to greater influence of photoelectric effect, can also be used to localize implanted radiopaque markers. Excellent translational (*x*-, *y*-, and z-axis) resolution. *Disadvantage* is that images are not collected from treatment beam, so there is an opportunity for misalignment between kV imager and treatment beam. Insensitive to rotational error. Vendors such as ExacTrac offer floor-to-ceiling noncoplanar imaging that can be compared to on-board imaging in real time to detect intra- or interfraction motion.

- **Ultrasound:** Allows for soft tissue imaging with the transducer calibrated and coregistered with the isocenter, both in the CT scanner and in treatment rooms. Most commonly transabdominal ultrasound used for prostate cancer treatment setup. Bladder ultrasounds can also be used to assess bladder fullness during treatment for pelvic malignancies (uterus, prostate, cervix, and bladder cancers). *Advantages* are that it is relatively inexpensive and shows soft tissue contrast for targets that do not reliably align to bone. *Disadvantages* are that it requires technical skill, pressure may displace target or OARs, and that it cannot image through bone or air cavities.
- **Cone beam CT (CBCT):** Allows for volumetric imaging on conventional linac using onboard orthogonal x-ray tube and detector. CT reconstructions are acquired in the treatment position just prior to treatment. Images may be acquired in whole-fan or half-fan mode. FOV can approach 50 cm in the transverse plane ×25 cm in the craniocaudal plane but may not include full thickness of patient. Total dose delivered is usually <3 cGy. *Advantages* include the ability to align soft tissue with good contrast in the treatment position, can see inter- and intrafractional changes in tumor and patient anatomy, and six-directional image verification. *Disadvantages* include limited FOV, which may not show patient to surface; slow image acquisition, making it susceptible to motion artifact and difficult to use with respiratory gating; and relatively high radiation dose delivered.
- **CT on rails:** Conventional CT scanner located in treatment room moves over patient and treatment table "on rails" to acquire images. Typically, treatment table is rotated 180 degrees from treatment position for scanning. Treatment table is made of special low-attenuation material. *Advantages* include faster CT imaging, allowing for verification of intrafractional immobilization (eg, breathhold). *Disadvantages* include the need for extra equipment, relative scarcity of CT on rail-enabled treatment vaults (which generally requires a larger vault), and requirement to rotate table out of treatment position for verification scans, introducing a potential new source of error.
- **Tomotherapy imaging:** Tomotherapy devices include MV CT image system that uses a fan beam and helical acquisition. Images are acquired using a 3.5-MV x-rays with suppressed photon output. Typically imaging administers dose of 0.5-3 cGy. *Advantages* include images collected in treatment position and MV imaging not susceptible to artifact. *Disadvantages* include low contrast in MV images.
- **Electromagnetic 4-D tracking:** Electromagnetic transponders implanted in the target tissue for improving both intrafraction motion of the tissue and interfraction setup error. Includes beacons, electromagnetic console, receiver array, and three ceiling-mounted infrared optical cameras. Currently in use for prostate radiotherapy (Calypso) with <2 mm accuracy
- **Optical (surface) imaging:** Optical, often infrared camera system tracks patient surface during actual treatment. Used to monitor intrafraction motion. Current systems include AlignRT and C-Rad Sentinel. *Advantages* include speed, ability to monitor respiratory motion, and absence of ionizing radiation. *Disadvantages* include inability to use for tumors that poorly correlate to patient surface.
- **Magnetic resonance imaging:** Uses hybrid MRI/radiation units to provide continuous real-time assessment of internal soft tissue anatomy and motion. *Advantages* include excellent soft tissue contrast, no ionizing radiation exposure, and excellent resolution. *Disadvantages* include inability to use for patients with metal implants or pacemakers and susceptibility to motion artifact.
- **Incorporating IGRT into margination:** ICRU 50 & 62 define target (PTV) and avoidance (PRV) volumes to account for setup and organ positional uncertainty. IGRT can be used to minimize magnitude of both random and systematic error, allowing reduced PTV margin.

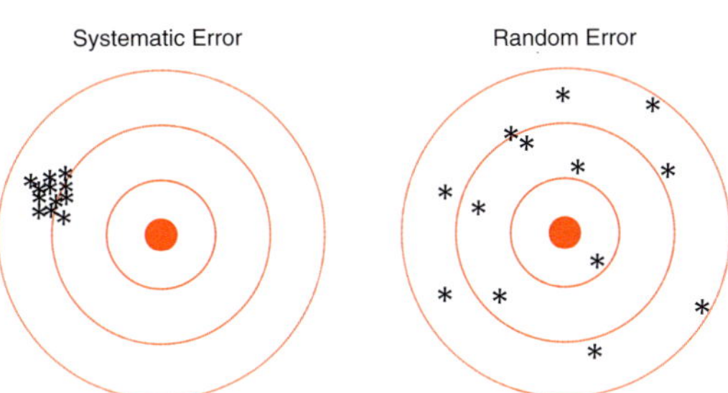

- **Random error, σ:** Fluctuations in patient position due to unknown and unpredictable factors (eg, changes in organ positions, bladder filling, minor fluctuations in immobilization devices). *Execution Errors*. Equal in all directions
  - Root mean square of SDs of measured fluctuations from all patients = σ
- **Systematic error, Σ:** Error in patient setup due to incorrect positioning information (eg, inaccurate isocenter determination, laser positioning, or setup documentation). *Preparation Errors*. Typically in a specific direction
  - SD of means per patient of observed fluctuations = Σ
  - Require 3-4× more margin than random errors
  - Can be minimized using multimodality imaging, clear delineation protocols, and electronic portal imaging with decision rules
- **Margin recipes**

  CTV *Margin* = $2.5 \times \Sigma + 0.7 \times \sigma$ (*van Herk et al. IJROBP* 2000)

  *Minimum dose to CTV is 95% for 90% of patients.

  OAR *Margin* = $1.3 \times \Sigma + 0.5 \times \sigma$ (*McKenzie et al. Radiother Oncol* 2002)

  *DVH of PRV will not underrepresent high dose to OAR for 90% of patients.

CHEMOTHERAPY AND IMMUNOTHERAPY

STEPHANIE DUDZINSKI • AARON GROSSBERG • CHAD TANG • SHANE STECKLEIN

Concurrent Chemoradiation

- Chemotherapy delivered concurrently with radiotherapy to increase efficacy
- Preclinical synergy with XRT: Gemcitabine, cisplatin, bleomycin, 5-FU, MMC, bevacizumab, cetuximab, PARP inhibitors, doxorubicin, dactinomycin, dacarbazine
- Associated with increased and earlier toxicity
- Rule of thumb: OAR dose constraints often **reduced by ~10%**

Head and Neck—*NPX, OPX, Supraglottic Larynx, Post-op*			
Drug	**Dose**	**XRT Rx**	**Notes**
Cisplatin	40 mg/m^2 qwk ×6 or 100 mg/m^2 q3wk ×2	70 Gy/33 fx	Total dose goal >200 mg/m^2
Cetuximab	400 mg/m^2 loading→ 250 mg/m^2 qwk ×6	70 Gy/33 fx	OPX, p16+, <N2b, <10 pk-yr G2+ acneiform rash = ↑ OS
Small Cell Lung Cancer (Limited Stage)			
Cisplatin	60 mg/m^2 d1 q3wk	45 Gy/30 fx *bid*	Start XRT during 1st two cycles of chemo (*De Ruysscher Ann Oncol* 2006)
Etoposide	120 mg/m^2 d1-3 q3wk		
Non–Small Cell Lung Cancer			
Cisplatin	50 mg/m^2 d1, 8, 29, 36	66 Gy/30 fx	Other platinum doublets used as well
Etoposide	50 mg/m^2 d1-5 and 29-33		
Esophageal			
Cisplatin 5-FU	20 mg/m^2 d1, 8, 15, 22, 29 300 mg/m^2/d CI	50.4 Gy in 28 fx	Oxaliplatin or capecitabine may be used as well
Carboplatin Paclitaxel	AUC2 mg/m^2 d1, 8, 15, 22, 29 50 mg/m^2	50.4 Gy in 30 fx	Other platinum doublets used as well
Gastric			
Capecitabine	825 mg/m^2 bid	45 Gy in 25 fx	Pre-op or post-op
5-FU	200 mg/m^2/d CI	45 Gy in 25 fx	

Pancreatic			
Capecitabine	825 mg/m² bid	50.4 Gy/28 fx	Pre-op or post-op
Gemcitabine	400 mg/m² qwk	50.4 Gy/28 fx	
Bladder Cancer			
Cisplatin and 5-FU	75 mg/m² d1 1000 mg/m² d1, 4	50-58 Gy at 2 Gy/fx	Many other concurrent bladder cancer regimes
MMC 5-FU	12 mg/m² d1 500 mg/m²/d CI given on 1-5 fx, 16-20 fx	55 Gy at 2.75 Gy/fx or 64 Gy at 2 Gy/fx	
Anal			
Cisplatin 5-FU	20 mg/m² d1, 8, 15, 22 300 mg/m²/d CI	50-58 Gy at 2 Gy/fx	XRT dose depends on T- and N-stage
MMC 5-FU	10 mg/m² d1, 29 300 mg/m²/d CI	50-58 Gy at 2 Gy/fx	
Rectal			
Capecitabine	825 mg/m² bid	50.4 Gy in 28 fx	Boost to 54 Gy post-op
5-FU	225 mg/m²/d CI	50.4 Gy in 28 fx	
Gynecologic Cancers (Cervix/Uterine/Vulvar/Vaginal)			
Cisplatin	40 mg/m² qwk	Variable	Final cycle with 2nd ICBT when giving PDR
Glioblastoma			
Temozolomide	75 mg/m² daily	60 Gy/30 fx	Adjuvant dose 150-200 mg/m² d1-5 q4wk × 6c (or indefinitely)
Medulloblastoma (Pediatric)			
Vincristine	1.5 mg/m² qwk	54 Gy/30 fx	Followed by adjuvant PCV
Rhabdomyosarcoma (Pediatric)			
Vincristine	1.5 mg/m²	36-50.4 Gy/30 fx	XRT dose and timing depends on risk stratification. Complex timing of concurrent chemo
Cyclophos-phamide	1.2 g/m²		
Irinotecan	50 mg/m²		

CHEMOTHERAPY AGENTS AND TOXICITIES

Underline = dose-limiting toxicity

Alkylating agents: Add alkyl group to 7-N guanine → DNA cross-link and strand breaks. Inhibit DNA repair and/or synthesis.

Cisplatin (Platinol) (20-100 mg/m² d1-5 q3-4wk; 40 mg/m² qwk—CCRT): N/V, nephrotox, ototoxicity (irreversible), neuropathy (reversible), ↓PLT, anemia, taste changes

Carboplatin (Paraplatin) (AUC 3-7.5 q3-4wk; AUC2 qwk—CCRT): Myelosuppression (nadir 3-4 weeks), N/V, nephrotox, ototoxicity, neuropathy, ↑LFTs

Oxaliplatin (Eloxatin) (85-140 mg/m² q2-3wk): Neurotox, neuropathy, fever, ↑LFTs, nephrotox

Bendamustine (Treanda, Bendeka) (70-120 mg/m² ×2d q3-5wk): Myelosuppression (nadir 3 weeks), N/V, fever, edema, rash, diarrhea

Cyclophosphamide (Cytoxan) (1-5 mg/kg/d po or 250-1800 mg/m² q3-4wk): Myelosuppression (recovery 1 week), hemorrhagic cystitis, nephrotox, N/V, cardiotox, infertility, alopecia

Chlorambucil (Leukeran) (0.1-0.2 mg/kg/d): Myelosuppression (nadir 3 weeks), hepatotox, rash, CNS tox, 2° malignancy

Melphalan (Alkeran) (2-10 mg/d po): Myelosuppression (nadir 4 weeks), mucositis, diarrhea, pulm fibrosis, 2° malignancy

Ifosfamide (Ifex) (1200-3000 mg/m²/d ×3-5d q2-3wk): Myelosuppression (nadir 1-2 weeks), hemorrhagic cystitis, nephrotox, reversible neurotox N/V, alopecia

Mechlorethamine (Mustargen, Valchlor) (0.1-0.4 mg/kg/d): Myelosuppression, N/V, alopecia, mucositis, infertility, CNS tox

Carmustine (BCNU, Gliadel) (150-200 mg/m² q6-8wk): Myelosuppression (nadir 4 weeks), N/V, hepatotox, hypotension, pulm fibrosis

Lomustine (CCNU, Gleostine) (100-130 mg/m^2 q6wk): Myelosuppression (nadir 4 weeks), N/V, hepatotox, nephrotox, pulm fibrosis ***Crosses BBB*

Busulfan (Busulfex, Myleran) (1.8 mg/m^2/d): Myelosuppression, N/V, diarrhea, anorexia, mucositis, infertility

Dacarbazine (375 mg/m^2 d1 and 15 q4wk): *N/V*, myelosuppression, flulike symptoms, inj site pain

Temozolomide (Temodar) (100-200 mg/m^2 d1-5 q4wk; 75 mg/m^2/d—CCRT): Myelosuppression (nadir 3 weeks), N/V, HA, fatigue, constipation, edema

Antimetabolites: Replace building blocks in DNA synthesis. Groups include nucleotide analogues (5-FU, -MP, Ara-C, fludarabine), folate antagonists (MTX, pemetrexed), ribonucleotide reductase inhibition (hydroxyurea)

5-FU (Adrucil) ([IVP] 325-425 mg/m^2 × 5d q4wk or [CI] 750-1000 mg/m^2 ×5d q4wk): Diarrhea, mucositis, N/V, marrow suppression, alopecia, nail changes, hand-foot

6-MP (Purinethol) (1.5-2.5 mg/m^2/d): Myelosuppression, jaundice, N/V, diarrhea, infxn

Capecitabine (Xeloda) (1000-1250 mg/m^2 bid ×2wk q3wk; 825-1000 mg/m^2 bid-CCRT): diarrhea, hand-foot, mucositis, neurotox, coronary vasospasm, XRT recall

Cytarabine (Ara-C) ([CI] 100-200 mg/m^2/d ×5-7d; high dose: 1500-3000 mg/m^2/d ×3d): Myelosuppression (nadir 7-9 days/15-24 days), N/V, diarrhea, neurotox, ↑LFTs ***Crosses BBB*

Fludarabine (20-30 mg/m^2/d ×3-5d q4wk): Myelosuppression (nadir 10-14 days, recovery 5-7 weeks), fever, infxn, weakness, cough, anorexia

Gemcitabine (Gemzar) (1000 mg/m^2 qwk or 800-1250 mg/m^2 d1, 8 q3wk): Myelosuppression, edema, flulike symptoms, fever, fatigue, N/V pneumonitis, ↑LFTs

Hydroxyurea (Droxia, Hydrea) (20-30 mg/kg/d): Myelosuppression (2-5 days), GI ulcer, rash, squamous cell ca., XRT recall

Methotrexate (MTX, Trexall) (range from 30-40 mg/m^2/wk to 100-12 000 mg/m^2 × 1): Myelosuppression, mucositis, N/V, neurotox, nephrotox, ↑LFTs

Pemetrexed (Alimta) (500 mg/m^2 q3wk): Myelosuppression, mucositis, hand-foot, anorexia, fatigue, ↑LFTs

Plant alkaloids: Inhibit enzymes used in DNA replication, mitosis, or cell division. Includes antimicrotubular agents (docetaxel, paclitaxel, vincristine, vinblastine, vinorelbine) and topoisomerase inhibitors (irinotecan, etoposide, topotecan, belotecan)

Docetaxel (Taxotere) (60-100 mg/m^2 q3wk): Myelosuppression (7 days), neuropathy, edema, alopecia, nail changes, N/V, XRT recall

Paclitaxel (Taxol) (60-250 mg/m^2 q1-3wk; 50 mg/m^2 qwk—CCRT): Myelosuppression (11 days), alopecia, neuropathy, arthralgias, N/V, diarrhea

Nab-paclitaxel (Abraxane): Myelosuppression, alopecia, ECG changes, neuropathy, arthralgias, N/V, weakness, fatigue

Vincristine (Oncovin) (0.5-1.5 mg/m^2 qwk; 1.5 mg/m^2 qwk—CCRT): Neuropathy, alopecia, constipation, N/V, weight loss ***Crosses BBB*

Vinblastine (Velban) (3.7-6 mg/m^2 qwk): Myelosuppression (~1 week), constipation, HTN, alopecia, bone pain, N/V

Vinorelbine (Navelbine) (25-30 mg/m^2 qwk): Myelosuppression (~1 week), N/V, alopecia, diarrhea, neuropathy

Etoposide (Toposar) (50-120 mg/m^2 ×3d q3-4wk): Myelosuppression (1-2 weeks), menopause, infertility, N/V, hypotension, rash, ↑LFTs, XRT recall

Irinotecan (Camptosar) (240-350 mg/m^2 q3wk): Diarrhea, abdominal cramping, myelosupp, N/V, alopecia, wt. loss, weakness

Topotecan (Hycamtin) (1.5 mg/m^2 ×5d q3wk): Myelosuppression (1-2 weeks), N/V, alopecia, diarrhea, fever, rash, weakness

Antibiotics: *Streptomyces* antibiotics that interfere with cell cycle or DNA replication. Anthracyclines (-rubicin) and actinomycins inhibit topoisomerase II by intercalation. Bleomycin and mitomycin generate free radicals causing DNA breaks. Commonly cause radiation recall.

Actinomycin D (Cosmegen) (400-600 μg/m^2/d ×5d): Myelosuppression (nadir 14-21 days), alopecia, N/V, fatigue, mucositis, hepatotox, diarrhea, infertility, *XRT recall*

Daunorubicin (Cerubidine) (30-60 mg/m^2/d ×3d): Myelosuppression (nadir 10-14 days), alopecia, dark urine, N/V, mucositis, pain, cardiotox. *Max lifetime cumulative dose = 550 mg/m^2*

Doxorubicin (Adriamycin) (20 mg/m^2 qwk or 40-60 mg/m^2 q3wk): Myelosuppression (nadir 10-14 days), cardiotox, N/V, mucositis *XRT recall,* 2ndary leukemia, tumor lysis. *Max lifetime cumulative dose = 500 mg/m², less if >65, mediastinal XRT, heart disease or cyclophosphamide*

Epirubicin (Ellence) (100-120 mg/m²/d q3-4wk, 50 mg/m² q3wk): Myelosuppression (nadir 10-14 days), alopecia, hot sweats, N/V, diarrhea, cardiotox. *Max lifetime cumulative dose = 1000 mg/m²*

Bleomycin (Blenoxane) (5-15 units/m²/wk ×3wk): Pulmonary tox/pneumonitis, skin rxn, mucositis, hypotension, hypersensitivity rxn, *XRT recall*

Mitomycin-C (Mutamycin) (10-15 mg/m² q6-8wk or 20-40 mg qwk or 10-15 mg/m² q4wk-CCRT): Myelosuppression (nadir 4-6 weeks), mucositis, rash, interstitial pneumonitis, HUS

Targeted Therapies

Naming Guide	
Monoclonal antibodies (-mab)	
Target	*Source*
• cir(r), circulatory system	• ximab, chimeric human-mouse
• li(m), immune system	• zumab, humanized mouse
• t(u), tumor	• mumab, fully human
Small molecules (-ib)	
• tinib, tyrosine kinase inhibitor (TKI)	
• zomib, proteasome inhibitor	
• ciclib, cyclin-dependent kinase inhibitor	
• parib, PARP inhibitor	

Adapted from: Abramson, 2017 Overview of Targeted Therapies for Cancer.

Common Nonchemotherapy Systemic Agents

Drug	Target	Indications	Side Effects
Erlotinib (Tarceva) **Afatinib (Gilotrif)** **Gefitinib (Iressa)** **Osimertinib (Tagrisso)** **Amivantamab**	EGFR	Lung adenoca, PDAC *EGFR ex19del; ex21mut; ex20mut*	**Rash**, **diarrhea**, fatigue, anorexia, neutropenia (osimertinib)
Cetuximab (Erbitux)	EGFR	HNC, mCRC	**Acneiform rash**, infusion rxn, anaphylaxis, N/V, ↓BP
Panitumumab (Vectibix)	EGFR	mCRC	Rash, N/V, diarrhea, hypoMg, keratitis
Bevacizumab (Avastin)	VEGF-A	mColorectal, lung adenoca, mBreast, GBM, RCC	Weakness, pain, N/V, GI perf, hypertensive crisis, nephrotic syndrome, CHF
Ramucirumab (Cyramza) **Apatinib (Aitan)**	VEGFR2	Gastric/GEJ, NSCLC, mColorectal, esophageal, DTC	HTN, diarrhea, HA, bleeding, GI perf
Lenvatinib (Lenvima)	VEGFR, FGFR, RET, KIT, & PDGFRa	HCC, cholangiocarcinoma, DTC, RCC, endometrial	HTN, fatigue, myalgias, Stomatitis, N/V, proteinuria, hand-foot syndrome
Temsirolimus (Torisel) **Everolimus (Afinitor)**	mTOR	RCC, GI NETs	Lymphopenia, anemia, fatigue, rash, mucositis, hyperglyc, ↑TGs
Sunitinib (Sutent)	PDGFR VEGFR c-KIT RET	GIST, RCC, meningioma, neuroendocrine	Fatigue, diarrhea, N, hand-foot syndrome, stomatitis, rash

Drug	Target	Indications	Side Effects
Sorafenib (Nexavar)	PDGFR VEGFR RAF	RCC, HCC, thyroid, desmoid	Lymphopenia, diarrhea, rash, hand-foot syndrome, N/V, fatigue
Pazopanib (Votrient)	PDGFR VEGFR c-KIT FGFR	RCC, sarcoma	N/V, diarrhea, changes in hair color, rash, myelosupp
Cabozantinib (Cabometyx, Cometriq)	VEGFR2 c-Met AXL RET	RCC, MTC	GI perf/fistula, bleeding, hand-foot syndrome, PRES, stomatitis
Regorafenib (Stivarga)	c-KIT PDGFR RAF RET VEGFR1-3	CRC, GIST, HCC	Anemia, ↑LFTs, fatigue, proteinuria, electrolyte abnl, ↓PLT, ↓WBC, wt loss
Axitinib (Inlyta)	VEGFR1-3 PDGFR c-KIT BCR-ABL	RCC, CML, ALL	Diarrhea, fatigue, hand-foot syndrome, N/V, fatigue, wt loss
Imatinib (Gleevec) **Dasatinib (Sprycel)** **Nilotinib (Tasigna)** **Bosutinib (Bosulif)**	BCR-ABL	CML, ALL, GIST, MDS	V, Diarrhea, muscle pain, edema, GI bleed, myelosuppr.
Trastuzumab (Herceptin), Ado-trastuzumab emtansine (Kadcyla), Margetuximab (Margenza)	Her2	Her2+ breast	Flulike, nausea, diarrhea, heart failure
Pertuzumab (Perjeta)	Her2	Her2+ breast	Diarrhea, joint pain, neutropenia, rash
Neratinib (Nerlynx), Tucatinib (Tukysa)	Her2	Her2+ breast	Diarrhea, N/V, rash, abdominal pain
Lapatinib (Tykerb), Pyrotinib (Irene)	Her2	Her2+ breast	Hand-foot syndrome, N/V, diarrhea, lapatinib-↑LFTs, heart failure, ↓RBC
Abemaciclib (Verzenio), Palbociclib (Ibrance), Ribociclib (Kisqali)	CDK4/CDK6 inhibitor	HR+, Her2-breast	Nausea, diarrhea (abemaciclib), fatigue, marrow suppression-neutropenia (Palbociclib/ribociclib)
Alpelisib (Piqray)	PIK3CA	PIK3CA-mutated HR+, HER2- breast cancer (in combination with fulvestrant)	Hyperglycemia, pneumonitis, diarrhea/colitis
Crizotinib (Xalkori) **Ceritinib (Zykadia)** **Alectinib (Alecensa)** **Brigatinib (Alunbrig)**	ALK ROS1- (crizotinib)	ALK-mutated NSCLC, anaplastic thyroid	Blurred vision, photophobia, N/V, diarrhea, pneumonitis, renal/hepatotox, marrow suppression, electrolyte abnl
Dabrafenib (Tafinlar)	BRAF	BRAFV600E mut melanoma and NSCLC	Hyperglycemia, hyperkeratosis, HA
Cobimetinib (Cotellic)	MEK	BRAFV600E mut melanoma, thyroid cancer	Nephrotoxic, myositis, ↑alk phos, N, diarrhea, lymphopenia, ↓Na

Drug	Target	Indications	Side Effects
Trametinib (Mekinist)	MEK	BRAFV600E mut NSCLC, melanoma, thyroid	↑LFTs, rash, diarrhea, anemia, lymphedema
Olaparib (Lynparza) Niraparib (Zejula)	PARP	Ovary, peritoneal, prostate BRCA-mut	↓RBC, ↓PLT, ↓WBC, URI, N/V, fatigue, myalgia, ↑Cr
Talazoparib (Talzenna)	PARP	BRCA-mut breast, prostate	↓RBC, ↑LFTs, ↓PLT, N, neutropenia, ↑glucose
Vismodegib (Erivedge)	PTCH,SMO	Basal cell ca	Muscle spasms, wt loss, alopecia, abnl taste, N
Vorinostat (Zolinza)	HDAC	CTCL	Fatigue, diarrhea, nausea, dysgeusia, ↓PLT
Belzutifan (Welireg)	HIF-2alpha	CNS heman-gioblastoma, pNET, VHL-RCC	Anemia, dizziness, fatigue, headache, N, ↑glucose
Dinutuximab (Unituxin)	Ganglioside GD2	Neuroblastoma	Fever, pain, hypotension, N/V, diarrhea
Erdafitinib (Balversa)	FGFR2,3	Bladder, FGF2/3 mutations	Hyperphosphatemia, soft tissue mineralization, eye disorders

Hormonal Therapy

Androgen

Enzalutamide (Xtandi) Androgen receptor signaling inhibitor
Indications: Metastatic castrate-resistant prostate cancer (mCRPC)
Dose: 160 mg po daily
Side effects: Edema, fatigue, HA, hot flashes, diarrhea, arthralgia, gynecomastia

Bicalutamide (Casodex) Nonsteroidal androgen receptor antagonist
Indications: Intermediate- to high-risk prostate cancer
Dose: 50 mg po daily × ≥14d w/ LHRH analogue or 150 mg daily (monotherapy)
Side Effects: Edema, constipation, hot flashes, diarrhea, bone pain, gynecomastia

Flutamide (Eulexin) Nonsteroidal androgen receptor antagonist
Indications: Intermediate- to high-risk prostate cancer; PCOS, congenital adrenal hyperplasia
Dose: 250 mg po tid
Side Effects: Hepatotoxicity (black box warning), hot flashes, bone pain, gynecomastia, N/V, diarrhea

Nilutamide (Nilandron, Anandron) Nonsteroidal androgen receptor antagonist
Indications: Intermediate- to high-risk prostate cancer; transgender hormone therapy
Dose: 300 mg po daily ×30d, then 150 mg po daily
Side Effects: Interstitial pneumonitis (black box warning), HA, hot flashes, insomnia, gynecomastia, impotence, breast tenderness, hepatitis

Apalutamide (Erleada) Nonsteroidal androgen receptor antagonist
Indications: Metastatic prostate cancer
Dose: 240 mg PO daily
Side Effects: Fatigue, nausea, vomiting, rash, bone fractures, seizures

Darolutamide (Nubeqa) Nonsteroidal androgen receptor antagonist
Indications: Metastatic prostate cancer
Dose: 600 mg PO bid
Side Effects: Fatigue, nausea, vomiting, rash, bone fractures, seizures

Abiraterone (Zytiga) decreases production of androgen precursors by inhibiting CYP17A1
Indications: Used in combination with prednisone (5 mg daily) in mCRPC
Dose: 1000 mg po daily
Side Effects: Edema, HTN, hypokalemia, fatigue, ↑glucose, ↑TG, ↑LFTs, joint swelling, hot flashes, cough insomnia, UTI, diarrhea

Estrogen

Anastrozole (Arimidex) aromatase inhibitor; blocks conversion of androgens to estrogens in extragonadal tissues
Indications: Hormone receptor–positive breast cancer in postmenopausal women; breast cancer prophylaxis
Dose: 1 mg po daily
Side Effects: Decreased bone mineral density, flushing, HTN, fatigue, HA, hot flashes, mood disturbance, arthralgia, ↑CV risk, ↑cholesterol

Letrozole (Femara) aromatase inhibitor
Indications: Hormone receptor–positive breast cancer in postmenopausal women
Dose: 2.5 mg po daily
Side Effects: Decreased bone mineral density, flushing, weakness, edema, fatigue, HA, hot flashes, mood disturbance, arthralgia, ↑cholesterol

Exemestane (Aromasin) aromatase inhibitor
Indications: Hormone receptor–positive breast cancer in postmenopausal women
Dose: 25 mg po daily
Side Effects: HTN, fatigue, insomnia, HA, decreased bone mineral density, flushing, hot flashes, diaphoresis, mood disturbance, arthralgia

Fulvestrant (Faslodex) selective estrogen receptor degrader (SERD): Binds to ER and causes degradation
Indications: Hormone receptor–positive breast cancer in postmenopausal women
Dose: 25 mg po daily
Side Effects: Hot flashes, ↑LFTs, joint disorders, bone pain fatigue, HA, nausea, pharyngitis

Tamoxifen (Nolvadex, Tamifen, Genox) selective estrogen receptor modulator (SERM): Competitive inhibitor of ER
Indications: Hormone receptor–positive breast cancer in premenopausal women
Dose: 20 mg po daily
Side Effects: ↑uterine cancer, ↑VTE risk, flushing, hot flashes, nausea, wt loss, vaginal discharge, weakness arthralgia, amenorrhea

Raloxifene (Evista, Optruma) SERM: Competitive inhibitor of ER
Indications: Breast cancer prophylaxis
Dose: 60 mg po daily ×5y
Side Effects: ↑VTE risk, ↑CVA risk, edema, hot flashes, arthralgia, leg cramps

Elacestrant (Orserdu) selective estrogen receptor degrader (SERD): induces degradation of ERα
Indications: ESR1-mutant advanced or metastatic ER+, HER2-breast cancer
Dose: 345 mg PO daily
Side Effects: ↑VTE risk, ↑CVA risk, edema, hot flashes, arthralgia, leg cramps

Gonadotropin-releasing hormone (GnRH)

Goserelin (Zoladex) GnRH agonist: Chronic activation leads to ↓LH/FSH and ↓steroidogenesis
Indications: Prostate cancer, breast cancer
Dose: 3.6 mg SC q4wk or 10.8 mg q12wk
Side Effects: Edema, fatigue, HA, hot flashes, mood disturbance, acne, ↓bone mineral density, ↓libido, vaginal dryness, ↑glucose

Leuprolide (Lupron) GnRH agonist
Indications: Prostate cancer, breast cancer
Dose: 7.5 mg q4wk/22.5 mg q12wk/30 mg q16wk/45 mg q24wk
Side Effects: Edema, fatigue, HA, hot flashes, mood disturbance, ↓bone mineral density, ↓libido, vaginal dryness, ↑glucose

Degarelix (Firmagon), Relugolix (Orgovyx) GnRH antagonist
Indications: Prostate cancer; especially *h/o CV disease*
Dose:
Degarelix: 240 mg loading dose SC × 1; then 80 mg SC q4wk
Relugolix: 360 mg loading dose PO × 1; then 120 mg PO qday
Side Effects: Hot flashes, ↑LFTs, wt gain, arthralgia

Bone-Modifying Agents

Bisphosphonates inhibit bone resorption by osteoclasts

Drugs: **Alendronate (Fosamax), etidronate (Didronel), ibandronate (Boniva), risedronate (Actonel), pamidronate (Aredia), zoledronate (Zometa)**

Indications: Reduce risk of fracture and bone pain in metastatic solid tumors or multiple myeloma. May reduce mortality in MM, breast, prostate ca

Side Effects: Osteonecrosis of the jaw, GI irritation, esophageal erosion, muscle pain, ↓Ca

Denosumab RANKL inhibitor; inhibits osteoclasts

Drugs: **Xgeva, Prolia**

Indications: Prevention of bone loss and skeletal events in solid tumors

Dose: Xgeva—120 mg SC q4wk (prevention of skeletal events); Prolia—60 mg SC q6mo (bone loss)

Side Effects: Osteonecrosis of the jaw, rash, fatigue, peripheral edema, GI irritation, ↓Ca

Hematology Systemic Agents

Drug	Target/ Mechanism	Indications	Side Effects
Arsenic trioxide (Trisenox)	PML-RAR alpha fusion protein	Mantle cell lymphoma	↑QT, chest pain, edema, ↑glucose
Belinostat (Beleodaq)	HDAC inhibitor	Cutaneous T-cell lymphoma	N/V, anemia, fever, SOB
Blinatumomab (Blincyto)	Bispecific T-cell engager (BiTE antibody) targeting CD19	DLBCL	Anemia, fever, cytokine release syndrome, ↑BP
Bortezomib (Velcade)	26S proteasome	Follicular lymphoma, mantle cell lymphoma, MM	Diarrhea, rash, peripheral neuropathy
Brentuximab vedotin (Adcetris)	Anti-CD30 with cleavable liner to chemo agent MMAE	DLBCL	N/V, alopecia, ↓RBC/ PLT/WBC, neuropathy
Cladribine (Leustatin)	Purine analog	Mantle cell lymphoma	BM depression, fever, infection
Duvelisib (Copiktra)	PI3K delta/gamma	Follicular lymphoma	↑K^+, ↓Na^+, ↓Ca^{2+}, ↓RBC/PLT/ WBC
Ibrutinib (Imbruvica)	Bruton's tyrosine kinase (BTK)	DLBCL, follicular/ mantle cell/ marginal zone lymphomas	↓RBC, neutropenia, lymphocytosis, edema, cough, ↑infection, fever
Lenalidomide (Revlimid)	Immunomodulatory	Follicular lymphoma, mantle cell lymphoma, MM	Pruritus, diarrhea, rash, muscle spasm, N/V/D
Mogamulizumab (Poteligeo)	CCR4	Cutaneous and peripheral T-cell lymphoma	↓albumin, ↓T cells, ↓PLT, ↑LFTs, MSK pain
Mosunetuzumab (Lunsumio)	CD3/CD20 bispecific engaging antibody	Follicular lymphoma	Cytokine release syndrome, fatigue, rash, fever, headache

Drug	Target/ Mechanism	Indications	Side Effects
Obinutuzumab (Gazyva)	CD20	DLBCL, mantle cell lymphoma	↓RBC/PLT/WBC, ↑K^+, ↓phos
Polatuzumab vedotin (Polivy)	CD79B	DLBCL	BM suppression, neuropathy, diarrhea/ vomiting, body aches, diarrhea, ↓K^+
Procarbazine (Matulane)	Alkylator	CNS lymphoma, follicular/ Hodgkin/mantle cell lymphoma	BM suppression, neuropathy, N/V, hearing loss
Selinexor (Xpovio)	Chromosome region maintenance 1 protein or exportin 1	DLBCL, transformed lymphoma	↓RBC/PLT/WBC, ↓appetite, N/V/D, ↑AST/ ALT, infection, fever
Tisagenlecleucel (Kymriah)	Anti-CD19 with TCR/CD3	Follicular lymphoma	↓RBC/PLT/WBC, hemorrhage, cytokine release

IMMUNOTHERAPY

Basic immunology

- **Innate immunity:** Immunogenic pattern recognition by macrophages, dendritic cells, and NK cells. Respond to pathogen-associated molecular patterns and damage-associated molecular patterns. Activation leads to cytokine production, recruitment of other immune cells, and phagocytosis. Antigen-presenting cells then present antigens, leading to activation of adaptive immune system
- **Adaptive immunity:** Predominantly lymphocyte-mediated (B and T cells) immune "memory" via activation of B-cell and T-cell receptors. B-cell activation leads to humoral immunity (mediated by antibody production) in response to a Th2 response; T cells mediate cellular immunity in response to Th1 response (thought to be more important for cancer surveillance).
- **Cell types**
  - **Macrophages (MΦ):** Monocyte derived. Function as antigen-presenting cells (APCs), phagocytes (in response to Fc, complement, or mannose), and innate immune surveillance/activation (activated by PAMPs, DAMPs). Often resident in tumor tissue (TAMs), where they can promote invasion and metastasis. Two subtypes with prognostic implications in cancer:
    - **M1:** "Antitumor"; produce tumoricidal TNF and NO; improved prognosis
    - **M2:** "Protumor"; produce IL-10, arginase, TGF-β; prevent Th1 response
  - **Dendritic Cells:** APCs that respond to PAMPs, cytokines. Play role in activating tumor-specific cytotoxic T cells.
  - **B Cells:** Lymphocytes that produce antibodies in response to B-cell receptor activation via Th2 response to antigens. Found in circulation, lymph nodes, spleen, MALT lymphoma
  - **T Cells:** Thymus-conditioned lymphocytes that recognize antigen-MHC complex. Mediate cellular immunity
    - **CD4:** Helper T cells; activate immune depending on cytokine and antigen context. Required for activation of cytotoxic responses that underlie cancer immune surveillance. HIV immunosuppression via CD4 depletion → increased cancer incidence
    - **CD8:** Cytotoxic T cell; activated by MHC class I; produce IFNγ, IL-2. Can directly kill infected/tumor cells via Th1 cytokine response to tumor-expressed MHC class I. Tumor down-regulation of MHC-I is a common means of immune evasion. Activation requires coincident TCR-MHC and CD-28/B7 signals. Immune checkpoint receptors can inhibit or stimulate CD-8 activation. **Immunotherapeutics target checkpoint ligands/receptors**.

- **Th17:** Produce IL-17 in response to IL-1, IL-6, and TGF-β. Regulate mucosal immunity and modulate inflammation. Pro- and antitumor effects
- **Treg:** Maintain self-tolerance by inhibiting anti-self lymphocyte expansion. May play a role in suppressing antitumor immunity. Activated by IL-10 and TGF-β
- **MDSCs:** Myeloid-derived suppressor cells. Immunosuppressive myeloid cells that can be found in tumor microenvironment and are associated with poor prognosis and outcome

• **NK Cells:** Cytotoxic innate immune lymphocytes activated by Mϕ cytokines. Important for containing viral infections during adaptive immune activation. Key role in preventing relapse after BMT

Common Immunotherapy Agents

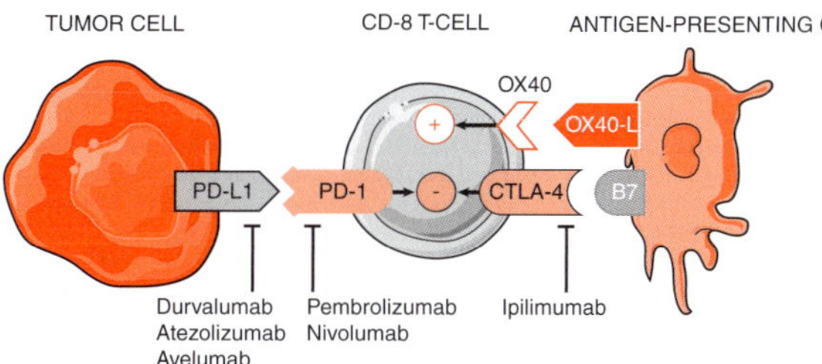

Drug	Target	Indications	Side Effects
Ipilimumab (Yervoy) **Tremelimumab (Imjudo)**	CTLA-4	Melanoma and combination with PD-1 for other cancers	**Diarrhea, colitis, hypophysitis**
Pembrolizumab (Keytruda) **Nivolumab (Opdivo)**	PD-1	Melanoma, NSCLC, HNC, HL, RCC, **MMR or MSI tumors**	**Pneumonitis,** colitis, hypophysitis, thyroiditis, vitiligo
Durvalumab (Imfinzi) **Atezolizumab (Tecentriq)** **Avelumab (Bavencio)**	PD-L1	Metastatic urothelial, NSCLC, Merkel	Rash, thyroiditis, hepatitis
Tiragolumab	TIGIT	In combination with atezolizumab for PD-L1 high NSCLC	Weakness, nausea, cough, SOB
Relatlimab	LAG3	In combination with nivolumab for melanoma	Fatigue, arthralgia, rash, diarrhea

Immunotherapy and Radiation

Several trials evaluated safety and effectiveness of radiation with immunotherapy.

- **XRT → ipilimumab**: Improved OS (not SS) in metastatic CRPC phase 3 trial (*Kwon Lancet Oncol* 2014)
- **Concurrent chemoRT → durvalumab**: **Increased PFS and OS** in stage III NSCLC in phase 3 PACIFIC trial (*Antonia NEJM* 2017 and *Antonia NEJM* 2018)
- **Concurrent WBRT or SRS + ipilimumab**: Phase I safe for melanoma patients with brain mets (*Williams IJROBP* 2017)
- **SBRT and ipilimumab**: Concurrent or sequential XRT/ipilimumab safe in metastatic solid cancers in phase I (*Tang Clin Cancer Res* 2017)
- **SBRT and nivolumab (I-SABR):** Phase II RCT demonstrating I-SABR to significantly improve EFS vs SABR alone among patients with early-stage treatment naive, node-negative, NSCLC (*Chang Lancet* 2023)

Several ongoing studies are evaluating possible synergy between radiation and immunotherapy in localized and metastatic solid cancer.

- Radiation may act as a "tumor vaccine," exposing neoantigens after radiation-induced immunogenic cell death
- Thought to be most effective in the context of hypofractionated or stereotactic XRT

Immune Checkpoint Inhibitor–Associated Adverse Events

Side effects much different from cytotoxic therapy. Due to stimulation of autoimmunity.

General management principles:

- **Grade 1**: Local/symptomatic treatment (topical steroids, antidiarrheal)
- **Grade 2**: Rule out infection/disease progression; oral steroids (eg, dexamethasone 4 mg every 6 hours). Treat symptoms.
- **Grade 3-4**: Hold or discontinue Rx; IV steroids +/− additional immunosuppressants (eg, infliximab 5 mg/kg single dose)

Hypophysitis: Clinical hypopituitarism and radiographic pituitary enlargement. Symptoms—Headache, fatigue/weakness. Decreased thyroid, adrenal, gonadal hormones. DI and vision Δ rare. Rule out brain mets with MRI; full endocrine workup. Can resume immunotherapy with hormone replacement.

Pneumonitis: Rule out infection and hold treatment with G1. G2—add steroids; G3-4—d/c Rx; hospitalize with high-dose IV steroids

Diarrhea/Colitis: Diarrhea and radiographic changes such as diffuse bowel thickening or colitis. First rule out *Clostridium difficile* or other infection. In severe instances, colonoscopy may help to diagnose. Treat diarrhea with antidiarrheal agents (eg, loperamide and atropine) and anti-immune medications (eg, steroids and infliximab).

Rash: Most common adverse event, occurring with 40-50% of Pd-1 and CTLA-4 inhibitors. G1-2—supportive treatment with cold compresses, topical corticosteroids, and hydroxyzine, G3—hold treatment until return to G1. If G4 consider infliximab, mycophenolate mofetil, or cyclophosphamide. Rarely Stevens-Johnson syndrome/toxic epidermal necrolysis has been reported.

Adoptive T-cell Therapy

Transplantation of more effective antitumor T cells to induce direct tumor killing

- **Chimeric antigen receptor (CAR-T cells)** autologous or allogeneic T cells genetically engineered to express a chimeric T-cell receptor that includes tumor antigen–specific monoclonal Ab variable regions fused with the TCR and a costimulatory receptor (CD28). Activation is MHC independent, and response to antigen is supraphysiologic.
  - **Indications (FDA approved):** Pediatric ALL; refractory large B-cell lymphoma
  - **Adverse effects:** Cytokine release syndrome, off target effects (B-cell aplasia), cerebral edema, neurotoxicity; GVHD (if allogeneic T cells are used)
- **Engineered TCR** T cells are isolated from blood or tumor tissue and tumor antigen–responsive T cells are selected TCR from these cells are cloned, and autologous lymphocytes are engineered to express selected tumor-specific TCR and infused into patient. Activation is MHC dependent.
- **Tumor-infiltrating lymphocytes (TIL)** lymphocytes are isolated from tumors, expanded in vitro in the presence of IL-2, and infused back into the patient after lymphodepletion with TBI or chemotherapy.
- **Donor lymphocyte infusion** Adoptive transfer of lymphocytes from a donor to a patient who has already received an HLA-matched transplant from the same donor. The goal is to augment antitumor immune response or ensure durable engraftment. Used to treat relapse after allogeneic SCT for CML, AML, and ALL
  - **Adverse effects:** Acute and chronic GVHD; bone marrow aplasia, immunosuppression

Oncolytic Viruses

Modified viruses that replicate preferentially in cancer cells. Many designed to stimulate immune system and induce antitumor immunity. Primary mechanism of action is virus replication in tumor cells causing oncolysis.

- **T-Vec (Imlygic)** modified HSV-1 expressing GM-CSF. Approved for inoperable melanoma. Delivered by intratumoral injection
- **Reolysin** unmodified human reovirus systemically administered oncolytic virus. Replicates in cells with activated Ras. Currently in phase III for HNSCC and CRC
- **JX-594 (Pexa-Vec)** attenuated vaccinia virus that expresses GM-CSF. Selectively replicates in cells with high levels of thymidine kinase (eg, p53 or Ras mutation). Currently in phase I-III clinical trials
- **DNX-2401 (Delta-24-RGD)** replication-competent adenovirus that selectively replicates in tumor cells with nonfunctional Rb pathway. Expresses RGD that enables uptake in tumor cells expressing integrins $\alpha_v\beta_3$ or $\alpha_v\beta_5$. Currently in phase I/II.
- **PVSRIPO**: Polio-rhinovirus chimera that recognizes the poliovirus receptor CD155, which is widely expressed in neoplastic cells of solid tumors. Recent phase I/II trial highlighted its use in recurrent glioblastoma, as it improved survival to 24-36 months, which is improved relative to historical controls (*Desjardins et al. NEJM* 2018).

Cytokines and Immune Stimulators

- **GM-CSF (sargramostim)**
  - *Indications:* Chemo-induced neutropenia; myeloid reconstitution for HSCT
  - *Mechanism:* Stimulate expansion of myeloid cells (PMNs, DCs, Mφ)
  - *Side Effects:* Bone pain, myalgias, arthralgias, injection site rxn
- **G-CSF (filgrastim)**
  - *Indications:* Chemo-induced neutropenia; myeloid reconstitution for HSCT
  - *Mechanism:* Stimulate expansion of myeloid cells (PMNs)
  - *Side Effects:* Bone pain, myalgias, arthralgias, injection site rxn
- **IL-2 (aldesleukin)**
  - *Indications:* RCC, melanoma, adjuvant for autologous BMT
  - *Mechanism:* Expansion of lymphocytes (↑CD4, CD8, Treg, B cells, NK cells)
  - *Side Effects:* Capillary leak, shock, flulike symptoms
- Bacillus Calmette-Guérin (BCG)
  - *Indications:* Bladder cancer (Intravesical)
  - *Mechanism:* Live mycobacteria that induces an immune response
  - *Side Effects:* Hematuria, fever, dysuria, urinary frequency, myalgias, fatigue

Vaccines

Induce immune response to shared or unique tumor antigens

Preventive vaccines: Vaccinate against cancer-causing viruses

- **HPV vaccines**: Inoculation of viruslike particles assembled from recombinant HPV coat proteins. Elicit virus–neutralizing antibody responses. 100% protection vs cervical CIN (*Harper Lancet* 2006)
  - **Gardasil and Cervarix** HPV types 6, 11, 16, and 18
  - **Gardasil-9** HPV types 6, 11, 16, 18, 31, 33, 45, 52, and 58
- **HBV vaccines**: Contain HBsAg, produced by yeast cells. Three vaccinations ~85-90% protection
  - **Engerix-B and Recombivax HB**: HBV infection only (all ages)
  - **Twinrix** HAV and HBV (18 and older)
  - **Pediarix** infants whose mothers are negative for HBsAg (as early as 6 weeks old)

Therapeutic vaccines: Vaccinate against tumor-specific antigens to induce a T-cell response.

- Can be made from whole cells, modified whole cells (eg, express immunostimulatory molecules), peptides (HLA-restricted), DNA, DC conditioning, or Ag presentation in vectors (eg, virus) containing immunostimulatory molecules
- **Sipuleucel-T (Provenge)**: Dendritic cell vaccine FDA approved for metastatic prostate cancer. Stimulate immune response to prostatic acid phosphatase. Patient's DCs collected and cultured with PAP-GM-CSF, then reinfused. ↑OS in mCRPC by 4 months (*Kantoff NEJM* 2010)
- **Prostvac-VF**: Recombinant vaccinia virus encoding PSA and costimulatory molecule. ↑OS in mCRPC by 4 months in phase II (*Kantoff JCO* 2010)

Radiopharmaceutical Therapy

Systemic delivery of radioactive atoms to tumor-associated targets using an antibody or other conjugate. The efficacy of the targeted radiopharmaceutical depends on numerous factors including antigen/receptor variables including affinity, avidity, density, availability, shedding, and heterogeneity of expressions as well as tumor factors including vascularity, blood flow, and permeability. For some antibody targets, they have an anti-tumor component in addition to the radionuclide. Additionally, when the antibody is internalized, cell death mechanisms may be induced including apoptosis, complement-dependent cytotoxicity, and antibody-dependent cell-mediated cytotoxicity.

- **Emission:** Primarily β-particles or potent α-particles
  - β-Particle emitters: Samarium-153, luteitium-177, yttrium-90, and iodine-131
  - α-Particles emitters: Astatine-211, bismuth-212, lead-212, bismuth-213, actinium-225, radium-223, and thorium-227

Radionuclide	Therapeutic Emission	Approximate Emission Range in Tissue (mm)	Radionuclide Half-Life
Strontium-89	β^-	2.4	50.5 d
Yttrium-90	β^-	5.30	64.1 h
Iodine-131	β^-	0.8	8.0 d
Samarium-153	β^-	0.4	46.5 h
Lutetium-177	β^-	0.62	6.6 d
Astatine-211	α	0.05	7.2 h
Lead 212/Bismuth-212	β^-/α	$<0.1/0.05$	10.6 h/1.0 h
Radium-223	α	0.05-0.08	11.4 d
Actinium-225	α	0.05-0.08	10.0 d
Thorium-227	α	0.05-0.08	18.7 d

With permission from Sgouros et al. *Nat Rev Drug Discov* 2020.

- **Commercially available radiopharmaceuticals:**
  - ^{223}Ra dichloride (Xofigo)—Metastatic castration-resistant prostate cancer
  - ^{90}Y-loaded glass/resin microspheres (SIR-Spheres)—Hepatic malignancies
  - ^{131}I radioiodine—Thyroid cancer
  - ^{153}Smlexidronam (Quadramet)—Cancer bone pain
  - ^{89}Sr (Metastron)—Cancer bone pain
  - ^{177}Lu-labelled dotatate (Lutathera)—Neuroendocrine tumors
  - ^{131I}mIBG (Azedra)—Adrenergic receptor tumors and neuroblastoma
  - ^{177}Lu-labeled PSMA (Pluvicto)—Prostate cancer
  - ^{90}Y ibritumomab tiuxetan (Zevalin)—Follicular lymphoma

CLINICAL STATISTICS

LAUREN ELIZABETH COLBERT • CLIFTON DAVID FULLER

Basic Biostatistics

- **Statistical testing** requires defining a study hypothesis and thus a null hypothesis (H_o) to be tested. Applying the appropriate statistical test to this null hypothesis results in a ***P*-value** (α) → the probability of a result equal to or beyond that observed assuming H_o is true.
- The test, H_o, and thus, the α can all be either **one sided** (only tests data on one side of the H_o) or **two sided** (tests data on both sides of the H_o).
- **Type I (or α) error** occurs when we conclude there is a difference when none exists; **Type II (or β) error** occurs when we conclude there is no difference when one exists; **Power (1-β)** is the probability of correctly rejecting H_o.
- **Sensitivity** and **specificity** are used to evaluate diagnostic tests. **Sensitivity** is ratio of True Positives/Actual Positives. Actual Positives includes True Positives + False Negatives. **Sensitivity** is the ratio of True Negatives/Actual Negatives. Actual Negatives includes True Negatives + False Positives.

Refer to Figure 5.1: Sensitivity = $A / (A + C)$

$$\text{Sensitivity} = A / (A + C)$$

- **Positive predictive value (PPV)** and **negative predictive value (NPV)** predict the likelihood of accuracy of a given test result. They both depend on the frequency of the disease in the underlying population. **PPV = True Positives/(True Positives + False Positives); NPV = True Negatives/(True Negatives + False Negatives).**

Refer to Figure 5.1: PPV = A / (A + C)

$$NPV = A / (A + C)$$

	Condition True	Condition False
+ Test	*A* (True Positive)	*B* (False positive, Type 1 error)
- Test	*C* (False Negative, Type 2 error)	*D* (True Negative)

Figure 5.1 2 × 2 contingency table showing expected test and condition results and their combinations.

Choosing a Statistical Test

Univariate analyses (one independent variable)

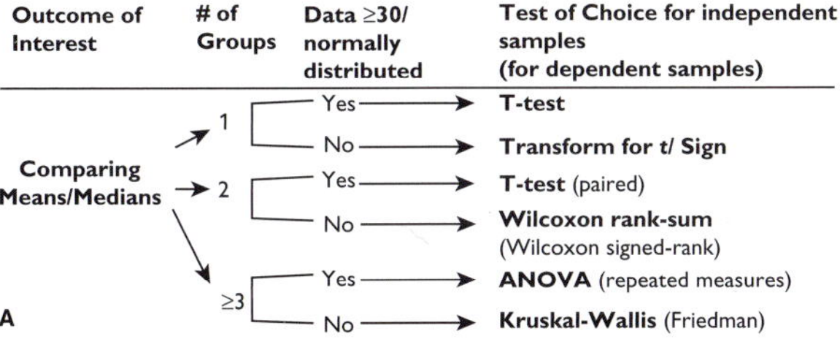

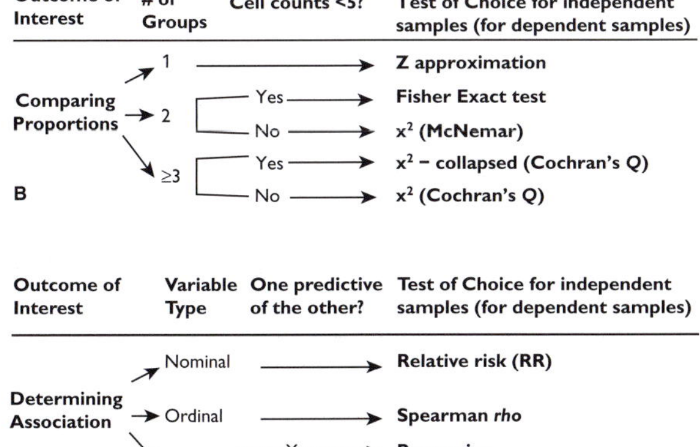

Multivariate analyses (two or more independent variables)

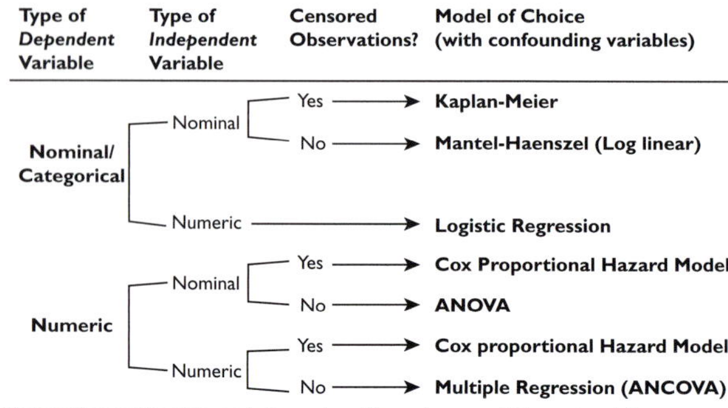

Note: A Cox multivariate analysis requires 10 events per variable analyzed. For example, if there are 100 local failures, then a total of 10 variables can be analyzed.

Clinical Trial Design

Phase 0	Proof of concept; first in human; testing pharmacokinetics, etc.
Phase I	Primary objective is toxicity; can test pharmacokinetics, dose finding, toxicity, MTD studies
Phase II	Primary objective is efficacy; can also continue to test safety; can be single-arm or small multi-arm (either randomized or nonrandomized) trials; IIA often demonstrate clinical efficacy and IIB find optimum dose
Phase III	Primary objective is determining efficacy when compared against gold standard; often multi-institutional and/or randomized/controlled; typically, single disease and well-defined patient population

Important Concepts—Clinical Studies

Phase I study designs

- **Traditional rule-based designs** (Classical 3 + 3, pharmacologically guided, accelerated titration)
  - **3 + 3 Design:** Based on traditional Fibonacci sequence. Cohorts of 3 patients are treated at a time and followed until specified time period (DLT window) before escalating. Once there is one patient with a dose limiting toxicity (DLT), a total of 6 are entered at that dose level. If a total of 2 or more the 6 have grade 3+ toxicity, then that dose level is the maximal tolerated dose (MTD). The recommended dose level (RDL) for the phase II is one dose level below the MTD. **Advantages:** Simple and easy to follow/implement. **Disadvantages:** can be slow due to DLT window and treat unnecessary patients at subtherapeutic doses below the MTD
  - **Accelerated titration (AT):** Allows escalating to next dose levels within cohort due to <3 patient cohorts (1 or 2). Only requires 3 patient cohort if a prespecified toxicity occurs. **Advantages:** Can increase pace of accrual and escalation. **Disadvantages:** Excessive/unsafe dose escalation may occur before toxicity is realized. May expose too many patients to toxic dose, particularly with radiation toxicities that may occur later
- **Model-based designs** (continual reassessment method [CRM, TITE-CRM], EffTox, Time to event, TriCR)
  - **Continual reassessment model (CRM):** Bayesian-based adaptive modeling accounts for *known prior probabilities* of toxicity including previously available data and previously accrued patients; adjusts dose as prior probabilities change. **Advantages:** May be more likely to treat patients at appropriate dose levels, does not throw out known data, may escalate more quickly. **Disadvantages:** Requires intensive statistical support and appropriate/trustworthy prior data.

- **TITE-CRM** is a variety of CRM that incorporates time-to-event rather than only dichotomous toxicity data.
- **EffTox** is a variety of CRM that incorporates both efficacy and toxicity into decision-making for dose assignment. Investigators set "rules" for requirements for efficacy and toxicity in order to escalate/de-escalate dose. **Advantages:** More efficient in diseases where some toxicity trade-off may be acceptable for increased efficacy (ie, pancreatic cancer, glioblastoma, diffuse intrinsic pontine glioma, etc.) or for extremely low toxicity studies (some RT studies). The Late Onset EffTox model (LOET) can be effective in radiation studies, where onset of toxicity may be later than in drug studies, for example.

- Phase I/II trials are designed to initiate a phase II trial at a prespecified criterion within the phase I trial. Often the MTD identified in the phase I component of the trial is utilized in the phase II component.

Phase II study designs

- **Single-arm designs** generally compare only to known historical outcomes, with no built-in comparison arm. Outcomes may be response/no response, recurrence-free survival, or overall survival. **Advantages:** These require small sample size and allow for choice of comparison arm. **Disadvantages:** Historical comparisons are limited; comparisons may be biased.
- **Randomized phase II:** Two-arm studies that may be either comparative, with the intent to choose a winner for a phase III trial, or noncomparative. **Advantages:** Avoids limitations of historical comparison. **Disadvantages:** Require a much larger sample size. Allowed type I and type II error rates may be clinically futile given limitations in sample size.

Randomized phase II/III study designs

Patients are entered on the phase II portion and if an interim analysis meets a prespecified criterion (eg, does not show a difference between treatment arms), the trial continues as a phase III. The patients entered on the phase II become part of the phase III. **Advantages:** More efficient since there is only one trial. **Disadvantage:** The primary endpoint of the phase II must be different than the phase III. For example, the primary endpoint of the phase II could be local control, whereas the primary endpoint of the phase III would be survival.

Phase III study designs

- **Randomized controlled trial (RCT)** represents "gold standard" of clinical testing. A double-blinded trial involves both the investigators and patients being blinded to treatment arm. Randomization can occur in many methods but involves randomly assigning patients to treatment arms. **Advantages:** Chance is only source of potential imbalance (eliminates selection and time biases), and randomization lends validity to statistical testing. **Disadvantages:** May require very large patient sample; not acceptable to some patients; administratively and financially complex. Placebo controls can be used for the control arm; this is difficult in radiation trials.
- **Superiority trials** are intended to show efficacy of a test treatment to be superior to that of a control (generally standard of care).
- **Noninferiority trial** is considered positive if efficacy is similar to a known effective treatment and involves a one-sided statistical test (ie, an experimental arm is *not worse* by an allowable amount determined by investigators). **Equivalence trials** are similar but require two-sided statistical tests. In general, an equivalence (and most noninferiority) trial requires about twice as many patients as a superiority trial.
- **Crossover design** trials allow patients to "cross over" from assigned arm to other arm. **Advantages:** Each patient can be his/her own control; more palatable to patients. **Disadvantages:** Difficult to interpret statistically; disease must be stable over time; one arm must not affect the other arm. Lastly, a crossover trial cannot use overall survival as the primary endpoint.
- **Two-by-two or "Factorial" design** involves more than one randomization or treatment arm assignment. **Advantages:** Allows testing of more potential treatments within one trial. **Disadvantages:** Difficult to analyze statistically; interactions between randomization factors may complicate interpretation; requires large patient sample sizes for reliability

---

Important Concepts

- **Odds ratio (OR)** represents the ratio of odds of an event (# currently with event/# currently without event) for the "exposed" cases divided by the "nonexposed" cases; often used in a case-control study.

- **Risk ratio or relative risk (RR)** is a measure of *incidence* (over time) and is expressed as ratio of cases who have or will develop an event in "exposed" group vs those in the "nonexposed" group.
- **Absolute risk reduction (ARR)** is the absolute difference between the RR in the experimental arm and the baseline RR of an event.
- **Number needed to treat (NNT)** is calculated as 1/absolute risk reduction and represents the number of patients that would need to be treated to avoid one event.
- **Hazard ratio (HR)** is an odds ratio that compares risk over time instead of at a static time. It can be interpreted as the ratio of hazard of time in the "experimental" arm vs "baseline" arm.
- **Median overall survival (OS)** is calculated using actuarial methods and represents the time at which <50% of patients remain alive. It accounts for "time contributed" of patients lost to follow up.
- **Recurrence/relapse-free survival (RFS)** is calculated based on patients who survive without *either* recurring or dying.
- **Selection bias** occurs when the studied population does not represent the population of interest. **Classification bias** occurs when the variables are not clearly measured (have subjectivity) and misclassification affects outcome. **Confounding bias** occurs when the factor and outcome are erroneously linked, when they may be a confounding factor.
- **Randomization** attempts to eliminate selection bias by randomly assigning patients to groups. Clearly defining outcomes and variables up front can help eliminate classification bias. Some trials from the NSABP as well as the German Rectal Cancer Trial used "prerandomization." This approach increased enrollment; however, due to ethical concerns, it is no longer allowed.
- **Inclusion and exclusion criteria** are used to determine eligibility. Patients must meet all inclusion criteria and not meet exclusion criteria to be eligible.
- **An Institutional Review Board (IRB)** is generally institution specific and is responsible for ensuring that trials are safely and ethically conducted.
- **Intention-to-treat** analysis indicates that results were evaluated based on treatment arms originally assigned, even if patients change arms or do not complete therapy. An intention-to-treat analysis should be used whenever possible in a superiority study. **Per protocol analysis** analyzes only patients who were treated according to intended protocol arm (and completed therapy).
- **CONSORT guidelines** were designed to simplify and standardize reporting of parallel group-controlled trials.

Levels of Evidence (per USPSTF)

Level I	Evidence from ≥1 properly designed RCT
Level II-1	Evidence from well-designed, nonrandomized trials
Level II-2	Evidence from well-designed cohort or case-control studies
Level II-3	Evidence from multiple time-based studies with or without intervention
Level III	Opinion-level evidence

BRACHYTHERAPY

AARON SEO • ANNA LIKHACHEVA • CHAD TANG

BACKGROUND

- **Definition:** Brachytherapy is a type of radiotherapy in which radioactive sources are placed inside or near target tissues.
- **Rationale:** Brachytherapy is arguably the most conformal form of radiotherapy. It can deliver ablative doses to the target while sparing adjacent uninvolved tissues.
- **Critical considerations:** Correct source placement is of utmost importance in brachytherapy. As opposed to EBRT where dose distribution is relatively homogenous, brachytherapy dose distribution is heterogeneous with maximum doses inside the target being orders of magnitude higher than the prescription. 3D treatment planning is imperative.

DOSE RATE DEFINITIONS

LDR: 0.4-2 Gy/h
MDR: 2-12 Gy/h
HDR: >12 Gy/h
PDR (pulsed dose rate): HDR delivered in small fractions over a period of time typical for LDR implants. It is thought to mimic the radiobiological quality of LDR, while providing the radiation safety of a remote afterloader and the 3D planning benefit of a stepping source. Generally requires inpatient admission

HDR BED calculation (*Nag and Gupta IJROBP* 2000): $N \times d\left(1+\frac{d}{\alpha/\beta}\right)$

LDR BED calculation (*Stock et al. IJROBP* 2006): $R/\lambda\left(1+\frac{R}{(\mu+\lambda)\times\alpha/\beta}\right)$

R (initial dose rate) = D90 × λ
λ (radioactive decay constant) = $0.693/t_{1/2}$
N = number of fractions, d = dose per fraction, and $t_{1/2}$ = half-life
μ = sublethal damage repair constant (typical values: prostate cancer = 0.693 h^{-1}, cervix cancer = 0.55 h^{-1})
α/β = characteristic parameter of the cell survival curve from the linear quadratic model (typical values: normal tissues = 2-4 Gy, tumors = 2-10 Gy)

COMMON BRACHYTHERAPY ISOTOPES

	^{125}I	^{103}Pd	^{131}Cs	^{192}Ir	^{137}Cs	^{226}Ra	^{198}Au
Half-life	59.4 d	17 d	9.7 d	73.8 d	30 y	1600 y	2.7 d
Energy (kV)	27	21	29	380	662	830	412
HVL (mm-lead)	0.025	0.0085	0.022	2.5	6.2	14	3.3

CONSIDERATIONS FOR INVASIVE PROCEDURES

- Labs <7 days prior to procedure or after last cycle of chemo: Hct > 25, Plt > 50k for intracavitary and >100k for interstitial and for epidural/spinal anesthesia; coag panel
- NPO after midnight for conscious/deep sedation
- Anticoagulation management guidelines (the timing of anticoagulation pause needs to be weighed against the risks and benefits of brachytherapy in conjunction with patient's multidisciplinary team):

Drug (Generic Name)	Class of Drug	Recommended Hold Interval
Aspirin 81 mg	NSAID	Do not hold unless PLT < 50k or per surgery instruction
Aspirin 325 mg	NSAID	7-10 d prior to procedure
Indocin (Indomethacin) Voltaren (Diclofenac)	NSAID	1 d prior to procedure

Drug (Generic Name)	Class of Drug	Recommended Hold Interval
Heparin Lovenox (Enoxaparin)	Heparin/low molecular weight heparin	12-24 h prior to procedure
Fragmin (Dalteparin)	Low molecular weight heparin	24-48 h prior to procedure
Xarelto (Rivaroxaban)	Direct factor Xa inhibitor	24 h prior to procedure
Eliquis (Apixaban)	Direct factor Xa inhibitor	24-48 h prior to procedure
Arixtra (Fondaparinux)	Direct factor Xa inhibitor	48 h prior to procedure
Pradaxa (Dabigatran)	Direct thrombin inhibitor	3-5 d prior to procedure
Coumadin (Warfarin)	Vitamin K antagonist	5-7 d prior to procedure
Brilinta (Ticagrelor) Plavix (Clopidogrel)	P2Y12 platelet inhibitor	5-7 d prior to procedure
Effient (Prasugrel)	P2Y12 platelet inhibitor	7 d prior to procedure
Pletal (Cilostazol)	PDE inhibitor	7 d prior to procedure
Ticlid (Ticlidopine)	Platelet aggregation inhibitor	7-10 d prior to procedure
Persantine (Aggrenox)	PDE5 inhibitor, platelet aggregation inhibitor	7-10 d prior to procedure
Mobic (Meloxicam)	Extended release NSAID	10 d prior to the procedure

Prostate Treatment Algorithms

- Screening colonoscopy within 3 years prior to prostate brachytherapy procedures
- 1× antibiotic at procedure (eg, Ancef) with gram-negative coverage if preexisting orthopedic hardware (eg, gentamicin). Discharge with 1-2 weeks of oral antibiotics (eg, fluoroquinolone).
- Bowel prep: Clear liquid diet in the PM prior to procedure, two tabs of bisacodyl at 2 PM, bisacodyl suppository at night, saline Fleet Enema in AM
- **Contraindications:** IPSS > 15-20 and postvoid residual >100 cc, large median lobe, gross ECE, seminal vesicle involvement, large-volume TURP, prostate volume >60 cc, IBD, or unable to undergo anesthesia

• Low risk: cT1c-T2a, PSA < 10, Gleason Grade Group 1 • Favorable intermediate risk: only 1 intermediate risk factor, <50% cores positive (strongly recommend staging MRI to exclude patients with T3 disease)	Brachytherapy monotherapy
Unfavorable intermediate risk	Brachytherapy monotherapy or EBRT* (to prostate + SVs) + brachytherapy boost (in select high-risk patients)
High risk	EBRT* (to prostate + SVs ± pelvic LNs) + brachytherapy boost 12-24 months of concurrent and adjuvant ADT

*EBRT typically administered using standard fractionation or moderate hypofractionation.

LDR Prostate Planning Metrics

Isotope	Loading Technique	Planning Metrics (PTV)	Monotherapy Prescription	Boost Prescription
I-125	Modified uniform	D90 > 140 Gy, V100 > 95%, V150 < 60%, V200 < 20%	144 Gy	100-110 Gy
Pd-103	Modified peripheral	D90 > 125 Gy, V100 > 95%, V150 < 75%, V200 < 45%	125 Gy	90-100 Gy
Cs-131	Modified peripheral with rectal modification	D90 > 115 Gy, V100 > 95%, V150 < 50%, V200 < 15%	115 Gy	75-85 Gy

- **Normal tissue constraints:** Urethra: V125 < 1 cc, Max 150%. External urethral sphincter (EUS): V200 < 0.04 cc (urethra and EUS constraints based on MRI simulation). Rectum: V100 < 1 cc (consider placement of a rectal wall spacer).
- **D0 evaluation metrics:** Consider the location of disease identified on pretreatment biopsy and MRI. Otherwise, D90 > 90% prescription dose and V100 > 90%. Immediate postimplant CT and/or MRI to evaluate dose distribution and confirm high-quality implant. Postoperative day 30 evaluation if concern identified on day 0 dosimetry. Consider additional seed placement if inadequate coverage.
- **SIM:** 2-4 weeks prior to implant with MRI or endorectal US: (1) Identify the base and apex; (2) Obtain length; and (3) Evaluate pubic arch interference. If PAI, consider cytoreduction with 3 months Casodex + Lupron; obtain LFTs prior to initiation of Casodex
- **Target:** PTV depends on risk of ECE and imaging uncertainties. General expansion from CTV: 2-5 mm in all directions except 0-2 mm posterior (Fig. 6.1)

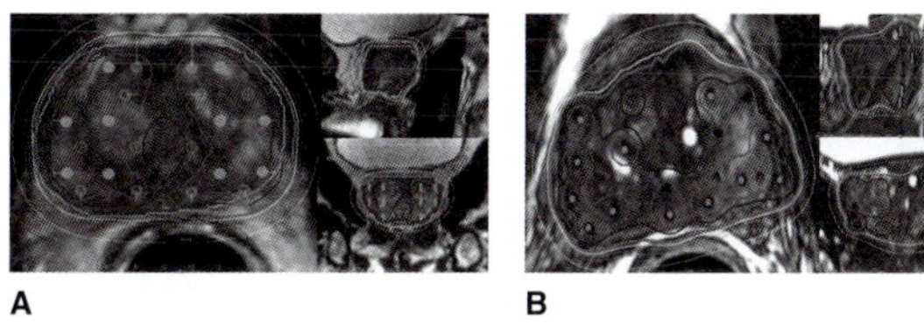

Figure 6.1 Example MRI LDR preplan **(A)** and D0 **(B)** plan for 144 Gy I-125 brachytherapy monotherapy implant to treat intermediate-risk prostate cancer. Showing the 100%, 150%, and 200% isodose lines. **See color insert.**

- **Side effects and management:**
  Infection: IV cefazolin and discharge home with PO ciprofloxacin
  Urinary (dysuria, hematuria, polyuria): Prophylactic use of alpha-blockers, discharge home with a Medrol Dosepak. If continued dysfunction, consider 2-week trial of ibuprofen 400 mg bid, increase alpha-blocker dose, or another Medrol Dosepak.
  Urinary retention: If unable to urinate, prompt placement of a Foley catheter is imperative. Consider other causes specifically postanesthesia (opioid-induced) retention.
  Erectile dysfunction: Consider daily Cialis prior to and after treatment.
  Proctitis and bleeding: steroid suppository/soften stools/reduce or eliminate anticoagulants if possible → steroid enema → referral to gastroenterology → hyperbaric oxygen → Argon plasma coagulation
- **Follow-up:** 1-month symptom phone call (and reevaluation if D0 implant concerns) → 6-month follow-up → regular intervals in first 5 years with PSA and EPIC QOL. PSA bounce can happen 12-30 months after implant.

High-Dose Rate (HDR)

- **Common indications:** Same as low dose rate
- **Contraindications:** IPSS > 20; prostate volume >60 cc can overcome with a freehand technique. Proximal seminal vesicles can be implanted if involved. HDR is an option for patients with prior TURP if done >6 months prior and TURP defect can be well visualized. IBD is a relative contraindication.
- **SIM:** Typically, no preplan is required. CT-based, US-based, or MR-based planning used.
- **Target:** Same as LDR, except can include ECE and proximal SV disease. No expansion from CTV to PTV if using real-time US planning (Fig. 6.2)
- **Evaluation metrics:** V100 > 97%, 105% < D90 < 115%; V150 < 35%; urethra V125% = 0; rectum V75% < 1 cc
- **Dose:**
  Boost: 15 Gy/1 fx or 19 Gy/2 fx.
  Monotherapy: 42 Gy/6 fx (two implants, 1 week apart), 38 Gy/4 fx (two implants, 1 week apart), 27 Gy/2 fx (one implant). All bid treatments should be delivered >6 hours apart.

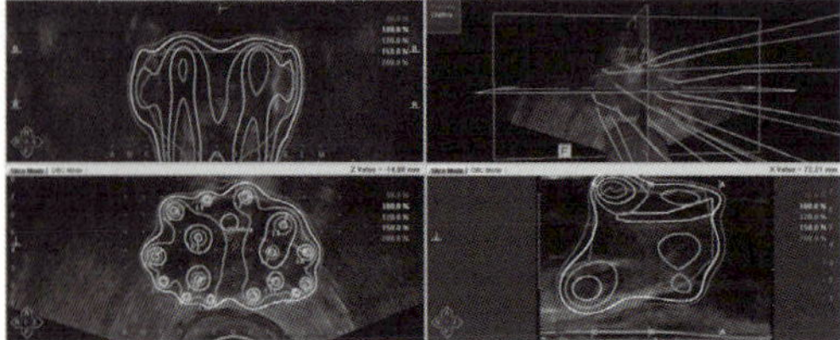

Figure 6.2 Example ultrasound HDR brachytherapy 15-Gy boost plan in a patient with high-risk prostate cancer after receiving 46 Gy/23 fx pelvic radiation.

- **Loading technique:** Start on a midgland slice. Peripheral catheter placement techniques are common (~2/3 peripheral, 1/3 central).
- **Side effects and management:** Same as LDR
- **Follow-up:** Regular intervals in the first 5 years with PSA and EPIC QOL. PSA bounce can happen 12-30 months after implant.

Gynecologic

Endometrial (see Endometrial chapter)

- **Timing:** Start 4-12 weeks postoperatively for brachy alone, within 2 weeks after EBRT.
- **Technique:** Vaginal cuff dome HDR (Fig. 6.3) for postoperative treatment. Endocavitary endometrial applicators (Rotte Y applicator or modified Heyman capsules) for definitive treatment of inoperable endometrial cancers.

Vaginal cuff brachytherapy

- **SIM:** During CT simulation, size dome for largest diameter cylinder that patient can tolerate, and verify dome positioning with CT scan. Alternatively, fiducial seed can be placed at vaginal cuff to be used for cylinder positioning verification with x-ray.
- **Target:** Top 2-4 cm of upper vagina
- **Dose:** 6 Gy × 5 fx (prescribed to mucosal surface) treated qod. for brachy alone; 5 Gy × 2 fx if post-EBRT
- **Dose constraints:** None if prescribing to the surface with above fractionation.
- **Follow-up:** q3mo for 2 years; q6mo until 5 years, then annually. Follow CA-125 if initially elevated

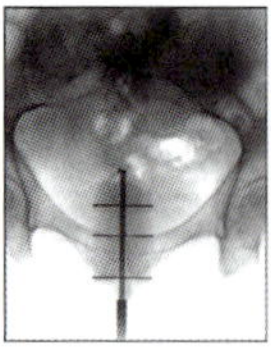

Figure 6.3 X-ray image of dome inserted in the vaginal cuff of an endometrial cancer patient ~6 weeks postoperatively. Note how the dome is up against the fiducial confirming adequate placement prior to HDR treatment.

Cervical (see Cervix chapter)

- **Indications:** Definitive treatment combined with EBRT and concurrent chemotherapy (total package time <8 weeks). Adjuvant/salvage
- **Technique:** Types of implants: intracavitary, interstitial, or hybrid.
- **SIM:** X-ray film immediately after device placement if CT unavailable in (tandem bisects ovoids, tandem 1/3 of the distance between the sacrum and pubic symphysis) CT simulation after device placement. MRI with in situ applicator for at least first implant
- **Target:** (per EMBRACE)
  GTV = T2 lesion on MRI
  HR-CTV = Entire cervix and gross disease/GTV at time of brachytherapy
- **Dose: 3D planning**
  EQD2 dose to HR-CTV D90 = >87 Gy, ideally >90 Gy but <95 Gy; D98 = >75 Gy
  PDR: 40-45 Gy/0.5 Gy/h in two implants of 44-48 hours each
  HDR: initial prescription 5.5-6 Gy × 5 fx (adjusted with subsequent fractions to achieve HR-CTV D90 coverage goals); 7 Gy × 4 fx (in resource constrained environment)

- **Dose constraints:** Per EMBRACE I and II. ABS provides online Excel form for calculating combined EQD2 at https://www.americanbrachytherapy.org/ABS/assets/file/public/consensus-statements/LQ_spreadsheet.xls
  Rectum/rectovaginal D2cc < 65 Gy (limit <75 Gy)
  Sigmoid and small bowel D2cc < 70 Gy (limit <75 Gy)
  Bladder D2cc < 80 (limit <90 Gy)
- **Follow-up:** 1 month after treatment; q3mo for 2 years; q6mo until 5 years, then annually. PET/CT at 3 months; cervical cytology annually

Breast

- **Indications:** see **ESBC** chapter.
- **Target/technique:**
  - Multicatheter interstitial brachytherapy: PTV_EVAL = (surgical cavity + 15 mm), limited by 5 mm from skin surface and posterior breast tissue (excludes CW + pectoralis)
  - MammoSite brachytherapy: PTV_EVAL = (balloon + 10 mm) – balloon volume, limited 5 mm from skin surface and limited by posterior breast tissue
  - Conformal external beam APBI: PTV_EVAL = (surgical cavity + 25 mm), limited 5 mm from skin surface and limited by posterior breast tissue (see **ESBC** chapter)
  - Contura MLB: PTV_EVAL = (balloon + 10 mm) – balloon volume, limited 5 mm from skin surface and limited by posterior breast tissue
  - SAVI: PTV_EVAL = (SAVI device + 10 mm) – lumpectomy cavity volume, limited 2 mm from skin surface (or periphery of SAVI device if closer than 2 mm from skin surface) and limited by posterior breast tissue
- **SIM:** Thin-slice CT scan <3 days prior to first fraction
- **Dose:**
  HDR primary treatment: 34 Gy in 10 fractions; boost is 10 Gy in 2 fractions.
  LDR primary treatment: 45-50 Gy/0.5 Gy/h; boost is 15-20 Gy/0.5 Gy/h.
- **Evaluation metrics/dose constraints:**

	Interstitial	MammoSite	Contura MLB	SAVI
% of dose covering % of PTV_EVAL	≥90%/90%	≥90%/90%	≥95%/95%	≥95%/95%
V150	<70 cc	<50 cc	<30 cc	<50 cc
V200	<20 cc	<10 cc	<10 cc	<20 cc
Max skin dose	≤100%	<125%	<125%	<100%
Max rib dose	NA	<125%	<125%	<125%

Skin

- **Indications:** Early-stage nonmelanoma skin cancer (BCC and SCC). Contraindications, PNI (>0.1 mm), depth >3-4 mm, young age (<50), genetic disorders predisposing to skin cancer, previous RT or burn at treatment site
- **Technique:** Variable, including Ir-192 interstitial brachytherapy and superficial kV contact radiation.
- **SIM:** Clinical setup for fixed geometry applicators; thin-slice CT SIM for custom applicators
- **Target:** CTV = GTV + 4-10 mm (depending on size and histology)
- **Dose:**
  LDR: 60-70 Gy over 5 days
  HDR: 40 Gy (5 Gy/fx); 44 Gy (4.4 Gy/fx) delivered twice or thrice per week, at least 48 hours apart (Fig. 6.4)
- **Dose constraints:** D_{min} > 95% and D_{max} < 135%
- **Follow-up:** H&P q3-12mo for 2 years, then q6-12; clinical photograph of treatment site at every visit

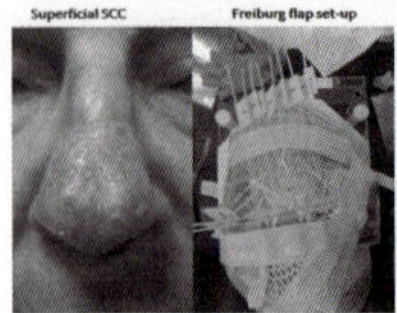

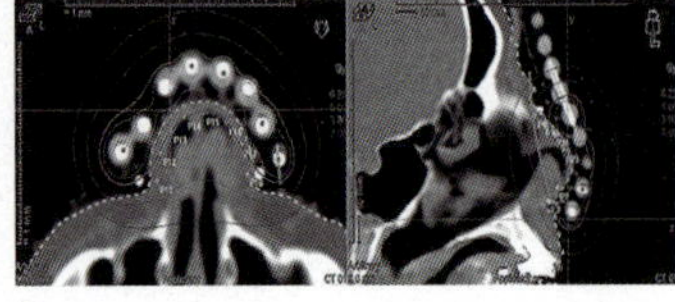

A B

Figure 6.4 Example HDR brachytherapy monotherapy plan utilizing a "Freiburg Flap" **(A)** to treat superficial cutaneous squamous cell carcinoma involving the nose and bilateral ala. Patient was treated to 40 Gy **(B)** in 8 fractions given twice a week.

NOTABLE PAPERS

Name/Inclusion	Arms	Outcomes	Notes
Prostate			
Randomized Data			
RTOG 0232 (*Michalski et al. JCO* 2023) 588 men with cT1c-T2b and GS2-6/PSA 10-20 OR GS7/PSA < 10	45 Gy partial pelvis EBRT + brachytherapy boost Boost dose: I-125: 110 Gy OR Pd-103: 100 Gy Brachytherapy alone Monotherapy dose: I-125: 145 Gy OR Pd-103: 125 Gy	89% of patients with GS7/PSA < 10. GS3+4 in 70% and GS4+3 in 18% of patients 5-y PFS EBRT + brachytherapy vs brachytherapy alone: 86% vs 83% (HR 0.84, $P = .18$). no difference in LP, DM, OS	No difference in outcomes for GS3+4 vs 4+3 patients Overall late 5- and 10-y cumulative grade 2+ GU/GI toxicities was 43% and 48% for combination vs 26 and 31% for brachytherapy mono. No difference in acute toxicities
ASCENDE-RT (*Morris et al. IJROBP* 2017; update: *Oh et al. IJROBP* 2023; *Rodda et al. IJROBP* 2017) 398 intermediate- and high-risk Excluded if PSA > 40, ≥cT3b, prior TURP, pre-ADT prostate volume >75 cc	EBRT (46 Gy pelvic, 78 Gy prostate) + 12 mo ADT EBRT (46 Gy pelvic) + LDR BT boost (I-125 115 Gy) + 12 mo ADT	Brachy boost improved *10-year TTP (85% vs 67%)* but not DM (88% vs 86%), PCSM (95% vs 92%), or OS (80% vs 75%)	Approx. 69% high risk. Brachy boost associated w/ worse 5-y grade ≥3 GU toxicity (18% vs 5%) w/ half of events being urethral strictures requiring dilatation
Nonrandomized Data			
Kishan et al. JAMA 2018 1809 patients with GS 9-10 treated in 12 tertiary centers between 2000 and 2013	Retrospective, multi-institution study comparing: RP, EBRT with ADT, EBRT + BT with ADT	5-y CSS better for EBRT + BT (97%) vs RP (88%) vs EBRT (87%) 5-y DM rates were lower for EBRT + BT (8%) vs RP (24%) vs EBRT (24%) Adjusted 7.5-y all-cause mortality rates were lower for EBRT + BT (10%) vs RP (17%) vs EBRT (18%)	

Name/Inclusion	Arms	Outcomes	Notes
RTOG 0526 (*Crook et al. IJROBP 2022*) 92 patients with low/intermediate-risk prostate cancer before EBRT, PSA < 10, no regional/distant disease	Single-arm phase 2 multicenter clinical trial Salvage LDR prostate brachytherapy after prior EBRT	10-y OS: 70% 10-y local failure rate: 5% 10-y distant failure rate: 19% 10-y biochemical failure rate: 46% 5-y DFS: 61% 10-y DFS: 33%	
	Cervix—Nonrandomized Data		
RetroEMBRACE (*Sturdaza et al. Radiother Oncol* 2016)	Retrospective cohort study. 731 patients from 12 tertiary cancer centers treated with EBRT + concurrent chemotherapy followed by image-guided brachytherapy (IGBT) for locally advanced cervical cancer	Excellent LC (91%), PC (87%), OS (74%), CSS (79%) with limited morbidity The 3/5-y actuarial LC, PC, CSS, OS were 91%/89%, 87%/84%, 79%/73%, 74%/65%, respectively Actuarial LC at 3/5 years for IB, IIB, IIIB was 98%/98%, 93%/91%, 79%/75%, respectively	Actuarial PC at 3/5 years for IB, IIB, IIIB was 96%/96%, 89%/87%, 73%/67%, respectively Actuarial 5-y G3-G5 morbidity was 5%, 7%, and 5% for the bladder, gastrointestinal tract, and vagina, respectively
EMBRACE I (Pötter *Lancet Oncol* 2021) MRI-based image-guided adapted BT (IGABT) in locally advanced cervical cancer 1341 patients, FIGO Stage IB-IVA or Stage IVB restricted to paraaortic LN metastasis below L1-L2 interspace	Prospective, observational, multicenter cohort study	Median minimum dose to 90% of HR-CTV was EQD2 90 Gy Actuarial 5-y LC, PC, nodal control, OS, and DSS were 92%, 87%, 87%, 74%, and 68%, respectively Post-hoc analysis of outcomes by nodal status: 5-y nodal control 93% in N0 vs 81% in N1 patients	Actuarial cumulative 5-y incidence of grade 3-5 toxicities was 6.8% for GU events, 8.5% for GI events, 5.7% for vaginal events, and 3.2% for fistulas Conclusion: MRI-based IGABT is the new gold-standard for IGABT of locally advanced cervical cancer

PT 2-8

Name/Inclusion	Arms	Outcomes	Notes
Breast—Randomized Data			
GEC-ESTRO (*Strnad et al. Lancet 2016; Strnad et al. Lancet 2023*) Randomized, noninferiority trial 1184 patients with low-risk invasive and ductal carcinoma in situ treated with breast-conserving surgery	Whole-breast irradiation (50-50.4 Gy in 25-28 fx) APBI using multicatheter BT (32 Gy/8 fx or 30.3 Gy/7 fx treated BID)	5-y local recurrence rates similar between APBI (1.4%) and whole-breast irradiation (0.9%) No difference in 5-y late skin toxicity, fibrosis, DFS, or IS	At 10 y, local recurrence rate with APBI was 3.51% compared to 1.58% in whole-breast irradiation though not statistically significant (*P* = .074). Significantly lower incidence of treatment-related grade 3 late side effects with APBI (1%) compared to whole-breast radiation (4%) (*P* = .021)

PROTON THERAPY

AARON SEO • DAVID GROSSHANS

Background

- **Brief history:**
  - 1946: First description of therapeutic protons
  - 1954: First patient treated with proton therapy at UC Berkeley synchrocyclotron
  - 1990: First hospital proton facility at Loma Linda University Medical Center, CA
  - 2008: MD Anderson Proton Therapy first in United States to offer scanning beam capability
  - 2014: 15 active proton therapy facilities in the United States
  - 2023: 42 active proton therapy facilities in the United States, >170 000 patients treated worldwide, with >75 000 of those in the United States
- **Principles of proton therapy:**
  - *Interactions with matter*:
    - Bragg peak: Protons lose energy at an increasing rate as particles slow, with peak in dose deposition known as the Bragg peak just prior to stopping. Singular peak is referred to as "monoenergetic" or "pristine" Bragg peak (Fig. 7.1, next page).
    - Higher-energy protons travel farther in tissues.
    - Spread-out Bragg peak (SOBP): Superposition of monoenergetic proton beams with differing intensities to sufficiently cover target volume (Fig. 7.2, next page)
    - Linear energy transfer (LET): Stopping power or average rate of energy loss of particle per unit path length ($-dE/dx$); inversely proportional to square of particle speed
  - *Relative biological effectiveness (RBE)*:
    - Protons are estimated to have 10% higher average biological effectiveness relative to photons (RBE = 1.1) for a given absorbed dose of radiation.
    - Clinical *approximation*: Proton dose (Gy [RBE]) = 1.1 × photon dose (Gy)
    - Limitations of using fixed RBE 1.1:
      - RBE varies with LET and therefore increases with depth.
      - RBE varies with fraction size and tumor cell line (*Spiotto et al. Semin Radiat Oncol* 2021; *Wang et al. IJPT* 2021).
      - RBE varies with oxygen concentration of irradiated tissue.

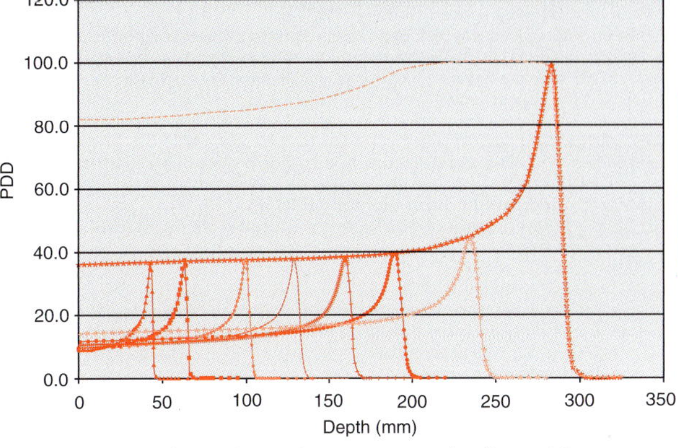

Figure 7.1 Summation of pristine Bragg peaks to generate a spread-out Bragg peak for proton therapy.

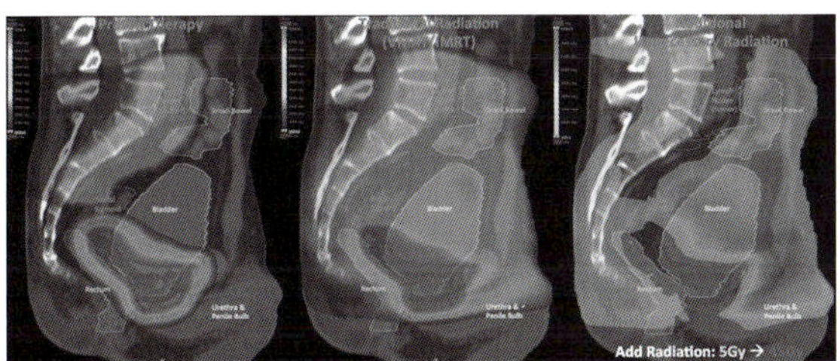

Figure 7.2 Comparative plan showing intensity-modulated proton therapy (*left*) vs a VMAT/IMRT plan (*middle*). Excess radiation dose (*right*) is calculated by subtracting the proton therapy plan from the VMAT/IMRT plan. **See color insert.**

- RBE underestimates complexity of proton-tissue interactions.
- Values are based on limited in vitro and in vivo experiments under varied conditions and cell lines.
- At the end of range (the distal portion of beam), LET increases and hence RBE may be higher than expected. This uncertainty necessitates consideration of proton beams direction to ensure that the end of range is not within a critical structure.
- Currently planning strategies, using scanned proton beams, which incorporate LET and variable RBE models, are in development.

- *Proton accelerators*:
  - Cyclotron:
    - Produces a continuous stream of fixed-energy protons
    - More compact, higher beam intensity
    - Uses energy degraders of varying widths in the beam path to create lower-energy beams for SOBP
  - Synchrotron:
    - Produces batches of protons at variable energies
    - Better energy flexibility and lower power consumption
    - Produces SOBP at any depth without energy degraders

Proton Therapy Technique

- **Passive scattering proton therapy (PSPT):**
  - Beam is spread laterally and longitudinally in the treatment head (nozzle).
    - Longitudinal: Using range modulators (ie, rotating modulator wheel) to create SOBP over the target volume; range compensator (eg, Lucite) to conform dose to distal edge of target
    - Lateral: Using dual scattering foils of high-Z materials; brass apertures to laterally conform dose to target and create a sharp penumbra
  - Limitation: SOBP is constant across field → little control of dose distribution proximal to target (*Mohan and Grosshans Adv Drug Deliv Rev* 2017)
- **Intensity-modulated proton therapy (IMPT):**
  - Beamlets (pencil beams) of differing energies (depths) are magnetically swept across the target.
  - Two categories of IMPT:
    - *Single-field optimization (SFO)*
      - Individual beams optimized to conform dose to the entire target volume
      - Each field optimized separately to deliver uniform dose to target
      - Less sensitive to uncertainties
      - Integrated boost possible
    - *Multifield optimization (MFO)*
      - All beams simultaneously optimized to deliver homogeneous target dose
      - Multiple fields required to cover target
      - More sensitive to uncertainties
      - Integrated boost is routinely used
      - QA more demanding
      - Potential to place higher LET/RBE regions of proton beam within tumor volume for dose escalation with improved normal tissue sparing
- **Proton treatment planning and treatment**
  - Protons more sensitive to anatomy changes and beam direction due to (1) sharp distal dose falloff and (2) range uncertainty
  - *Simulation*:
    - Position must be reproducible and provide adequate patient comfort.
    - Use proton-compatible immobilization devices.
    - Special considerations for high-Z materials. Generally, try to avoid placing these materials in the beam's path.
    - Use dual-energy CT for more accurate stopping power mapping of tissues.
  - *Target delineation*: Use beam directions with short path to distal edge of target, minimal transit through heterogeneous tissue intensities, and avoidance of distal edge close to critical normal structures (increased RBE at end of proton beam).
    - Conventional "PTV" definitions for photons have its limitation to protons due to range uncertainty (related to target depth and beam direction). Therefore, use of these terms in proton therapy literature should be interpreted with this understanding that PTV is more for lateral setup uncertainties for proton. In the beam direction, the proton beam range uncertainties are used.
    - Beam-specific PTVs with different distal margins in each beam direction. See below for PTV margins in representative disease.
  - *Beam selection*: Use energy absorber (attached to the snout) if target depth <3 cm for scanning beam, and avoid high-Hounsfield Unit materials.
  - *Dose and fractionation*: Use RBE adjustment as described above; RBE may vary from <1.0 to >1.7, but variable RBE models are not currently part of clinical treatment planning.
  - *Image guidance*: Daily kV imaging and/or volumetric imaging to minimize setup variation, similar to conventional photon-based treatment
    - Prompt gamma imaging (PGI): Formation of gamma-emitting nuclear isotopes after proton therapy used to approximate dose deposition; using "Compton cameras" or single gamma ray detectors is being studied.
  - *Adaptive planning*: Consider verification simulation during 1st and 4th week of therapy and/or if any drastic changes in patient volume is noted during treatment.
    - Deformable registration with planning CT
    - Monitor weight loss and other anatomical changes that can alter dose distribution and DVH data.

Clinical Indications

- **Standard indications (selected):**
  - *Craniopharyngioma* (*Bishop et al. IJROBP* 2014; *Boehling et al. IJROBP* 2012)
    - Target: GTV, operative cavity and residual disease; CTV, 5-mm customized margin
    - Intent: Postoperative, definitive, salvage
    - Adverse effects: Endocrinopathy (hypopituitarism)
    - Considerations: PTV margin for lateral border especially close to optic apparatus and brainstem and CTV for proximal/distal borders
  - *Rhabdomyosarcoma* (*Ladra et al. JCO* 2014)
    - Intent: Postoperative or definitive
    - Adverse effects: Radiation dermatitis, mucositis
    - Considerations: Dose dependent on extent of residual tumor and primary site of disease (COG protocols)
  - *Atypical teratoid/rhabdoid tumor* (*McGovern et al. IJROBP* 2014)
    - Target: GTV, operative cavity and residual disease; CTV, anatomically constrained 1-cm margin; PTV, distal/proximal 3-mm margin
    - Intent: Postoperative
    - Adverse effects: Erythema, alopecia, cytopenia (with concurrent chemotherapy)
  - *Craniospinal* (*Barney et al. Neuro Oncol* 2014; *Brown et al. IJROBP* 2013)
    - Target: CTV, entire CSF space (brain; upper, middle, and lower spine); entire vertebral bodies are included in target volume for pediatric patients in order to avoid growth asymmetries.
    - Intent: Postoperative
    - Adverse effects: Myelosuppression, nausea, vomiting, dermatitis
    - Considerations: For PSPT, junction shift 1 cm every 5 fractions; feather junctions for scanning beam; block anterior orbit (lens) and spare anterior structures: bowel, heart, lungs, pancreas, and thyroid.
  - *Nasopharynx, oropharynx, larynx* (*Alterio Acta Oncol* 2020; *Blanchard Radiother Oncol* 2016; *Frank et al. IJROBP* 2014; *Holliday et al. IJROBP* 2014; *Holliday IJROBP* 2016; *Lee Int J Part Ther* 2021; *Li JAMA Netw Open* 2021; *Manzar Radiother Oncol* 2020; *McDonald Radiat Oncol* 2016; *Patel Lancet Oncol* 2014; *Romesser Radiother Oncol* 2016; *Smith Int J Part Ther* 2021; *Zhang Radiother Oncol* 2017); Proton therapy is a standard treatment option for most tumor subsites of the head and neck as supported by consensus guidelines, ASTRO model policy for proton beam therapy, and a current NRG trial for nasopharyngeal carcinoma (NRG HN-001).
    - Target: CTV1, gross disease; CTV2, high-risk nodal volume; CTV3, subclinical disease; PTV, 3- to 5-mm margin outside of critical structures
    - Intent: Definitive
    - Adverse effects: Xerostomia, mucositis, dysgeusia, dermatitis, nausea, malnutrition, dysphagia
    - Considerations: Consider IMPT in nonlateralized treatments. Use three to five fields to treat bilateral neck (3-field: LAO and RAO with distal Bragg peaks lateral to the spinal cord and single posterior beam with distal Bragg peak posterior to the parotid).
  - *Prostate* (*Pugh et al. IJROBP* 2013; *Sosa et al. IJROBP* 2022; *Zhu et al. Radiat Oncol* 2014)
    - Target: CTV, prostate +/− seminal vesicles; ETV, uniform radial 6-mm margin except 5 mm posteriorly, 9-12 mm proximal/distally; STV, 12 mm lateral, 5 mm posterior, 6 mm all others to CTV
    - Intent: Definitive
    - Adverse effects: Bowel and urinary function, sexual function
    - Considerations: Use opposed R/L lateral beams.
  - *Skull base—Chordoma/Chondrosarcoma* (*Grosshans et al. IJROBP* 2014)
    - Target: GTV, gross residual disease; CTV, 5- to 8-mm margin (to include areas of gross disease before resection) (CTV1—higher risk, CTV2—lower risk/surgical path); PTV, 2-3 mm
    - Intent: Postoperative, progression, recurrence
    - Adverse effects: Fatigue, nausea
    - Considerations: Use multiple CTVs: CTV1 = GTV + 5- to 8-mm margin (higher risk, higher dose), CTV2 = additional expansion to cover lower risk and surgical pathway; PTV with small margin to avoid optic chiasm, brainstem, temporal lobes
  - *Seminoma* (*Haque et al. PRO* 2015; *Pasalic et al. IJPT* 2020)
    - Target: CTV (para-aortic and ipsilateral iliac vessels + 7 mm); GTV (involved LN + 10 mm); STV, uniform 5-mm margin for both CTV and GTV

- Intent: Definitive
- Adverse effects: Nausea
- Considerations: Consider extended SSD technique and gantry rotation.

- **Sites under study (selected):**
  - *Esophageal* (*Lin et al. IJROBP* 2012; *Lin et al. JCO* 2020)
    - Target: GTV, all disease present on PET and EGD; CTV, areas of potential spread; PTV, 1- to 1.5-cm margin
    - Intent: Preoperative, definitive
    - Adverse effects: Fatigue, esophagitis, nausea, anorexia, dermatitis
    - Considerations: Use 4DCT for simulation/planning. AP/PA, PA/LLO, or 3-beam brass blocks/Plexiglas compensators for SOBP to cover treatment volume
  - *Lung* (*Chang et al. Cancer* 2011; *Koay et al. IJROBP* 2012; *Liao et al. JCO* 2017)
    - Target: iGTV, envelope of motion of GTV on MIP image; iCTV, 8-mm isotropic margin
    - Intent: Definitive (with chemotherapy)
    - Adverse effects: Dermatitis, esophagitis, pneumonitis
    - Considerations: Use 4DCT for simulation/planning.
  - *Breast* (*Strom et al. IJROBP* 2014; *Strom et al. Pract Radiat Oncol* 2015)
    - Target: CTV, 15 mm expansion of tumor bed (including clips/seroma) with 5 mm contraction from skin and edited to exclude chest wall/muscle; PTV, radial 5 mm
    - Intent: APBI postoperative (see ESBC chapter)
    - Adverse effects: Radiation dermatitis
    - Considerations: Proximal/distal beam margins 3.5% of range + 1 mm from CTV
  - *Liver—unresectable hepatocellular carcinoma and intrahepatic cholangiocarcinoma* (*Hong et al. JCO* 2016)
    - Target: CTV, 10 mm expansion on GTV (depending on proximity of normal tissues); PTV, 5-10 mm expansion
    - Intent: Definitive
    - Adverse effects: Thrombocytopenia, transaminitis, and liver failure
    - Considerations: Use 4DCT for simulation/planning.
  - *Postoperative prostate*
    - Target: CTV, prostate, and seminal vesicle fossa; ETV, uniform radial 7-mm margin except 5 mm posteriorly, 9-12 mm proximal/distally; STV, 12 mm lateral, 5 mm posterior, 6 mm all others to CTV
    - Intent: Postoperative/salvage
    - Adverse effects: Bowel and urinary function, sexual function
    - Considerations: Use opposed R/L lateral beams.

MRI-GUIDED RADIOTHERAPY

AARON SEO • JINZHONG YANG • CLIFTON DAVID FULLER

Background

- **Definitions:**
  - *Magnetic resonance (MR) simulation registration*: The process of registering an MRI at time of simulation to the planning CT simulation scan for CT-based RT planning
  - *MRI-guided adaptive radiotherapy (MRgART)*: Utilization of on-board MR imaging integrated within a linear accelerator (linac) for the purpose of adapting radiation treatment
  - *Offline adaptation*: Adaptation outside the treatment session
  - *Online adaptation*: Adaptation during the treatment session
  - *Adapt-to-position (ATP)*: Adaptation workflow where the isocenter is shifted on the CT simulation plan based on a rigid registration followed by either dose recalculation or plan reoptimization
  - *Adapt-to-shape (ATS)*: Adaptation workflow that utilizes deformable image registration to project target and organ-at-risk contours from CT simulation onto daily setup MR image followed by a full plan reoptimization on MR
- **Potential Benefits of MR guidance compared to CT-based image guidance:**
  - Superior soft tissue contrast to delineate both clinical targets and organs-at-risk to aid in treatment adaptation, potentially eliminating the need for fiducial placement

    - Potential for real-time beam-on motion tracking
    - In the future, functional MRI-based markers of response may guide additional radiation dose selection and adaptation
- **Limitations of MR guidance:**
    - Current limited data on the significance of visualized differences with MR guidance on affecting clinical outcomes; many clinical studies are ongoing (see below).

PRINCIPLES OF MRGART

- **Commercially available hybrid MR-linac devices:**

Device Name (Manufacturer)	MRI Field Strength	Bore Diameter	Beam Configuration
ViewRay MRIdian (ViewRay Technologies, Inc.; Oakwood, OH)	0.35 Tesla	70 cm	6 MV (linac) or Cobalt-60 source, perpendicular
Elekta Unity (Elekta AB; Stockholm, Sweden)	1.5 Tesla	70 cm	7 MV, perpendicular
MagnetTx Aurora (MagnetTx Oncology Solutions Ltd; Edmonton, Canada)	0.5 Tesla	110 × 60 cm	6 MV, in-line

- **Preferred MRI sequences by anatomical region**

Anatomical Region	Preferred Sequence
CNS (high-grade glioma)	T1+C T2 FLAIR
Head and neck (general)	T2 TSE
Nasopharynx	DWI
Oropharynx	T2 FS T1+C
Esophagus, lung	T1 3D mDIXON TFE
Breast, chest wall	T1 3D mDIXON TFE
Abdomen	T2 TSE
Pelvis (female)	T2 3D TSE
Pelvis (male)	T2 TSE

- **Physics and Dosimetric Considerations:**
    - *Electron-return effect*: X-ray interaction with matter generates charged particles such as secondary electrons, which then deposit the energy of the initial beam downstream. Within a magnetic field, electrons travel in a circular pattern in heterogeneous anatomic locations such as air-tissue interfaces, allowing the electron to travel back to the original tissue from air. This phenomenon is known as the electron-return effect. These effect increases in magnitude with increasing magnetic field strength.
    The current commercially available MR-linacs lack more advanced IMRT features found in CT-based linacs such as noncoplanar beams, arc-based radiation delivery, more versatile couch positions.
- **Practical considerations:**
    - *Patient factors*:
        - MRgART contraindicated if patient has contraindications or cannot tolerate MR imaging (eg, pacemaker, implanted ferrous metal objects, significant claustrophobia)
        - Body habitus, weight, and size requirements for the MR-linac based on MR bore diameter and field size limitations
        - Ability to hold treatment position for extended duration of time
        - Overall mobility (ability to walk to and from treatment vault)
    - *Treatment team factors*:
        - Presently, there is substantial time commitment over traditional CT-based linac RT related to imaging review and physician-based plan adaptation decision-making.
        - Additional staffing requirements for online adaptive planning

MR-Linac: Treatment Planning and Adaptation

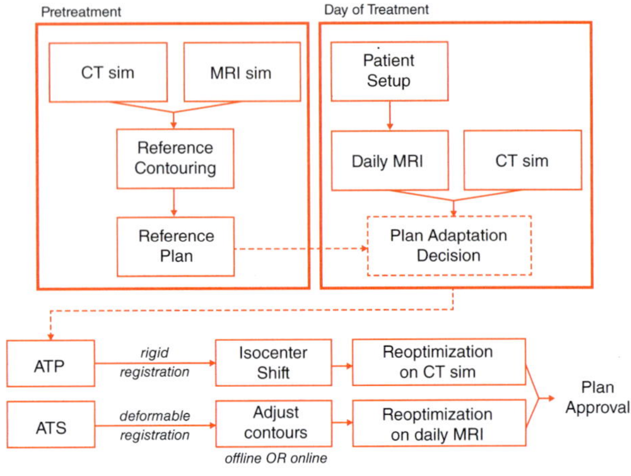

Clinical Evidence

- At this time, there is overall lack of clinical data, especially randomized controlled clinical trials, describing the efficacy of MRgART.
- The R-IDEAL conceptual framework has been developed by the MR-Linac Consortium for timely systematic clinical evaluation of MRgART (*Verkooijen et al. Front in Oncol* 2017).

Treatment Site Considerations

Site	Potential Benefit of MRgART	Potential Challenge of MRgART
Central nervous system	MRI is the standard for evaluating brain parenchyma	
Head/neck	• Some tumors regress quickly during RT = great candidate for plan adaptation • MR soft tissue resolution superior to CT in setting of patient weight loss	
Thorax Esophagus	MR soft tissue resolution may be useful in central lung tumors, esophageal tumors	• Electron-return effect (lung) • MRI less established in staging, diagnostic evaluation of primary lung cancers
Upper GI	• Abdominal structures often difficult to visualize with CT imaging • Upper abdominal structures can have significant motion in close proximity to radiosensitive OARs	
Prostate	• MR delineation of prostatic tumor may potentially guide RT dose boost to dominant nodules • MR soft tissue resolution of surrounding OARs to spare dose	

Site	Potential Benefit of MRgART	Potential Challenge of MRgART
Gynecology	• MR visualization of small pelvis lymph nodes for boost treatment • MR visualization of primary target for boost treatment • MR soft tissue resolution of surrounding OARs to spare dose	

NOTABLE PAPERS

Study	Details	Results	Notes
		Head/Neck	
***Chen et al. Adv Radiat Oncol* 2017** 13 patients with recurrent or new primary cancers in previously irradiated field	Retrospective ViewRay Co-60 source Median dose 66 Gy conventional fx OR SBRT 7-8 Gy fractions to median dose 40 Gy	2-y in-field control: 72% 2-y OS: 53% 2-y PFS: 59% No treatment-related fatalities or hospitalizations	Conclusion: MRgART feasible for reirradiation
***Fu et al. IJROBP* 2022** Randomized controlled trial 260 patients with stage III-IVa nasopharyngeal carcinoma	Group A: Induction chemo → chemoRT with DWI-guided dose-painting IMRT Dose to GTV DWI: 75.2 Gy/32 fractions for T1-T2 disease and to 77.55 Gy/33 fractions for T3-T4 disease Group B: Induction chemo → conventional MRI-based IMRT Dose 70.4-72.6 Gy/32-33 fractions	CR rates after chemoRT: 99.2% vs 93.8% (*P* = .042) in groups A and B, respectivelyMedian follow-up 25 mo 2-y DFS: 93.6% vs 87.5% (*P* = .015) in groups A and B, respectively 2-y LRRFS: 95.8% vs 91.3% 2-y DMFS: 97.8% vs 90.9% 2-y OS: 100% vs 94.5%	No statistically significant differences in acute and late toxicities
		Thorax	
***Finazzi et al. IJROBP* 2020** 29 patients with primary lung cancer, 21 patients with lung metastases with high-risk factors for possible toxicity (eg, central tumor location, previous thoracic RT, interstitial lung disease)	Retrospective SBRT dosing Gated SBRT	BED > 100 Gy to 95% PTV delivered in 93% of tumors 1-y LC: 95.6% 1-y OS: 88.0% 1-y DFS: 63.6%	Any grade ≥2 toxicity: 30% Any grade ≥3 toxicity: 8% Conclusion: MR-guided SBRT to thoracic tumors feasible
		Pancreas	
***Rudra et al. Cancer Med* 2019** 44 patients with inoperable, nonmetastatic pancreatic cancer	Retrospective 40-55 Gy/25-28 fx (13 patients) 30-52 Gy/5 fx (22 patients) 50-67.5 Gy/10-15 fx (9 patients)	• High-dose RT improved 2-y OS: 49% vs 30% (*P* = .03) • High-dose vs standard-dose RT FFLF: 77% vs 57%, respectively	Grade 3 GI toxicity: 3/44 patients (all standard-dose patients)

Study	Details	Results	Notes
Hassanzadeh et al. Adv Radiat Oncol 2020 44 patients with locally advanced pancreatic cancer	Retrospective 50 Gy/5 fx	• Median OS: 15.7 mo • 1-y LC: 84.3% • Late grade 3 GI toxicity: 4.6%	
SMART (*Parikh et al., IJROBP* 2023) 136 patients with locally advanced pancreatic cancer	Single-arm, phase II trial SBRT 50 Gy/5 fx delivered with ViewRay MRIdian utilizing gating	Incidence of acute grade 3+ GI toxicity possible or probably related to RT: 8.8% including 2 postoperative deaths	1-y LC: 82.9% 1-y DPFS: 50.6% 1-y OS: 65%
Chuong et al. Front Oncol 2022	Retrospective Induction chemo → ablative stereotactic MRI-guided RT (A-SMART) with ViewRay MRIdian	Median induction chemo duration: 4.2 mo Median prescribed dose: 50 Gy 2-y LC, PFS, and OS: 68.8%, 40.0%, and 45.5%, respectively	Acute and late grade 3+ toxicity rates: 4.8% and 4.8%, respectively
	Gynecology		
Lakomy et al. PRO 2022 10 patients with gynecological malignancies, 7/10 patients treated for isolated recurrent disease	Single institution, prospective implementation series (R-IDEAL stage 1 and 2a) Median total dose: 22.5 Gy (range: 10.2-60.5 Gy) Median 6 fractions (range: 3-28)	Fractions shorter with ATP than with ATS (30 min vs 42 min, *P* < .0001) Average extent of isocenter shift: <0.5 cm in each axis	Accumulated dose to GTV was within 5% of the reference plan for all ATP cases
	Prostate		
MIRAGE (*Kishan et al. JAMA Oncol* 2023) Randomized controlled trial 156 patients with localized prostate cancer receiving SBRT for localized prostate cancer	CT-guided SBRT to 40 Gy/5 fx using 4-mm planning margins MR-guided SBRT to 40 Gy/5 fx using 2-mm planning margins	Acute toxicity significantly reduced with MR-guided SBRT including grade >2 GI (43.4% vs 24.4%, *P* = .01) and >2 GI (10.5% vs 0%, *P* = .003)	IPSS urinary and EPIC-26 bowel domain scores significantly better with MR-guided SBRT at 1 mo but resolved 3 mo post-SBRT

Ongoing Studies

Study	Details
MOMENTUM (NCT04075305) (*de Mol van Otterloo et al. Front Oncol* 2020)	Prospective international registry led by the MR-Linac Consortium in partnership with Elekta
Head/Neck	
MR-ADAPTOR (NCT03224000) (*Bahig et al. CTRO* 2018)	R-IDEAL stage 2a-2b/Bayesian phase II trial MR-based response assessment and dose adaptation in HPV+ oropharynx tumors treated with RT
Pancreas	
LAP-ABLATE (NCT05585554)	Phase III RCT induction chemo +/− A-SMART (50 Gy/5 fx) on ViewRay MRIdian

LOW-GRADE GLIOMAS

MIKE ROONEY • MARTIN TOM • SUBHA PERNI • D. NANA YEBOA

Background

- **Incidence/prevalence:** There are numerous subtypes of low-grade adult and pediatric gliomas. This chapter will focus primarily on adult-type diffuse grade 2 gliomas, of which there are estimated to be 2000 cases diagnosed per year.
- **Outcomes:** Median survival for grade 2 oligodendrogliomas (IDH mutant, 1p/19q codeleted) is >14 years, and *IDH* mutant astrocytomas is >11 years.
- **Demographics:** The median age of diagnosis for grade 2 gliomas is estimated to be between 35 and 40 years. Males > females
- **Risk factors:** Gliomas are largely sporadic without any clear risk factors aside from exposure to ionizing radiation.

Tumor Biology and Characteristics

- **Genetics:** Increased risk of developing low-grade astrocytomas in patients with NF1 and NF2. Tuberous sclerosis is associated with increased risk of developing subependymal giant cell astrocytomas. Increased risk is also seen in patients with Li-Fraumeni syndrome.
- **Pathology:** Historically, gliomas were classified based upon the histopathologic grade, but diagnosis now integrates molecular features (*WHO 2021 update; Louis et al. Neuro-Oncology* 2021). The newest 2021 CNS Classification uses an integrated histopathologic and molecular classification system. Oligodendrogliomas are defined by the presence of an IDH mutation and 1p/19q codeletion (can be grades 2-3). IDH-mutant astrocytomas are defined by the presence of IDH mutation, 1p/19q noncodeletion, ATRX loss, and/or TP53 mutation (can be grades 2-4). Presence of CDKN2A/B homozygous deletion upgrades an oligodendroglioma to grade 3, and an IDH-mutant astrocytoma to grade 4. IDH wild-type status typically upgrades to a glioblastoma (grade 4).
- **Imaging:** Grade 2 diffuse gliomas are typically lobar in location (most commonly in frontal or temporal lobes) and are contrast nonenhancing, unlike high-grade gliomas. Due to the infiltrative nature of grade 2, they are associated with a hyperintense signal on T2 sequences, best seen on the T2/FLAIR sequence (Fig. 9.1).

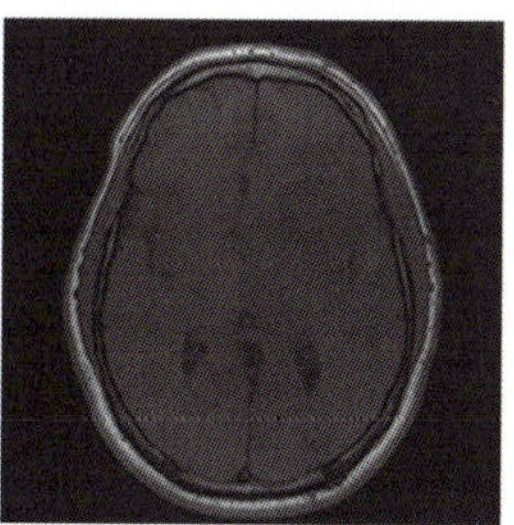

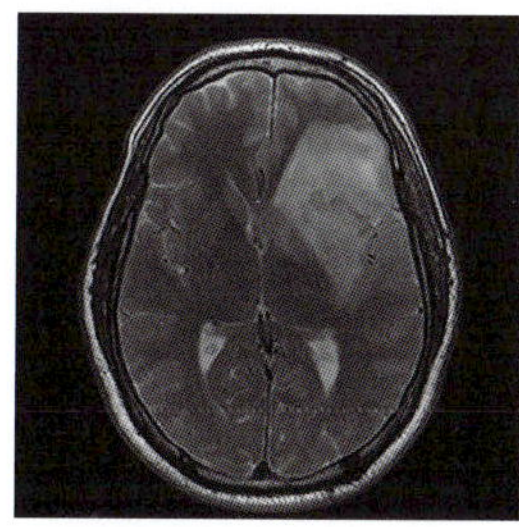

Figure 9.1 T1 + contrast MRI image **(left)** shows an ill-defined non–contrast-enhancing hypointense lesion in the left frontal lobe without any necrotic features. The lesion is associated with a significant edematous component seen on T2-FLAIR sequence **(right)**, indicating associated edema and infiltrative pattern of spread.

Anatomy

LGGs typically arise from supratentorial cortex.

- **Frontal lobe:** Functions in regulating personality, behavior, emotions, and decision-making. Precentral gyrus (motor strip) lies anterior to central sulcus. Speech (Broca's)
- **Parietal lobe:** Interprets language, words, and sensory information. Postcentral gyrus (sensory cortex) lies posterior to central sulcus.

- **Occipital lobe:** Vision
- **Temporal lobe:** Language comprehension (Wernicke's), memory, hearing, sequencing
- **Cerebellum:** Balance, movement, and spatial positioning

WORKUP

- **History and physical:** Including presenting symptoms, history of seizures (most common presenting symptom), and family history. Assessment of neurologic deficits and performance status important. Establish preoperative neurocognitive evaluation if applicable.
- **Labs:** CBC, CMP
- **Procedures/biopsy:** Neurosurgery evaluation for maximal safe resection or biopsy
- **Imaging:** MRI of the brain with and without contrast is the gold standard (Fig. 9.1) to evaluate location, grade, and extent of disease. Obtain postoperative MRI within 3 days of surgery to determine extent of resection and whether there is any residual disease. After 3 days, blood products make MRI interpretation difficult.

STAGING/GRADING

- Grade 2 oligodendroglioma is defined by the presence of IDH mutation and 1p/19q codeletion, absent CDKN2A/B homozygous deletion, absent/low mitotic activity, and lacking histopathologic features of anaplasia, necrosis, or microvascular proliferation.
- Grade 2 IDH-mutant astrocytoma is defined by the presence of an IDH mutation, TP53 mutation, ATRX loss, 1p/19q noncodeletion, absent CDKN2A/B homozygous deletion, absent/low mitotic activity, and lacking histopathologic features of anaplasia, necrosis, or microvascular proliferation.

TREATMENT ALGORITHM

Grade 1 glioma	Maximal surgical resection → observation for all patients (RT only if clinical progression)
Grade 2 glioma <40 y of age[a]	Maximal surgical resection → RT + adjuvant PCV or TMZ if STR, observation if GTR (RT at progression)
Grade 2 glioma >40 y of age[b]	Maximal surgical resection → RT + adjuvant PCV or TMZ

[a]Low-grade gliomas have multiple options and are managed with institutional variation. Important considerations for early radiation therapy may include large size (>5 cm), crossing midline, neurologic symptoms/seizures, or astrocytoma histology (Pignatti criteria).

[b]Intitutional variations may include a range of ages above 40 years rather than a strict cut-off.

RADIATION TREATMENT TECHNIQUE

- **SIM:** Supine, holding A-bar, Aquaplast mask with isocenter placed at midbrain. MRI fusions—T1 + C sequence and T2 FLAIR sequences
- **Dose:** 50.4-54 Gy in 28-30 fractions at 1.8 Gy/fx (can consider 2 Gy/fx)
- **Target:**
  GTV—surgical cavity + residual T2/FLAIR-hyperintense signal concerning for tumor
  CTV—GTV + 1 cm
  PTV—CTV + 0.3 cm (daily kV)
  Considerations: Limit CTV expansions to anatomic boundaries of disease spread (eg, bones, falx, tentorium, and ventricles; brainstem is not an anatomic boundary when there is anatomic contiguity with tumor).
- **Technique:** IMRT/VMAT. Consider individualized use of protons on trial.
- **IGRT:** Daily kV imaging
- **Planning directive:**
  Brainstem: V30Gy < 33%. Max < 54 Gy. If necessary, may allow point max <60 Gy
  Brain: V30Gy < 50%
  Optic chiasm: Max ≤ 54 Gy
  Cochlea: Max < 54 Gy. Mean < 30 Gy
  Lens: Max < 5 Gy
  Optic nerves: Max ≤ 54 Gy
  Pituitary: Mean < 36 Gy
  Eyes: Max < 40 Gy. Mean < 30 Gy
  Spinal cord: Max ≤ 45 Gy

Chemotherapy

- **Adjuvant:**
  Procarbazine, lomustine, vincristine (PCV) regimen (as per RTOG 9802)—procarbazine 60 mg/m^2 on days 8-21, lomustine 110 mg/m^2 on day 1, and vincristine 1.4 mg/m^2 on days 8 and 29. Cycle length is 8 weeks. Data suggest that oligodendrogliomas derive a greater benefit with PCV than astrocytomas.
  Temozolomide (TMZ)—150-200 mg/m^2 daily for 5 days, every 28 days for 6-12 cycles. If given concurrently with RT as per RTOG 0424, the dose is 75 mg/m^2.

Side Effect Management

- Nausea: First-line Zofran (4 mg q8h prn)
- Headaches/worsening neuro deficits: Likely due to increased edema. Consider treatment with dexamethasone at low dose (2 mg bid) with taper following resolution of symptoms.
- Scalp irritation/dryness/dermatitis: Aquaphor (OTC)
- Thrombocytopenia/lymphopenia/neutropenia: Likely due to PCV or TMZ. Refer to medical oncologist.

Follow-up

- Every 2-3 months with MRI of the brain w/ and w/o contrast for the first year following treatment, q4mo during years 2-4, and q6mo thereafter. Patients with age >40 years, large size (>5 cm), incomplete resection, astrocytic histology, and high proliferative index (MIB > 1-3%) at high risk for recurrence (*Pignatti et al. JCO* 2002). Consider reirradiation on protocol or enrollment in investigational clinical trials at progression.

Notable Trials

Name/Inclusion	Arms	Outcomes	Notes
EORTC 22844 ("Believer's Trial"), *Karim et al. IJROBP* 1996 379 patients with LGG after maximal safe resection	Adjuvant RT 45 Gy in 25 fx Adjuvant RT 59.4 Gy in 33 fx	5-y OS 58% for low-dose RT, 59% for high-dose RT (ns). No difference in 5-y PFS (47% vs 50%)	Conclusion: No benefit to dose escalation for adjuvant RT (confirmed also on NCCTG 86-72-51 trial testing 64.8 Gy vs 50.4 Gy)
EORTC 22845 ("Non-Believer's Trial"), *Van den Bent et al. Lancet* 2005 311 patients with LGG after maximal safe resection	Adjuvant RT 54 Gy in 30 fx Observation (with RT at tumor recurrence)	RT was associated with improved PFS, median 5.3 vs 3.4 y, $P < .001$ but no significant difference in OS. RT improved seizure control at 1 y (41% vs 25%)	Conclusion: Adjuvant RT improves PFS and seizure control but does not improve OS Of patients undergoing observation, ~65% ultimately received RT after tumor recurrence No high-grade transformation secondary to RT
RTOG 9802, *Shaw et al. JCO* 2012 and *Buckner et al. NEJM* 2016 251 patients with LGG age >40 yo and/or subtotal resection	Adjuvant RT alone 54 Gy in 30 fx Adjuvant RT + PCV (6 cycles)	Median OS 13.3 y in RT + PCV vs 7.8 years in RT-alone arm (HR 0.59, $P = .003$). Median PFS 10.4 y in RT + PCV vs 4.0 y in RT alone (HR 0.5, $P < .001$)	Conclusion: Adjuvant RT + PCV improves PFS and OS compared to adjuvant RT alone

Name/Inclusion	Arms	Outcomes	Notes
RTOG 0424, *Fisher et al. IJROBP* **2015** 129 high-risk (defined by ≥3 high-risk factors) patients with LGG Single-arm study	Historical controls RT (54 Gy in 30 fx) + concurrent and adjuvant TMZ	3-y OS was 73.1%, significant improved compared to historical control of 54% ($P < .001$). 3-y PFS was 59.2%	Conclusion: Adjuvant TMZ may offer similar OS and PFS benefit compared to PCV, but RCT comparing them is pending (see HGG chapter, CODEL trial)

HIGH-GRADE GLIOMAS

MIKE ROONEY • MARTIN TOM • SUBHA PERNI • D. NANA YEBOA

Background

- **Incidence/prevalence:** Historically, "high-grade gliomas" referred to grade 3 and grade 4 gliomas as defined by histopathology alone, and many earlier clinical trials of glioblastoma included grade 3 astrocytomas due to similarly poor prognoses. However, in the integrated histopathologic/molecular classification era, grade 3 gliomas (as well as grade 2 gliomas) are defined by an IDH mutation and have a substantially improved prognosis compared to glioblastomas, which are IDH wild type. There are ~2000 grade 3 glioma and 13 000 glioblastoma cases per year diagnosed in the United States. Of all malignant brain tumors, glioblastomas constitute ~50%.
- **Outcomes:** Median survival rates are 14.7 years for grade 3 oligodendroglioma (RTOG 9402) and 9.7 years for grade 3 IDH-mutant astrocytoma (CATNON). Patients with glioblastoma with good performance status have a median survival of 1.4 years if MGMT unmethylated and 2.6 years if MGMT methylated (*Stupp et al. JAMA* 2017); if elderly (>65-70) and/or poor performance, survival is typically <1 year.
- **Demographics:** The mean age at diagnosis of high-grade gliomas is 65 years. Males > females
- **Risk factors:** Gliomas are largely sporadic without any clear risk factors aside from prior exposure to ionizing radiation and genetic syndromes as noted below. There is no evidence that cell phone use leads to increased risk of developing gliomas.

Tumor Biology and Characteristics

- **Genetics:** Associated with various familial genetic syndromes including Li-Fraumeni (germ-line mutations in *TP53*), neurofibromatosis type 1, and Turcot syndrome. Glioblastoma was the first cancer type to be systematically studied via The Cancer Genome Atlas (TCGA). P53, RB, and receptor tyrosine kinase (RAS) signaling pathways were found to be abrogated across nearly all glioblastomas (*Cancer Genome Atlas Network Nature* 2008). *TERT* promoter mutations, leading to increased expression and activity of telomerase, are also found in ~80% of glioblastoma (*Killela et al. Proc Natl Acad Sci* 2013). Methylation of the *MGMT* promoter has improved prognosis, as well as improved response to concurrent chemoradiation with temozolomide (*Hegi et al. NEJM* 2005). Historically, diagnosis was based upon histopathologic grade, although the diagnosis integrates molecular data (*WHO* 2016 update; *David et al. Acta Neuropathol* 2016). IDH wild-type gliomas, regardless of histopathologic features, are typically treated as aggressive high-grade gliomas due to their aggressive nature and poor outcomes. Grade 3 astrocytomas and grade 4 GBMs are highly cellular and infiltrative. Classically, glioblastomas are characterized by foci of microvascular proliferation and pseudopalisading necrosis.
- **Imaging:** High-grade gliomas are typically contrast-enhancing on T1 scans with an associated edematous component best seen on T2-FLAIR sequences (Fig. 10.1). Additionally, glioblastomas commonly show a centrally necrotic pattern on imaging and can routinely cross midline ("butterfly" pattern).
- **Anatomy:** Commonly present in the frontal lobe compared to parietal/temporal and occipital lobes. Infratentorial tumors are uncommon. See **LGG** chapter for review of neuroanatomy.

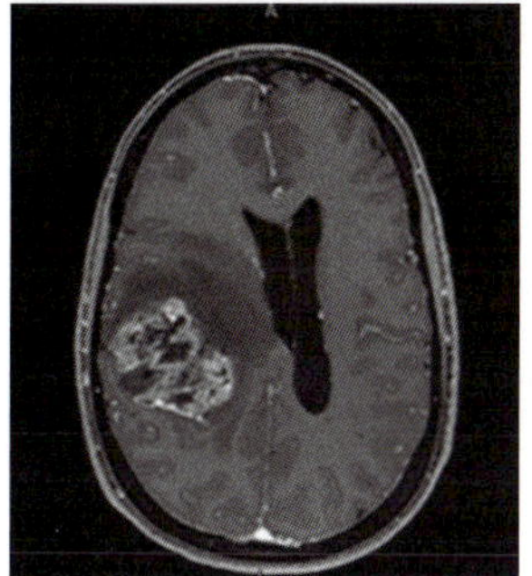
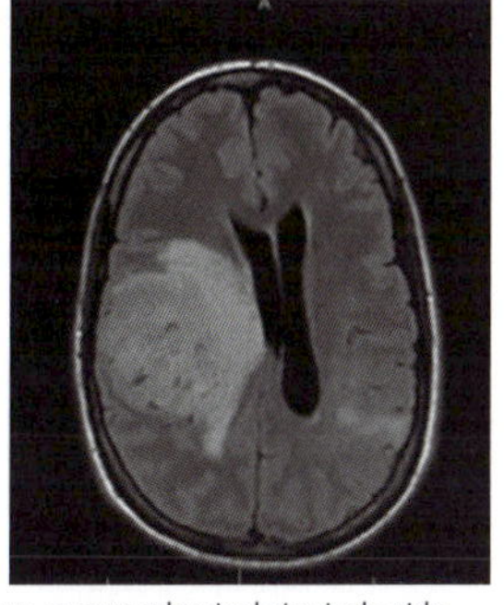

Figure 10.1 T1 + contrast MRI image **(left)** shows large contrast-enhancing lesion in the right frontoparietal lobe with necrotic features consistent with glioblastoma. The lesion is associated with a significant edematous component seen on T2-FLAIR sequence **(right)**.

Workup

- **History and physical:** Including presenting symptoms, history of seizures, and family history. Assessment of neurologic deficits and performance status is important. Important to ask whether they are on steroids and whether their symptoms have improved
- **Labs:** CBC, CMP
- **Procedures/biopsy:** Neurosurgery evaluation for biopsy and/or maximal safe resection of enhancing tumor. Some data suggest "supramaximal resection" inclusive of nonenhancing tumor is associated with improved outcomes.
- **Imaging:** MRI of the brain with and without contrast is the gold standard (Fig. 10.1) to evaluate location, grade, and extent of disease.

Staging/Grading

- **Grade 3 oligodendroglioma:** Presence of IDH mutation and 1p/19q codeletion. Grade 3 if anaplastic features or significant mitotic activity. Presence of CDKN2A/B homozygous deletion is associated with worse outcomes and can upgrade to grade 3 (from an otherwise grade 2 oligodendroglioma).
- **Grade 3 astrocytoma, IDH-mutant:** Presence of IDH mutation, 1p/19q noncodeletion, ATRX loss, and/or TP53 mutation. Grade 3 if anaplasia or significant mitotic activity. Absence of CDKN2A/B homozygous deletion (upgrades to grade 4)
- **Grade 4 astrocytoma, IDH-mutant:** Presence of IDH mutation, 1p/19q non-codeletion, ATRX loss, and/or TP53 mutation. Grade 4 if microvascular proliferation, necrosis, and/or CDKN2A/B homozygous deletion. Often treated similar to glioblastoma
- **Grade 4 glioblastoma, IDH wild type:** Astrocytic glioma lacking an IDH mutation (ie, IDH wild type), with any one or more of the following: microvascular proliferation, necrosis, TERT promoter mutation, EGFR gene amplification, and/or +7/−10 chromosome copy number changes

Treatment Algorithm

Grade 3 oligodendroglioma	Maximal surgical resection → RT → adjuvant PCV. Can consider concurrent and/or adjuvant TMZ as an alternative to PCV
Grade 3 astrocytoma	Maximal surgical resection → RT → adjuvant TMZ
Grade 4 glioblastoma*	Maximal surgical resection → concurrent chemoRT with TMZ → adjuvant TMZ + alternating electrical tumor-treating fields (TTF)

Grade 4 glioblastoma Elderly with good PS*	Maximal surgical resection → concurrent hypofractionated chemoRT with TMZ → adjuvant TMZ +/− alternating electrical tumor-treating fields (TTF)
Grade 4 glioblastoma Elderly with poor PS or MGMT methylation*	Maximal surgical resection → TMZ

*Elderly patients with glioblastoma have a multitude of options and can be treated with any of the above options. Important considerations include life expectancy, PS, methylation, and comorbidities.

Radiation Treatment Technique

- **SIM:** Supine, holding A-bar, Aquaplast mask with isocenter placed at the midbrain. MRI fusions (unless obtaining MRI SIM)—T1 + C sequence and T2/FLAIR sequences.
- **Dose and target:** See below for various delineation strategies.

Considerations:

- GTV includes cavity + residual contrast enhancement. Limit CTV expansions to anatomic boundaries of disease spread (eg, bones, falx, tentorium; brainstem is not an anatomic boundary if the tumor is in anatomic contiguity), unless T2 hyperintense signal spreads beyond these barrier areas indicating probable disease.
- For all high-grade gliomas, PTV expansions on CTV1 and CTV2 are generally 0.3 cm (daily kV) or 0.5 cm (weekly kV), at our institution.
- Can consider hypofractionated courses 50 Gy/20 fx, 40 Gy/15 fx, 34 Gy/10 fx, or 25 Gy/5 fx for patients that are elderly or with poor PS.

Histology	Approach (Boost Timing)	Target Definitions	Prescribed Dose/ Fractionation
Grade 3 glioma	MDACC (SIB)	CTV1: GTV	57 Gy in 30 fractions
		CTV2: GTV + 1.5 cm and additional FLAIR hyperintensity	50 Gy in 30 fractions
	RTOG (Sequential)	CTV1: GTV + T2/FLAIR + 2 cm	50.4 Gy in 28 fractions
		CTV2: GTV + 1 cm	Sequential boost 9 Gy in 5 fractions
	EORTC (Sequential)	CTV1: GTV + T2/FLAIR +1.5 cm	45 Gy in 30 fractions
		CTV2: GTV +1.5 cm	Sequential boost 14.4 Gy in 8 fractions
Glioblastoma	MDACC (SIB)	CTV1: GTV	60 Gy in 30 fractions
		CTV2: GTV + 2 cm and additional FLAIR hyperintensity	50 Gy in 30 fractions
	RTOG (Sequential)	CTV1: GTV + T2/FLAIR + 2 cm	46 Gy in 23 fractions
		CTV2: GTV + 2 cm	Sequential boost 14 Gy in 7 fractions
	EORTC	CTV: GTV + 2 cm	60 Gy in 30 fractions

- **Technique:** IMRT/VMAT. Consider use of protons on trial depending on anatomy and age.
- **IGRT:** Daily kV imaging
- **Planning directive:**

Brainstem: V30Gy < 33%. Max < 54 Gy. If necessary, may allow point max <60 Gy
Brain: V30Gy < 50%
Optic chiasm: Max ≤ 54 Gy
Cochlea: Max < 54 Gy. Mean < 30 Gy
Lens: Max < 5 Gy
Optic nerves: Max ≤ 54 Gy
Pituitary: Mean < 36 Gy
Eyes: Max < 40 Gy. Mean < 30 Gy
Spinal cord: Max ≤ 45 Gy (Fig. 10.2)

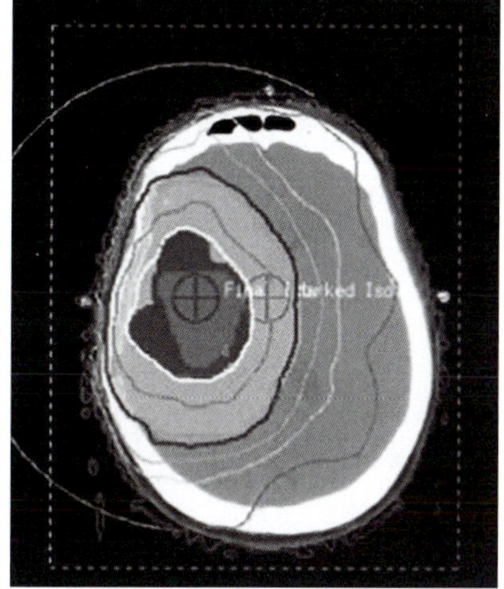

Figure 10.2 Representative plan for a patient with a grade 4 glioblastoma. The 60-Gy isodose line (*white*) can be seen surrounding the red GTV/resection cavity (*red color wash*). The 50-Gy isodose line (*blue*) covers GTV + 2 cm (*tan color wash*), which is expanded to include hyperintense signal on T2-FLAIR sequence. **See color insert.**

Chemotherapy

- **Concurrent:** Temozolomide (TMZ) 75 mg/m^2 daily during RT, 7 days a week
- **Adjuvant:** TMZ 150-200 mg/m^2 daily for 5 days, every 28 days for 6 cycles (or indefinitely). Procarbazine, lomustine, vincristine (PCV) regimen appears to be more effective for oligodendrogliomas than astrocytomas and is being compared to TMZ on the CODEL for patients with oligodendroglioma.

Side Effect Management

See **LGG** chapter.

Follow-up

Every 2-3 months with MRI of the brain w/ and w/o contrast for the first year following treatment, q4mo during years 2-4 and q6mo thereafter. Offer NovoTTF to glioblastoma patients after they have completed RT if they are willing. Many glioblastoma patients will recur in the first year following treatment. Consider reirradiation on protocol or enrollment in investigational clinical trials.

Notable Trials

Glioblastomas

Name/Inclusion	Arms	Outcomes	Notes
EORTC 26961/22981-NCIC ("Stupp Trial") *Stupp et al. NEJM 2005; Stupp et al. Lancet Oncol 2009* 573 patients w/ GBM s/p maximal safe resection	Adjuvant RT alone 60 Gy in 30 fx Adjuvant RT 60 Gy in 30 fx with current and adjuvant TMZ	Median OS for RT alone of 12.1 mo vs 14.6 mo for RT +TMZ G3/4 hematologic toxicity with TMZ of 7%	Conclusion: Adjuvant and concurrent TMZ improves OS after resection with RT Notes: 40% of patients had GTR. MGMT methylation status was predictive of response to TMZ
EF-14 NovoTTF *Stupp et al. JAMA 2015* 695 patients with GBM s/p maximal safe resection followed by adjuvant RT + TMZ	Adjuvant RT + TMZ Adjuvant RT + TMZ + tumor-treating fields (TTF)	Median OS 20.5 mo in TTF arm vs 15.6 mo in control (HR 0.64, $P = .004$)	Conclusion: TTF in addition to adjuvant RT + TMZ improves OS Note: TTF required continuous delivery (>18 hours/day) on a shaved scalp

Grade 3 gliomas

Name/Inclusion	Arms	Outcomes	Notes
EORTC 26951 *Van den Bent et al. JCO 2006, 2013* 368 patients with anaplastic astrocytoma and oligodendroglioma s/p maximal safe resection	Adjuvant RT alone 59.4 Gy in 33 fx Adjuvant RT 59.4 Gy in 33 fx + PCV × 6 cycles	RT + PCV was associated with improved median OS (42.3 vs 30.6 mo, $P < .05$)	Conclusion: Adjuvant PCV after RT increased OS and PFS Notes: 82% of patients in observation arm received chemo at progression. 1p/19q codeleted tumors derived more benefits from PCV
RTOG 9402 *Cairncross et al. JCO 2013* 291 patients with anaplastic oligodendrogliomas or mixed anaplastic oligo/astrocytomas randomized after maximal safe resection	PCV + RT (59.4 Gy in 33 fx) RT alone	For the entire cohort, no difference in median survival by treatment (4.6 y for PCV + RT vs 4.7 y for RT alone)	Importantly, the median survival of patients *with codeleted tumors treated with PCV + RT was twice that of those treated with RT alone (14.7 y vs 7.3 y, HR 0.59, P = .03)*

Name/Inclusion	Arms	Outcomes	Notes
CATNON *Van den Bent et al. Lancet Oncol 2021* 751 patients with 1p/19q noncodeleted (cat"NON") anaplastic glioma s/p maximal safe resection	2 × 2 factorial design randomizing to: 1. RT alone (59.4 Gy in 33 fractions) 2. RT + TMZ 3. RT → TMZ 4. RT + TMZ → TMZ	2nd interim analysis declared the futility of concurrent TMZ (median OS 66.9 mo w/ concurrent vs 60.4 mo w/o concurrent; HR 0.97, $P = .76$). Adjuvant TMZ, however, improved OS. Median OS 82.3 mo vs 46.9 mo (HR 0.64, $P < .0001$)	Adjuvant TMZ, but not concurrent TMZ, was associated with a survival benefit in patients with 1p/19q noncodeleted anaplastic glioma
CODEL **Initial report** *Jaeckle et al. Neuro Onc 2021* Ongoing trial at time of writing, interim report of 36 patients with G3 1p/19q codeleted oligodendrogliomas/p maximal safe resection	RT alone 59.4 Gy in 33 fx RT with concurrent and adjuvant TMZ TMZ alone	Interim analysis: TMZ alone was associated with inferior PFS (17% TMZ alone vs 63% in RT arms) at median 7.5 y. TMZ alone arm was closed and other arms remained recruiting	Conclusion: Omission of RT in patients with 1p/19q gliomas is associated with worse outcomes. Updated trial design will clarify impact of TMZ

MENINGIOMA

MIKE ROONEY • MARTIN TOM • SUBHA PERNI • D. NANA YEBOA

Background

- **Incidence/prevalence:** Meningioma is the most common benign brain tumor (1/3 of primary intracranial neoplasms), ~25-30 000 cases per year in the United States.
- **Outcomes:** Typically long natural history. Recurrence rate is strongly correlated with WHO grade (~10% for G1, 40% for G2, 70% for G3).
- **Demographics:** Female > male (2:1), incidence peaks in sixth to seventh decades
- **Risk factors:** Prior radiation at long interval (~20 years) from even low dose (1-2 Gy), NF2, MEN1, and long-term hormonal replacement usage are all identifiable risk factors.

Tumor Biology and Characteristics

- **Genetics:** Loss of chromosome 22 is the most common alteration, associated with NF2 mutation (50%). Less common alterations include AKT1 (~10%), SMO, TRAF7 (~25%), and PI3KA.
- **Pathology:** WHO grading based on mitotic activity—grade 1 (85-90% of cases, benign histology), grade 2 (5-10%, atypical, clear cell, choroid), and grade 3 (<5%, anaplastic, papillary, rhabdoid). Characteristically, psammoma bodies and calcifications are seen in grade 1 meningioma. Grade 2 is defined by ≥4 mitoses/10 HPF and/or brain invasion. And grade 3 is defined as ≥20 mitoses/10 HPF or the presence of

carcinomatous, sarcomatous, and melanomatous features. Subset expresses hormone receptors (progesterone and/or estrogen).

- **Imaging:** Contrast-enhanced MRI is preferred as a dural tail can be seen on 2/3 of cases (Fig. 11.1), typically T1 isointense, T2 hyperintense, and strongly enhancing. CT shows extra-axial mass displacing normal brain, isodense, with ~25% having calcification. Consider DOTA-TATE-PET/CT.

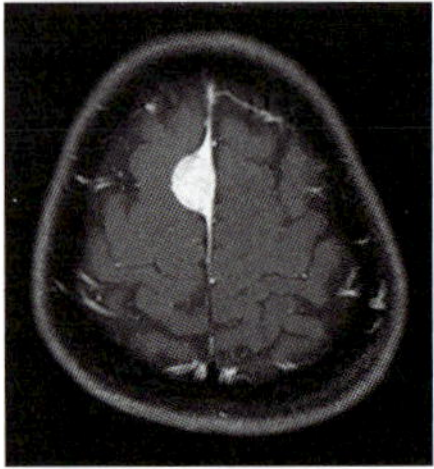

Figure 11.1 T1 + C MRI sequence showing enhancing lesion with dural origin, consistent with meningioma. Note enhancing dural tail seen in ~2/3 of cases.

Anatomy

- Meningiomas have dural origin, most commonly within the skull (90%) at sites of dural reflection (falx cerebri, tentorium cerebelli, venous sinuses) but can also present in the optic nerve sheath and choroid plexus. Common sites of presentation include cerebral convexity and parafalcine/parasagittal regions.

Workup

- **History and physical:** History with careful attention to neurologic deficits and exam
- **Labs:** CBC, CMP
- **Procedures/biopsy:** Neurosurgery evaluation for maximal safe resection and/or biopsy
- **Imaging:** Head CT and MRI of the brain to evaluate extent of disease. Evaluate for perilesional edema and/or bony invasion. G1 tumors typically grow ~1 mm/year. G2-3 tumors more likely to have faster growth rate, perilesional edema, and/or brain invasion.

Staging and Grading (see Table 11.1)

Table 11.1 Simpson Grading System for Meningioma

Grade	Description	10-Year Recurrence
1	GTR, including dural attachment and any abnormal bone	9%
2	GTR, with coagulation instead of resection of dural attachment	19%
3	GTR of meningioma without resection or coagulation of dural attachment	29%
4	Subtotal resection	44%
5	Tumor debulking or decompression only	N/A

Treatment Algorithm

Incidental/asymptomatic	Observation with MRI at 3, 6, and 12 mo (2/3 will stay stable)
Progressive/symptomatic At diagnosis	Surgery ± RT depending on grade

G1 GTR or STR	Observe
G1 recurrent	Adjuvant RT with either conventional, SRS, or fractionated SSRS as per below
G2 GTR	54-59.4 Gy adjuvant RT as per below; SRS for select small tumors is reasonable
G2 STR/recurrent or any G3	54-60 Gy RT adjuvant RT as per below

Radiation Treatment Technique

- **SIM**: Supine, thermoplastic mask, scan vertex to shoulders. Isocenter placed at midbrain. MRI fusions (unless obtaining MRI SIM)—T1 + C sequence and T2-FLAIR sequences
- **Dose and target:**

WHO Grade	Dose	Target
Grade 1	50.4-54 Gy in 28-30 fx at 1.8 Gy/fx **or** SRS 12-14 Gy	Residual enhancing tumor
Grade 2 (or recurrent G1)	54-59.4 Gy in 30-33 fx at 1.8 Gy/fx **or** SRS 14-16 Gy	Tumor and/or resection bed + 0.5-1 cm CTV (restrain to dura unless brain invasion)
Grade 3 (or recurrent G2)	CTV1: 60 Gy in 30 fx CTV2: 50-54 Gy in 30 fx (SIB with CTV1)	CTV1: Tumor and/or resection bed + 1 cm CTV2: Tumor and/or resection bed + 2 cm

- **Technique:** IMRT/VMAT. PTV 3 mm if daily kV, 5 mm if weekly kV. Consider SRS if G1, <3 cm size, with sufficient distance from critical structures, that is, optic apparatus (>2 mm). For SRS, prescribe 12-16 Gy or 25 Gy/5 fx FSRS for larger G1 tumors
- **IGRT:** Daily kV
- **Planning directive:**

  Fractionated EBRT
  Brainstem: V30Gy < 33%. Max < 54 Gy. If necessary, may allow point max < 60 Gy
  Brain: V30Gy < 50%
  Optic chiasm: Max ≤ 54 Gy
  Cochlea: Max < 54 Gy. Mean < 30 Gy
  Lens: Max < 5 Gy
  Optic nerves: Max ≤ 54 Gy
  Pituitary: Mean < 36 Gy
  Eyes: Max < 40 Gy. Mean < 30 Gy
  Spinal cord: Max ≤ 45 Gy

For single-fraction SRS, limit dose to optic apparatus to 8 Gy (can push up to 10 Gy point dose). Can consider dose escalation to 16 Gy in single fraction if grade 2. We do not recommend SRS for grade 3 tumors as upfront treatment.

Chemotherapy

Experience with systemic therapy are primarily studies in the recurrent setting with limited efficacy. Studied options include Sutent, hydroxyurea, somatostatin analogs (octreotide), and various inhibitors (progesterone, estrogen, PDGF, EGFR, VEGF).

Follow-up

Grade 1: MRI at 6 months and then annually
Grade 2: MRI q3-6mo × 1 year and then annually
Grade 3: MRI q3-6mo × 5 years and then q6-12mo

Depending on location of RT, important to assess for potential hormonal deficiencies (ie, pituitary hormones)

Notable Studies

Name/Inclusion	Arms	Treatment	Early Outcomes
RTOG 0539 *Rogers et al. J Neurosurg* 2018; *IJROBP* 2020 Phase II nonrandomized trial of risk adapted treatment of meningioma based on grade and extent of surgical resection	Low risk: Grade 1, GTR or STR	Observation	60 patients with low risk, the median follow-up was 9.1 y. 10-y PFS was 85% and 93.8% for OS 52 patients with Intermediate-risk disease treated per protocol had excellent 3-y PFS (93.8%) and OS (96%) at first report 53 patients with high-risk disease had a 3-y PFS of 58.8% at first analysis despite surgery + RT at higher dose. Additional investigations are needed to further improve outcomes for this cohort
	Intermediate risk: Grade 2, GTR or recurrent grade 1	RT 54 Gy in 30 fractions	
	High risk: Any grade 3 or recurrent grade 2 or new grade 2 s/p STR	RT 60 Gy in 30 fractions	

BENIGN CNS

KATHRYN MARQUEEN • MARTIN TOM • SUBHA PERNI • D. NANA YEBOA

Vestibular Schwannoma

Background

- **Incidence/prevalence:** Vestibular schwannoma (acoustic neuroma) accounts for 8% of adult intracranial tumors and 85% of cerebellopontine angle tumors. Incidence is ~1 per 100 000 person-years, although true rate may be higher based upon incidental findings on autopsy and MRI studies. Almost always presents with unilateral involvement except for patients with NF2
- **Outcomes:** Typically slow-growing with long natural history. 40% will show no growth.
- **Demographics:** Median age of diagnosis 50 years. 1:2 M/F ratio
- **Risk factors:** NF1 and NF2 (bilateral lesions), acoustic trauma (loud noise), childhood exposure to low-dose radiation

Tumor biology and characteristics

- **Genetics:** Inactivation of *NF2* gene (produces tumor suppressor schwannomin) is found in most sporadic schwannomas.
- **Pathology:** Benign (WHO grade 1) tumor arises from perineural elements of Schwann cell of the 8th CN with S-100+ on IHC. Malignant transformation is rare.
- **Imaging:** MRI with contrast is the gold standard and preferred, including mm sections through internal auditory canal (IAC), seen as well-circumscribed, homogenously contrast-enhancing lesions (Fig. 12.1).

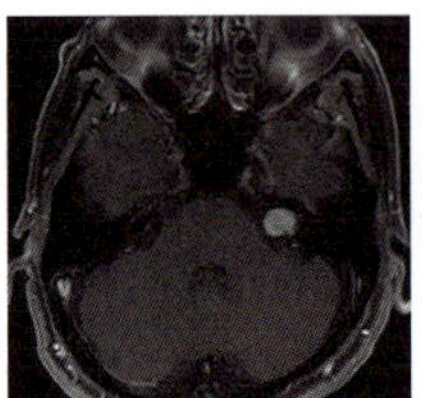

Figure 12.1 T1 + C MRI sequencing showing a 1.3 × 1.0 cm schwannoma on the left intracanalicular space. The tumor extends slightly into the left cerebellopontine angle.

Anatomy

Schwannomas are the most common peripheral nerve sheath tumor and can involve other extracranial or intracranial (trigeminal, facial, jugular foramen) nerves. The internal acoustic canal is a short segment (~1 cm) in the temporal bone that contains CN VII and VIII; vestibular schwannomas typically affect the intracanalicular segment of the vestibular portion of CN VIII.

Workup

- **History and physical:** History with careful attention to neurologic deficits and exam (Weber and Rinne tests). If facial/trigeminal involvement, patients may present with altered taste and facial paresis.
- **Procedures/biopsy:** Audiometry should be done to establish baseline. Neurosurgical evaluation for resection/biopsy
- **Imaging:** MRI of the brain w/ contrast

Koos grading scale for vestibular schwannoma

Grade	Description
I	Intracanalicular
II	Tumor extending into posterior fossa without touching brainstem
III	Tumor extending into posterior fossa, touching brainstem, no midline shift
IV	Tumor extending into posterior fossa, touching brainstem, with midline shift

Treatment algorithm

Small (<2 cm), no symptoms, no growth, elderly patients with comorbidities	Audiometry and MRI scans every 6 mo to 1 y
Large (>4 cm), symptomatic, recurrent or progressive after XRT	Surgical resection
Large, symptomatic, not surgical candidate	Definitive radiation

Radiation treatment technique

- **SIM:** Supine, thermoplastic mask. MRI fusions (unless obtaining MRI sim)—T1 + C sequence
- **Dose, target, technique, IGRT:**

Technique	Dose	Target	IGRT*
Standard fractionation preferred for lesions >2-3 cm	50.4 Gy in 28 fx	GTV + 3 mm PTV	Daily kV
Stereotactic radiosurgery (Fig. 12.2) preferred for smaller lesions, <3 cm in diameter	12-13 Gy	GTV only	
Hypofractionation (*Kapoor IJROBP* 2011) is preferred for larger lesions that are not ideal SRS candidates owing to anatomic constraints	18 Gy in 3 fx 25 Gy in 5 fx	GTV only	

*IGRT for conventional, hypofractionated, and SRS cases are institution dependent and also on what PTV margins are used.

- **Planning directive:**
  SRS
  Brainstem: 0.01 cc ≤ 12 Gy; max < 15 Gy
  Optic nerves and chiasm: Max < 8-10 Gy
  Cochlea: Limit central cochlear dose to <4.2 Gy (*Kano et al. Neurosurgery* 2009)
- **Fractionated radiotherapy (1.8 Gy/fx):**
  Spinal cord: Max < 45 Gy
  Brainstem: Max < 54 Gy
  Optic nerves and chiasm: Max < 54 Gy
  Cochlea: Max < 35 Gy
  Pituitary: Max < 40 Gy

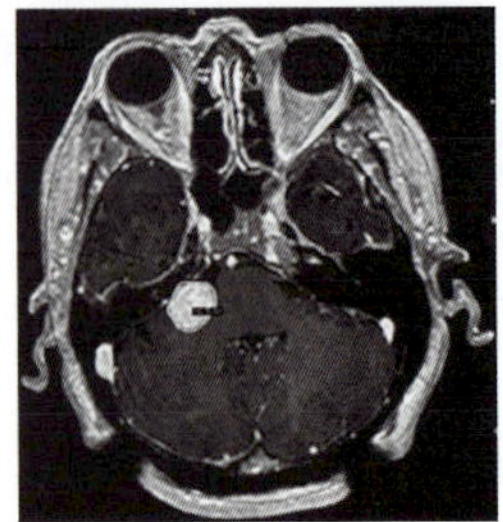

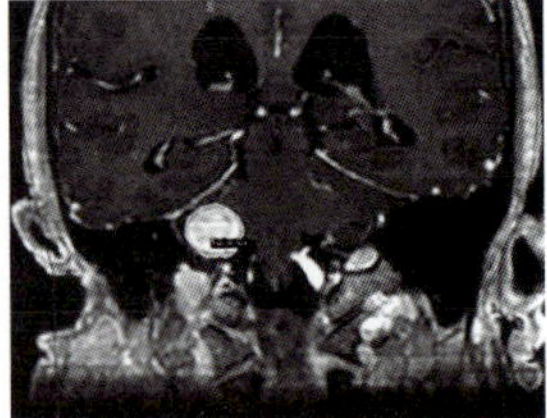

Figure 12.2 Axial and coronal sections demonstrating treatment of an acoustic neuroma with Gamma Knife SRS. A dose of 12.5 Gy was prescribed with 50% isodose.

Follow-up

- First follow-up at 3-6 months and then annual MRI is typically recommended for 10 years with less frequent studies if no evidence of tumor progression.
- All patients should undergo baseline audiology evaluation prior to treatment and regularly with follow-up posttreatment.

Surgery

- **Technique:**
  - Middle cranial fossa approach: Best suited for small tumors with focus on hearing preservation
  - Translabyrinthine approach: Usually reserved for larger tumors in patients who have already lost functional hearing, as this approach sacrifices hearing in the operated ear
  - Retrosigmoid (keyhole) approach: Most often used for moderate or large tumors in patients with functional hearing with the goal of hearing preservation
- **Outcomes:** Excellent if GTR, but about 15% LR if STR

Notable Studies

Study	Population/Treatment	Results
German retrospective (*Combs et al. Int J Radiat Oncol Biol Phys* 2010)	Prospective cohort study of 200 patients treated to median dose of 57.6 Gy at 1.8 Gy/fx or Linac-based SRS	No difference in 10-y LC of 96%. Hearing preservation of 78% at 5 y for standard fractionation and patients with SRS < 13 Gy
Japan retrospective (*Hasegawa et al. Int J Radiat Oncol Bio Phys* 2013)	Single-institution review of 440 patients using Gamma Knife SRS	Median marginal dose of 12.8 Gy showed 10-y PFS of 92% and <5% rate of CN palsy

Paraganglioma (Jugulotympanic)

Background

- **Incidence/prevalence:** Rare, typically benign, neuroendocrine tumor, which most commonly presents during the fifth to sixth decade of life
- **Clinical presentation:** Less than 5% of all paragangliomas are present in the head and neck. Most symptoms result from the mass effect of the tumor and may include pulsatile tinnitus, hearing loss, and cranial nerve palsies. Paragangliomas of the head and neck are more often noncatecholamine secreting compared with other organ sites.
- **Pathology:** Mutations in the succinate dehydrogenase enzyme complex have been shown to predispose to the development of head and neck paragangliomas (*Neumann et al. Cancer Res* 2009).
- **Imaging:** Reliably imaged with both CT and MRI angiography. CT is beneficial for visualizing the destruction of the temporal bone. Octreotide imaging has demonstrated a sensitivity of 94% in patients with head and neck paragangliomas (*Telischi et al. Otolaryngol Head Neck Surg* 2000).

Treatment

Observation

- Initial observation and close follow-up may be considered for small asymptomatic tumors.
- The median growth rate for head and neck paragangliomas is ~1 mm/y (*Jansen et al. Cancer* 2000).

Surgery

- Typically preferred for small tumors in which there is felt to be a low risk of serious complications or functional deficits
- Resection is also preferred for immediate relief of symptomatic tumors or catecholamine-secreting tumors.
- Local control rates with surgery alone exceed 80-90% following gross total resection.
- Needs negative biochemical workup or alpha-blockade before surgery to avoid catecholamine crisis.

Radiotherapy

- Stereotactic radiosurgery:
  - Provides excellent local control (>95% at 3 years; *Guss et al. IJROBP* 2011) and is a good option for smaller tumors that are at high risk of potential surgical complications
  - Typically prescribed as 12-16 Gy to the 50-80% isodose
  - Fractionated SRS 25-30 Gy in 5 fractions may be used for larger tumors in critical locations
- Fractionated radiotherapy:
  - Useful for larger tumors, which cannot be safely treated with SRS due to tumor volume and/or potential dose to critical structures
  - Doses of 45-50.4 Gy in 1.8 Gy/fx are associated with local control similar to surgical series.

Dose constraints

See dose constraints for vestibular schwannomas.

Follow-up

- Imaging every 6-12 months for 3 years and then annually for 10 years
- Serum markers should be tested in secretory tumors.

Trigeminal Neuralgia

Background

- **Incidence/prevalence:** Annual incidence is ~5 per 100 000 person-years. Approximately 50% more prevalent among females vs males. Most commonly seen in patients aged 50 years and older.
- **Clinical presentation:** Brief, recurrent episodes of severe unilateral shooting/stabbing pain localized to one or more divisions of the trigeminal nerve in the absence of other neurologic deficits
- **Pathology:** Majority of cases are thought to be caused by compression of the trigeminal nerve root, which leads to demyelination and disrupted neuronal signaling.
- **Imaging:** Volumetric acquisitions with thin slice MRI/MRA are useful in the detection of neurovascular compression.

Treatment

Medical management

- Preferred as upfront treatment prior to consideration of surgery or radiotherapy
- Carbamazepine is the most commonly used agent for front-line therapy. Others shown to be efficacious include oxcarbazepine, baclofen, and lamotrigine.

Surgery

- Usually reserved for patients with medically intractable symptoms. Very effective for initial pain relief, although efficacy tends to fall over time
- Surgical options include the following:
  - Microvascular decompression to relieve the pressure of vascular structures off the trigeminal nerve
  - Rhizotomy with destruction of the gasserian ganglion by RF ablation, mechanical compression, or chemical lysis

Radiosurgery

- Mechanism of pain relief remains poorly understood, although animal models have demonstrated axonal degradation, fragmentation, and edema following ablative SRS doses to the trigeminal nerve root (*Kondziolka et al. Neurosurgery* 2000).

- When performed using Gamma Knife SRS, a maximum point dose of 70-90 Gy is delivered using a single 4-mm isocenter targeting the proximal ipsilateral trigeminal nerve (Fig. 12.3). Several institutional series have also demonstrated efficacy of CyberKnife/Linac modalities with acceptable rates of toxicity.
- Prospective data demonstrate pain relief in a proportion of patients with low rates of toxicity (*Regis et al. J Neurosurg* 2006). However, the efficacy over time also declines similar to reported surgical series.

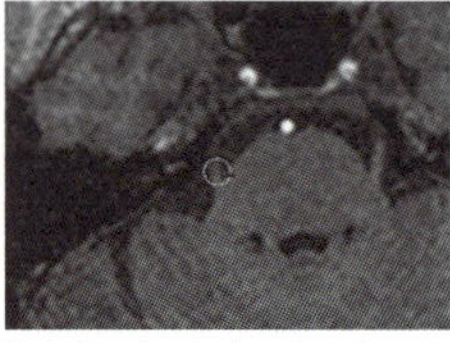

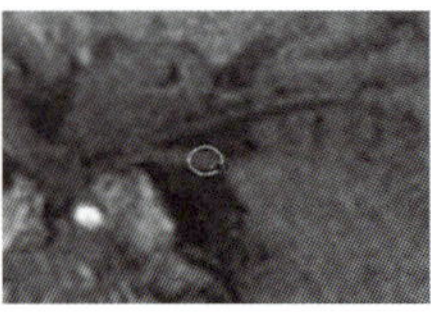

Figure 12.3 Axial and sagittal sections demonstrating treatment of a right-sided trigeminal neuralgia using Gamma Knife SRS. A maximum point dose of 80 Gy was delivered using a single shot with a 4-mm collimator.

Arteriovenous Malformation

Background

- **Incidence/prevalence:** Annual incidence of ~1 per 100 000 person-years. Median age at diagnosis of 30 years
- **Clinical presentation:** Wide range of initial presentation from detection as an incidental finding to intracranial hemorrhage, seizures, headaches, and focal neurologic deficits. Most are supratentorial (90%) and present with a single lesion (90%). The presence of multiple AVMs is strongly associated with Osler-Weber-Rendu syndrome (hereditary hemorrhagic telangiectasia).
- **Pathology:** Abnormal communication between arteries and veins without usual intervening capillary network. The high flow rates can create vessel enlargement and both arterial and venous aneurysms.
- **Imaging:** Cerebral angiography is the gold standard for evaluating the location of feeding vessels and drainage patterns. Contrast-enhanced CT and MRI angiography can also be useful for initial diagnosis.

Treatment

Medical therapy

- Historically, interventional therapy for AVMs has been favored due to the 2% annual rate of hemorrhage in patients with untreated lesions.
- The role of routine interventional therapy in asymptomatic patients is controversial and requires a multidisciplinary approach. The ARUBA trial demonstrated a significantly elevated risk of stroke and death following intervention as compared with those receiving medical management alone, though criticisms of this study include the small number of patients, nonstandardized interventional treatment approach, and early stopping (*Mohr et al. Lancet* 2014).

Microsurgery

- Treatment of choice for patients felt to be at high risk of hemorrhage, as it provides immediate treatment of symptomatic AVMs and immediately reduces risk of hemorrhage postprocedure
- The Spetzler-Martin grading system is used to assess the risk of postoperative neurologic complications and aids in treatment modality decision-making (*Spetzler and Martin J Neurosurg* 1986).

Embolization

- Endovascular embolization is commonly used to reduce the size of large AVMs prior to treatment with radiotherapy or surgery, but it can result in complete obliteration of the nidus in few instances.

Radiosurgery

- Usually reserved for lesions that are inaccessible or felt to be at very high risk with surgical intervention due to operative complications or medical comorbidities.
- The mechanism of action is thought to be via induction of progressive thrombosis and fibrosis.

- Approximately 80-90% of patients will have eventual obliteration of the nidus, although the mean time to obliteration following SRS is ~2-3 years. The elevated risk of hemorrhage is not eliminated until complete obliteration of the AVM, although risk of hemorrhage decreases 50% during latency period after radiosurgery.
- A prescription dose of 16-20 Gy covering the nidus is associated with in-field obliteration rates in excess of 90% (*Flickinger et al. IJROBP* 1996).
- Large AVMs (eg, >10-15 cc) can be treated with a volume-staged approach, whereby a portion (eg, half) of the AVM is initially treated with SRS, and the rest is treated with SRS 3-6 months later.
- MRI/MRA can be used for posttreatment surveillance with cerebral angiography used to confirm resolution.

PITUITARY ADENOMA AND CRANIOPHARYNGIOMA

KATHRYN MARQUEEN • MARTIN TOM • SUBHA PERNI • D. NANA YEBOA

Background

- **Incidence/prevalence:** The most common sellar mass is pituitary adenoma (90-95%), which accounts for 10% of intracranial tumors. 12 000 cases per year in the United States (*Ostrom et al. Neuro Oncol* 2017). Male to female 1:1, although females are more likely to have symptoms. There are ~350 craniopharyngioma cases annually, accounting for 1-3% of brain tumors.
- **Outcomes:** Long natural history as incidental imaging finding, endocrine abnormality, or local compressive symptoms; RT provides 90+% LC.
- **Demographics:** Pituitary adenoma presents at 30-50 years, craniopharyngioma bimodal (1/3 at 0-14 years, 2/3 at 50-75 years).
- **Risk factors:**
  - Pituitary adenoma: MEN-1 (parathyroid, pancreas, pituitary)
  - Craniopharyngioma: No identified risk factors

Tumor Biology and Characteristics

- **Pituitary adenoma:** Classified by size (<1 cm microadenoma vs >1 cm macroadenoma, >4 cm giant adenoma), functional vs nonfunctional, and cell origin. 75% of pituitary adenomas are secretory (50% PRL, 25% GH, 20% ACTH, <1% TSH).
- **Craniopharyngioma:** Epithelial tumor derived from Rathke pouch, the embryonic precursor to anterior pituitary; adamantinomatous (Wnt activation; *CTNNB1* mutation) vs papillary (*BRAF* mutation; more common in adults). Usually arise along the pituitary stalk, less frequently within the sella, third ventricle, or optic system.
- **Pathology:** Mallory trichrome staining helps differentiate functional vs nonfunctional adenomas.
- **Imaging:** Craniopharyngioma often presents with calcification (60-80%) and mixed solid-cystic (75%) components. Adenomas appear hypointense in the early phase of dynamic contrast-enhanced MRI (due to poor vasculature relative to normal tissue).

Anatomy

- **Sella:** Located within the sphenoid bone, bounded by hypothalamus and optic chiasm (superior), sphenoid sinus (inferior), and cavernous sinus (lateral)
- **Pituitary gland:** Divided into anterior (GH, PRL, TSH, ACTH, FSH, LH) and posterior (oxytocin, ADH)

Workup

- **History and physical:** History with careful attention to potential endocrinopathies. Presenting symptoms may include visual symptoms (including bitemporal hemianopsia), headache, and signs of hypopituitarism.
- **Procedures/biopsy:** Neurosurgical evaluation for resection/biopsy. Endocrine evaluation if medical management desirable. Visual field evaluation
- **Labs:** CBC, CMP, endocrine function tests (TSH, ACTH, cortisol, prolactin, IGF-1)
- **Imaging:** MRI of the brain w/ contrast

Treatment Algorithms

- **Pituitary adenoma:**
  - Observation can be considered for small asymptomatic lesions without mass effect
  - First line: Medical management for prolactinoma or if functional (see "Medical Management")
  - For all others, surgery is the first treatment. Consider adjuvant RT for STR or persistent hormone elevation.
  - Consider medical management for persistent hormone elevation.
- **Craniopharyngioma:**
  - Maximal safe resection (shunt if hydrocephalus) → consideration for RT (if STR, recurrent disease)

Radiation Treatment Technique

- **SIM:** Supine, thermoplastic mask, bite block, scan vertex to shoulders
- **Dose, target, and technique:**

	Target	External Beam	SRS*
Nonfunctional pituitary adenoma	GTV or postoperative bed + 0.3 cm PTV (CTV institutionally dependent)	45-50.4 Gy in 25-28 fx	14-18 Gy
Functional pituitary adenoma		50.4-54 Gy in 28-30 fx	20-25 Gy
Craniopharyngioma		50.4-54 Gy in 28-30 fx	12-14 Gy

*If difficulty in achieving chiasm single fx constraint, ok to consider FSRS regimens including 21/3, 20/4, 25/5, although prospective long-term follow-up from these regimens is lacking.

- **IGRT:** Daily kV, weekly-biweekly reimaging with MRI for craniopharyngioma to monitor changes in cyst shape/size, which may necessitate replanning
- **Considerations:** We favor fractioned EBRT for larger (>3 cm) tumors or for tumors close (<2 mm) to critical structures (ie, optic chiasm). Repeat imaging during treatment of craniopharyngioma to assess cyst volume changes. See **LGG** chapter for normal tissue constraints. Hold antisecretory medications for several weeks prior to RT, during RT, and 1 month after RT, especially for prolactinomas.

Surgery

- **Transsphenoidal resection:** >95% of cases. Endoscope inserted through one nostril and opening made in the nasal septum and sphenoid sinus to access the sella. Fat graft placed in resection bed and cartilage craft to seal sella hole. Complications include diabetes insipidus, CSF leaks, and hemorrhage.
- **Pterional craniotomy:** Temporal craniotomy may be required to access extrasellar disease, particularly for craniopharyngioma.

Medical Management

Hormone	Labs	Symptoms	Medical Tx
PRL	Serum PRL	Galactorrhea, amenorrhea	Dopamine agonist (eg, cabergoline, bromocriptine)
GH	Serum GH, IGF-1	Acromegaly	Somatostatin analog (eg, octreotide) or GH antagonist (pegvisomant)
ACTH	24-h urine free cortisol	Cushing syndrome	Steroid synthesis inhibitor (eg, ketoconazole, etomidate)
TSH	TSH, T4	Hyperthyroidism symptoms	Carbimazole, methimazole, somatostatin, propylthiouracil

Follow-up

- Endocrine evaluation and MRI q6mo, normalization of hormones can take years.

Notable Studies

Study	Population	Results
Pituitary adenoma UVA retrospective (*Sheehan et al. J Neurosurg* 2011)	Review of 418 patients treated with Gamma Knife	LC 90%, median time to endocrine remission 48 minutes, new pituitary hormone deficiency in 24% of patients. Smaller adenoma volume correlated with improved endocrine remission rates
Craniopharyngioma UCSF retrospective (*Shoenfeld et al. J Neurooncol* 2012)	Review of 122 patients treated with GTR vs STR + XRT	No difference in PFS ($P = .54$) and OS ($P = .74$) when treated with GTR vs STR + XRT but significantly shorter PFS if STR alone ($P < .001$). Additionally, GTR was associated with greater risk of DI (56% vs 13%, $P < .001$) and panhypopituitarism (55% vs 27%, $P = .01$) vs STR + XRT
Craniopharyngioma retrospective (*Bishop et al. Int J Radiat Oncol* 2014)	Review of 52 children treated with protons (21) or IMRT (31) at two institutions	Of 24 patients with imaging during RT, 10 (42%) had cyst growth and 5 (21%) required change in treatment plan. Outcomes similar with IMRT and protons

MEDULLOBLASTOMA

ADAM GRIPPIN • ARNOLD PAULINO

Background

- **Incidence/prevalence:** Second most common pediatric brain tumor. Most common malignant tumor in the posterior fossa. There are ~500 cases per year in the United States.
- **Outcomes:** 5-Year survival 80-85% for average-risk disease and 60-65% for high-risk disease
- **Demographics:** Bimodal age distribution; peak incidence 6 years in children and 25 years in adults
- **Risk factors:** Gorlin syndrome (nevoid basal cell carcinoma syndrome, due to mutations in *PTCH*, which regulates Sonic Hedgehog [SHH] signaling), Turcot syndrome (familial adenomatous polyposis [FAP] with brain tumors, due to mutations in *APC*, which regulates Wnt signaling)

Tumor Biology and Characteristics

- **Pathology:** Small, round, blue cell tumor. Primitive neuroectodermal tumor (PNET) of the superior medullary velum (germinal matrix) of the cerebellum or cerebellar vermis. Classic histologic finding is the Homer-Wright pseudorosette (tumor cells concentrically arranged around a lumen containing neuropil).
- **Imaging:** Typically, hypointense to isointense on T1-weighted images and generally shows avid enhancement on postcontrast sequences

Anatomy

Tumors most commonly arise from the cerebellar vermis and often protrude into the 4th ventricle and may grow through the lateral foramina of Luschka and the posteromedial foramen of Magendie into the subarachnoid space. Midline tumors are most commonly associated with Wnt subtype, extensive anterior growth (including into the brainstem) is seen in group 3/4 tumors, and lateral tumors are most likely to be SHH subtype. Obstruction of the cerebral aqueduct can cause obstructive hydrocephalus.

Subtypes of Medulloblastoma (*Taylor et al. Acta Neuropathol* 2012)

Molecular Subtype	Histologic Subtype	Age*	Prognosis
Wnt	Classic, rarely large cell/anaplastic	C, A	Very good
SHH	Desmoplastic/nodular, medulloblastoma with extensive nodularity (MBEN)	I, C, A	Good (I)/intermediate (C, A)
Group 3 (MYC+++, SMARCA4)	Classic, large cell/anaplastic	I, C	Poor
Group 4 (MYCN+)	Classic, large cell/anaplastic	I, C, A	Intermediate

*I, infants; C, children; A, adults.

Workup

- **History and physical:** Baseline evaluations by endocrinology, ophthalmology, audiology, and neuropsychology. Neurologic examination may reveal cerebellum deficits including gait or truncal ataxia, cranial nerve deficits, or signs of increased intracranial pressure including papilledema and loss of vision. Postoperatively, surgical resection associated with posterior fossa syndrome, which appears 1-2 days after surgery and includes mutism and emotional lability
- **Labs:** General labs and CSF evaluation 10-14 days after surgery
- **Procedures/biopsy:** Lumbar puncture often contraindicated prior to surgery secondary to risk of herniation. Perform lumbar puncture 10-14 days after surgery
- **Imaging:** Contrast MRI is the preferred examination. Preoperative and postoperative (within 48 hours of surgery) contrast-enhanced brain MRI. Spine MRI (if not done preoperatively) 10-14 days after surgery

Staging and Risk Stratification

Modified Chang Staging	
M0	No subarachnoid or hematogenous metastases
M1	Microscopic tumor cells in the CSF
M2	Gross intracranial nodular seeding
M3	Gross spinal subarachnoid seeding
M4	Metastases outside the neuroaxis (rare; bone and bone marrow most common sites of extraneural spread)
Risk Stratification	
Average risk	≤1.5 cm^2 residual tumor after surgery, M0 by craniospinal MRI and lumbar puncture
High risk	Subtotal resection (>1.5 cm^2 residual tumor), M+

MB 4-2

Treatment Algorithm

Average risk	Maximal safe resection; standard-dose craniospinal irradiation (CSI) with tumor bed boost; adjuvant chemotherapy
High risk	Maximal safe resection; high-dose CSI with tumor bed boost and boost to other sites of gross disease; adjuvant chemotherapy
Infants <3 y	Maximal safe resection; consideration of chemotherapy intensification and deferment of CSI until age 3 or later

All patients should be considered for a clinical trial.

Radiation Treatment Technique

- **SIM:** Supine on foam board, thermoplastic mask. Anesthesia often required for young children.
- **Dose:**
  - Average risk: CSI to 23.4 Gy in 17 fractions (1.8 Gy/fx), sequential boost to tumor bed plus margin to 54.0 Gy
  - High risk: CSI to 36.0 Gy in 20 fractions (1.8 Gy/fx), sequential boost to tumor bed plus margin to 54.0 Gy
- **Target:**
  - CSI:
    - Entire craniospinal axis
    - Ensure coverage of cribriform plate and thecal sac
  - Tumor bed boost:
    - Collapsed tumor bed and gross residual disease if present
    - 1.0-1.5 cm anatomically constrained expansion for CTV
- **Technique:** Passive scatter proton radiotherapy to spare anterior structures. RAO and LAO cranial fields (10-15 degrees from horizontal plane to reduce dose to contralateral lens; do not compromise cribriform plate coverage to spare lenses) and posterior spinal fields. Multiple ways to handle junctions, including junction shifts every 4-5 fractions to feather overlap at brain-spine and spine-spine junctions. For growing children, ensure coverage of entire vertebral body to prevent asymmetric growth and reduce risk of lordosis.
- **IGRT:** Daily kV
- **Dose constraints:**

Spinal cord	Max < 50 Gy
Brain stem	Max < 57 Gy, V54 < 10%
Optic nerves	Max < 54 Gy
Optic chiasm	Max < 54 Gy
Retinas	Max < 45 Gy
Cochleae	Max < 45 Gy, mean < 26 Gy (can tolerate mean dose of 38 Gy for high risk)
Parotids	Mean < 10 Gy

Lacrimal glands	Mean < 26 Gy
Kidneys	V20 < 30%, V12 < 55%
Pituitary	Mean < 36 Gy

Chemotherapy

- Standard adjuvant regimens include cisplatin, vincristine, and lomustine (CCNU) or cyclophosphamide.
- Use of targeted agents (eg, vismodegib [Erivedge] for SHH medulloblastoma) emerging.
- Some protocols (COG) include weekly vincristine given during radiotherapy.

Treatment of Medulloblastoma in Children <3 Years of Age

- Goal is to delay radiotherapy as long as possible to mitigate long-term toxicity.
- Standard approach is maximal safe resection followed by intensive chemotherapy (high-dose methotrexate followed by carboplatin, thiotepa, and etoposide) with autologous stem cell rescue.
- Focal radiotherapy to tumor bed may be considered in select cases, but patients are at significantly higher risk for failure at nontumor bed-irradiated sites.

Follow-up

- MRI of the brain and spine 4-6 weeks after radiotherapy, then every 3 months for the 1st year, every 4 months for the 2nd year, every 6 months until year 5, and then annually thereafter
- Patients should have periodic evaluations by endocrinology, ophthalmology, audiology, and neuropsychology to detect and manage long-term sequelae of treatment.

Notable Trials/Papers

Name/Inclusion	Randomization Arms	Outcomes	Notes
CCG 9892 (*Packer et al. JCO* 1999) 65 children 3-10 yo w/ nondisseminated MB (medulloblastoma)	CSI (23.4 Gy) with PF boost to 55.8 Gy with concurrent vincristine followed by lomustine/vincristine/cisplatin	3-y PFS: 86%, 5-y PFS: 79%	Low-dose CSI + adj chemo is comparable to high-dose CSI
ACNS0331 (*Michalski et al. JCO* 2021) 549 children 3-21 yo w/ average-risk MB	LDCSI + PFRT (3-7 y) LDCSI + IFRT (3-7 y) SDCSI + PFRT (3-21 y) SDCSI + IFRT (3-21 y)	5-y EFS: 82.5% (IFRT) vs 80.5% (PFRT) 5-y EFS: 71.4% (LDCSI) vs 82.9% (SDCSI)	Boost to involved field (IFRT) is safe and does not compromise survival compared to posterior fossa (PFRT). Low-dose CSI (LDCSI) (18 Gy) reduces EFS but improves neurocog outcomes vs standard dose (SDCSI) (23.4 Gy)
Kahalley et al. JCO 2020 79 children w/ MB, any risk group retrospective review	Photon radiation (n = 42) Proton radiation (n = 37)	Photon radiation is associated with worse IQ, reasoning, memory compared to proton therapy	Proton XRT improves neuropsychological outcomes relating to photons, including working memory, perceptual reasoning, and global IQ

Name/Inclusion	Randomization Arms	Outcomes	Notes
Leary et al. JAMA Oncol 2021 294 children 3-21 yo w/ high-risk MB	36 Gy CSI + weekly vincristine → maintenance chemo 36 Gy CSI + weekly vincristine → maintenance chemo + Isotretinoin 36 Gy CSI + weekly vincristine + daily carboplatin → maintenance chemo 36 Gy CSI + weekly vincristine + daily carboplatin → maintenance chemo + isotretinoin	5-y EFS: 73% w/ vs 54% w/o carboplatin in group 3 patients 5-y OS: 100% for WNT, 54% for SHH, 74% for group 3, and 77% for group 4	Randomized clinical trial in high-risk MB patients. Isotretinoin arms closed early due to futility. Carboplatin extended EFS only in group 3 patients. 5-y OS varied by molecular subgroup
Baby POG 1 (*Duffner NEJM* 1993; *Duffner Neuro-oncology* 1999) 193 children <3 yo w/ malignant brain tumor	Postoperative chemotherapy and delayed radiation in 198 children <3 y of age with malignant brain tumors	Medulloblastoma 5-y PFS: 32%, OS 40%	RT can be delayed by 1 or 2 y in children <3 yo, but PFS is not as good as in children >3 y where upfront CSI is used

EPENDYMOMA

ADAM GRIPPIN • ARNOLD PAULINO

BACKGROUND

- **Incidence/prevalence:** The third most common childhood brain tumor. Bimodal distribution with peaks at 4 and 35 years old. Approximately 200 cases per year in the United States
- **Outcomes:** Degree of resection most important predictor of outcomes. 5-Year overall survival ~75% with gross total resection (GTR) and ~35% with subtotal resection (STR)
- **Demographics:** Infratentorial lesions occur more commonly in younger children. Supratentorial lesions are more common in adolescents and adults. In children, 90% of tumors are intracranial.
- **Risk factors:** Spinal cord ependymomas are associated with neurofibromatosis type 2.

TUMOR BIOLOGY AND CHARACTERISTICS

- **Genetics:** Greater than 2/3 of supratentorial ependymomas have oncogenic fusions between *RELA* (which drives NF-κB) and *C11orf95*, leading to uncontrolled activation of NF-κB signaling pathway, which drives tumorigenesis (*Parker et al. Nature* 2014). Among posterior fossa tumors, a poor prognostic subgroup is one which exhibits a CpG island methylator phenotype, which silences genes that prevent neuronal differentiation. This is prognostic of PFS and OS (*Mack et al. Nature* 2014).
- **Pathology:** Origin is the ependymal cells lining the ventricular system and spinal canal. Classic features are ependymal and perivascular pseudorosettes. GFAP, S100, and vimentin stain positive. Subependymomas are rare tumors that are found in adults in the 4th or lateral ventricles. These tumors appear benign histologically and

grow slowly. Similarly, myxopapillary ependymomas are slow-growing and are found in adults almost exclusively within the conus and filum terminale of the spinal cord.

- **Imaging:** Classically hypointense on T1 MRI sequences and hyperintense on T2. Tumors enhance with gadolinium contrast. On CT, tumors will enhance with contrast and calcifications are commonly seen.

Anatomy

Tumors can occur throughout the entire cranial spinal axis. If the tumor is in the posterior fossa, the most common site is the fourth ventricle and often involves the foramen of Luschka. Supratentorial tumors also arise in the ventricular system and spread through intraparenchymal extension. Direct extension through the foramen magnum into the upper cervical spinal canal is common. Subarachnoid seeding occurs in ~12% of children.

Workup

- **History and physical:** Common presenting symptoms include those resulting from increased ICP (headaches, nausea, vomiting) due to obstruction of CSF flow. For adults with myxopapillary ependymomas, chronic back pain is typically reported with or without neurologic deficits. Perform thorough neurologic exam.
- **Labs:** CBC, CMP
- **Procedure/biopsy:** CSF sampling with cytology (unless contraindicated due to obstructive hydrocephalus)
- **Imaging:** MRI of the brain and spine is essential. After resection, MRI should be obtained <24 hours to evaluate degree of resection. CSF cytology and MRI of the spine should be obtained ~2 weeks after surgery to avoid false-positive result.

Ependymoma Grade

WHO I	Subependymoma
WHO II	Classic ependymoma, myxopapillary ependymoma
WHO III	Anaplastic ependymoma

Treatment Algorithm

Localized ≥1 yo	Maximal safe surgical resection followed by postoperative radiation therapy (RT) for infratentorial lesions. For supratentorial tumors, postoperative RT is given if STR or anaplastic (grade III). Observation after a GTR is a valid option for supratentorial, grade II tumors.
Localized <1 yo	Maximal safe surgical resection followed by adjuvant chemotherapy until patient is at least 12 mo and then consider RT
Disseminated ≥3 yo	Maximal safe surgical resection of the primary tumor followed by craniospinal irradiation (CSI) and tumor bed boost
Disseminated <3 yo	Maximal safe resection of the primary tumor followed by chemotherapy
Recurrent ependymoma	No prior RT: Maximal safe surgical resection followed by adjuvant XRT Prior RT: Maximal safe surgical resection. Consider reirradiation
Spinal/myxopapillary ependymoma	Maximal safe resection, if GTR can be observed. If STR or biopsy, follow with postoperative RT

Radiation Treatment Dose/Target/Technique

Infratentorial tumor

- **SIM:** Supine, arms at side, Aquaplast mask over head. For spinal tumor or CSI, use full body Vac-Lok. Sedation with general anesthesia may be required for children. Scan from the vertex of the skull through coccyx.
- **Dose:** 54-59.4 Gy in 30-33 fractions at 1.8 Gy/fx

- **Target:** CTV margin = preoperative GTV + 1 cm. Consider 3- to 5-mm CTV to PTV margin depending on IGRT and setup.
- **Technique:** Proton beam therapy or intensity-modulated radiation therapy for primary intracranial tumor. Treatment planning for CSI will require feathering of junctions to avoid potential hot spots at field borders (Fig. 15.1).

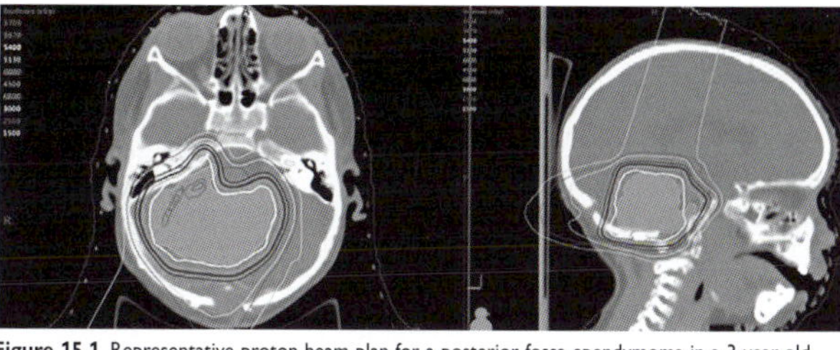

Figure 15.1 Representative proton beam plan for a posterior fossa ependymoma in a 3-year-old child. 54-Gy isodose line is represented by the *white line*.

Supratentorial tumor

- **Dose:** 54-59.4 Gy in 30-33 fractions at 1.8 Gy/fx for anaplastic tumors, if WHO grade I or II can be observed if completely resected
- **Target:** Same as above
- **Technique:** Same as above

Spinal tumor

- **Dose:** 45 Gy in 25 fractions at 1.8 Gy/fx, including two vertebral bodies/sacral nerve roots above and below tumor. Cone down to 50.4-54 Gy if safely below cord.
- **Target:** Same as above. May consider <3-mm PTV margins
- **Technique:** Same as above

PTV as per institutional standards and image guidance (we do 0.3-0.5 cm)

- **IGRT:** Daily kV imaging
- **Planning directive:**
  Spinal cord D_{max} < 50 Gy
  Brain stem D_{max} < 57 Gy, V54 Gy < 10%
  Chiasm D_{max} < 54 Gy
  Lt and Rt cochlea mean < 38 Gy, D_{max} < 45 Gy
  Lt and Rt eye D_{max} < 40 Gy
  Lt and Rt lens D_{max} < 5 Gy
  Lt and Rt parotid mean < 10 Gy
  Lt and Rt lacrimal gland mean < 26 Gy

SIDE EFFECT MANAGEMENT

- Nausea/vomiting: First-line Zofran → second-line Compazine
- Decline in IQ: More prominent in patients treated with CSI and in children <10 years old treated with localized fields, referral to neuropsychology and counsel parents
- Growth deficiency: Rule out growth hormone deficiency. Can occur with CSI secondary to irradiation of vertebral bodies and supporting musculature. Counsel parents.

FOLLOW-UP

- Follow-up period is long, ~10 years as ependymomas can recur very late following completion of treatment.
- History/physical with MRI: q3-4mo for year 1 → q4-6mo for year 2 → then q6-12mo thereafter
- If CSI, check growth hormone and TSH labs at least once per year.
- Consistent follow-up with neuropsychologist, especially with CSI

Notable Trials

Adjuvant radiation

Name/Inclusion	Arms	Outcomes	Notes
ACNS0121 (*Merchant et al. JCO* 2019) 356 children 1-21 yo. Nonrandomized study	GTR (classic supratentorial ependymoma only)	5-y EFS: 61%	Children age 3 yo or younger had RT delayed by 1-2 y or until tumor progressed. This did not compromise EFS. Aggressive surgery and immediate postoperative RT results in good outcomes. 1q gain is poor prognostic factor
	STR → chemo → second surgery → CRT	5-y EFS: 37%	
	GTR → CRT	5-y EFS: 68.5%	
St. Jude (*Merchant et al. JCO* 2004; *Merchant et al. Lancet Oncol* 2009) 153 children 0-23 yo. Nonrandomized study	GTR → CRT STR → chemo → surgery → CRT	3-y PFS: 74% IQ stable after 2 y 7-y OS: 81% 7-y LC: 87.3% 7-y EFS: 69.1%	Immediate postoperative radiation be safely reduced to 59.4 Gy in patients ≥18 mo (*n* = 73) and 54 Gy in patients <18 mo (*n* = 15)
Barrow (*Rogers et al. J Neurosurg* 2005) 45 children w/ posterior fossa ependymoma <u>Retrospective review</u>	GTR	10-y OS: 67% 10-y PFS: 50%	Retrospective study demonstrating benefit of postoperative radiation in patients with posterior fossa ependymoma
	GTR + RT	10-y OS: 83% 10-y PFS: 100%	
	STR + RT	10-y OS: 43% 10-y PFS: 36%	

INTRACRANIAL GERM CELL TUMOR

ADAM GRIPPIN • SUSAN L. MCGOVERN • ARNOLD PAULINO

Background

- **Incidence/prevalence:** Intracranial germ cell tumor (GCT) accounts for 1-2% of pediatric CNS tumors, higher in Asian/Pacific Islander populations, including those of Asian/Pacific Islander descent living in Western countries.
- **Outcomes:** Modern trials report 5-year PFS for pure germinoma >90%, for both localized and disseminated disease. Nongerminomatous GCT (NGGCT) 5-year PFS is poorer, ~70-80% for localized NGGCT and ~50-70% for disseminated NGGCT.
- **Demographics:** Median age of diagnosis 10-12 years old, male > female (2-3:1), as above Asians and those of Asian descent have 2-3× higher incidence of GCT.
- **Risk factors:** No major risk factors known

Tumor Biology and Characteristics

- **Genetics:** Aberrations in KIT/RAS and/or AKT/mTOR pathways in majority of intracranial GCTs
- **Pathology:** Histologic division of GCT into germinoma vs NGGCT. Germinomas are more RT sensitive and have better prognosis than NGGCT. Approximately 65% of intracranial GCTs are germinoma ("pure" germinoma). NGGCT includes

embryonal carcinoma, yolk sac tumor (aka endodermal sinus tumor/endodermal sinus tumor), choriocarcinoma, teratoma, or mixed GCT. Mixed GCT may include germinoma components, but any NGGCT component makes tumor "mixed" and therefore treated as NGGCT (25% of NGGCT are mixed GCT). Helpful markers for GCT: B-hCG and alpha-fetoprotein (AFP)
- B-hCG and AFP can be examined on IHC, as well as in serum and CSF.

Serum/CSF B-hCG and AFP Differentiation of Tumor Histology		
Histology	**B-hCG**	**AFP**
Embryonal carcinoma	Wnl	Wnl
Yolk sac tumor	Wnl	Increased (can be marked)
Choriocarcinoma	Increased (can be marked)	Wnl
Teratoma	Wnl	Wnl
Germinoma	<50-100 IU/L	Wnl*

*Elevated AFP in serum (>10 ng/mL), in CSF, or on IHC **rules out** pure germinoma.

- Origin: Extragonadal GCT occurs intracranially, as well as in the sacrococcygeal region and the retroperitoneum, among other sites. Extragonadal GCT may arise from primordial germ cells that exhibit aberrant or incomplete migration during embryonal development.
- Location: Primary locations of intracranial GCT are the pineal gland and suprasellar region, pineal gland more common than suprasellar (2:1). Rare to occur at other intracranial sites. Approximately 5-10% of cases have both pineal and suprasellar tumors, which are known as "bifocal" GCT.
- Imaging: GCT is usually iso/hypointense on T1, and hyperintense on T2 (similar to MB), and like medulloblastoma shows postcontrast enhancement. No radiographic factors reliably differentiate germinomas from NGGCTs.

Workup

- **History and physical:** Recommend baseline evaluations by endocrinology, ophthalmology, audiology, and neuropsychology. Consideration should be made for baseline neurocognitive studies (for GCTs as well as other intracranial pediatric tumors). Clinical presentation varies by primary tumor site:
  - **Pineal tumors:** Increased ICP (headaches, N/V, papilledema, lethargy/somnolence, due to obstructive hydrocephalus); ~40% of pineal GCTs present with increased ICP. Parinaud syndrome presents in 40-50% of cases. This syndrome consists of upward gaze paralysis and sluggish pupillary reflex, as well as convergence nystagmus. This syndrome is thought to be due to compression of superior colliculus.
  - **Suprasellar tumors:** Neuro-endocrinopathies/hypothalamus axis disruption, especially diabetes insipidus, precocious/delayed puberty, and bitemporal hemianopia (chiasm compression). Complete a neurologic exam including cranial nerve exam + funduscopy to evaluate papilledema.
  - **Historical note:** Decades prior, germinoma was empirically diagnosed w/ initiation of RT. If response after ~20 Gy of radiation, it was considered an empirical diagnosis (w/o histologic/pathologic confirmation) of germinoma and RT continued.
  - **Differential diagnosis:** Pineal tumor differential diagnosis includes GCT (germinoma/NGGCT), glioma, pineoblastoma, pineocytoma, PNET, ependymoma, pineal parenchymal tumor of intermediate differentiation (PPTID), papillary tumor of the pineal region, meningioma, lymphoma, and hamartoma. Suprasellar tumor differential diagnosis includes craniopharyngioma, Langerhans cell histiocytosis, glioma, GCT (germinoma/NGGCT), pituitary adenoma, meningioma, and aneurysm.
- **Procedures/biopsy:** LP and CSF analysis, including CSF AFP and B-hCG levels, as well as CSF cytology. CSF AFP and B-hCG are more sensitive than serum markers. Prefer LP for markers + cytology rather than ventricular CSF (ie, if shunt already placed for hydrocephalus). LP for CSF analyses 10-14 days after procedure (shunt placement, surgery). Biopsy mandatory for patients w/ normal serum and CSF markers (AFP and B-hCG). Biopsy only is appropriate for germinoma (no role for extent of resection), whereas data suggest possible role for maximal safe resection in NGGCT.
- **Labs:** CBC, CMP (including BUN/Cr and LFTs), serum AFP, serum B-hCG
- **Imaging:** MRI brain + entire spine w/ gadolinium contrast. MR spine critical as ~10% of patients will have spinal/leptomeningeal seeding at diagnosis.

STAGING

M staging per modified Chang system as below used for intracranial GCTs as well as medulloblastoma (see "Medulloblastoma" chapter).

Modified Chang Staging	
M0	No metastases (bifocal GCT [pineal + suprasellar tumors] w/o evidence of other metastasis = treated as localized/M0)
M1	Microscopic tumor cells in the CSF/positive CSF cytology
M2	Gross intracranial seeding
M3	Gross spinal seeding
M4	Metastases outside neuroaxis

TREATMENT ALGORITHM

- **Germinoma:** RT alone or neoadjuvant chemotherapy → RT. Chemotherapy-only approaches for germinomas have yielded inferior outcomes, with >50% rates of relapse, even after CR from chemotherapy (*Balmaceda et al. JCO* 1996).
- **NGGCT:** Several approaches, but in general, maximal safe resection → chemotherapy (6 cycles) → possible second-look surgery (if restaging after chemotherapy demonstrates sufficient residual tumor to warrant second-look surgery before CSI) → consolidative RT (including CSI)

RADIATION TREATMENT TECHNIQUE

- **SIM:** Supine, thermoplastic mask. Sedation (anesthesia) may be required for younger patients.
- **Dose:**
  - Generally, treat at 1.5 Gy/fx for germinoma and 1.8 Gy/fx for NGGCT, unless otherwise specified.
  - Localized germinoma: If RT alone, whole-ventricle RT (WVRT) to 24 Gy → boost gross disease to 40-45 Gy
  - Localized germinoma: If RT after chemotherapy, then treat per COG ACNS1123 RT dose depending on tumor response on repeat imaging after chemotherapy.
    - ACNS1123: If PR/SD after chemotherapy: 24 Gy WVRT → 12 Gy boost to primary site
    - ACNS1123: If CR after chemotherapy: 18 Gy WVRT → 12 Gy boost to primary site
  - Bifocal germinoma: Treat as above for localized germinoma but boost both primaries (suprasellar and pineal). Cannot have other tumors beyond these two sites to be classified as bifocal
  - Disseminated (M+) germinoma: CSI to 24-30 Gy → boost to primary to total dose ~40-45 Gy
  - NGGCT: Off protocol, current standard of care is CSI to 36 Gy and boost primary to 54 Gy. ACNS2021 is evaluating reducing dose to 30.6 Gy and reducing volumes to primary site, whole-ventricular and spinal RT, instead of CSI.
- **Target:**
  - Whole-ventricular RT (WVRT): Outlined in ACNS1123 atlas online
    - WVRT includes targets: Lateral, 3rd, and 4th ventricles, as well as suprasellar and pineal cisterns. Cover prepontine cistern if history of 3rd ventriculostomy (ie, done previously for obstructive hydrocephalus from tumor) or large suprasellar tumor. WVRT target well defined using T2 MRI fusion (or MRI simulation, if available)
    - Contour WV-CTV = ventricles/ventricular space, and then expand 5 mm (depending on IGRT) to generate WV-PTV
  - Tumor bed boost:
    - Collapsed tumor bed and gross residual disease if present
    - 1-cm expansion from tumor bed for tumor CTV, then expand 3-5 mm for PTV (dependent on IGRT)
  - CSI:
    - Ensure coverage of cribriform plates, middle cranial fossae, and thecal sac.
- **Technique:** Similar to medulloblastoma, especially with regard to CSI. IMRT and proton beam therapy reasonable options. See **Medulloblastoma** chapter for CSI—considerations if CSI indicated.
- **IGRT:** Daily kV
- **Planning directive:** See **Medulloblastoma** chapter (Fig. 16.1).

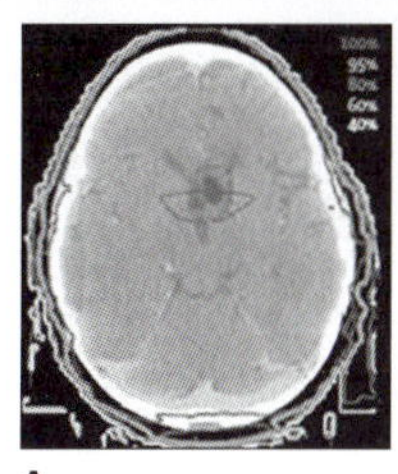
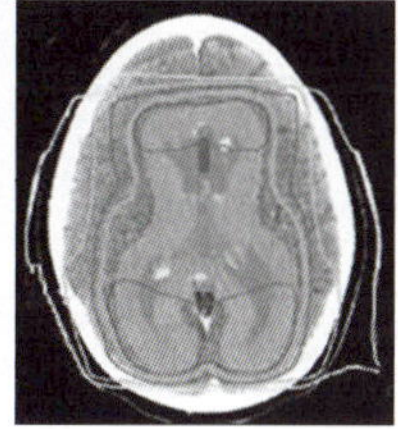
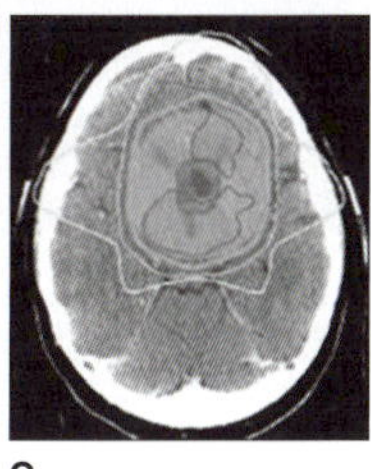

A B C

Figure 16.1 Axial imaging showing dose distribution with whole brain radiation **(A)** as part of CSI. WVRT **(B)** and focused radiation of a primary target, as would be conducted in a sequential boost **(C)** (With permission from *Rogers Lancet Oncol* 2005).

Chemotherapy

- Carboplatin/etoposide ×4 cycles typical for induction chemotherapy for germinoma (ACNS1123). Platinum-based chemotherapy ×6 cycles for NGGCT. Other regimens may include bleomycin and cisplatin for intracranial GCTs.

Notable Trials/Papers

Radiation for localized intracranial germinomas

Name/Inclusion	Arms	Outcomes	Notes
SFOP Involved Field RT Experience (*Alapetite et al. Neuro Oncol* 2010) Analysis of 10 of 60 patients treated with chemo → IFRT	Induction chemo → 40 Gy IFRT	10-y EFS: 82% 10-y OS: 96%	80% of relapses after IFRT were periventricular. This retrospective review supports the use of WVRT for germinoma patients
SIOP CNS GCT96 (*Calaminus et al. Neuro Oncol* 2013) 190 patients 4-42 yo w/ localized germinoma Nonrandomized study	24 Gy CSI + 16 Gy tumor bed boost	5-y PFS: 97% 5-y OS: 95%	Prospective study demonstrating reduced PFS with chemo + local radiation. All failures were ventricular, supporting WVRT even w/ CR
	Carbo/etop ×2 cycles alternating with ifox/etop → 40 Gy local RT	5-y PFS: 88% 5-y OS: 96%	
ALTEO7C1 (*Bartels et al. Neuro Oncol* 2022) 137 children w/ localized germinoma Nonrandomized study	Carbo/etop → CR → 18 Gy WVRT + 12 Gy boost to tumor bed (*n* = 74)	3-y PFS: 94.5% 3-y OS: 100%	Noninferiority trial failed to meet primary end point due to study design but suggests equivalent outcomes and improved neurocognitive function with 18 Gy whole ventricular and 30 Gy total dose to primary site for complete responders. 2-drug chemotherapy regimen resulted in high response rates
	Carbo/etop → PR → 24 Gy WVRT + 12 Gy boost to tumor bed (*n* = 16)	3-y PFS: 93.75% 3-y OS: 100%	

Treatment strategy of NGGCT

Name/Inclusion	Arms	Outcomes	Notes
ACNS0122 (*Goldman et al. JCO* 2015) 104 children w/ NGGCT or high-risk germinoma Nonrandomized study	Induction chemo → CR → 36 Gy CSI + 54 Gy tumor/tumor bed boost Induction chemo → near CR → encouraged second-look surgery → 36 Gy CSI + 54 Gy tumor/tumor bed boost	3-y PFS: 92% 3-y OS: 94%	Phase II demonstrating excellent survival outcomes in NGGCT patients with CR or near CR after induction chemotherapy +/− second-look surgery treated with 36 Gy CSI and 54 Gy tumor/tumor bed boost
ACNS1123 (*Fangusaro et al. JCO* 2019; *Murphy et al. IJROBP* 2022) 107 children w/ localized NGGCT	30.6 Gy WVRT + 54 Gy tumor bed boost	3-y PFS: 87.8% ± 4.04% 3-y OS: 92.4% ± 3.3%	Increased spine recurrences with WVRT compared to CSI from ACNS0122. CSI remains standard of care

WILMS TUMOR

ADAM GRIPPIN • ARNOLD PAULINO

Background

- **Incidence/prevalence:** Approximately 600 cases per year in the United States, about 7% of childhood malignancies (SEER)
- **Outcomes:** Markedly improved survival with the addition of radiation therapy (RT) and chemotherapy (CHT) over the last century; all-comers Wilms tumor (WT) overall survival (OS) ~10% in the 1920s to >90% by 2000. 4-Year OS for favorable histology (~90% of total) patients ≥90% for stages I-IV and 85-90% for stages V. Worse outcomes if unfavorable histology (UH) (stage IV UH 4-year OS ~45-50%).
- **Demographics:** Median age at diagnosis is 44 months for unilateral cases and 31 months for bilateral cases. Sex predilection higher in girls (F:M = 1.1:1 for unilateral WT)
- **Risk factors:** Approximately 10% WT cases have a congenital syndrome, including WAGR (**W**T, **A**niridia, **G**U malformations, **R**etardation [mental]; deletion 11p13), Beckwith-Wiedemann syndrome (hemihypertrophy, visceromegaly, macroglossia, macrosomia, anterior abdominal wall defects; duplication 11p15), and Denys-Drash syndrome (nephrotic syndrome, XY pseudohermaphroditism; mutation 11p13).

Tumor Biology and Characteristics

- **Pathology/genetics:** Intrinsic renal tumor derived from nephrogenic blastemal cells, also known as nephroblastoma. 90% of WT are favorable histology (FH), classically "triphasic" including epithelial, blastemal, and stromal components. 10% of WT are unfavorable histology (UH), including tumors w/ focal anaplasia (FA) or diffuse anaplasia. UH tumors have higher rates of nodal and distant metastasis. Combined LOH 1p and LOH 16q is poor prognostic indicator (*Grundy et al. JCO* 2005). Other pediatric renal tumors (not WT family members) include clear cell sarcoma of the kidney (CCSK) and rhabdoid tumor of the kidney (RTK). RTK histologically not discernable from AT/RT of the brain (both show loss of nuclear INI1 staining).
- **Imaging:** Radiographic differentiation of WT vs NB: WT arises within the kidney (claw sign); rare calcifications in WT (~10%); WT rarely crosses midline (WT occasionally "overhang" onto contralateral side).

Workup

- **History and physical:** Patients typically present with painless abdominal mass, without constitutional symptoms. Approximately 33% of WT patients have abdominal pain, weight loss, or N/V. 25% have secondary HTN (elevated renin). 30% present with hematuria and 10% with coagulopathy. Evaluate family history and assess for congenital syndromes, including GU malformations, macroglossia, hemihypertrophy, aniridia, and intellectual disability.
- **Labs:** CBC, CMP, UA, and urine catecholamines (HVA/VMA)
- **Procedures/biopsy:** No biopsy unless unresectable or stage V (bilateral). North American approach is staging after surgical resection, w/ nephrectomy as first step in treatment paradigm for most patients.
- **Imaging:** Abdominal US w/ Doppler (assess vessel patency), usually followed by CT chest/abdomen/pelvis, w/ contrast, as well as CXR. Additional workup for uncommon histologies: CCSK = bone scan, BMBx, and MRI brain (assess for brain mets); RTK = MRI brain (assess for synchronous AT/RT)

Staging

- **Surgery:** In North America, upfront radical nephrectomy and LN sampling via transabdominal or thoracoabdominal incision, with en bloc removal of the kidney. Inspect contralateral kidney and assess for preoperative and intraoperative spill. Discussion between the surgeon and radiation oncologist is crucial for site(s) of intraoperative spill in particular.

Staging—WT	
I	Tumor confined to kidney, completely resected (R0)
II	Tumor completely resected (R0), with extension beyond the kidney through vessel involvement and/or penetration of renal capsule/sinus
III	R1 or R2 resection (+margins or STR), preoperative or intraoperative tumor spill, tumor biopsy, piecemeal resection (not en bloc), peritoneal implants, LN involvement in abd/pelvis, tumor penetration of peritoneal surface
IV	Hematogenous mets (lung, liver, bone, etc.) or LN outside abd/pelvis
V	Bilateral renal involvement

Treatment Algorithm

For favorable histology patients

Stage I and II	Surgery → chemotherapy (omit RT for FH patients)
Stage III	Surgery → RT[a] → chemotherapy
Stage IV	Surgery → RT[b] → chemotherapy
Stage V	Neoadjuvant chemotherapy → surgery

[a]Flank RT for all "local" stage III FH patients; whole abdomen irradiation (WAI) indicated if preoperative rupture or diffuse intraoperative spill. Discuss with surgical team if intraoperative spill occurred to better delineate extent/location of spill, which will inform adjuvant treatment with flank RT vs WAI.
[b]Whole lung irradiation (WLI) for WT patients w/ lung mets if no radiographic complete response on CT after 6 weeks of VAAdr (regimen DD4A; *Dix et al. JCO* 2018).

Generally, recommend flank/abdominal RT within 14 days postoperatively after nephrectomy. However, for sequencing, can delay flank/abdominal RT for stage IV WT patients w/ lung mets until after 6 weeks of CHT; importance of early RT for WT patients appears to matter in the nonmetastatic setting (*Stokes et al. IJROBP* 2018). This allows flank RT/WAI to be delivered concurrently w/ WLI if needed for stage IV patients.
For unfavorable histology and RTK patients: At least flank RT regardless of stage (I-IV)
For CCSK: At least flank RT for stages II-IV. No RT for stage I if adequate nodal sampling

Radiation Treatment Technique

- **SIM:** Supine, Vac-Lok, most will require sedation (anesthesia)
- **Dose (for FH):**
  - Flank (hemiabdomen) RT to 10.8 Gy in 6 fx (1.8 Gy/fx)
    - If PA nodes involved, include PA chain in flank field from T11-L4.
    - If gross residual disease >3 cm, boost additional 10.8 Gy (in 6 fx).
  - WAI to 10.5 Gy in 7 fx (1.5 Gy/fx)
  - WLI to 12 Gy in 8 fx (1.5 Gy/fx); if patient <12 months, drop 1 fx (10.5 Gy in 7 fx).

- Additional dosing specifications:
  - Undissected (gross) LNs—19.8 Gy/11 fx
  - Flank RT for stage III diffuse anaplasia or RTK I-III—19.8 Gy/11 fx
  - Boost gross residual lung dz 2 weeks after WLI—7.5 Gy/5 fx
  - Bone mets: 25.2 Gy/14 fx (30.6 Gy/17 fx if age >16 years old)
  - Liver mets: Sx if local, whole liver if diffuse mets (19.8-21.6 Gy)
  - Brain mets: 21.6 Gy/12 fx WBRT or 30.6 Gy/17 fx if >16 years old
- **Target/technique (flank RT, Fig. 17.1 below):**
  CTV: Preoperative tumor + kidney + 1 cm + entire vertebral body if block edge touches VB w/ AP/PA technique
  Technique: Generally, AP/PA: Sup/Inf = 1 cm expansion off disease/kidney. Med = 1 cm lateral to whole VB (include whole VB in field, generally). Lat = body wall (no flash)

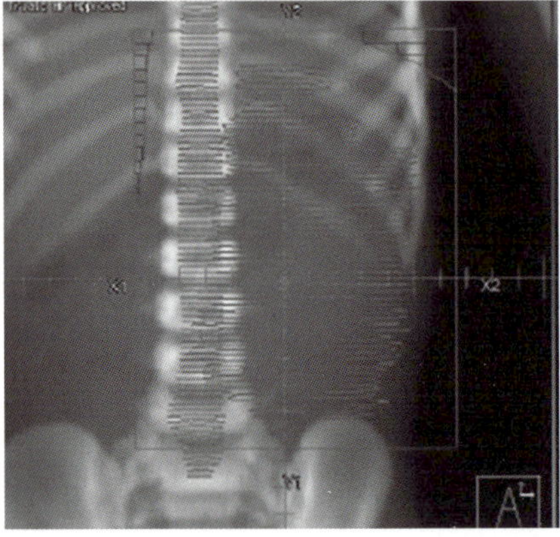

Figure 17.1

- **Target/technique (WAI, Fig. 17.2 below):**
  CTV: As above
  Technique: Generally AP/PA: Sup = 1 cm above diaphragm. Inf = bottom of obturator foramen (therefore, more accurately this is whole "abdominopelvic" RT not just the abdomen). Lat = body wall (no flash)

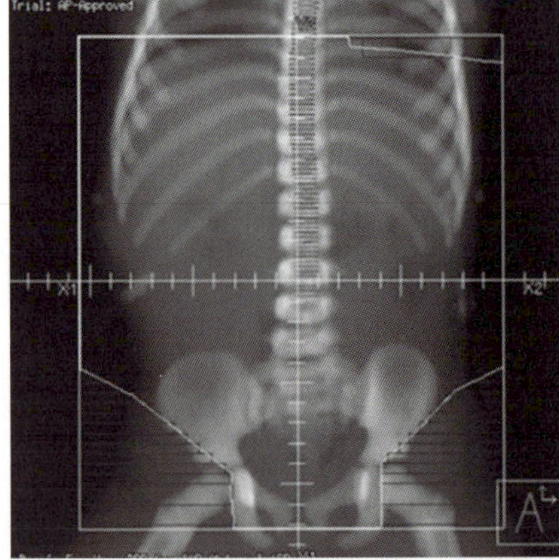

Figure 17.2

- **Target/technique (WLI, Fig. 17.3):**
  CTV: Includes bilateral lungs, mediastinum, and pleural recesses
  Technique: AP/PA or IMRT (cardiac-sparing IMRT warrants 4D-CT simulation; see *Kalapurakal et al. IJROBP* 2012). If AP/PA: Sup = 1 cm above clavicle/lung apex (flash SCV fossa). Inf = below diaphragm. Lat = chest wall

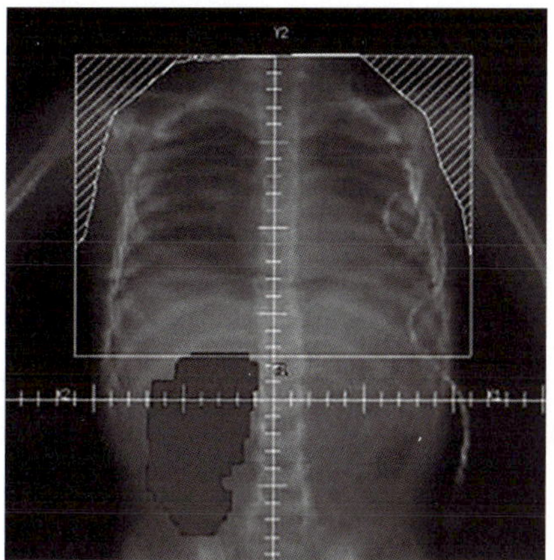

Figure 17.3

- **Planning directive:**
  Contralateral kidney: V14.4 < 33%
  Liver: V19.8 < 50%

Chemotherapy

- Generally, vincristine/actinomycin D/Adriamycin (VAA; regimen DD4A); with addition of cyclophosphamide/etoposide (with VAA; regimen M) for higher-risk stage III/IV

Side Effect Management

Acute: Skin reaction, nausea/vomiting, indigestion, diarrhea, esophagitis, pneumonitis
Late (varies by treatment field, age, among others): Height loss, kyphosis/lordosis/scoliosis, chronic renal insufficiency (rare <1%, unless bilateral Wilms tumor), muscular hypoplasia, pneumonitis (4% with whole lung irradiation), pulmonary fibrosis, infertility, malabsorption, SBO, VOD, increased risk of cardiac morbidity, second malignancy (1-2% at 15 years)

Follow-up

- Follow-up with imaging recommended q3mo for 2 years, then q6mo for 2 more years. Imaging recommend alternating between CXR + abdominal US and CT C/A/P. Most relapses occur w/in first 2 years; some question regarding role of further imaging beyond 2 years (*Brok et al. Lancet Oncol* 2018).
- Long-term monitoring for late effects, which may include echocardiography, height/growth abnormalities/bone density, hypogonadism, chronic renal insufficiency, pulmonary function testing, screening for second malignancies (breast, colon)

Notable Trials

Name/Inclusion	Arms	Outcomes	Notes
NWTS (*D'Angio et al. Cancer* 1989) 1439 children, any stage or histology	Multifactorial design with plan adapted by stage and histology. Stage II FH received 0 or 20 Gy and stage III FH received 10 or 20 Gy	Equivalent outcome w/o radiation for stage II FH and w/ 10 Gy for stage III FH	Established 10 Gy dose for flank RT for stage III
COG AREN0533 (*Dix et al. JCO* 2018) FH stage IV patients <30 yo w/ isolated lung mets Nonrandomized study	Incomplete response or 1p16Q LOH → lung RT + DD4A + cyclophosphamide	4-y EFS: 88.5% 4-y OS: 95.4%	Lung RT can be safely avoided in patients without 1p16Q LOH and with lung nodule CR after 6 wk of chemotherapy
	CR w/o LOH → DD4A	4-y EFS: 79.5% 4-y OS: 96%	

NEUROBLASTOMA

ELAINE CHA • ARNOLD PAULINO

Background

- **Incidence/prevalence:** Accounts for ~8% of all childhood cancers in the United States. Approximately 650 new cases per year diagnosed in the United States, overall, 10 cases per million children (SEER data)
- **Outcomes:** 5-Year OS for low- and intermediate-risk patients is >90%. For high-risk neuroblastoma, the 5-year OS is between 40% and 50%. Neuroblastoma is a rare cancer that has the potential to spontaneously regress without any treatment.
- **Demographics:** Most common extracranial tumor of childhood. Median age at diagnosis is ~17 months. Most common malignancy of infants (~50%). No sex predilection, M:F is 1.2:1.
- **Risk factors:** Majority of cases (>98%) sporadic due to chance mutations. However, in 1-2% of cases, neuroblastoma develops due to a hereditary mutation in either the *ALK* or *PHOX2B* genes (*Mosse et al. Nature* 2008).

Tumor Biology and Characteristics

- **Genetics:** *MYCN* is a DNA-binding transcription factor, which can cause malignant transformation due to downstream effects. Amplified in 25% of all neuroblastoma and is associated with rapid progression and poor prognosis (*Chan et al. Clin Can Res* 1997; *Seeger et al. NEJM* 1985). *ATRX* mutations were recently identified in adolescents and young adults with neuroblastoma and are associated with an indolent disease course (*Cheung et al. JAMA* 2012).
- **Pathology:** Arise from primitive neural crest sympathetic ganglion cells. Small, round, blue cell tumor of childhood (like Ewing's, medulloblastoma, rhabdomyosarcoma, and PNET). Shimada pathologic classification dependent on degree of differentiation, mitosis-karyorrhexis index, stromal component, and nodularity (*Shimada et al. Cancer* 1999). Classically stains positive for synaptophysin, chromogranin A, and neurofilaments
- **Imaging:** X-rays may demonstrate calcifications in ~80% of neuroblastomas (in comparison with Wilms tumors, which classically do not have calcifications). CT of the abdomen with contrast is typically performed, which can help identify extent of tumor and presence or absence of regional or distant metastatic disease. Importantly, nuclear medicine meta-iodobenzylguanidine (MIBG) radionuclide scans can be used to identify distant sites of disease and response to systemic therapy (Fig. 18.1).

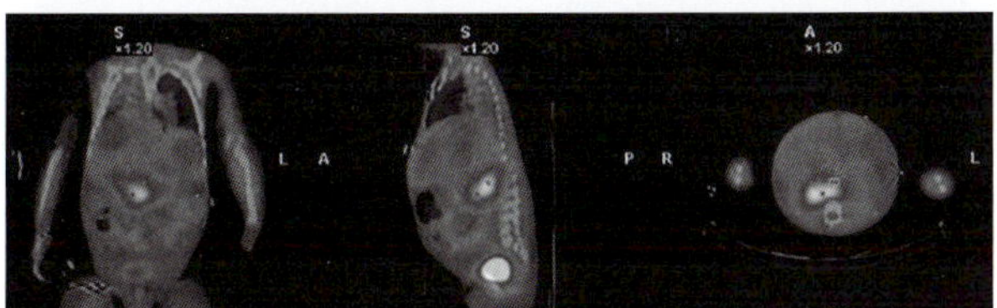

Figure 18.1 Representative coronal, sagittal, and axial (*left* to *right*) MIBG scans in a patient presenting with a right adrenal neuroblastoma. The avidity can be seen in his right suprarenal area, consistent with the primary malignancy. There were no additional MIBG-avid sites, suggesting absence of distant metastases.

ANATOMY

- May arise from any site in the sympathetic nervous system. Most common sites are adrenal gland in the abdomen and paraspinal ganglia along the abdomen, thorax, and head and neck.

WORKUP

- **History and physical:** Patients typically present with an abdominal mass with additional symptoms such as malaise, irritability, and pain. Evaluate for Horner syndrome (meiosis, ptosis, anhidrosis) due to involvement of the sympathetic chain on the ipsilateral affected side. Evaluate for back pain due to possible bony involvement. Important to do careful skin examination as metastatic disease can present with a bluish tinge ("blueberry muffin" sign) and may be indicative of stage 4S disease. Opsoclonus-myoclonus syndrome—presenting as truncal ataxia and/or cerebellar encephalopathy—may be seen.
- **Labs:** CBC, CMP. Include measurement of urinary catecholamines HVA and VMA, which are found to be elevated in >90% of patients with stage IV disease
- **Procedures/biopsy:** Can obtain tissue from primary site or from gross lymph nodes. **Bone marrow aspirate and biopsy are required for appropriate staging of neuroblastoma**.
- **Imaging:** Abdominal x-rays may show calcification in up to 80-85% of neuroblastomas. Obtain CT of the abdomen with contrast and MIBG nuclear medicine scan at diagnosis to determine extent of metastatic disease. Consider MRI of the abdomen w/ and w/o contrast if equivocal findings on CT scan.

STAGING/GRADING

International Neuroblastoma Risk Group Staging System (INRGSS) (*Monclair et al. JCO* 2009)

Stage L1: localized tumor not involving vital structures as defined by the list of image-defined risk factors* and confined to one body compartment

Stage L2: locoregional tumor with the presence of one or more image-defined risk factors

Stage M: distant metastatic disease (except stage MS)

Stage MS: metastatic disease in children younger than 18 months with metastases confined to skin, liver, and/or bone marrow (<10%)

*Image-defined risk factors: ipsilateral tumor extension within 2 body compartments (neck-chest, chest-abdomen, abdomen-pelvis); tumor in neck/cervicothoracic junction—encasing carotid a./vertebral a./internal jugular v./brachial plexus roots/subclavian vv., extending to skull base, compressing trachea; tumor in thoracoabdominal region—encasing aorta/major branches of aorta/vena cava, compressing trachea/principal bronchi, lower mediastinal tumor infiltrating costovertebral junction between T9 and T12; tumor in abdomen/pelvis—infiltrating porta hepatis/hepatoduodenal ligament, encasing SMA origin or branches at the mesenteric root/origin of the celiac axis/aorta/vena cava/iliac vv., invading renal pedicles, crossing sciatic notch; intraspinal tumor—extension such that >1/3 of spinal canal in axial plane is invaded/perimedullary leptomeningeal spaces are not visible/spinal cord signal is abnormal; tumor infiltration of adjacent organs/structures.

Treatment Algorithm

Low risk	Surgery If unresectable: preoperative chemo → surgery
Intermediate risk	Surgery → chemotherapy
High risk	Induction chemotherapy → surgery → myeloablative therapy and ABMT → consolidative RT to tumor bed and residual MIBG-avid sites → maintenance therapy with isotretinoin and immunotherapy

Radiation Treatment Technique

- **SIM:** Supine, Vac-Lok, nearly all will require anesthesia.
- **Dose:** 21.6 Gy in 12 fractions
- **Target:**
  GTV: Define tumor bed using postinduction and chemotherapy preoperative CT or MRI. Treat postinduction residual MIBG sites as well (*Mazloom et al. IJROBP* 2014).
  CTV: Tumor bed + 1- to 1.5-cm margin, limiting to anatomic barriers of spread (bone, etc.)
  PTV: 0.5-1 cm depending on institutional standards and image guidance
  Considerations: Different than other pediatric tumors, the GTV is not based upon the initial tumor volume. Consider shorter RT course. Consider 4.5 Gy/3 fx regimen for palliation of liver metastases.
- **Technique:** IMRT typically used, especially if tumor extended past midline. Consider AP/PA techniques if well-lateralized tumor (may spare dose to contralateral kidney). Proton therapy can be considered if dosimetric advantage.
- **IGRT:** Daily kV imaging
- **Planning directive:**
  Kidneys—D_{mean} < 14.4 Gy

Chemotherapy

Commonly used induction and myeloablative chemotherapy regimens include cyclophosphamide or ifosfamide, cisplatin/carboplatin, vincristine, doxorubicin, etoposide, topotecan, and busulfan or melphalan (for stem cell transplant).

Side Effect Management

Acute: Skin reactions, mucositis, diarrhea, and fatigue are commonly seen. Prescribe Aquaphor for mild skin reactions; consider Silvadene if worse.

Late: Spinal deformities are commonly seen due to RT to the bony structures. Children may be shorter than their peers. Chronic renal insufficiency rarely seen in survivors. Risk of secondary malignancies about 1-2% per decade of life

Follow-up

Typically, will resume care with medical oncologist following completion of RT for maintenance therapy (for stage IV patients). Follow-up with abdominal and whole-body imaging is recommended q3mo for 1 year, q6mo for 2-4 years, and then every year.

Notable Trials

Name/Inclusion	Arms/Design	Outcomes	Notes
CCG 3891 (*Matthay et al. NEJM* 1999) 539 high-risk stage IV or stage III with MYCN amplification patients	Myeloablative therapy and autologous bone marrow transplant (ABMT) with TBI (2nd randomization: 6 cycles 13-cis-retinoic acid vs no therapy)	3-y EFS was 34% (ABMT) vs 22% (no ABMT) (*P* = .034) and 46% (retinoic acid) vs 29% (no retinoic acid) (*P* = .027)	Conclusions: Myeloablation with AMBT and treatment with 13-cis-retinoic acid improve EFS

Name/Inclusion	Arms/Design	Outcomes	Notes
	Intensive nonmyeloablative chemotherapy (2nd randomization: 6 cycles 13-cis-retinoic acid vs no therapy)		
COG ANBL0032 (*Yu et al. NEJM* 2011) 226 high-risk patients who responded to induction therapy + SCT	Standard maintenance therapy (6 cycles isotretinoin)	2-y EFS improved with immunotherapy (66% vs 46%, *P* = .01) 2-y OS improved with immunotherapy (86% vs 75%, *P* = .02)	Conclusions: Immunotherapy (dinutuximab) improves EFS and OS
	Immunotherapy (Ch14.18/ dinutuximab with GM-CSF and IL-2) and 6 cycles of isotretinoin		
COG ANBL0532 (*Park et al. JAMA* 2019) 355 high-risk patients who received induction chemotherapy	Tandem transplant with thiotepa/ cyclophosphamide followed by dose-reduced carboplatin/ etoposide/ melphalan	3-y EFS superior with tandem transplant (61.6% vs 48.4%, *P* = .006)	Conclusions: Tandem transplant has better EFS compared to single transplant
	Single transplant with carboplatin/ etoposide/ melphalan		
COG ANBL0532 (CONTD) (*Liu et al. JCO* 2020) 355 high-risk patients (same cohort as prior table row)	COG ANBL0532 patients (*subset analysis of single transplant patients who had a STR and received RT (21.6 Gy + 14.4 Gy boost)	No difference in 5-y CILP, EFS, or OS	*Patients underwent tumor resection between cycles 4 and 5 (if not performed at dx) and RT following SCT. All received 21.6 Gy to the preoperative GTV, with 14.4 Gy boost to any gross dz Conclusions: No benefit with increased dose RT boost to gross residual disease
	COG A3973 patients (single transplant, received 21.6 Gy)		

EWING SARCOMA

ELAINE CHA • ARNOLD PAULINO

BACKGROUND

- **History:** Described in 1921 by James Ewing as a bone tumor sensitive to radiation. Ewing family of tumors (EFT) includes Ewing sarcoma (EWS) (both osseous and extraosseous), as well as malignant small cell tumor of the chest well (Askin tumor), and primitive neuroectodermal tumor (PNET). Osseous EWS accounts for ~85% of EFT; 8% of EFT are extraosseous EWS.
- **Incidence/prevalence:** Approximately 200 cases per year dx in the United States of EFT including EWS ~3% of adolescent malignancies. Second most common pediatric malignant bone tumor after osteosarcoma
- **Outcomes:** 5-Year OS for localized EWS ~70% (~60% for pelvic primaries, 80% for extremity primaries). 5-Year OS for metastatic EWS ~30% (~40% for lung mets only)

- **Demographics:** Median age at diagnosis is 14 years. 20-30% of EFT occur in patients <10 years old, and another 20-30% occur in patients >20 years old. Higher incidence in M (M:F = 1.5:1 for EFT) and in Caucasians (very uncommon among African Americans)
- **Risk factors:** No known/established congenital syndrome associated w/ EFT. Rare reports of EWS as a second malignancy after treatment with chemotherapy
- **Prognostic factors:** Better prognosis w/ extremity tumors vs axial tumors. Larger size has worse prognosis (both those treated definitively with surgery and RT). Also prognostic: extent of viable tumor after neoadjuvant chemotherapy (≥5% residual viable tumor is a poor prognostic marker) and older age. Better prognosis for fusion of exon 7 of *EWS* to exon 6 of *FLI*

TUMOR BIOLOGY AND CHARACTERISTICS

- **Pathology/genetics:** Proposed neuroectodermal origin of EFT, though other hypotheses exist. Histologically, EFT are small round blue cell tumors, differentiated by expression of vimentin, c-myc, and CD99 (CD99 being sensitive for EWS but not specific as it is also expressed in rhabdomyosarcoma). Most cases involve breakpoints clustered within *EWSR1* gene on chromosome 22. 80-90% of EFT have t(11;22), generating an *EWS-FLI* fusion protein, which has been shown to function as a transcription regulator. An additional 5-10% of EFT have other translocations involving *EWSR1*, including t(21;22) and t(7;22) and less commonly t(17;22) and t(2;22).

ANATOMY

For osseous EWS, pooled data from European Intergroup Cooperative Ewing Sarcoma Studies (EI-CESS) trials demonstrated that 54% of tumors had primary axial skeletal sites and 42% had primary appendicular skeletal sites (*Cotterill et al. JCO* 2000). Pelvic primary tumors = 25% of osseous EWS, and femoral primary tumors = 16% of osseous EWS. Primary location is typically diaphyseal.

WORKUP

- **History and physical:** Patients typically present with pain and swelling at the primary tumor site; often, minor trauma can precipitate pain/swelling at the site, which worsens over weeks. Pain associated with primary tumor is often worse at night and w/ exercise. Patients can present with pathologic fracture as well. Constitutional symptoms, including fevers and weight loss, occur in ~10-20% of EWS patients at presentation and can portend metastatic dz + poorer prognosis.
- **Imaging:** Plain x-ray of primary site ("onion skin" appearance in EWS vs "sunburst" in osteosarcoma). Contrasted MR or CT of primary site (MRI preferred due to soft tissue delineation and involvement of neurovascular structures, surgical planning/considerations). Metastatic workup outlined per guidelines (*Meyer Pediatr Blood Cancer* 2008) generally includes PET/CT and radionuclide bone scintigraphy (bone scan). Also, note that repeat imaging prior to local therapy is recommended (usually MRI of primary site) to guide surgical planning and/or RT volumes.
- **Labs:** CBC, CMP (including BUN/Cr and LFTs), LDH, ESR
- **Procedures/biopsy:** Core needle biopsy (often CT guided) or incisional biopsy. Ensure surgeon is involved before biopsy, especially for cases where limb salvage is being considered (extremity EWS cases). At least unilateral bone marrow biopsy is recommended due to a significant risk of bone marrow metastases from EFT as well.

STAGING

- No commonly used staging systems are present for EFT; rather the primary categorization of EWS (osseous and extraosseous) is localized or metastatic.
- Notably, 25% of EWS patients p/w metastatic disease, most commonly in the lungs (50%), bones (30%), and bone marrow (25%). Rare spread (<10%) to LNs, brain, and liver. If mets to other bones, vertebral column most often involved. Patterns of relapse mirror de novo sites of metastatic disease, w/ lung as most common site of relapse.

TREATMENT ALGORITHM

Conceptually, even localized EWS patients should be regarded as having occult systemic disease.

- **General treatment algorithm:** VDC/IE × 12 weeks → local therapy → VDC/IE through week 48 (~14-17 total cycles of VDC/IE)
- **Local therapy:** Surgery (+adj RT if needed) vs definitive RT
- **Surgery:** Favored if possible, to decrease risk of second malignancy and often less morbidity of resection in developing child than RT. Often, surgery is favored if limb reconstruction/sparing approach is possible. Resectable/dispensable bones (generally amenable to surgery): fibula (proximal), ribs, portions of hands/feet (esp small tumors), and distal clavicle, among others. To avoid exposing patients to both surgery and adjuvant RT, definitive surgery should generally be pursued if complete resection is feasible.
- **Radiation:** Concurrent non–doxorubicin-containing chemotherapy is often delivered with RT during local therapy. Common indications for adjuvant RT include +margin/incomplete resection (R1 or R2), >10% viable tumor after induction chemotherapy (12 weeks of VDC/IE), or tumor spill. Per COG AEWS0031, adequate surgical margins are >1 cm for bone and >5 mm for soft tissue. Also, for bulky tumors in challenging sites, preoperative or postoperative RT can be utilized in conjunction with surgery. Similarly, adjuvant hemithoracic RT can be indicated in high-risk chest wall primary tumors (especially those w/ pleural infiltration or intraoperative contamination of pleural space). Whole lung irradiation (WLI) is generally recommended for pulmonary metastases, especially for those with good response to initial chemotherapy.

Radiation Treatment Technique

- **SIM:** Dependent on primary tumor site; some pediatric patients may require sedation (anesthesia).
- **Dose (primary EWS site):**
  - Definitive RT: 55.8 Gy (lower if paraspinal EWS w/ respect to cord tolerance)
  - Adjuvant RT: 55.8 Gy for gross residual, 50.4 Gy for microscopic residual
  - Doses in 1.8 Gy fractions (55.8 Gy in 31 fractions, for instance)
- **Target (primary EWS site):**
  - Definitive:
    - GTV1 = pre-CHT bone and pre-CHT soft tissue involved
    - GTV2 = pre-CHT bone and post-CHT soft tissue involved
    - GTV1 + 1.5 cm = CTV1
    - GTV2 + 1.5 cm = CTV2
    - CTV1 + 5 mm (generally) = PTV1 → treat to 45 Gy in 25 fractions
    - CTV2 + 5 mm (generally) = PTV2 → treat to additional 10.8 Gy in 6 fractions (total to 55.8 Gy/31 fx)
  - Adjuvant:
    - As per definitive, but GTV2 = postoperative residual/site of positive margins
    - CTV2 = GTV2 + 1.5 cm
    - CTV2 + 5 mm (generally) = PTV2 → treat to additional 5.4 Gy if microscopic residual or additional 10.8 Gy if macroscopic residual
  - Paraspinal EWS considerations:
    - Challenge with respect to cord tolerance. Often dose limited to 45 Gy or 50.4 Gy for tumors w/ proximity to cord
- **Technique (primary EWS site):**
  Proton beam therapy and intensity-modulated radiation therapy (IMRT) are reasonable options. For certain pelvic tumors, consideration can be given to bladder filling, if full bladder displaces bowel from the treatment field. Daily bladder scanning may be helpful if this is the case. For hands/feet, use bolus/compensators. Consider bolus to scar/drain sites if adjuvant RT.
- **WLI/hemithorax RT:**
  Dose: 15 Gy/10 fx
  CTV: Includes the bilateral lungs, mediastinum, and pleural recesses for WLI. For hemithorax RT (ie, due to pleural effusion), include the ipsilateral lung + pleural recess.
  Technique: AP/PA or IMRT (cardiac-sparing IMRT warrants 4DCT simulation; see *Kalapurakal IJROBP* 2012). If AP/PA borders are as follows: Superior = above the clavicle/lung apex (flash SCV fossa). Inferior = below the diaphragm. Lateral = chest wall. See **Wilms Tumor** chapter for representative fields.
- **Planning directive constraints:**
  Specific constraints are largely dependent on the primary site, but in general:
  - Cord D_{max} < 45 Gy (though consideration can be given to a D_{max} < 50.4 Gy, depending on circumstances)

- Avoid circumferential limb irradiation (see "Soft Tissue Sarcoma" section for more information), sparing 1- to 2-cm strip of skin to reduce lymphedema risk.
- Extra care should be given to avoid unnecessary bladder dose, given cystitis associated w/ EWS CHT agents cyclophosphamide and ifosfamide, which are often given concurrent w/ RT.
- Avoid premature epiphyseal closure by avoiding RT to uninvolved epiphyseal growth plates.

Chemotherapy

- VDC/IE = Vincristine + doxorubicin + cyclophosphamide (VDC) alternating with ifosfamide + etoposide (IE)

Side Effects

- **Acute:** Varies by treatment field/primary site
- **Late:** Varies by treatment field/primary site, but in general: height loss, premature epiphyseal closure/decreased bone growth (and therefore skeletal asymmetry in some cases), kyphosis/lordosis/scoliosis, fracture, cystitis, pneumonitis, pulmonary fibrosis, infertility, and second malignancy (SMN). Note the relatively high rate of SMN for EWS survivors, w/ CCSS report of 24% cumulative SMN risk at 35 years (*Marina et al. Cancer* 2017).

Follow-up

- End-treatment imaging with PET/CT at completion of chemotherapy and MRI of primary site ~3-4 months after definitive local treatment (*Meyer Pediatr Blood Cancer* 2008)
- Follow-up q3mo for first 2 years, then q6mo for years 2-5, then annually for another 5 years, and likely longer than that. Includes H&P, labs, as well as primary + chest imaging, generally plain films unless concerning/focal sxs present, or abnormality detected on XR
- Late relapses not uncommon w/ EWS, per CCSS occurring in 13% of 5-year EWS survivors by 20 years. Site-specific monitoring for late effects should also be pursued (relevant site-specific guidelines available from COG).

Notable Trials

Name/Inclusion	Arms/Design	Outcomes	Notes
POG 8346 (*Donaldson et al. IJROBP* 1998) 178 children with EWS (79% localized dz) who achieved PR/CR after induction VDC/dactinomycin and with primary tumors involving nonexpendable bone	Whole-bone RT field Involved field RT (GTV + 2 cm)	53% LC in both arms	Conclusions: established involved field RT for EWS (compared to whole-bone RT)
INT-0991 (*Grier et al. NEJM* 2003) 518 EFT patients	Induction VDC + dactinomycin Induction VDC + dactinomycin alternating with IE	For patients with localized EFT: alternating VDC + dactinomycin with IE improves 5-y OS (72% vs 61%, $P = .01$) and LC (95% vs 85%, $P < .001$)	Conclusions: Adding IE improves EFS and OS for localized EFT

Name/Inclusion	Arms/Design	Outcomes	Notes
R2Pulm (*Dirksen et al. JCO* 2019) 287 EWS patients with only pulmonary/pleural mets who underwent induction chemo (VIDEx6 + VAIx1)	Standard chemotherapy (VAIx7) with whole-lung irradiation (WLI) High-dose busulfan-melphalan (BuMel) with SCT	No difference in OS or 8-y EFS More severe toxicities in BuMel arm (4 toxicity-related deaths, none in standard arm)	Conclusions: In setting of lung mets, no clear benefit to replacing WLI with BuMel
Tata Memorial Centre RCT (*Laskar et al. IJROBP* 2022) 95 nonmetastatic, unresectable EWS/PNET patients who underwent induction chemotherapy (VDC/IE)	Standard dose RT (SDRT, 55.8 Gy/31 fx) Escalated dose RT (EDRT, 70.2 Gy/39 fx)	5-y EFS improved with EDRT (76.4% vs 49.4%, *P* = .02) No difference in DFS or OS	Site: 63% pelvic tumors, 30% extremities Conclusions: EDRT improves LC in unresectable EWS/PNET

RHABDOMYOSARCOMA

ELAINE CHA • ARNOLD PAULINO

Background

- **Incidence/prevalence:** Rhabdomyosarcoma (RMS) is the most common pediatric soft tissue sarcoma, with ~350-400 cases per year in the United States. Accounts for ~3-4% of pediatric malignancies
- **Outcomes:** Varies by primary tumor site, histology, translocation status, and risk stratification, among others. The 5-year overall survival (OS) by COG risk stratification: low risk = 92%, intermediate risk = 65%, and high risk = 14%.
- **Demographics:** Male predominance; M:F = ~1.4:1. Slight racial trends in RMS incidence: African Americans > Caucasians > Asians. Incidence peaks at 2-6 years old (embryonal histology) and 10-14 (alveolar histology). However, 7% of RMS is in infants (<1 year old), and 13% of RMS is in patients 15+ years old, including cases in adults.
- **Risk factors:** Limited knowledge, w/ most RMS cases being sporadic. RMS has been associated w/ some genetic syndromes including Li-Fraumeni, NF-1, and Beckwith-Wiedemann.

Tumor Biology and Characteristics

- **Pathology:** Small round blue cell tumor. IHC helpful to distinguish from other small blue round cell tumors. RMS positive for muscle-specific proteins including myoglobin, Z-band protein, myogenic differentiation 1 (MyoD1), actin, myosin, and desmin.
- **Cell of origin:** Hypothesized to arise from primitive mesenchymal cells, though emerging data suggest nonmesenchymal origin may be possible for fusion-negative RMS (*Drummond et al. Cancer Cell* 2018).
- **Histology:** Multiple histologic subtypes with prognostic importance. From the best to the worst prognosis: botryoid, spindle cell, embryonal, alveolar, and pleomorphic/undifferentiated. Botryoid and spindle cells are variants of embryonal histology and confer excellent prognosis. Botryoid is common in infants and tumors of the GU tract (ie, vaginal RMS in infants, typically botryoid histology, which has "bunch of grapes" appearance on physical exam). Embryonal histology displays patchy myogenin staining, with appearance similar to embryonal skeletal muscle; RMS of head and neck enriched for embryonal histologies (especially orbital tumors). Alveolar histology, with a worse prognosis, occurs in older children (10+) and has diffuse myogenin staining. Furthermore, alveolar tumors occur in more unfavorable sites, especially the extremities, perineum, and trunk. Approximately 50-55% of RMS are embryonal, and ~25% are alveolar.

- **Genetics:** Translocations involving *FOX01* on chromosome 13 have been shown to be associated with alveolar RMS. Approximately 80% of alveolar RMS have either *PAX3-FOX01* or *PAX7-FOX01* fusion transcripts, corresponding to t(2;13) and t(1;13), respectively. Of those w/ fusion transcripts, majority are *PAX3-FOX01* fusions. *PAX-FOX01* is a negative prognostic indicator (*Sorenson et al. JCO* 2002). Moreover, fusion-negative alveolar RMS has comparable outcomes to embryonal RMS (*Williamson et al. JCO* 2010). Therefore, there is a trend toward fusion status for risk assignment and trial design (including ongoing COG trials).

Anatomy

Approximately 20% GU, ~15% H&N parameningeal, ~10% orbital, ~10% H&N non-parameningeal, ~20% extremity, and ~15% other (including trunk, retroperitoneum)

*Parameningeal H&N includes MMNNOOPP mnemonic = Middle ear, Mastoid, Nasal cavity, Nasopharynx, infratemporal fOssa, pterygopalatine fOssa, Paranasal sinuses, and Parapharyngeal space

Classify primary site into favorable and unfavorable prognostic categories:

- **Favorable sites:** Orbit, nonparameningeal H&N, biliary, nonprostate/nonbladder GU
- **Unfavorable sites:** All other sites

Diagnostic Evaluation

- **History and physical:** Clinical presentation varies by primary site. Orbital: proptosis, ophthalmoplegia. Parameningeal H&N: nasal/aural/sinus obstruction, CN deficits, and altered mental status (consider intracranial extension). Other H&N: painless enlarging mass. Extremities: mass (+/− pain associated with mass), swelling. GU: hematuria/urinary obstruction (bladder), discharge (vagina), scrotal/inguinal enlargement (paratesticular)

  Nodal metastasis rates, including at presentation, vary by primary site/histology; highest risks of LNs involved by site are prostate, paratesticular, and extremity tumors. H&N alveolar tumors may also have increased risk of LN mets.

  Distant mets in ~20% of RMS patients at diagnosis, usually the lung, bone marrow, and bone. Mets within the CNS can occur in parameningeal RMS patients w/ intracranial extension (seeding within CSF).
- **Imaging:** Assess primary site: MRI preferred. Assess for LN + distant mets: PET/CT; can omit chest CT and bone scan if PET/CT performed. Bone marrow biopsy recommended, though bilateral BMBx not required for embryonal RMS patients and clinically node-negative patients.
  - **Parameningeal RMS:** These tumors have high risk of extension into the CNS (intracranial extension, as well as cranial bone erosion and CN deficits). Therefore, for parameningeal RMS, CSF cytology (LP) as well as MRI of the brain is needed.
- **Labs:** CBC, CMP (including BUN/Cr and LFTs), uric acid
- **Procedures/biopsy:** Core needle or incisional Bx. As above, for parameningeal RMS, LP is needed for CSF cytologic analysis.
  - **Nodal evaluation:** Biopsy any suspicious LNs to confirm nodal status. Sentinel LN biopsy indicated for extremity tumors. Males >10 years old w/ paratesticular RMS are recommended for ipsilateral nerve-sparing retroperitoneal LN dissection.
- **Miscellaneous:** Sperm banking/fertility consult, as indicated

Risk Stratification/Staging

- Risk stratification guides treatment; 4-step process

1. **Site: favorable vs unfavorable:** See above re: dividing primary sites into favorable vs unfavorable categories.
2. **Stage:** Start by site, and then determine the stage (I-IV) as below:

Stage	Site	Size	L Nodes	Mets
I	Favorable	Any	Any	M0
II	Unfavorable	≤5 cm	N0	M0
III	Unfavorable	>5 cm OR N1 (any size)		M0
IV	Any	Any	Any	M1

Favorable site: Orbit, non-PM H&N, nonbladder/prostate GU, biliary tract
Unfavorable site: PM, everything else

3. **Group (extent of surgery):** IRS grouping based on the extent of surgery

Group	Definition
1	R0 (complete) resection
2	R1 resection and/or LN+ (with R0-1)
3	R2 resection or unresectable/Bx only
4	Metastatic disease

4. **Risk stratification:** Combination of stage + group, as well as histology (now fusion status; *Pappo et al. JCO* 2017). See above for OS rates for each risk category.
   - **Low risk:** Fusion-negative: Stage 1 Group 2, Stage 2 Groups 1 and 2, and orbital Stage 1 Group 3
   - **High risk:** All Stage 4 Group 4 except fusion-negative patients <10 years old
   - **Intermediate risk:** All others

TREATMENT ALGORITHM

- Overarching Tx paradigm: maximal safe resection (or biopsy) → chemotherapy, start RT as indicated during chemotherapy, timing noted below
- RT used as definitive local therapy for sites w/ limited options for primary resection w/o significant morbidity, including orbital as well as other H&N (esp parameningeal).
- RT dosing, timing, and indications vary by stage/group/risk stratification as above.

RADIATION TREATMENT TECHNIQUE

- **SIM:** Primary site dependent; sedation (anesthesia) may be required in children <8 years old, for both sim and treatment.
- **Dose:** All in 1.8 Gy fractions, generally
  - Group I fusion negative = no RT
  - Group I fusion positive = 36 Gy to prechemo site
  - Group II N0 (microscopic residual after surgery) = 36 Gy to prechemo site
  - Group II N1 (resected LN involvement) = 41.4 Gy to prechemo site and nodal region
  - Group III nonorbital = 50.4 Gy
  - Group III orbital = 45 Gy (if CR after induction chemo) and 50.4 Gy (if non-CR after induction chemo)
- **RT timing:** Relative to start of chemotherapy, generally by risk stratification
  - Low risk = week 13 (per ARST0331)
  - Intermediate risk = week 13 (per ARST1431)
  - High risk = week 20
  - Emergent RT should be initiated as soon as indicated, regardless of the above.
  - Parameningeal RMS w/ intracranial extension conventionally treated weeks 0-2. ARST1431 delaying RT start to week 13.
- **Target:**
  - In general: GTV = prechemotherapy volume and CTV = GTV + 1 cm
  - PTV margin depends on site(s) being treated, IGRT utilized, etc.
- **Technique:** Varies by treatment site, but in general proton beam therapy and IMRT are reasonable options, w/ multiple series utilizing both techniques across primary sites.
- **IGRT:** Primary site dependent, usually at least daily kV-IGRT
- **Planning directive dose constraints:** Primary site dependent

CHEMOTHERAPY

- Commonly utilized: VAC (vincristine/dactinomycin/cyclophosphamide), VI (vincristine/irinotecan), and IE (ifosfamide/etoposide)

SIDE EFFECTS

- **Acute:** Varies by treatment field/primary site
- **Late:** Varies by treatment field/primary site. For orbital tumors, for instance, xerophthalmia, cataracts, decreased visual acuity H&N RT leads to dentofacial abnormalities, facial asymmetry/hypoplasia, endocrinopathies, and neurocognitive deficits. Other late risk factors include premature epiphyseal closure and decreased bone growth (and therefore skeletal asymmetry), fracture, cystitis, urinary incontinence, infertility (especially w/ cyclophosphamide), and second malignancy (SMN).

NOTABLE TRIALS/PAPERS

Name/Inclusion	Arms/Design	Outcomes	Notes
IRS I (*Maurer et al. Cancer* 1988) 686 patients with RMS or undifferentiated sarcoma	Group I: VAC vs VAC + RT Group II: VA + RT vs VAC + RT Group III/IV: pulse VAC + RT vs pulse VAC + doxorubicin + RT	Group I: no diff in OS Group II/III: coverage of whole muscles vs involved fields results in no diff in LC For patients >6 yo, LR 32% for RT < 40 Gy and LR 12% for RT > 40 Gy (*P* > .4); no dose response	*Group I: localized dz, completely resected *Group II: regional dz, grossly resected *Group III: STR *Group IV: mets Conclusions: no RT for clinically favorable patients; no need to cover whole muscle when irradiating
IRS IV (*Crist et al. JCO* 2001) 883 post-op RMS patients a group III subset (see prior row)	50.4 Gy/28 fx 59.4 Gy/54 fx bid	No diff in FFS (*P* = .85) or LC (*P* = .9). Increased mucositis in bid arm	Conclusions: conventional daily fractionation remains the SOC
MDACC Proton Beam Therapy (PBT) protocol (*Buszek et al. IJROBP* 2021) 94 RMS patients	Prospective protocol, patients treated with combo chemotherapy and PBT (36-50.4 cGE)	4y OS, PFS, and LC was 71%, 63%, 85% respectively. Worse OS, PFS, and LC with increasing tumor size (*P* = .01, *P* = .02, *P* = .007) and > 13wk delay in RT from chemo start (*P* = .03, *P* = .04, *P* = .01)	Protons can safely be used when consolidating RMS with RT. Important to start RT in a timely manner after chemo and to limit delays.

OSTEOSARCOMA/RETINOBLASTOMA/ BRAINSTEM GLIOMA

ELAINE CHA • ARNOLD PAULINO

OSTEOSARCOMA

- **Background:**
  - Most common pediatric bone tumor (2nd most is Ewing sarcoma [EWS]), w/ ~400 pediatric cases per year. Bimodal distribution w/ peak in teenage years and another peak >65 years old. M > F and African American > Caucasian
  - Increased risk of osteosarcoma in patients w/ history of germline *RB* mutation as well as h/o RT for retinoblastoma (irrespective of germline *RB* mutation presence)
  - Presents with local symptoms including pain, swelling, palpable mass, and fracture. Less common for systemic symptoms at presentation than EWS. "Sunburst" pattern on films vs "onion skin" appearance in EWS
  - 80% of cases in appendicular skeleton, majority of which originate in metaphysis (distal femur > tibia)
  - 90% of osteosarcoma patients have radiographically localized disease at dx, but w/ symptoms alone, ~80% of patients will develop lung mets within 12 months. Therefore, like w/ EWS, osteosarcoma is an "occult systemic" disease.
- **Treatment paradigm:**
  Neoadjuvant chemotherapy → surgery* → adjuvant chemotherapy (usually double doxorubicin/cisplatin)
  *Pathologic response to neoadjuvant chemotherapy on surgical specimen is prognostic, with >90% necrosis resulting in ~80% relapse-free survival.

- **Role of RT:**
  - Unlike EWS, osteosarcoma is generally considered radioresistant (variant histologies of osteosarcoma are to some extent more radiosensitive).
  - Beyond palliative indications, RT may be used in the definitive setting for inoperable patients (inoperable due to patient and/or disease factors) in the adjuvant setting for those with close or positive margins or in treatment of oligometastatic bone met disease.
  - Definitive RT, or RT after R2 resection (gross residual dz), is thought to require high doses of RT (60-70 Gy, usually at least 66 Gy in 2 Gy fractions).
  - Data suggest no role for prophylactic WLI despite high risk of lung metastases.

Retinoblastoma (RB)

- **Background:**
  - Most common primary intraocular pediatric malignancy, with ~300 cases per year. Occurs usually in infants/toddlers (~2 years median age at dx). 95% of cases in those <5 years old
  - 60% of Rb cases are sporadic, and 40% are heritable (germline *RB* mutation). Most heritable *RB* mutation is via de novo germline mutations, since <10% of *RB* patients have family history of *RB* mutation.
  - Approximately 1/3 of Rb cases are bilateral, generally suggestive of germline *RB* mutation. However, 15% of unilateral Rb patients have germline mutation, so genetic testing should be considered even in unilateral cases. Trilateral retinoblastoma cases refer to bilateral retinoblastoma with a concordant pineoblastoma. Occurs in 5% of patients with *RB* mutation
  - Earlier age of presentation (~1-1.5 years old) for bilateral Rb patients and patients w/ germline *RB* mutation
  - Usually p/w leukocoria, although can p/w strabismus, nystagmus, and others
  - Multiple classification systems; COG currently using the International Classification of Intraocular Retinoblastoma system, where the eyes are risk stratified from A through E.

    A: Small tumors (3 mm), limited to the retina and not near important structures
    B: All other tumors, limited to the retina
    C: Well-defined tumors with small amount of spread under the retina or vitreous seeding
    D: Large or poorly defined tumors with widespread vitreous or subretinal seeding
    E: Large tumor, extending near the front of the eye. Bleeding, causing glaucoma, or have almost no chance the eye can be served
- **Treatment paradigm:**
  - Variable but includes both systemic therapy (usually VCE = vincristine/carboplatin/etoposide) and focal therapies w/ the goal of sparing the eye from enucleation if possible
  - Array of local treatment options available, including intra-arterial chemotherapy, intravitreous chemotherapy, cryotherapy, laser photocoagulation, external beam RT, and plaque brachytherapy
  - EBRT may be indicated in adjuvant setting after enucleation as well, if positive margin or nodal involvement is identified; enucleation is often indicated for advanced (very high risk = group E) tumors, among others.
- **Role of EBRT and brachytherapy:**
  - EBRT was developed as the first technique to allow globe sparing. However, it is used less now due to concerns for second malignancy. Roarty et al. examined bilateral Rb patients; 35% had second malignant neoplasm after EBRT vs 6% for those who didn't have EBRT (*Roarty et al. Ophthalmology* 1988). Data support field and dose dependence of second malignant neoplasm incidence after RT for Rb. Second malignant neoplasm after RT for Rb includes osteosarcoma of bones within the treatment field around the orbit.
  - EBRT (usually with concurrent chemotherapy) is often indicated in adjuvant setting after enucleation w/ +margin or +LN. Doses 36-45 Gy.
  - Plaque brachytherapy provides a custom-design shielded source that decreases RT dose to bones and therefore reduces risk for developing secondary malignant neoplasms.
  - Usually I-125 or Ru-106 sources for plaques, **prescribing** 45 Gy to 1 mm beyond the apex of the tumor
  - Logistically challenging, as plaques remain in place for ~2 days in these young children before returning to the operating room for plaque removal. Similarly,

technically challenging; therefore not used often in the frontline setting, but rather considered in the setting of persistent dz after other local therapies exhausted

Brainstem Glioma

- **Background:**
  - 80% of pediatric brainstem gliomas arise from pons. Most pontine tumors are diffuse intrinsic pontine gliomas (DIPGs). Approximately 20% of pediatric brainstem gliomas = focal, predominantly at cervicomedullary jxn (low medulla) and tectum (upper midbrain). Usually present with CN palsies, especially CNs VI and VII, as well as ataxia, incr ICP (H/A, N/V, lethargy/somnolence). Pontine gliomas are primarily infiltrative, high-grade, and aggressive and portend poor prognosis.
  - Nondiffuse nonpontine lesions include dorsally exophytic lesions, usually low-grade gliomas including JPA (WHO grade I tumors).
  - Incidence: DIPGs usually present at 4-9 years old, ~300 cases per year. No gender predilection for DIPG
  - Pathology: Emerging understanding of molecular pathogenesis of DIPG, including high incidence of mutations in *H3F3A* (histone H3 gene). Approximately 80% of DIPG in one study found to have *H3F3A* mutation (*Wu et al. Nat Genet* 2012). These *H3 K27M* mutations have been identified as portending poor prognosis. 2016 WHO classification includes "H3 K27M-mutant diffuse midline glioma" as a diagnostic entity.
  - DIPG on MRI demonstrates characteristic T1-hypointense and T2-hyperintense expansile infiltrative pattern within the pons, w/ variable rates of Gd contrast enhancement.
- **Treatment paradigm:**
  - Management of peritumoral edema (steroids) and management of hydrocephalus (shunt) as indicated. Biopsy of tumor only indicated if atypical appearance on imaging questioning DIPG dx. Emerging studies/protocols are demonstrating safety of biopsy of DIPG, but outside of protocol, do not biopsy due to risks of injury to the brainstem.
  - The only standard antitumor therapy is RT. Despite this, median survival ~1 year, w/ minimal (<5%) survival at 5 years. Of note, non-DIPG brainstem gliomas, such as dorsal exophytic brainstem gliomas, have better prognosis (~75% 10-year OS)
  - Limited role for conventional chemotherapeutics, though increasingly HDAC inhibitors/inhibitors of histone demethylation are being utilized on the protocol
- **Role of RT:**
  - Dose: RT for DIPG involves treatment to 54 Gy in 30 fractions (1.8 Gy/fx)
  - Target: Tumor volume (MRI fusion helpful) + 1-1.5 cm for CTV. Additionally, 5 mm PTV w/ daily kV-IGRT
  - Technique: Photon-based RT (IMRT/VMAT) rather than proton beam therapy, owing to theoretical considerations regarding the higher risk of brainstem injury w/ protons.
  - Alternative RT dose via hypofractionation, using 39 Gy at 3 Gy/fx (13 daily fractions) or 44.8 Gy at 2.8 Gy/fx (16 daily fractions). Matched cohort analysis (*Janssens et al. IJROBP* 2013) suggested comparable outcomes with shorter treatment time/burden. However, RCT from Egypt (see table below) randomized DIPG patients to 54 Gy/30 fx vs 39 Gy/13 fx found similar results between 2 arms, but w/ PFS differences exceeding prespecified noninferiority assumption (PFS favoring conventional arm).
  - Therefore, we continue to utilize conventional fractionation at MDACC at present.
  - RT usually results in response and symptom improvement in the majority (~65-75%) of patients, but virtually all will recur 1 year after RT

Name/Inclusion	Arms/Design	Outcomes	Notes
Cairo University RCT (*Zaghloul et al. IJROBP* 2022) 253 patients with DIPG	HF1 (39 Gy/13 fx)	No diff in OS between arms	Conclusions: emerging alternative HF option, however CF remains SOC (reflected in consensus guidelines)
	HF2 (45 Gy/15 fx)	HF1 and HF2 noninferior to CF at 18 months	
	CF (54 Gy/30 fx)	Younger age (2-5 yo) associated with improved OS in all groups, except HF2	

LATE EFFECTS

ELAINE CHA • ARNOLD PAULINO

Background

- **Overview:**
  - Late toxicity from radiotherapy, especially in pediatric patients, informs treatment choices and risks.
  - Increasing concern regarding late toxicity given improved survival of pediatric patients across disease sites over the last 50 years.
  - Top causes of mortality in 5-year survivors of childhood cancers are recurrent disease (57%), secondary malignancies (SMNs; 15%), and cardiac toxicities (7%) (*Mertens et al. JCO* 2001).
- **Factors affecting late effects:**
  - Factors may affect risk of late toxicity to different organ systems/sites.
  - Host factors, including age, gender, comorbidities, ethnicity/race, and genetic predisposition, may affect late toxicity.
  - Age of patient is particularly important for OARs, given differential rates of maturation. For example, early development of brain vs teenage development of reproductive system; conceptually, brain more sensitive to RT during development in early childhood, whereas gonads more sensitive to RT during puberty
  - Genetic effects are also important: NF1 patients after RT for optic pathway gliomas had ~50% risk of second malignancy (*Sharif et al. JCO* 2006). Similarly, increased risk for moyamoya syndrome for NF1 patients after RT and also increased risk of cutaneous basal cell carcinomas in field after RT in patients w/ Gorlin syndrome (see *Happle JAAD* 1999). Secondary neoplasm risk in Rb patients markedly increased if hereditary Rb vs nonhereditary after RT (33% vs 13%; *Marees et al. JNCI* 2008)
  - Gender is also critical, as discussed below; there is evidence for increased sensitivity for RT toxicity in females, including neurocognitive deficits and height impairments after cranial RT for leukemia, hypothyroidism, and secondary malignancies after mediastinal RT for Hodgkin lymphoma (specifically breast).
  - Treatment parameters also influence toxicity: radiation dose, fraction size, volume treated, concurrent chemotherapy, as well as timing of chemotherapy and radiation; also important are other oncotherapeutics employed, including surgery and chemotherapy. Multiple modalities may synergize to increase the risk of toxicity.

Late Effects by Organ Site

- **CNS:**
  - Neurocognitive effects due to brain radiation; most sensitive in utero and then for the first few years of life. Synaptogenesis, axonal growth, dendritic arborization, and maturation of neural networks over these early years are thought to be central to RT neurotoxicity in the very young.
  - Neurocognitive changes affected by age of RT; IQ scores for pediatric low-grade glioma patients show more significant long-term IQ deficits w/ younger age at RT (*Merchant et al. JCO* 2009).
  - CSI + posterior fossa boost for medulloblastoma patients is shown to affect both verbal and nonverbal IQ (*Ris et al. JCO* 2001).
  - The above study suggested that female patients are more likely to have verbal IQ deficits after RT; possible gender sensitivity to IQ changes in females in study w/ ALL patients s/p CSI: 50% of girls vs 14% of boys had IQ < 90 on follow-up (*Waber et al. JCO* 1992).
  - Cranial RT may also cause leukoencephalopathy, though unlikely (<1%) in the absence of methotrexate (IV or intrathecal).
- **Musculoskeletal:**
  - RT injury to bone is dependent on portion of bone treated; for example, epiphyseal RT arrests chondrogenesis.
  - Skeletal effects are observed across multiple series, including scoliosis, kyphosis/lordosis, and iliac wing hypoplasia, among others. The most common of these (dependent on RT fields) is scoliosis.
  - Height deficits after RT are also noted, dependent on both dose and age at RT. Example is Wilms tumor patients treated w/ RT: 8-year-old patients s/p 10 Gy had only 0.8 cm height loss, whereas 2-year-old patients s/p 30 Gy had 7.2 cm height loss (*Hogeboom et al. Med Pediatr Oncol* 2001).

- Prior to puberty, if a vertebral column or growth plate cannot avoid radiation, then it is better to treat the entire column or growth plate to avoid asymmetric growth.
- Similarly thought to have gender bias w/ female more sensitive to RT-related height loss
- Growth abnormalities d/t both direct RT to developing bones and cranial RT (GH deficits). Short stature risk for patients s/p cranial RT > 20 Gy for ALL patients (*Chow et al. J Pediatr* 2007).

- **Second malignancy:**
  - Secondary breast cancer ~9-10% incidence after RT for Hodgkin's
  - Increased sensitivity for secondary breast cancer if patient is pubescent (~12-16 years old) at RT vs younger (<12 years old; *Constine IJROBP* 2008).
  - After RT for Hodgkin lymphoma, secondary thyroid cancer is also observed with comparable frequency to SBC (*O'Brien JCO* 2010).
  - Secondary malignancy is risk linked closely to RT use, among other factors (including certain chemotherapeutics such as procarbazine, anthracycline, and etoposide); secondary sarcoma is largely related to prior RT, and secondary GI malignancies are similarly related to prior abdominal RT.
  - Differential secondary malignancy rates by primary tumor histology (see **Ewing Sarcoma** chapter; high secondary malignancy incidence for EWS). Other reports describe low secondary malignancy risk for other lesions, including ~1-2% at 10-15 years for Wilms tumor, ALL, and rhabdomyosarcoma.
  - SMN studies are challenging due to time lapse between RT, treatment, and tumor-causing events; modeling suggests modern techniques have decreased risk of RT-related secondary malignancies. Emerging data suggest trend toward decreased secondary malignancies with progressive era of treatment (Turcotte et al. *JAMA* 2017).

STRATEGIES TO REDUCE LATE TOXICITY

- **Delaying/omitting RT**
  - Utilized in young children, especially <3-year-old patients w/ brain tumors. CSI delayed to >3 years old for MB and other CNS patients. Approach of deferring/delaying RT supported infants w/ ependymoma (*Merchant et al. JCO* 2004).
- **Hyperfractionated RT**
  - Relying on radiobiological principles, hyperfractionation is thought to decrease late effects, supported by a few series. Examples include decreased fracture and muscle atrophy in Ewing sarcoma patients w/ hyperfractionation and decreased hypothyroidism with RT for medulloblastoma w/ hyperfractionation.
  - Trials across multiple disease sites, however, have found limited to no difference w/ fractionation (IRS-IV, EWS CESS-86, MB HIT-SIOP PNET 4).
- **Decreasing RT dose and volume**
  - Decreased RT dose is successfully applied in NWTS-3, the results of which decreased adjuvant RT dose for stage III favorable histology Wilms tumor patients from 20 to 10 Gy w/ addition of doxorubicin to chemo regimen. Used additional chemotherapy to offset decreased RT dose.
  - In medulloblastoma patients, ACNS0031 demonstrated that involved field boost is equivalent to posterior fossa boost, which translated into a significant reduction in total brain doses.
  - Significant RT dose reductions for Hodgkin lymphoma, previously total nodal/subtotal nodal/mantle field RT to 36-44 Gy, now involved field/site/nodal RT to much lower doses (20-30 Gy generally).
  - May also attempt to eliminate RT for favorable subsets of patients: for example, in COG AREN0533, elimination of WLI for Wilms tumor patients w/ lung metastases w/ favorable chemo response. Also, see multiple Hodgkin lymphoma trials recommending RT for patients w/ PR after chemo vs observation for patients w/ CR after chemo.
- **Advanced RT technologies**
  - IMRT Example: Decreased ototoxicity in MB patients w/ IMRT vs 3DCRT (*Huang et al. IJROBP* 2002)
  - Proton beam therapy: see **Proton therapy** chapter, minimal exit dose via Bragg peak particularly advantageous for certain disease sites. Among the most notable examples, CSI, sparked 2013 debate in *IJROBP* whether proton beam therapy "only ethical" approach for pediatric patients needing CSI
  - Despite a concern for secondary neutron production/contamination w/ proton beam therapy, clinical data are not suggestive of increased risk of secondary malignancies with protons (*Sethi et al. Cancer* 2013).
  - PENTEC group, pediatric analog of the QUANTEC effort, developing quantitative, evidence-based guidelines for RT treatment planning and dose constraints, among others

ORAL CAVITY

ALAN SOSA • ADAM GARDEN

Background

- **Incidence/prevalence:** Approximately 34 470 cases diagnosed annually in the United States
- **Outcomes:** Subsite specific. 5-Year survival for oral tongue across all stages is estimated at 68% (SEER data).
- **Demographics:** M > F, older age
- **Risk factors:** Smoking, smokeless tobacco, alcohol, chronic dental inflammation, chronic sun exposure (lip), betel nut, and premalignant lesions (leukoplakia <5% risk of developing cancer at 10 years, erythroplakia 15-50% risk)

Tumor Biology and Characteristics

- **Genetics:** Majority associated with genetic alterations from external factors
- **Pathology:** Vast majority are SCC (<95%). Rare histologies include minor salivary cancers (adenoid cystic, mucoepidermoid, adenocarcinoma), sarcoma, and mucosal melanoma (typically upper lip).

Anatomy

- **Subsites:** Oral tongue, mucosal lip, floor of the mouth, alveolar ridges, retromolar trigone, buccal mucosa, hard palate
- **Extrinsic muscles of the tongue:** Genioglossus, hyoglossus, styloglossus, palatoglossus (alter position)
- **Lymph node drainage** (35% are cN+):
  - Primary drainage to level IB and IIA
  - The upper lip can drain to preauricular.
  - The lower lip and FOM can drain to IA.
  - About 15% of oral tongue cancers bypass level II and go directly to levels III-IV.
  - Levels IV-V can be involved with advanced nodal disease.

Oral Cavity Subsites	Anatomic Boundaries	Primary Lymphatic Drainage
Oral tongue	Mobile portion of tongue (anterior 2/3) from circumvallate papillae to dorsal surface of tongue • Sensation—lingual nerve (V3) ◦ Vagus nerve posteriorly ◦ CN IX posterolaterally • Taste—chorda tympani (CN VII) • Motor function—hypoglossal nerve (CN XII)	**3 routes of drainage:** • Tip of tongue—IA • Lateral tongue—IB • Medial tongue—deep cervical LN II-IV ◦ 15% drain to levels III-IV skipping II
Lip	Orbicularis oris muscle. Externally covered by skin and internally by mucous membrane Bordered by upper and lower lip vermillion • Sensation—V2 and V3 ◦ Upper lip—infraorbital nerve (V2) ◦ Lower lip—mental nerve (V3)	• All drain to **IB, II, III** • Upper lip—preauricular • Lower lip—IA
Floor of mouth	Area under the dorsal surface of tongue, which extends anteriorly from the gingiva to the undersurface of the tongue	• IA • IB • II-IV

Oral Cavity Subsites	Anatomic Boundaries	Primary Lymphatic Drainage
Alveolar ridges (gingiva or "gums")	Refers to the bone that houses the teeth as well as the adjacent overlying mucosa Posterior margin (upper) pterygopalatine arch Posterior margin (lower) ascending ramus of mandible	• IB • II-IV
Hard palate	Mucosa that covers the hard palate consisting of the palatine bone of the maxilla. It is bordered anteriorly by the palatal alveolar ridge and posteriorly by the posterior edge of the palatine bone	• II-IV
Retromolar trigone	Mucosal lining posterior to the last molar on each side. It includes the mucosa overlying the ascending mandibular ramus to the maxillary tuberosity	• IB • II-IV
Buccal mucosa	Mucosa of the inner cheek and lips that extends to the junction at the alveolar ridge mucosa medially and to the pterygomandibular raphe posteriorly	• IB • II-IV

HEAD AND NECK LYMPH NODE LEVELS

The neck is divided into six LN levels (Fig. 23.1). For all the remaining chapters in this section, please refer to the following definitions:

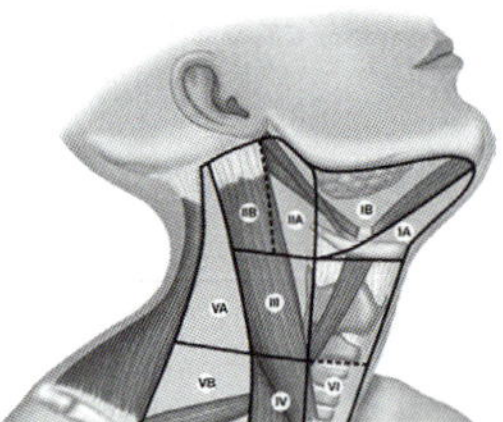

Figure 23.1 Diagram of LN stations of the neck. Used with permission of the American College of Surgeons, Chicago, Illinois. The original source for this information is the AJCC Cancer Staging System (2023).

Level I: Inferior to mylohyoid muscle and above the caudal border of the hyoid bone/carotid bifurcation:
- **IA (submetal):** Between anterior bellies of the bilateral digastric muscles
- **IB (submandibular):** Posterolateral to the anterior belly of the digastric muscle and anterior to the posterior border of the submandibular gland

Level II (internal jugular chain): Base of the skull to caudal border of the hyoid bone/carotid bifurcation. Anterior to the posterior border of SCM. Posterior to the posterior border of the submandibular gland:
- **IIA:** Anterior or immediately adjacent to (eg, inseparable from) the internal jugular vein
- **IIB:** Posterior to internal jugular vein with a fat plane separating node from vein (otherwise considered level IIA)

Level III (internal jugular chain): Caudal border of the hyoid to caudal border of the cricoid. Anterior to posterior border of SCM. Lateral to medial margin of the common/internal carotid artery

Level IV (internal jugular chain): Caudal border of the cricoid to clavicle. Anterior to posterior border of SCM. Lateral to the medial margin of the common carotid artery

Level V (posterior triangle/spinal accessory): Posterior to SCM and anterior to trapezius muscle:
- **VA:** Superior half, posterior to level II and III LN levels
- **VB:** Inferior half, posterior to level IV LN levels

Level VI (prelaryngeal/pretracheal/Delphian node): Caudal edge of hyoid bone to the manubrium, anterior to levels III and IV and visceral space (Fig. 23.2)

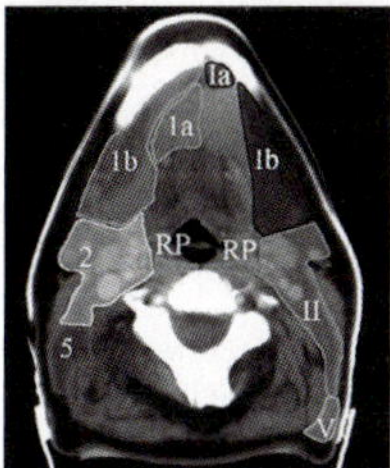

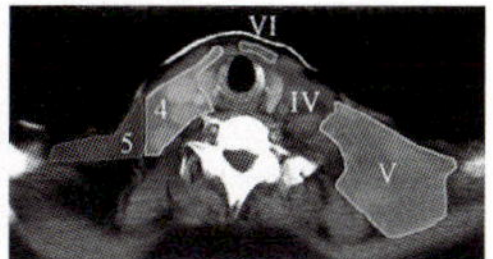

Figure 23.2 Axial CT images showing LN levels at the lower edge of the mandible **(left panel)** and low neck **(right panel)**. **See color insert**. (Reprinted from Grégoire V, Levendag P, Ang KK, et al. CT-based delineation of lymph node levels and related CTVs in the node-negative neck: DAHANCA, EORTC, GORTEC, NCIC, RTOG consensus guidelines. *Radiother Oncol*. 2003;69(3): 227-236. Copyright © 2003 Elsevier Ireland Ltd. With permission.)

Workup

- **History and physical:** Assess presenting symptoms including oral cavity function, cranial nerve deficits, otalgia, and trismus. Direct palpation and visualization of tumor and adjacent subsites with nasolaryngoscope and/or mirror exam useful to assess disease spread
- **Labs:** CBC, CMP
- **Procedures/biopsy:** Biopsy of primary and FNA of enlarged LNs as clinically indicated
- **Imaging:** CT or MRI with contrast of the head and neck. Consider CT of the chest for low neck nodes or extensive smoking history. FDG-PET/CT recommended for stage III/IV disease
- **Additional consultations:** Multidisciplinary evaluation with head and neck surgical oncology, radiation oncology, medical oncology, speech, nutrition, and dental (fluoride/extractions)

Treatment Algorithm

- **Surgery is the primary approach for oral cavity cancers. Radiation's role is therefore principally adjuvant.** Patients are assigned into one of three risk-based categories: low, intermediate, and high, with recommendations for observation, postoperative radiation or postoperative chemoradiation chosen based on each of the respective risk categories.
- Definitive radiation is an infrequently used modality. For the healthy patient, brachytherapy is a sole treatment or combined with external beam. For the medically inoperable, external beam may be an alternative. For the patient with very advanced local disease who has technically inoperable disease, radiation, either concurrent or sequential with chemotherapy, is often recommended, but as these patients have a low probability for cure, the goals of therapy and aggressiveness should be given consideration.

Surgery	
T1-T2, N0	Resection of primary ± ipsi neck dissection (>4 mm DOI, consider for DOI 2-4 mm) or SLNB
T3N0, T1-T4 N+	Resection of primary + ipsi or bilateral neck dissection + PORT
Adjuvant Radiation	
Intermediate risk[a]	Adjuvant RT
High risk[b]	Re-resection if possible; if not, then adjuvant chemoRT (cisplatin Category I)

[a]**Intermediate risk:** pT3/T4, N+, PNI, LVSI, level IV/V
[b]**High risk:** +margins, ENE

RADIATION TREATMENT TECHNIQUE

- **Timing:** Should be started within 4-6 weeks of surgery
- **Dose:**
  High risk (tumor bed): 60 Gy in 30 fractions
  Intermediate risk (operative bed and dissected neck): 57 Gy in 30 fractions
  Low risk (elective nodal coverage): 54 Gy in 30 fractions
  Consideration for boost to highest risk areas (close/positive margins/ECE): 63-66 Gy in 30-33 fractions
- **Target:** Tumor bed, operative bed, and draining lymphatics (levels I-IV, level V if node positive). Consider unilateral treatment for a well-lateralized retromolar trigone, buccal mucosa, or alveolar ridge without nodal disease.
- **Technique:** IMRT, IMPT
- **SIM:** Supine, consider mouth opening with the tongue forward (oral tongue), tongue lateralizing (buccal/alveolar/retromolar trigone) or ramp (FOM) dental stent, and Aquaplast mask. Wire scar. 3-mm bolus 2 cm around the scar (Fig. 23.3)
- **IGRT:** Daily kV with weekly CBCT or daily CBCT
- **Planning directive (for conventional fractionation):**

PTV	>95% coverage
Spinal cord	Max < 45 Gy
Brainstem	Max < 50 Gy
Brachial plexus	Max < 63-66 Gy (lower dose if fraction size to OAR > 2 Gy)
Mandible	Max ≤ to prescription dose to CTV_{HD} if PTV in mandible; V44 < 42%, V58 < 25%
Total lung	V20 < 20%
Cochlea	Max < 35 Gy
Lens	Max < 5 Gy
Parotids	Mean < 26 Gy, lower for contralateral
Larynx	Mean < 30 Gy
Cervical esophagus	Mean < 30 Gy

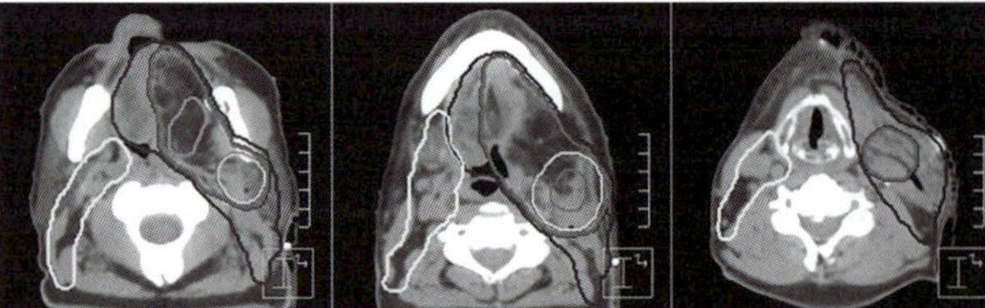

Figure 23.3 A 64-year-old patient with a resected pT2N2a (4.5 cm LN with ECE) SCC of the oral tongue reconstructed with a pectoralis flap treated with chemoRT. GTV (*green*), GTV-N (*forest green*), CTV63 (*aqua*), CTV60 (*red*), CTV57 (*blue*), and CTV54 (*yellow*) in 30 fractions. **See color insert.**

SURGERY

- Resection of the primary tumor, ranging from wide local excision to partial or total removal of the organ involved (ie, glossectomy, mandibulectomy)
  - Close margin is < 5 mm; positive margin < 1 mm
  - Advanced resections may need flap/graft reconstruction (soft tissue and/or bone).
- Neck dissection for node positive or DOI > 4 mm (tongue). Consider neck dissection if is DOI 2-4 mm.

Radical neck dissection	All LN groups I-V, CN XI, IJ vein, SCM
Modified radical neck dissection	All LN groups I-V, preserves at least one of CN XI, IJ, SCM
Selective neck dissection	Preservation of ≥1 LN group LN groups in levels IB-IV, with sparing of IJ, SCM, and CN XI

Supraomohyoid	SND of only I-III, considered for early oral cavity cases
Lateral neck dissection	SND II-IV, considered for oropharynx, hypopharynx, larynx
Central neck dissection	SND VI, considered for thyroid

Chemotherapy

- **Concurrent:** Cisplatin either high-dose (100 mg/m^2) weeks 1 and 4 or weekly cispatlin (40 mg/m^2); weekly carboplatin if cisplatin contraindicated

Side Effect Management

- Nausea/vomiting: First-line Zofran (4-8 mg q8h prn) → second-line Compazine (5-10 mg q6h prn) → ABH (lorazepam 0.34 mg, diphenhydramine 25 mg, and haloperidol 1.5 mg) 1 capsule q6h
- Anxiety: The thermoplastic immobilizing mask can cause anxiety; lorazepam 0.5-1 mg 30 minutes to 1 hour before simulation or treatment
- Oral infection: Candidiasis; if superficial—nystatin 500 000 units tid; if significant—Diflucan 100-mg tablet once daily. Bacterial superinfection: tongue VERY red, consult dental oncology for oral cultures and appropriate antimicrobial recommendations.
- Pain: Gabapentin starting dose 300 mg bid and can increase to 600 tid if tolerated. May consider starting with radiation as prophylaxis. Tramadol 50 mg q6h prn. If refractory, consider opiates including hydrocodone/acetaminophen (7.5/325) mg q6h prn and hydromorphone 2 mg q3-6h prn (can increase frequency) are common choices. If refractory, fentanyl 12.5- to 25-µg transdermal patch q72h with prn breakthrough narcotics. If pain is recalcitrant to the above, consider a pain management specialist.
- Skin: Dermatitis: Routine moisturizer use (ie, Aquaphor, coconut oil, Egyptian magic, NutriShield). Pruritus: Hypoallergenic soap and lotion and hydrocortisone 1% ointment. Moist desquamation: Mepilex dressing, Biafine cream. Crusting: Consider Domeboro soaks. Infectious dermatitis: Most likely MSSA can be treated with Bactroban 2% ointment 3× daily for 7-10 days. If infection does not clear, consider consult to infectious disease specialists.
- Thick secretions: Baking soda rinses, diet ginger ale gargles, papaya juice gargles, and guaifenesin. Glycopyrrolate, scopolamine patches, Hycodan (care advised if already on hydrocodone for pain), and/or a portable suction device can be tried for refractory cases.
- Xerostomia: Acupuncture and Biotene spray; encourage hydration

Follow-up

- History/physical exam and CT neck: Every 3 months for 1 year → every 4 months for the 2nd year → every 6 months for the 3rd year → yearly to 5 years
  Assess compliance with fluoride trays and neck range of motion/lymphedema exercises.

Randomized Evidence

Name/Inclusion	Arms	Outcomes	Notes
	Adjuvant ChemoRT vs RT		
RTOG 95-01 (*Cooper et al. NEJM* 2004; *Cooper et al. IJROBP* 2012) Phase III RCT 459 patients with completely resected OC, OPX, larynx, hypopharynx cancer w/ high risk fx (2+ LNs, ECE, +margins)	**RT alone** 60 Gy ± 6 Gy boost to high-risk areas **ChemoRT** 60 Gy ± 6 Gy Concurrent cisplatin 100 mg/m^2 q3wk	**Initial report:** Improved 2-y LRC (72% vs 82%) and DFS (HR = 0.78) with chemoRT **Long-term update:** 10-y DFS not significantly different	Unplanned subset analysis in long-term update demonstrated chemoRT improved 10-y LRF (33% vs 21%) and DFS (12% vs 18%) in patients with ECE and/or +margins

Name/Inclusion	Arms	Outcomes	Notes
EORTC 22931 (*Bernier NEJM* 2004) Phase II RCT 167 patients with completely resected OC, OPX, larynx, hypopharynx cancer w/ high risk fx (ECE, +margins, stage III/IV, OC/OPX w/ level IV/V, PNI/LVI)	**RT alone** 54 Gy/27 fx ± 12 Gy boost to high-risk areas **ChemoRT** 54 Gy/27 fx ± 12 Gy boost to high-risk areas Concurrent cisplatin 100 mg/m^2 q3wk	Combination chemoRT was associated with improved PFS (HR = 0.75) and OS (HR = 0.7)	
Meta-analysis of EORTC 22931/RTOG 95-01 (*Bernier et al. Head Neck* 2005)	Pooled data from EORTC and RTOG studies	Combined analysis showed chemoRT improved OS in patients with the high-risk features (+margins, ECE)	
		Optimal RT Dosing	
Dose-Response Relationship for PORT (*Peters et al. IJROBP* 1993; *Rosenthal IJROBP* 2017) Phase III RCT 302 patients with resected stage III/IV SCC of OC, OPX, larynx, hypopharynx cancer that required PORT. Risks assigned using 14-point scale based on margins, nerve invasion, and neck LN involvement	**Lower risk randomized to:** • Dose A (57.6/32) • Dose B (63/35) **Higher risk randomized to:** • Dose B (63/35) • Dose C (68.4/38)	Dose escalation did NOT appear to improve locoregional control (no benefit over 57.6 Gy for the lower risk and 63 Gy for the higher risk) MVA showed ECE and +margins were associated with worse LRC and OS	Patient with advanced H&N cancers were assigned a PORT dose based on a composite score from their surgical pathology results Treatment package time ≥ 85 days was also associated with worse outcomes
		Role for SLNB	
Senti-MERORL (*Garrel et al. JCO* 2020) Phase III RCT 279 patients with T1-T2 N0 OC/OPX	**Tumor resection + neck dissection (ND)** **Tumor resection + SLNB** Bx alone if negative, or followed by ND if positive	No significant differences in neck RFS (2/5 y 90%/90% vs 91%/89% [SLNB]) Furthermore, no significant differences in 2- or 5-y neck locoregional RFS, DSS, or OS	OC >> OPX There is oncologic equivalence of SLNB relative to ND with a neck failure rate of ~10% in the two arms NRG-HN006 currently open comparing SLNB to neck dissection

OROPHARYNX

RAMEZ KOUZY • JAY REDDY • ADAM GARDEN

Background

- **Incidence:** Approximately 12 000 cases annually in the United States
- **Outcomes:** 5-Year survival across all stages estimated at ~80% for HPV+ and 50% for HPV−
- **Demographics:** Incidence in men is greater than in women, 3:1 for HPV− and 8:1 for HPV+
- **Risk factors:** Age, HPV, tobacco, and alcohol (HPV−). Rise in HPV-associated OPC increased by 225% from 1988 to 2004 (SEER data)

Tumor Biology and Characteristics

- **Pathology:** Majority are squamous cell carcinomas (>95%) and HPV associated. Common HPV serotypes are 16, 18, 31, and 33. p16+ staining (via IHC) can be used as a surrogate marker of HPV+. In HPV+, EGFR can be amplified and is often associated with worse prognosis.

Clinical Presentation

- The most common presentation is a painless neck mass. Otalgia, dysphagia, or odynophagia are possible due to local invasion. Oral tongue fixation and trismus suggest more invasive/advanced disease. HPV-associated OPC tends to present with smaller primary disease and nodal, often cystic, disease.

Anatomy

- Sites: Base of the tongue, tonsil (subsites: anterior and posterior tonsillar pillars and tonsillar fossa), soft palate, and posterior/lateral pharyngeal wall
- Borders: Circumvallate papillae (anterior), pharyngeal wall (posterior), tonsillar fossa (lateral), soft palate (superior), vallecula (inferior)
- Lymph node drainage: 80-90% of patients are cN+:
  - Level II(a) is the most often involved level.
  - Skip metastases are uncommon, though level III can be involved infrequently without level II involvement.
  - Levels IB, IV, V, and the retropharyngeal (RP) nodes are at low risk of involvement especially in the absence of level II nodal disease.
  - See the Oral Cavity chapter for neck LN description (Fig. 23.1).

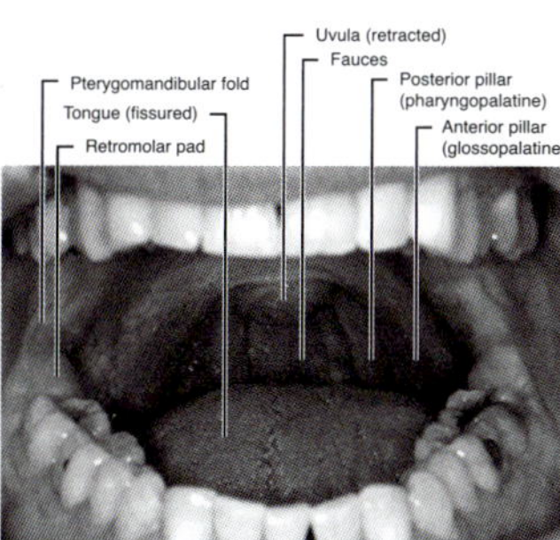

Figure 24.1 Sites of the oropharynx.

Workup

- **History and physical:** Assess presenting symptoms including oral function, cranial nerve deficits (especially XII), dentition, speech quality, otalgia, and trismus. Direct palpation and visualization of tumor and adjacent subsites with nasolaryngoscope and/or mirror exam to assess disease spread.
- **Labs:** CBC, CMP. Circulating HPV DNA can be obtained, but its role particularly at baseline is still under investigation.
- **Procedures/biopsy:** Biopsy of primary and/or FNA or core biopsy of abnormal LNs as clinically indicated, with tumor HPV testing
- **Imaging:** CT or MRI with contrast of the head and neck. Consider CT chest or chest x-ray, though FDG-PET/CT recommended for all but the earliest of stages.

- **Additional consultations:** Multidisciplinary evaluation with head and neck surgical oncology, radiation oncology, medical oncology, speech, nutrition, dental (fluoride/extractions)

Oropharynx Staging

Staging now depends on HPV status, though the main differences relate to N-category and overall group staging.

Treatment Algorithm

T-category, N-category, and HPV status drive the main treatment management algorithms.

	Treatment Options
T1/T2 N0	Transoral robotic surgery (TORS)/neck dissection (ND) is often preferred, if resection expected to significantly impact function, definitive RT is also an option (consider ipsilateral RT,[a] concurrent cetuximab or accelerated fx for bulky T2)
T1/T2 N+	TORS/ND ± adjuvant or concurrent CRT. Definitive RT alone for patients with small primary + low nodal burden
T3/T4	Concurrent chemoradiation with cisplatin
Bulky/low LN	Consider induction chemo[b] → RT or chemoRT
	Postoperative RT
+Margins or ECE	Adjuvant chemoRT
Other risk factors[c]	RT or consider chemoRT

[a]Criteria for ipsilateral RT: tonsil primary, <1 cm soft palate involvement, no BOT involvement, ipsilateral nodal disease. Risk of contralateral neck failure 0-3%

[b]Given recent data from randomized trials, there is little evidence to support the use of induction chemotherapy.

[c]Risk factors include pT3/T4, N2/N3, PNI, level IV/V, and LVSI.

- **Chemotherapy:** High- or low-dose cisplatin. Carboplatin/5-FU can be considered if contraindication to cisplatin. Cetuximab has inferior OS outcomes, similar toxicity but is an accepted sensitizer if cytotoxic chemotherapy contraindicated. Induction chemotherapy mainly cisplatin, 5-FU, and docetaxel

Radiation Treatment Technique

Definitive radiation therapy

- **Dose:**

	CTV_{HD}	CTV_{ID}	CTV_{ED}	Fx #
T1	66	60	54	30-33
T2	70	60-63	57	33 or 35*
T3/T4 (chemoRT)	70	60-63	57	33
PORT	60	57	54	30

*Finish in 6 weeks (DAHANCA, eg, 6 fx/wk) if cisplatin not given.
HD, high dose; ID, intermediate dose; ED, elective dose

- **Target:**
  - **General:** CTV_{HD} includes GTV + 8-mm margin, CTV_{ID} includes high-risk mucosal and nodal volumes, and CTV_{ED} includes uninvolved regions at risk for microscopic spread.
  - **Tonsil:** CTV_{ID} includes the entire tonsillar fossa from maxillary tuberosity to superior to hyoid. CTV_{ED} typically begins at pterygoid plates. Typically includes GP sulcus and parapharyngeal space. For well lateralized T1-T2/N0 can consider unilateral RT
  - **BOT:** CTV_{ID} includes generous coverage of the BOT beyond CTV_{HD}. The inferior extent covers the vallecula/hyoid, and anteriorly, a minimum of 2 cm of the posterior tongue is included.
  - **Nodal:** CTV_{ED} routinely covers levels II-IV on the N0 neck (each side individualized) and levels IB and V on involved side of the neck. The RP nodes (from the jugular foramen to C2) are frequently covered on the side of the tumor and

involved nodes, but consideration for omission can be given particularly for tumors confined to the tongue base.

- **Technique:** IMRT/VMAT or IMPT in experienced centers
- **SIM:** Supine, Aquaplast mask covering the head and shoulders, mouth-opening, tongue-depressing stent (for BOT/soft palate), and consideration for tongue displacing stent in tonsil cases where only the ipsilateral side will be treated. Pull straps for shoulder retraction, arms at sides. If the patient had neck dissection, wire scars and place 3-mm bolus on top of wired scars. Patient should be reminded not to swallow during simulation as this distorts anatomy. IV contrast can be used or fusion of CTsim with MRI/PET.

Postoperative

- **Target/Dose: Region of resected gross disease:** 60 Gy in 2 Gy fractions (high dose) and 66 Gy in 2 Gy fractions for positive margins
  Operative bed: 57 Gy (intermediate dose)
  Nondissected at-risk regions including nondissected at-risk nodal levels: 54 Gy (low dose)
- **Technique:** IMRT or VMAT. Scanning beam proton therapy can be used in experienced centers.
- **SIM:** See **Oral Cavity** chapter.

IGRT

- Daily kV imaging with weekly or daily CBCT

Planning directive

See **Oral Cavity** chapter.

Special circumstances

- **Indications for neck dissection after definitive XRT or chemoRT:** Persistent neck disease
- **Dose reduction** for HPV+ still pending trials
- **Transoral robotic surgery (TORS):** Increasingly common minimally invasive surgical technique utilizing robot arms controlled remotely to remove lesions in the tonsil, BOT, and soft palate. Neck dissection is typically performed during the same procedure. Risk-based decisions (usually based on the neck findings) are used to select observation, postoperative radiation (PORT), or postoperative chemoradiation.
  - Can be associated with life-threatening bleeding
- **Ipsilateral treatment:** Consider for T1-T2 tumors limited to the tonsillar fossa with N0-N1 (N2b per AJCC 7) ipsilateral neck involvement. Cover LN levels II-IV.

Chemotherapy, side effect management, and follow-up

See **Larynx** chapter.

Notable Studies

Name/Inclusion	Arms	Outcomes	Notes
HPV Status as a Positive Prognostic Marker in Oropharynx Patients			
RTOG 0129 (Ang et al. *NEJM* 2010) Phase III randomized Stage III/IV oral cavity, oropharynx, hypopharynx, or larynx cancer *N* = 743	Accelerated fractionation (72 Gy/42 fx in 6 wk) + concurrent cisplatin Standard fractionation (70 Gy/35 fx) + concurrent cisplatin	No difference in overall survival and toxicity between arms Post hoc analysis of this trial found that among oropharynx patients, 3-y OS was 82.4% in HPV+ vs 57.1% in HPV−	RPA was used to risk-stratify patients (with 3-y OS as end point): • Low risk (p16+ and <10 PY, 94%) • Intermediate risk (p16+ and >10 PY, or p16− and <10 PY, 67%) • High risk (p16− and >10 PY, 42%)
Accelerated Fractionation			
Fractionation issues are principally for patients receiving radiation without chemotherapy. The role of altered fractionation for patients receiving chemoradiation is poorly established, and standard fractionation is typically used.			

Name/Inclusion	Arms	Outcomes	Notes
RTOG 00-22 (*Eisbruch et al. IJROBP* 2010) Assess feasibility of modest acceleration Early-stage OPC (T1/T2 N0/N1) *N* = 69	**Single arm:** 66 Gy/30 fx	2-y LRF 9% Acceptable toxicity, frequent grade ≥2 toxicities were salivary (67%), mucosa (24%), esophagus (19%), skin (12%), and osteoradionecrosis (6%)	Modality: IMRT Parallel published data showed low rate of xerostomia with IMRT 6 mo = 55% 1 y = 25% 2 y = 16%
RTOG 90-03 (*Beitler IJROBP* 2014; *Fu et al. IJROBP* 2000) 4-arm RCT Stage III-IV OPC, oral cavity, hypopharynx, and larynx cancer *N* = 1113	Standard fx (70 Gy/35 fx) Hyperfractionated (81.6 Gy/68 fx [1.2 Gy bid]) Accelerated fx with split course (67.2 Gy/42 fx [1.6 Gy bid]) with a 2-wk break Accelerated fx with concomitant boost (54 Gy/30 fx + 18 Gy/12 fx bid boost to a total of 72 Gy)	2-y LRC: Arm 1, 46% Arm 2, 54% Arm 3, 47% Arm 4, 54% At 5 y, only the comparison of arm 1 vs arm 2 was significant for locoregional control (HR = 0.79, *P* = .05) and OS (HR = 0.81, *P* = .05)	<u>All arms did not receive concurrent chemotherapy</u>
DAHANCA 6/7 (*Overgaard et al. Lancet* 2003) 2 RCTs *N* = 1485 D6 enrolled glottic D7 enrolled OC + pharynx	5 fx per week 6 fx per week	6 fx a week improved local control (5-y LRC: 60% vs 70%, *P* = .0005) disease-specific survival (5-y DSS: 73% vs 66%, *P* = .01) No OS difference	<u>All patients received nimorazole and did not receive chemotherapy</u>
Cetuximab			
Bonner trial (*Bonner et al. NEJM* 2006; *Bonner et al. Lancet Oncol* 2010) Stage III/IV OPC, hypopharynx/larynx *N* = 424	Radiation + cetuximab Radiation alone	Arm 1: RT + cetuximab had a significantly better OS 5 y (46% vs 36%, *P* = .018) Benefit associated with development of grade 2 cetuximab-associated rash (HR = 0.49, *P* = .002)	Control arm was not SOC, later trials showed cisplatin with RT > cetuximab + RT
RTOG 1016 (*Gillison et al. Lancet* 2019) Randomized trial HPV+ oropharyngeal cancer patients *N* = 805	Accelerated IMRT with concurrent cisplatin (100 mg/m^2 days 1 and 22) Accelerated IMRT with concurrent cetuximab	Cetuximab was not noninferiority in OS (HR 1.45, *P* = .5) 5 y OS was 84.6% with cisplatin vs 77.9% with cetuximab (*P* = .016) 5 y LRF was 9.9% with cisplatin vs 17.3% with cetuximab (*P* = .0005)	Improved outcomes with concurrent cisplatin compared with concurrent cetuximab
De-escalate HPV (*Mehanna et al. Lancet* 2019) Randomized trial Low-risk HPV+ OPX *N* = 334	Radiation with concurrent cetuximab Radiation with concurrent cisplatin	2-y OS superior with cisplatin (89% vs 98%, *P* = .001) 2-y recurrence superior with cisplatin (16% vs 6%, *P* = .0007)	Improved outcomes with concurrent cisplatin compared with concurrent cetuximab even in a low-risk HPV+ population

Name/Inclusion	Arms	Outcomes	Notes
ARTSCAN III (*Gebre-Medhin et al. JCO* 2021) Stage III/IV SCC *N* = 298	Radiation with concurrent cetuximab	Terminated early 3-y OS superior with cisplatin (78% vs 88%, *P* = .086) 3-y locoregional failure reduced with cisplatin (23% vs 9%, *P* = .0036)	Cetuximab arm had higher locoregional failures and trended toward worse OS
	Radiation with concurrent cisplatin		
Unilateral RT in Tonsil Tumors			
MDACC (*Taku et al. IJROBP* 2022) Retrospective Tonsillar ca (98% HPV+) *N* = 403	Primary site and ipsilateral levels II-IV and VII for node negative Primary + ipsilateral levels IB-IV and VII for node-positive patients	Median follow-up of 5.8 y 3% w/ neck failure (1% ipsilateral, 2% contralateral) The 5-y LC = 97% RC = 96% N2b patients cont' recurrence = 3%	85% were node positive, with 14% N2a and 45% N2b. 52% received postoperative treatment, and 32.5% received concurrent chemotherapy
PMH study (*Huang et al. IJROBP* 2017) RR T1-T2N0-N2b stratified by HPV status *N* = 379	Unilateral RT	Median follow-up 5.03 Regional control not different between HPV+ or HPV− 5-y contralateral neck failures were 2%	Deeper invasion requires caution

SINONASAL AND NASOPHARYNX

RAMEZ KOUZY • JAY REDDY

BACKGROUND

Nasopharynx

- **Incidence/prevalence:** Estimated 3000-4000 cases per year in the United States annually with 0.5-2 cases per 100 000. Endemic in East Asia and North Africa with rates at 25 cases per 100 000
- **Outcomes:** 5-Year survival estimated 38-72% (stage I-IV) (SEER data)
- **Demographics:** Median age 55, endemic to Southern China, common in North Africa and the Middle East
- **Risk factors:** Endemic regions: Male sex (RR 2-3), EBV, and preserved and smoked foods; nonendemic: smoking and alcohol

Sinonasal

- **Incidence/prevalence:** Incidence 0.56 per 100 000, estimated 2000 cases per year in the United States annually, nasal cavity and maxillary sinus most common
- **Outcomes:** 5-Year survival estimated 35-63% (stage I-IV) (SEER data)
- **Demographics:** Median age 50-60; higher frequency of cases in Japan and South Africa
- **Risk factors:** Male sex, environmental/occupational exposures (eg, wood dust, glues, adhesives), smoking, HPV, retinoblastoma

TUMOR BIOLOGY AND CHARACTERISTICS

Nasopharynx

- **Pathology:**
  - Keratinizing (WHO I): Most common sporadic form (25% United States, 2% endemic)
  - Nonkeratinizing differentiated (WHO II): (12% United States, 3% endemic)

- Nonkeratinizing undifferentiated (WHO III): Commonly associated with endemic disease and has favorable prognosis (63% United States, 95% endemic)
- Basaloid: Rare with aggressive clinical course

Sinonasal

- **Pathology:** Squamous cell carcinoma is the most common, but adenocarcinoma, melanoma, adenoid cystic carcinoma, olfactory neuroblastoma (esthesioneuroblastoma), angiosarcoma, mucoepidermoid, and sinonasal undifferentiated carcinoma (SNUC) are also seen.

Anatomy

Nasopharynx

- Anterior border: Nasal cavity posterior to the choana
- Lateral border: Torus tubarius, pharyngeal recess (fossa of Rosenmüller)
- Superior border: Clivus
- Posterior border: Clivus/occipital bone, C1/C2 vertebral bodies
- Inferior border: Soft palate
- Lymph node drainage:
  - RP nodes
  - Jugular chain (levels II-IV)
  - Spinal accessory nodes (level V)
  - See the **Oral Cavity** chapter for neck LN description.
- Local invasion:

Extension	Potential Anatomical Invasion Site
Lateral	Eustachian tube occlusion (causing hearing loss), masticator space
Inferior	Oropharynx
Anterior	Nasal cavity
Superior	Base of the skull (clivus), sphenoid sinus, intracranial through clivus or adjacent foramina, foramen lacerum (easy access to intracranial), foramen ovale and rotundum (V3 and V2 deficits), cavernous sinus (abducens nerve (VI) and III), temporal lobe (very advanced cases)
Posterior	Prevertebral muscle, adjacent bone (inferior clivus, C1), brainstem impingement or adjacent posterior cranial nerves (IX-XII)

Sinonasal

- Includes the nasal cavity and the paranasal sinuses (maxillary, ethmoid, sphenoid, and frontal)
- The nasal cavity:
  - Anterior border: Limen nasi and nasal vestibule
  - Posterior border: Choana
  - Lateral border: Maxillary sinus
  - Inferior border: Hard palate of the oral cavity
  - Superior: Frontal sinus and cribriform plate
  - The borders of the sinuses are complex. The main point is that they all abut the orbit and also are in close proximity to the brain.
- Lymph node drainage:
  - Nasal vestibule: Submandibular, facial, preauricular, can be bilateral
  - Nasal cavity and ethmoid sinuses: Retropharyngeal and levels I-II
  - Maxillary sinus drains to levels I-II; tumors with premaxillary space or skin involvement can drain to buccal and facial nodes.
  - See **Oral Cavity** chapter for neck LN description.
- Local invasion:
  - Orbital structures, bones of the hard palate, nasal meatus, cribriform plate, dura, brain, clivus, and middle cranial fossa

Workup

- **History and physical:** Assess presenting symptoms including cranial nerve dysfunction. Direct visualization of tumor and adjacent subsites with nasolaryngoscope.
- **Labs:** CBC and CMP; consider EBV virus titers pre- and posttherapy.
- **Procedures/biopsy:** Biopsy of primary and FNA of enlarged LNs as clinically indicated

- **Imaging:** CT with contrast of the head and neck/skull base to evaluate bony invasion and LN involvement. MRI with contrast of the head and neck/skull base to evaluate soft tissue component and cranial nerve involvement. Consider CT of the chest. FDG-PET/CT is recommended for stage III/IV disease.
- **Additional consultations:** Multidisciplinary evaluation with head and neck surgical oncology, radiation oncology, medical oncology, nutrition, and dental (fluoride/extractions). Consider ophthalmologic and endocrine evaluation.

TREATMENT ALGORITHM

Nasopharynx

Stage I	Definitive RT alone
Stage II-IVa	Concurrent chemoRT ± adjuvant chemotherapy *OR* induction chemotherapy followed by concurrent chemoRT
Stage IVb	Chemotherapy alone or concurrent chemoRT

TREATMENT ALGORITHM

Sinonasal: ethmoid sinus and nasal cavity

T1-T2	Definitive RT alone or surgical resection followed by (RT ± chemo[a]) or (observation[b])
T3-T4a	ChemoRT or surgical resection followed by RT ± chemo
T4b	ChemoRT or RT alone

[a]Indications for postoperative chemoRT: positive margins, intracranial extension, ENE
[b]For select T1N0 tumors centrally located, low grade, and with negative margins

Consider systemic therapy for all patients with sinonasal undifferentiated carcinoma (SNUC), small cell neuroendocrine carcinoma (SNEC), or small cell tumors.

Sinonasal-maxillary sinus

T1-T2, N0	Surgical resection followed by (RT ± chemo[a]) or (observation) or (reresection[b])
T3-T4a	Surgical resection[c] followed by RT ± chemo
T4b, any N	ChemoRT or RT alone

[a]Indications for postoperative RT: PNI, positive margins, intracranial extension, adenoid cystic histology, ENE, T3/T4 disease. No phase III clinical trials to guide recommendations, follows other H&N SCC recommendations.
[b]For positive margins, if feasible. Follow with RT ± chemo
[c]Add neck dissection for any node-positive disease.

Consider systemic therapy for all patients with sinonasal undifferentiated carcinoma (SNUC), small cell neuroendocrine carcinoma (SNEC), or small cell tumors.

RADIATION TREATMENT TECHNIQUE

- **Dose/target:**
  - **Nasopharynx (Definitive, Fig. 25.1)**
  - *Gross disease* (CTV_{HD}):
    - *Dose:* 70 Gy in 33-35 fractions, daily
    - *Target:* GTV (tumor + involved nodes) + 5- to 8-mm margin (margins may be tighter if GTV abuts critical neural structures)
  - Intermediate risk (CTV_{ID}):
    - *Dose:* 59.4-63 Gy in 33-35 fractions
    - *Target nasopharynx*: Entire nasopharynx, RP nodes, clivus (anterior 1/2 if uninvolved, entire clivus if involved), pterygoid fossa, parapharyngeal space, sphenoid sinus (inferior 1/2 if uninvolved, entire if involved or cavernous sinus disease), posterior 1/3 of maxillary sinus and nasal cavity, cavernous sinus in locally advanced disease, and skull base (rotundum, ovale, lacerum)
    - *Target neck (excludes neck covered by CTV_{HD})*: In the positive neck, cover the remaining neck level in the axial plane not covered in CTV_{HD} and 2 cm cranially and caudally.

- Low risk (CTV_{ED}):
  - Dose: 54-56 Gy in 33-35 fractions
  - Target *(excludes neck covered by CTV_{HD} and CTV_{ID})*: In the N0, neck levels II-IV should be covered. In the involved neck levels IB-V, the bilateral RPs should be covered.
- *PTV expansion*: 3-5 mm depending on the setup and IGRT
- **Sinonasal**

Definitive:	***Postoperative:***
High-risk or gross disease (CTV_{HD}): • *Dose:* 66-70 Gy in 33-35 fractions • *Target:* GTV (gross tumor + involved LNs) + 5- to 8-mm margin unless constrained by critical normal tissues *Intermediate risk (CTV_{ID}):* • *Dose:* 60 Gy in 30 fractions, 63 Gy in 33-35 fractions • *Target:* entire disease subsite, include nerves to skull base if PNI or adenoid cystic histology, ipsilateral involved nodal levels if N+, cribriform plate if esthesioneuroblastoma or ethmoid sinus involvement *Low risk (CTV_{ED}):* • *Dose:* 54 Gy in 30 fractions, 56 Gy in 33-35 fractions • *Target:* Uninvolved neck nodal levels (see Anatomy section)	*High risk (CTV_{HD}):* • *Dose:* 60 Gy in 30 fractions to preoperative tumor bed with 1- to 2-cm margins • *Consider 3-6 Gy boost target:* Positive margins and gross nodal disease + 5- to 8-mm margin *Intermediate risk (CTV_{ID}):* • *Dose:* 57 Gy in 30 fractions • *Target:* operative bed including primary and LN operative areas. Include the entire flap if utilized *Low risk (CTV_{ED}):* • *Dose:* 54 Gy in 30 fractions • *Target:* Uninvolved neck nodal levels (if at risk, dependent on site and histology); cover nerve pathways to base of skull (or beyond) dependent on histology and extent of PNI

- *PTV expansion:* 3-5 mm depending on setup
- **Technique:** IMRT with 6-MV photons is preferred; option to consider matched low-neck field of 40 Gy in 20 fractions with larynx block, followed by 10 Gy in 5 fractions with full midline block; however, IMRT/VMAT plans with larynx avoidance may achieve excellent dosimetric results. Start postoperative cases within 6 weeks of surgery.
- **SIM:** Supine, thermoplastic mask, shoulder pull straps. Mouth-opening tongue-depressing stent (with space to fill cavities in maxillary sinus cancers, may optimize position to displace tissues that don't need treatment, posterior head cradle, isocenter at arytenoids). Consider adding MR simulation, and/or fuse previous MRI imaging.
- **IGRT:** Daily kV imaging, cone beam CT
- **Planning directive (for conventional fractionation)**
  Brainstem: General goal Max < 45 Gy; proximity of targets may require higher dose, and constraint can be set at 54 Gy.
  Spinal cord: Max < 45 Gy
  Parotids: Mean < 26 Gy
  Mandible: Less than prescribed dose to CTV_{HD}
  Brachial plexus: Max < 66 Gy if treating adjacent disease; otherwise Max < 60 max
  Larynx: Mean < 30 Gy or ALARA
  Esophagus: Mean < 30 Gy
  Oral cavity: Max < 40 Gy
  Optic nerves/chiasm: Max < 54 Gy

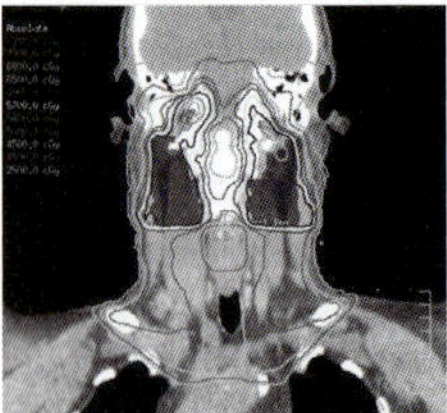

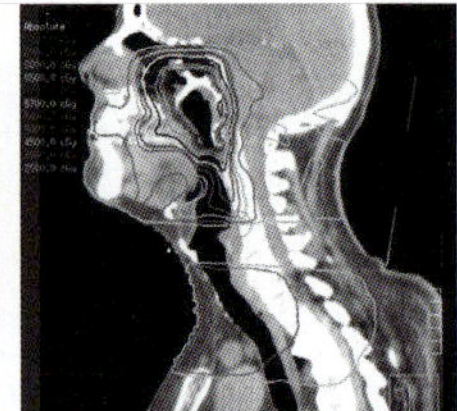

Figure 25.1 Definitive chemoradiation planning showing treatment IMRT treating to 70 Gy to CTV_{HD} and 59.4 Gy to CTV_{ID}. A 3D conformal field is treating 45 Gy to the low neck.

Chemotherapy

Nasopharynx

- **Concurrent:** Cisplatin 30-40 mg/m^2 weekly or 100 mg/m^2 on days 1, 22, and 43 (cumulative cisplatin dose goal 200 mg/m^2); carboplatin can be used in patients who cannot tolerate or have contraindication to cisplatin.
- **Adjuvant:** Cisplatin 80 mg/m^2 weekly + 5-FU 1000 mg/m^2 q4wk × three cycles
- **Induction:** No defined standard of care; possible regimens include
  Cisplatin + gemcitabine (Top choice)
  Docetaxel + cisplatin ± 5-FU
  Cisplatin + 5-FU
  Cisplatin + epirubicin + paclitaxel

Sinonasal

- **Concurrent:** Cisplatin 30-40 mg/m^2 weekly or 100 mg/m^2 on days 1, 22, and 43 (cumulative cisplatin dose goal 200 mg/m^2); carboplatin can be used in patients who cannot tolerate or have contraindication to cisplatin. Can consider cetuximab

Side Effect Management

See **Oral Cavity** chapter.

Follow-up

- First posttreatment follow-up at 8 weeks with MRI and/or CT imaging.
- Consider PET/CT at 12 weeks if suspicion for persistent disease or lack of response.
- Consider neck dissection for PET-positive lymph nodes with >1 cm of residual primary disease.
- History/physical with nasopharyngoscopy: Every 3-4 months for years 1-3 → every 6 months for years 4-5
- Thyroid function tests every 6 months
- Can consider EBV titer monitoring if initially positive pretreatment for nasopharyngeal
- Consider longer-term follow-up for esthesioneuroblastoma as recurrence can occur >15 years after primary treatment.

Notable Studies

Name/Inclusion	Arms	Outcomes	Notes
Nasopharynx			
Benefit of ChemoRT Over RT Alone			
Intergroup-0099 (*Al-Sarraf et al. JCO* 1998) Phase III RCT Stage III-IV NPC *N* = 147	Definitive RT Concurrent cisplatin/RT + adjuvant cisplatin	Concurrent cisplatin/RT + adjuvant cisplatin demonstrated improved 3-y PFS: 24% vs 69% ($P < .001$) and OS: 46% vs 78% ($P = .005$)	Established 70 Gy in 1.8-2 Gy/fx, 66 Gy for involved nodes, and 50 Gy for elective nodes as standard with concurrent chemo
Singapore phase II (*Wee et al. JCO* 2005) Phase II randomized controlled study Stage III-IV NPC *N* = 221	Definitive RT Concurrent cisplatin/RT + adjuvant cisplatin	Concurrent cisplatin/RT + adjuvant cisplatin demonstrated improved 2-y OS (78% vs 85%; HR = 0.51, $P = .0061$)	Confirmed the results of Intergroup-0099 in an endemic (Asian) population
MAC-NPC meta-analysis (*Blanchard et al. Lancet Oncol* 2015) 19 trials *N* = 4806	Concomitant CRT RT alone	Benefit with CRT: 10-y OS benefit 9.9% 10-y PFS benefit of 9.5% No OS benefit for induction or adjuvant	

Name/Inclusion	Arms	Outcomes	Notes
Benefit of IMRT for Nasopharynx Cancer			
Kam et al. JCO 2007 RCT T1-T2b N0-N1 M0 NPC *N* = 60	IMRT 2DCRT	1 y after RT, patients in the IMRT arm had lower rates of xerostomia (39.3% vs 82.1%, *P* = .001)	66 Gy in 33 fractions to gross tumor and 60-54 Gy to the node-negative regions
***Pow et al. IJROBP* 2006** RCT T2N0-1M0 NPC *N* = 51	IMRT Conventional RT	IMRT significantly improves quality of life (*P* < .001) Most significant improvement in xerostomia-related symptoms at 12 mo for IMRT group	
Induction Chemotherapy			
GORTEC NPC 2006 (*Huang et al. Eur J Cancer* 2015) RCT Advanced NPC *N* = 408	Induction followed by CRT Induction followed by RT	No OS benefit (50.4% vs 48.8% *P* = .71) No LRF benefit (79% vs 82.5%, *P* = .41) No distant failure-free survival benefit (67.7% vs 66.1%, *P* = .90)	No significant survival differences were found between the IC + CCRT and IC + RT arms at 10 y
***Sun et al. Lancet Oncol* 2016** Phase III multicenter RCT Locally advanced NPC *N* = 480	Induction TPF (cisplatin, fluorouracil, docetaxel) + chemoRT (cisplatin) ChemoRT alone	3-y failure-free survival improved in the induction group (80% vs 72%, *P* = .034)	Induction TPF + chemoRT may improve outcomes compared to chemoRT alone in locally advanced cases
***Cao et al. Eur J Cancer* 2017** Phase III multicenter RCT Locoregionally advanced NPC *N* = 476	Induction (cisplatin, fluorouracil) + chemoRT (cisplatin) ChemoRT alone	Induction chemotherapy improved 3-y DFS (82% vs 74%, *P* = .028), DMFS (86% vs 82%, *P* = .056) No difference in OS (88.2% vs 88.5%, *P* = .815) and locoregional relapse-free survival (94.3% vs 90.8%, *P* = .430)	There was a significant (*P* < .001) increase in grade 3-4 toxicity in the induction arm
***Zhang et al. NEJM* 2019** Phase III multicenter RCT Locoregionally advanced NPC *N* = 480	Induction gemcitabine-cisplatin + CRT Concurrent CRT	Improvement in 3-y RFS (85.3% vs 76.5%, *P* = 0.001) and OS (94.6% vs 90.3%) with an OS HR of 0.43 (*P* < .05) Higher G3-G4 toxicity in the induction arm	Median follow-up: 42.7 mo

Name/Inclusion	Arms	Outcomes	Notes
Adjuvant Chemotherapy			
***Chen et al. Eur J Cancer* 2017** Phase III multicenter RCT Locoregionally advanced NPC *N* = 251	CRT CRT + adjuvant chemo	No significant difference in 5-y failure-free survival (adjuvant 75% vs no adjuvant 71%, *P* = .45) Late grade 3 or 4 toxicity (adjuvant 27% vs no adjuvant 21%, *P* = .14)	Long-term outcomes Chemo: cisplatin
Sinonasal Proton Beam Therapy			
***Yu et al. Adv Radiat Oncol* 2019** Multi-institutional RR Sinonasal tumors *N* = 69	Comparison of 42 patients receiving initial treatment and 27 receiving retreatment	De novo RT had a 100% 3-y OS rate, 84% FFDP rate, and 77% FFLR rate Retreatment had a 3-y OS rate of 76.2%, a FFDP rate of 32.1%, and a FFLR rate of 33.8%	15% of patients with late toxicity, no severe toxicities or complications
Induction Chemotherapy in SNUC			
MDACC (*Amit et al. JCO* 2019) Prospective cohort SNUC *N* = 95	Induction chemo followed definitive locoregional therapy	5-y disease-specific survival (DSS) rate of 59% Patients who responded well to induction chemo had higher 5-y DSS rates with CRT vs surgery followed by RT or CRT (81% vs 54%, *P* = .001) Patient who did not respond well had lower 5-y DSS rates with CRT vs surgery followed by RT or CRT (0% vs 39%, adjusted hazard ratio 5.68, 95% CI 2.89-9.36)	

LARYNX AND HYPOPHARYNX

ALAN SOSA • AMY MORENO

BACKGROUND

- **Incidence/prevalence:** Approximately 12 470 laryngeal cancers and ~2000-4000 hypopharyngeal cancers annually in the United States in 2022
- **Outcomes:** 5-Year survival across all stages estimated at ~60% for larynx (45% for supraglottis, 77% glottis, 49% subglottis) and 37% for hypopharynx (SEER data)
- **Demographics:** Majority of patients are male and associated with advanced age (>60).
- **Risk factors:** Larynx cancer—smoking is associated with most cases; in nonsmokers, GERD is associated with larynx cancer. Hypopharyngeal cancer—in addition to smoking, alcohol abuse, chronic voice strain, vitamin C and iron deficiencies (Plummer-Vinson syndrome), and prior head and neck malignancy particularly if the patient received prior head and neck radiation

Tumor Biology and Characteristics

- **Pathology:** Majority are squamous cell carcinomas (>95%). Minority of cases are HPV associated (hypopharynx). In larynx cancer, invasive cancer can progress from leukoplakia or erythroplakia (premalignant lesions).
- **Symptoms:** Hoarseness, sore throat, dysphagia, odynophagia, globus sensation in the throat, referred otalgia from branch of cranial nerve X (Arnold nerve), and asymptomatic neck mass

Anatomy

- The larynx consists of three sites each with multiple subsites (Fig. 26.1):
  - *Supraglottis* (suprahyoid and infrahyoid epiglottis, aryepiglottic folds, arytenoids, false vocal folds, and ventricles)
  - *Glottis* (true vocal cords including anterior/posterior commissures, 5 mm inferior to free margin of true cords)
  - *Subglottis* (lower boundary of the glottis to the inferior aspect of the cricoid cartilage). Site incidence: Glottis (65-70%) > supraglottis (25-30%) > subglottis (2%)
- The hypopharynx consists of the pyriform sinuses, the posterior pharyngeal wall, and the postcricoid area (3 Ps). Site incidence: Pyriform sinus (75%) > posterior pharyngeal wall (20%) > postcricoid (5%) (Fig. 26.1)

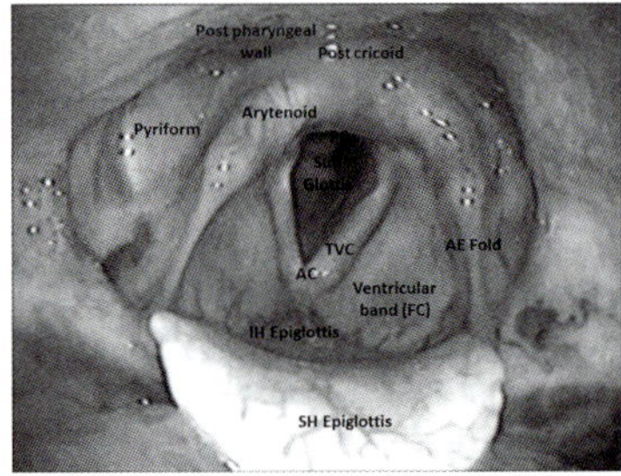

Figure 26.1 Larynx and hypopharynx structures. AC, anterior commissure; AE, aryepiglottic; FC, false cord; IH, infrahyoid; PC, posterior commissure; SH, suprahyoid; TVC, true vocal cord. (Reprinted by permission from Dr. Rahmat Omar.)

Workup

- **History and physical:** Assess presenting symptoms; assess voice quality, swallow function, breathing, and ability to protect airway. Visualization of tumor and adjacent subsites with nasolaryngoscope and/or mirror exam to assess disease spread. Consider videostroboscopy. Palpate the thyroid to evaluate for pain as it may be indicative of cartilage invasion.
- **Labs:** CBC, CMP
- **Procedures/biopsy:** Biopsy of primary and FNA of enlarged LNs as clinically indicated
- **Imaging:** CT or MRI with contrast with thin-angled cuts through the larynx. Evaluation of cartilage invasion and infiltration of adjacent subsites. Consider CT of the chest. FDG-PET/CT recommended for stage III/IV disease
- **Additional consultations:** Multidisciplinary evaluation with head and neck surgical oncology, radiation oncology, medical oncology, speech/swallow (swallowing exercise regime), nutrition, and dental (fluoride/extractions)

Larynx and Hypopharynx Staging (*AJCC 8th Edition* 2018)

- The different sites of the larynx have different T staging.

Larynx Treatment Algorithm

Stages I-II	Definitive RT[a], laser cordectomy, or partial laryngectomy Add concurrent chemotherapy if bulky T2
Stages III-V	Definitive CRT alone *or* Total laryngectomy + LND → RT[b] or CRT[c] Note: definitive CRT should not be offered to patients who have impaired larynx function.

[a]Consider altered fractionation (DAHANCA 70/35 in 6 weeks) for T2 treated with definitive RT.
[b]pT3/pT4, pN2/N3, PNI/LVSI, subglottic extension, thyroid cartilage invasion
[c]Positive margins, ENE

Hypopharynx Treatment Algorithm

T1-T2	Definitive RT or partial pharyngectomy Add concurrent chemotherapy if bulky T2
T3 and/or N+	Good glottis function (eg, no dysphagia or other symptoms): Definitive CRT alone *or* Induction chemotherapy → concurrent CRT or surgery if less than partial response to induction Poor glottis function (eg, dysphagia and other symptoms): Consider pharyngolaryngectomy → RT ± concurrent chemo
T4	Total pharyngoesophagectomy → RT or CRT

Radiation Treatment Technique

Early-stage glottic

- **Dose:**
  T1: 63 Gy in 28 fractions at 2.25 Gy/fx or 66 Gy in 33 fractions
  T2: 70 Gy in 35 fractions at 2 Gy/fx or 65.25 at 2.25 Gy/fx; mild acceleration for 35 fx (bid once per week to complete treatment in 6 weeks)
  Factors that influence local control (especially T2): (1) Fraction size 2.25 Gy > 2 >> 1.8 Gy (Le *et al. IJROBP* 1997), (2) overall treatment time ≤ 43 days (Le *et al. IJROBP* 1997), and (3) altered fractionation increases local control ~10% in T2N0 disease (Trotti *et al. IJROBP* 2014; DAHANCA—*Overgaard et al. Lancet* 2003).

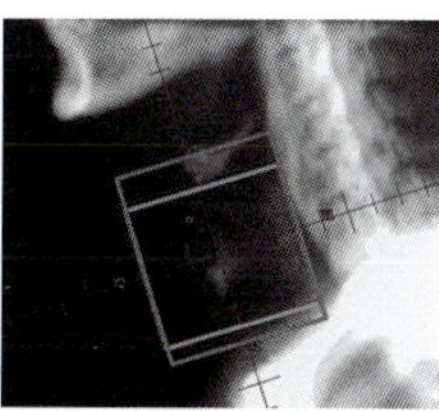

Figure 26.2 Classic early-stage glottic fields. *Smaller box* represents T1 lateral field. *Larger box* represents T2 lateral field.

- **Target:**
  3D Fields
  T1: Entire glottic larynx, anteriorly flash 1 cm, posteriorly cover to anterior edge of vertebral bodies, superiorly cover to top of thyroid cartilage, and inferiorly cover to bottom of cricoid cartilage (Fig. 26.2).
  T2: Same as T1 with adjustments superiorly and/or inferiorly if T2 based on supraglottic or subglottic extension. Typically, with conventional techniques field border 2 cm above or below GTV

IMRT Volumes
  - **Whole larynx:** CTV covers entire larynx including glottis (TVCs, anterior and posterior commissures), part of supraglottis (FVCs, arytenoids) down to caudal edge of cricoid.
  - **Narrow field (partial larynx)**: CTV covers partial larynx including involved TVC/FVC, anterior commissure, anterior half of contralateral TVC/FVC. Sup/inf borders are the same as whole larynx.
- **Technique**:
  - **3DCRT:** Right and left opposed laterals
  - **IMRT/VMAT: Can consider IMRT for carotid sparing** (Rosenthal *et al. IJROBP* 2010)

- **SIM:** Supine w/ neck neutral to hyperextended, Aquaplast mask covering the head and shoulders, isocenter in midlarynx. Pull straps for shoulder retraction. Consider thin bolus for patients with anterior disease. Patient should be reminded not to swallow during simulation or treatment as this can cause distortion of anatomy.
- **IGRT:** Daily kV imaging; daily CBCT for partial field larynx

ADVANCED STAGE GLOTTIC, SUPRAGLOTTIC, SUBGLOTTIC, AND HYPOPHARYNGEAL

- **Dose:**
  Primary tumor and involved nodes:
  70 Gy in 33-35 fractions (high dose, CTV_{HD}) (Fig. 26.3)
  - **Supraglottis/hypopharynx T1 | T2:** 66 Gy/33 fx | 70/35 (bid 1/wk)
  - **Larynx (advanced) T3-T4:** 70 Gy in 35 fractions chemoRT
    Intermediate-risk regions (involved nodal level and disease adjacent mucosa): 60-63 Gy (intermediate dose, CTV_{ID})
    Subclinical disease (at-risk nodal levels): 56-57 Gy in 33-35 fractions (low dose, CTV_{ED})
- **Target:** Primary tumor with 8-mm to 1-cm CTV margin, anatomically confined, and involved nodes (~5-mm margin) receive high dose (CTV_{HD}). Traditionally, majority of the larynx should be included in CTV_{HD}. Adjacent at-risk tissue and involved nodal levels receive intermediate-risk subclinical dose (CTV_{ID}). Uninvolved at-risk nodal levels receive low-risk subclinical dose (CTV_{ED}) (levels II-IV, VI, include IB and V in LN+ hemineck, include bilateral RP nodes in hypopharyngeal cancers).
- **Technique:** IMRT or VMAT. Scanning beam proton therapy can be used in experienced centers.
- **SIM:** Same as for early larynx
- **IGRT:** Daily kV imaging, consider weekly CBCT

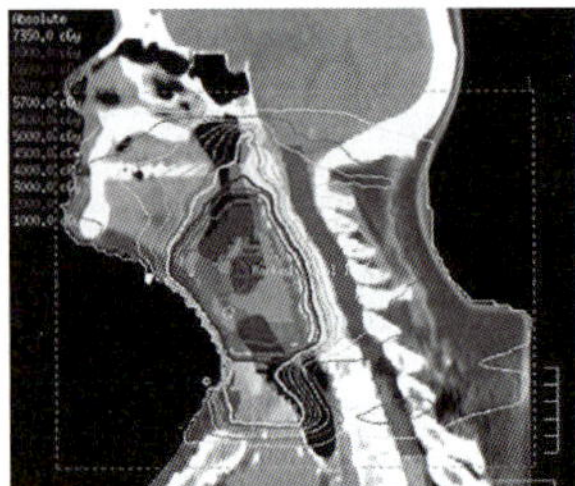
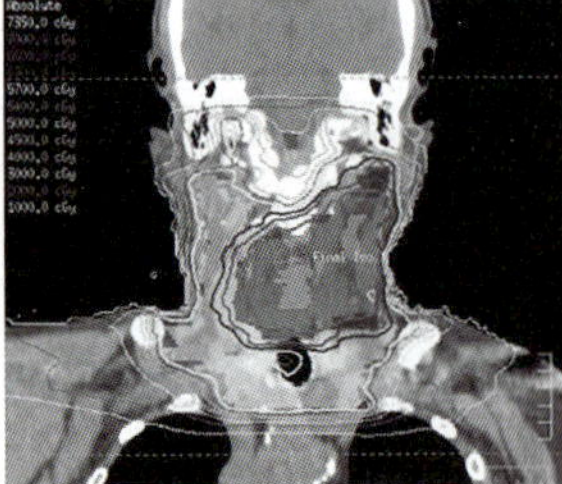

Figure 26.3 Representative VMAT treatment plan of patient with hypopharyngeal cancer involving structures of the larynx including epiglottis. Note extensive elective LN coverage. Inner RT field shows high-risk dose (CTV_{HD}) treated to 70 Gy and intermediate-dose CTV (CTV_{ID}) treated to 63 Gy. The outer RT field shows low-dose CTV treated to 57 Gy.

LYMPH NODE DRAINAGE

- Supraglottic cancers most commonly spread to levels II, III, and IV LNs. Glottic cancers have almost no LN drainage, so LNs are not covered for stage I disease and rarely in stage II disease. Subglottic cancers can involve level VI nodes (Fig. 26.4).
- Hypopharyngeal cancers are richly drained by lymphatics, and ~75% have nodal involvement at diagnosis. Levels II, III, IV, and V and RP LNs are most commonly involved and should be covered when planning RT. Will often cover level VI as well.
- See **Oral Cavity** chapter for neck LN description.

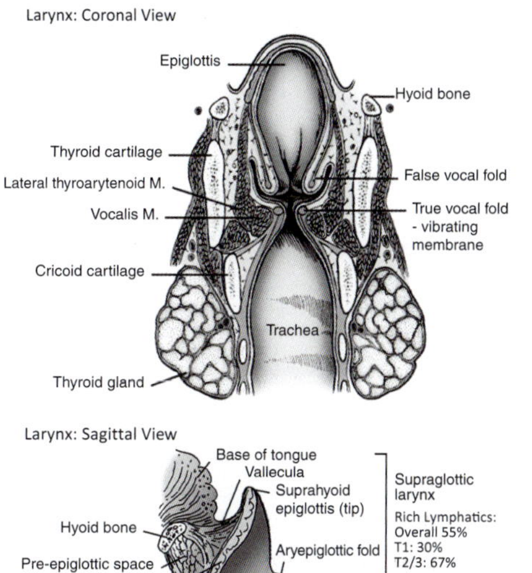

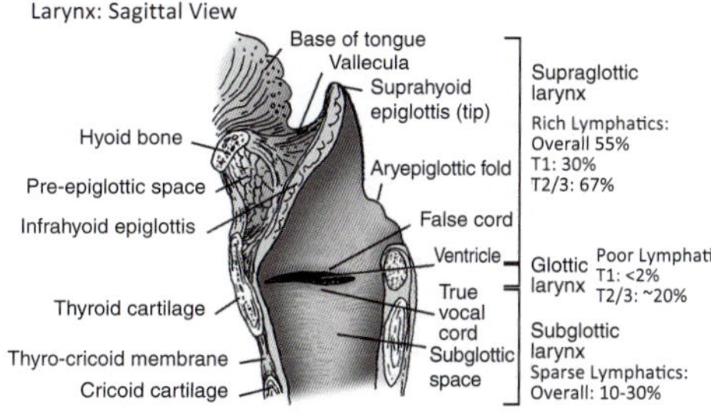

Figure 26.4 Lymph node involvement of laryngeal cancer based on site. (**Top:** Reprinted from Garrett CG, Ossoff RH. Hoarseness. *Med Clin N Am*. 1999;83(1):115-123. Copyright © 1999 Elsevier. With permission. **Bottom:** Reproduced with permission from Koch WM, Machtay M, Best S. Treatment of early (stage I and II) head and neck cancer: The larynx. In: UpToDate, Post TW, ed. *UpToDate*, Waltham, MA: Copyright © 2019 UpToDate, Inc. For more information visit www.uptodate.com.)

Postoperative

- **Target/dose: Region of resected gross disease:** 60 Gy in 2 Gy fractions (high dose, CTV_{HD}), 66 Gy in 2 Gy fractions for positive margins (+concurrent chemo) **Operative bed of primary and LNs:** 57 Gy (intermediate dose, CTV_{ID}) **Nondissected at-risk regions including nondissected at-risk nodal levels:** 54 Gy (low dose, CTV_{ED}). Include stoma if subglottic/anterior soft tissue extension or if emergent tracheostomy was performed.
- **Technique:** IMRT or VMAT. Scanning beam proton therapy can be used in capable centers.
- **SIM:** Same as above. Wiring scars helps define the operative bed. Especially if there was neck disease with ENE, consider bolus for scars, and consider bolus for stoma if at increased risk due to disease proximity.
- **IGRT**: Daily kV imaging, consider weekly CBCT
- **Planning directive (for conventional fractionation):**

PTV	>95% coverage
Spinal cord	Max < 45 Gy
Brainstem	Max < 54 Gy
Optic nerve	Max < 54 Gy
Temporal lobe	D_{max} < 60 Gy, D0.03 cc < 70 Gy
Brachial plexus	D_{max} < 66 Gy

Mandible	Max < 70 Gy or Max less than prescription dose to CTV_{HD}
Total lung	V20 < 30%; mean < 20 Gy
Cochlea	Max < 35 Gy
Lens	Max < 5 Gy
Parotids	Mean < 26 Gy, V30 < 50%, lower for contralateral
Larynx	Mean < 35 Gy (part of target for larynx cancer)
Cervical esophagus	Mean < 35 Gy

Special Circumstances

- **Indications for neck dissection after definitive RT or CRT:** Persistent neck disease. Avoid treatment of brachial plexus to doses >66 Gy. If nodal disease is adjacent to brachial plexus, consider treating disease to 60-64 Gy with a planned nodal dissection.

Surgery

- Endoscopic resection: For early-stage tumors—done either via a transoral laser microsurgery (TLM) technique or transoral robotic surgery (TORS) technique. Preserves the larynx. Compared to RT, results in equivalent oncologic outcomes, but voice outcomes may not be as good as RT (controversial).
- Total laryngectomy: Resection of the entire larynx including all three substructures (supraglottis, glottis, subglottis) and creation of a stoma to provide a method for the patient to breathe. Requires total thyroidectomy. Primary closure is usually possible.
- Pharyngolaryngectomy: Resection of the entire larynx including all three substructures (supraglottis, glottis, subglottis) and partial resection of the soft tissues of the pharynx. May include partial esophageal resection based on involvement. Performed for bulky hypopharyngeal cancers, used sparingly secondary to morbidity. Requires creation of a stoma, total thyroidectomy, and typically requires a flap resection of pharyngeal structures

Chemotherapy

- **Concurrent:**
  Weekly IV cisplatin at a dose of 40 mg/m^2 *or*
  IV cisplatin 100 mg/m^2 every 3 weeks (days 1, 22, and 43) of RT
  If the patient cannot tolerate cisplatin secondary to toxicity, weekly carboplatin or cetuximab can be considered.
- **Neoadjuvant:** Most common regimen is TPF (docetaxel, cisplatin, 5-fluorouracil). Consists of docetaxel at a dose of 75 mg/m^2, administered as a 1-hour infusion on day 1; followed by cisplatin at a dose of 75 mg/m^2, administered as a 1-hour infusion on day 1; and fluorouracil at a dose of 750 mg/m^2, administered by continuous infusion on days 1 to 5 (*Vermorken et al. NEJM* 2007). Can give up to 4 cycles every 3 weeks. Primarily used for downstaging prior to RT, *NO* survival advantages.
- **Adjuvant:** No role.

Side Effect Management

See **Oral Cavity** chapter.

Follow-up

- General: History/physical with nasolaryngoscopy, TSH, T4, BUN, Cr, CT, or MRI (use the same imaging as pretreatment): q3mo at year 1 → q4mo at year 2 → q6mo at years 3-5 → annually after year 5. PET/CT as baseline posttherapy evaluation ~12 weeks posttreatment, particularly in the node-positive patient treated definitively.
- Annual CXR: Screening for metastases and second primary
- For early-stage glottic cancers, imaging is not needed; just use videostroboscopy and regular follow-up with MD.
- If PEG tube is placed, follow-up with speech pathology and nutrition. Goal to achieve >3 weeks of full and adequate PO intake with no tube use prior to removal; verify with nutritionist for removal.

NOTABLE TRIALS

Name/Inclusion	Arms	Outcomes*	Notes
	Early-Stage Glottic		
Hypofrac T1N0 (*Yamazaki et al. IJROBP* 2006) PRT T1N0 glottic larynx carcinoma treated with definitive RT (N = 180)	**Definitive RT 2 Gy/fx** Tumor length < 2/3 glottis: 60 Gy Tumor length ≥ 2/3 glottis: 66 Gy **Definitive RT 2.25 Gy/fx** Tumor length < 2/3 glottis: 56.25 Gy Tumor length ≥ 2/3 glottis: 63 Gy	2 Gy/fx vs 2.25 Gy/fx 5-y LC: 77% vs 92% No difference in OS: 87% vs 88% No significant differences in acute mucosal reaction, skin reactions, or chronic toxicity Larger fraction sizes were associated with improved LC while maintaining similar rates of acute and late toxicity	80% were T1a Conventional arm had relatively low LC (77%) Technique: Parallel opposed fields, 4 MV
	Induction Chemotherapy for Larynx Preservation		
VA larynx trial (*Hong et al. Cancer Res* 1993; *Wolf et al. NEJM* 1991) Phase III RCT Stage III-IV laryngeal cancer, SCC (N = 332)	**Total laryngectomy → PORT** 60 Gy ± 5-14.2 Gy boost to any areas of presumed residual disease **Induction chemo 2C → + 1C chemo (if PR) → RT** Induction: cis/5-FU Primary: 66-76 Gy Nodes: 50-75 Gy (dosed according to size) Total laryngectomy if poor response	Tumor response after 2 cycles: • CR 31% • PR 54% (Surg vs def RT) **2-y OS:** 68% vs 68% **Primary site recurrence:** 2% vs 12% **DM:** 17% vs 11% **Overall larynx preservation**: 66% Induction chemo followed by definitive RT provides comparable OS and DFS with improved rates of larynx preservation (even at 5-y FU)	After definitive RT, patients with residual disease in the larynx underwent salvage TL Neck dissection for persistent disease in the neck T4 tumors had significantly higher salvage laryngectomy rates than < T4 tumors (56% vs 29%)

Name/Inclusion	Arms	Outcomes*	Notes
RTOG 91-11 (*Forastiere et al. NEJM* 2003; updates *JCO* 2006 and 2013) Phase III RCT Stage III glottis and supraglottis (*N* = 547)	**Arm 1** **Induction chemo 2C → + 1C chemo (if PR) → RT** Induction: cis/5-FU TL if poor response **Arm 2** **ChemoRT** Concurrent cisplatin **Arm 3** **RT alone**	Larynx preservation (LP) rate was improved with chemoRT vs induction arm (HR 0.58) **10-y LP:** 68% vs 82% vs 64% Both induction and chemoRT improved laryngectomy-free survival (LFS) over RT alone (HR 0.75 and HR 0.78, respectively) **10-y LFS:** 29%* vs 24%* vs 17% **10-y LRC:** Concurrent chemo improved LRC compared chemoRT and RT alone 49% vs 65% vs 47% **10-y OS** similar; slight trend toward better survival with induction over chemoRT 39% vs 28% vs 32%	All RT arms 70 Gy/35 fx 50 Gy/25 fx to elective neck and SCV Salvage total laryngectomy for Bx+ at 8 wk post RT Neck dissection for persistent disease in the neck

*Significant relative to RT alone.

SALIVARY GLAND NEOPLASMS

RAMEZ KOUZY • JACK PHAN

Background

- **Incidence/prevalence:** Malignant salivary gland tumors account for ~6% of all H&N malignancies. Annual incidence is ~1 per 100 000 (SEER). Peak incidence occurs during the sixth decade of life.
- **Outcomes:** 5-Year survival across all stages and sites is estimated at 70%.
- **Risk factors:** Prior radiation exposure, smoking (Warthin tumor), male sex, solvent exposure

Tumor Biology and Characteristics

- **Genetics:** t(11;19)(q21;p13) translocation creates a fusion oncogene (*CRTC1-MAML2*), which is associated with the development of mucoepidermoid carcinomas. t(6;9) translocations produce the *MYB-NFIB* fusion protein commonly observed in many adenoid cystic carcinomas. NTRK, EGFR, c-kit, and HER2 in salivary duct carcinomas
- **Pathology:**
  - 70% arise in the parotid gland; however, a majority of parotid tumors are benign.
  - Minor salivary glands are most likely malignant.

Histology	Characteristics
Mucoepidermoid	Most common, grade is prognostic
Adenoid cystic	Tubular is low grade, cribriform intermediate grade, while solid type is considered high grade. PNI common, high rate of distant lung met and known to have late recurrences

Histology	Characteristics
Acinic cell	Low grade
Adenocarcinoma	Low-grade polymorphous adenocarcinoma (aggressive) and salivary duct carcinoma
Salivary duct	High grade, M > F
Mixed malignant tumor (MMT)	Commonly have components resembling benign pleomorphic adenomas but despite this are often high grade

Anatomy

Gland	Borders	Associated Nerves
Parotid	Abuts the posterior mandibular ramus and is separated into superficial and deep lobes by the plane of the facial nerve	Sensory innervation by auriculotemporal nerve. Autonomic innervation by glossopharyngeal nerve (CN IX). Traversed by facial nerve (CN VII)
Submandibular	Located within the submandibular triangle and is bounded superiorly by the lower border of the mandible and inferiorly by the anterior belly of the digastric muscle	Innervation by chorda tympani via CN VII. The lingual nerve (CN V) passes superiorly over gland; the hypoglossal nerve (CN XII) passes inferiorly
Sublingual	Between mylohyoid and floor of mouth mucosa	Innervation by chorda tympani via CN VII, which unifies with lingual branch of mandibular nerve (CN V3)

- The intracranial facial nerve (four segments) arises from the base of the pons, traverses through internal auditory canal then through the temporal bone, and exits the skull base at the stylomastoid foramen. The extracranial facial nerve courses with the parotid gland providing motor supply to the face via the five major terminal branches but does not provide innervation to the gland.
- Lymph node involvement is less common for low- and intermediate-grade tumors compared to high-grade tumors. Primary drainage for parotid is to the periparotid nodes and ipsilateral submandibular and upper jugular nodes (primarily levels IB and II). See **Oral Cavity** chapter for neck LN description.

Workup

- **History and physical:** Head and neck evaluation with special attention to cranial nerve deficits particularly those involving CN V and CN VII. Direct palpation and visualization of tumor. Intraoral visualization for direct spread and to assess CN IX and XII. Consideration of nasolaryngoscope and/or mirror exam to evaluate for mucosal lesions. Major salivary gland masses may represent a lymph node metastasis from a separate primary site, specifically cutaneous squamous cell carcinoma of the skin; thus, consider a skin examination of the head and neck.
- **Labs:** CBC, CMP
- **Procedures/biopsy:** Biopsy of primary and FNA of enlarged LNs as clinically indicated
- **Imaging:** CT or MRI with contrast of the head/neck. MRI useful for evaluation of perineural spread and soft tissue component. CT useful for evaluation of bone invasion. Consider CT of the chest. Ultrasound can be useful for superficial tumors of the parotid or submandibular glands.
- **Additional consultations:** Multidisciplinary evaluation with head and neck surgical oncology, radiation oncology, medical oncology, nutrition, and dental (fluoride/extractions)

Minor Salivary Gland Staging (AJCC 8th edition)

Tumors arising in minor salivary glands are staged the same as a head and neck squamous cell carcinoma arising from the same anatomical location. For example, a minor salivary gland cancer arising from the tonsil region would be staged as an oropharynx cancer.

Surgery

- Surgical management is preferred with definitive radiotherapy reserved for patients who are not operative candidates or those with unresectable tumors.
- Patients with cN+ typically are treated with a planned neck dissection. While there is no consensus regarding the role of an elective neck dissection in all clinically N0 patients, it is generally recommended for those with high-grade histologies felt to be at highest risk of occult nodal disease.

Chemotherapy

- While the use of platinum agents is often extrapolated from other H&N sites, there is a lack of prospective data for use in salivary gland tumors (currently under investigation on RTOG 1008).
- Retrospective series have failed to demonstrate a survival benefit with adjuvant chemoradiotherapy vs radiotherapy alone in these patients (*Amini et al. JAMA Otolaryngol Head Neck Surg* 2016).

Indications for Postoperative Radiotherapy

- Extraglandular extension
- High-grade histology
- Close or positive surgical margins
- Perineural invasion
- Lymph node metastases
- Recurrent disease

Conventional Borders for Postoperative Radiation Fields

As a general rule of thumb, it is useful to use the contralateral intact gland as a reference in all patients. All borders listed below are contingent on tumor extent.

Parotid	
Superior	Zygomatic arch
Inferior	Hyoid
Anterior	Anterior edge of the masseter muscle
Posterior	Just behind the mastoid process
Submandibular	
Superior	Line extending from oral commissure to mandibular ramus just inferior to temporomandibular joint
Inferior	Thyroid notch; posterior belly of digastric muscle
Anterior	Determined by surgery. Shield oral commissure if possible
Posterior	Just behind the mastoid process
Medial	Anterior belly of digastric muscle

Modern Radiation Treatment Technique (Simultaneous Integrated Boost)

- **Dose: High risk** (CTV_{HD}): 60 Gy in 30 fractions at 2 Gy/fx (Fig. 27.1)
  **High-risk areas for residual disease (ECE, +margin) can be boosted to 66 Gy.*
  Intermediate risk (CTV_{ID}): 57 Gy (1.9 Gy/fx)
  Low risk/elective dose (CTV_{ED}): 54 Gy (1.8 Gy/fx)
- **Target:**
  CTV_{HD}: Primary and nodal tumor bed with 8- to 10-mm expansion
  CTV_{ID}: Remaining operative bed not included in CTV_{HD}
  CTV_{ED}: Ipsilateral neck levels II-IV in N0 patients with high-grade tumors, coverage of at-risk perineural tracks
- **Technique:** IMRT or IMPT
- **SIM:** Supine with head extended. Thermoplastic mask extending to the shoulders for immobilization. For parotid tumors, a tongue-lateralizing oral stent can help displace the tongue away from the target volume. Scan vertex to the carina.
- **IGRT:** Daily 2D kV orthogonal imaging or cone beam CT

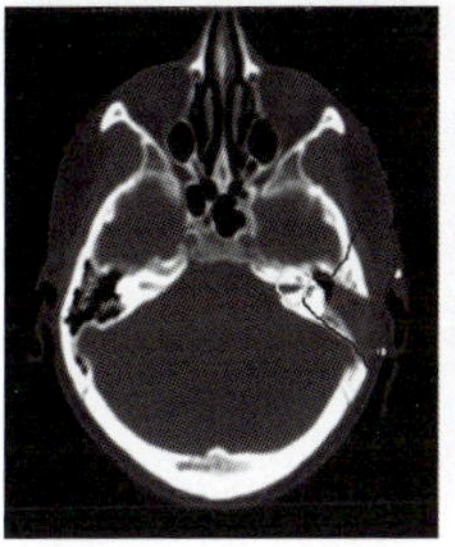

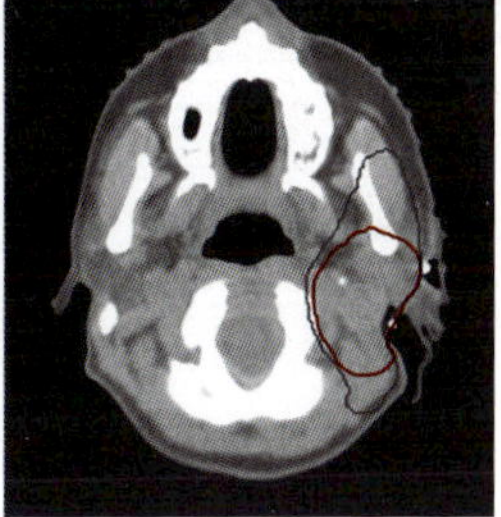

Figure 27.1 Adjuvant treatment for an early-stage adenoid cystic carcinoma of the left parotid gland with perineural invasion. *Maroon*, CTV_{HD} 60 Gy.

- **Dose constraints (at 2 Gy/fx):**
  Contralateral parotid: Mean < 10 Gy
  Oral cavity: Mean < 30 Gy
  Larynx: Mean < 30 Gy
  Spinal cord: Max < 45 Gy
  Brainstem: Max < 45 Gy
  Brachial plexus: Max < 66 Gy
  Optic nerves and chiasm: Max < 54 Gy. Can go to Max < 60 Gy if necessary (eg, PNS salivary gland cancer abutting optic structure)
  Cochlea: Max < 35 Gy; soft constraint if have to cover facial nerve through temporal bone
  Mandible: Max less than prescription dose for CTV_{HD}

Side Effect Management

See **Oral Cavity** chapter.

Follow-up

- Posttreatment clinical assessment at 4-6 weeks → if response/no recurrence, then PET/CT at 3 months
- History/physical with imaging: Every 3 months for 2 years → then every 6 months for 3 years → annual clinical exam thereafter
- TSH every 6-12 months if the neck was treated
- Dental evaluation every 6-12 months
- Audiology and speech/swallow assessment as needed

Notable Studies

Name/Inclusion	Arms	Outcomes	Notes
Risk Factors and Radiation Doses			
Dutch Cooperative Group (*Terhaard et al. IJROBP* 2005) RR Salivary gland treated with surgery *N* = 498	Surgery with or without adjuvant radiotherapy. 78% received adjuvant radiation	RT improved 10-y LC and 5-y LRC focusing on select subgroups with adverse risk factors (see notes)	• T3/T4 tumors (84% vs 18%, *P* < .001) • Close margins (95% vs 55%, *P* = .003) • Incomplete resection (82% vs 44%, *P* < .001) • Bone invasion (86% vs 54%, *P* = .04) • Perineural invasion (88% vs 60%, *P* = .01) For pN+ patients, adjuvant RT improved 5-y LRC (83% vs 57%, *P* = .04)

Name/Inclusion	Arms	Outcomes	Notes
UCSF (*Chen et al. IJORBP* 2007) RR cN0 salivary gland carcinoma *N* = 251	Surgery and adjuvant radiotherapy. 52% received elective nodal irradiation	10-y nodal relapse-free survival was significantly improved with elective nodal irradiation (26% vs 0%, *P* = .0001)	Histologies associated with the highest rate of nodal relapse: SCC (67%), undifferentiated carcinoma (50%), adenocarcinoma (34%), and mucoepidermoid carcinoma (29%) No nodal failures occurred with omission of elective neck RT in adenoid cystic or acinic cell
MD Anderson (*Garden et al. IJORBP* 1995) RR Adenoid cystic carcinoma patients *N* = 198	Surgery with adjuvant radiotherapy	Improved local control with doses ≥56 Gy in positive margins (88% vs 40%, *P* = .006)	Worse 10-Y local control with +margins vs close/− margin (77% vs 93%, *P* = .006); worse with named nerve involved vs not (80% vs 88%, *P* = .02); both +margins and nerve involved vs one vs none (70% vs 83% vs 93%, *P* = .002) Recommended doses: 60 Gy to tumor bed, 66 Gy for +margins
		Neutron-Based RT	
RTOG-MRC Neutron Trial (*Laramore et al. IJORBP* 1993) Two-arm prospective randomized phase III Inoperable/recurrent malignant salivary gland tumor *N* = 32	Fast neutron RT, 16.5-22 Gy in 12 fx Conventional RT, 55 Gy/4 wk or 70 Gy/7.5 wk	Improved 10-Y local control with neutrons (56% vs 17%, *P* = .009); no difference in OS (15% vs 25%, *P* = .5) 9 patients in neutron arm vs 4 patients in photon arm had "severe or greater" complications (*P* = .007)	Trial stopped early due to significant improvement in local control in neutron arm However, with no difference in OS and worse complications in neutron arm, photons remain standard of care

THYROID CANCER

RAMEZ KOUZY • GARY WALKER

BACKGROUND

- **Incidence/prevalence:** Approximately 56 000 cases diagnosed annually in the United States
- **Outcomes:** 5-Year survival for well differentiated across all stages estimated at 98% (SEER data). 5-Year survival for anaplastic histology is <5%.
- **Demographics:** F > M, 63% are age 35-65
- **Risk factors:** Family history, diet low in iodine, history of goiter, radiation exposure (diagnostic tests, previous cancer treatment, and nuclear fallouts), genetics (Cowden's, MEN2 for medullary), nodules (4% are malignant)

Tumor Biology and Characteristics

- **Genetics:** Papillary and follicular thyroid cancer associated with defects in the gene *PRKAR 1A*, familial adenomatous polyposis (FAP), Cowden disease, Carney complex, and familial nonmedullary thyroid carcinoma. Medullary thyroid cancer can be familial, either as part of the multiple endocrine neoplasia type 2 (MEN2) or isolated familial medullary thyroid cancer syndrome. Anaplastic thyroid cancers appear to arise from differentiated cancers.
- **Pathology:** Four major subtypes of thyroid cancer are papillary carcinoma (85%), follicular carcinoma (11%), medullary carcinoma (2%), and anaplastic carcinoma (1%). Papillary and follicular carcinomas are differentiated subtypes, while medullary carcinoma is derived from neuroendocrine C cells and anaplastic carcinoma is undifferentiated. Other thyroid pathologies include primary thyroid lymphomas and metastasis.

Anatomy

- The thyroid gland is a bilobed gland joined near the lower pole by an isthmus, crossing anterior to the trachea below the cricoid cartilage and behind to sternohyoid muscle. It consists of two lobes and isthmus.
- Lymph node drainage (35% are cN+)
  - Prelaryngeal (level VI, Delphian)
  - Pretracheal/paratracheal nodes/mediastinal
  - Levels II-IV and supraclavicular
  - See **Oral Cavity** chapter for neck LN description.

Workup

- **History and physical:** Assess presenting symptoms including symptoms of hyper/hypothyroidism. Direct palpation and visualization of the thyroid and vocal cords with nasolaryngoscope when advanced
- **Labs:** CBC, CMP, TSH, free T4/T3, T4/T3, calcitonin, CEA
- **Procedures/biopsy:** US-guided FNA of primary and enlarged LNs as clinically indicated
- **Imaging:** Ultrasound, ^{123}I thyroid uptake and scan, CT neck + C/A/P or MRI of the neck with contrast for locally advanced, PET/CT for anaplastic histology. For ATC, consider brain imaging.
- **Additional consultations:** Multidisciplinary evaluation with head and neck surgical oncology, endocrinology, nuclear medicine, radiation oncology, medical oncology, speech (evaluation of vocal cord mobility), nutrition, dental (fluoride/extractions)

Treatment Algorithm

Indications for Postoperative Radioiodine (RAI) Decision-Making*		
ATA Risk Stratification[a]	**TNM Stage**	**RAI Indicated?**
Low risk	T1a N0 M0	No
Low risk	T1b N0 M0	Not routine
Low risk	T2 N0 M0	Not routine
Low to intermediate risk	T3 N0 M0	Consider if age > 55 and large size or in patients with ETE
Low to intermediate risk	Any T, N+ M0	Strongly consider, especially if advanced age or clinically evident lymph nodes
High risk	T4 any N/M	Yes
High risk	Any T/N, M+	Yes

*Ref: *Haugen et al. Thyroid* 2016. Entire body is imaged ~1 week post-RAI administration to assess quality of treatment.

ATC (M0) (M1 or poor PS)	Consider Resection + Adjuvant EBRT ± Chemotherapy Palliative Radiation May Be Considered		
Indications for Adjuvant External Beam Radiation for Differentiated Disease			
	ATA	**BTA**	**ESMO**
Locally advanced	Yes	Yes	
>60 y with ETE	Consider		
Multiple reoperations	Consider	Yes	Yes
Residual gross disease		Yes	
No radioactive iodine uptake		Yes	Consider

ATA, American Thyroid Association; BTA, British Thyroid Association; ESMO, European Society of Medical Oncology

EXTERNAL RADIATION TREATMENT TECHNIQUE

- **Timing:** Should be started within 4-6 weeks of surgery
- **Dose:** Highest risk (close/positive margins/ECE): 63-66 Gy in 30-33 fractions (Fig. 28.1)
  High risk (tumor bed): 60 Gy in 30 fractions
  Intermediate risk (operative bed): 57 Gy in 30 fractions
  Low risk: 54 Gy in 30 fractions
- **Target: The principal target is the central compartment (hyoid to top of aortic arch and between the carotids).** This typically includes the tumor bed, operative bed, draining lymphatics (levels VI, III-V), paratracheal (consider level II, only if significant nodal disease with ECE), tracheal esophageal groove. Consider including previous operative beds.
- **Technique:** VMAT/IMRT and IMPT in experienced centers
- **SIM:** Supine, Aquaplast mask. Wire scar. Consider 3-mm bolus 2 cm around scar.
- **IGRT:** Daily kV with weekly CBCT or daily CBCT
- **Planning directive (for conventional fractionation):**

95% PTV coverage	
Spinal cord	Max < 45 Gy
Brain stem	Max < 45 Gy
Mandible	Max < 60 Gy
Total lung	V20 < 20%
Lens	Max < 5 Gy
Parotids	Mean < 20 Gy, lower for contralateral
Submandibular	Mean < 10 Gy if level II included, then <26 Gy
Larynx	Mean < 35 Gy
Esophagus	Max < 60 Gy (will often be in the CTV)

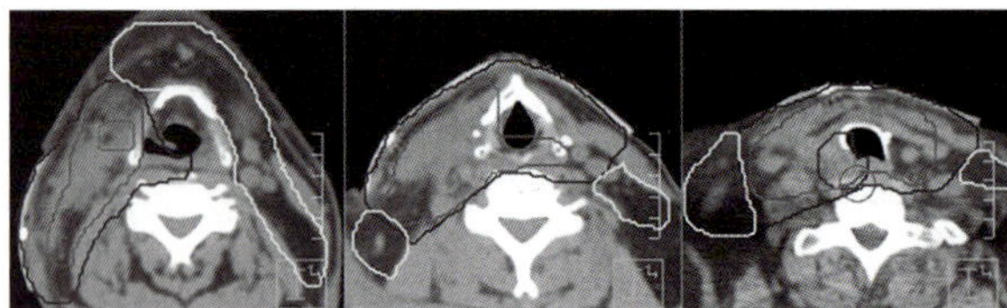

Figure 28.1 A 74-year-old patient with four previous resections for papillary thyroid cancer. Following surgery, he was found to have a 3-cm right level II node with ECE, 2/10 level right level III nodes up to 2 cm, as well as a right tracheal sidewall mass resected with SM+. Contours shown are GTV-LN (*green*), CTV63 (*purple*), CTV60 (*red*), CTV57 (*blue*), and CTV54 (*yellow*). Treatment was delivered utilizing simultaneous integrated boost in 30 fractions. **See color insert.**

Surgery

- Total thyroidectomy or ipsilateral thyroid lobectomy with central neck dissection
- Neck dissection for node positive
  - Radical neck dissection = I-V, CNXI, IJV, SCM
  - Modified radical neck dissection = I-V, preserve one of the above
  - Supraomohyoid = I-III
  - Lateral = II-IV
  - Selective neck dissection = LNs based on site

Chemotherapy

- **Limited role for traditional chemotherapy**
- **TKIs:** Lenvatinib, vandetanib, cabozantinib, pazopanib, sorafenib, etc.
- **Anaplastic thyroid cancer:** Current regimens are paclitaxel/carboplatin or docetaxel, doxorubicin. Targeted treatment includes BRAF, NTRK fusion, RET fusion agents. IO can be considered RTOG 0912 looked at paclitaxel/pazopanib with radiation, but no OS benefit was seen.

Side Effect Management

See **Oral Cavity** chapter.

Follow-up

- History/physical exam and ultrasound or CT of the neck: Every 3-6 months for 3 years → yearly to 5 years. Maintain follow-up with endocrinologist to evaluate thyroid supplementation and target TSH levels.
- Assess compliance with fluoride trays (if applicable) and neck/lymphedema exercises.

Notable Studies

Name/Inclusion	Arms	Outcomes	Notes
RT in Differentiated Thyroid Cancer			
MDACC Matched Pair Analysis (*Tam et al. JAMA Otolaryngol* 2017) Retrospective matched pair analysis *N* = 88 surgically resected T4a-differentiated thyroid cancer patients	RAI with or without external beam radiation therapy. 44 (50%) received external beam radiation	5-y DFS: 43% in RAI alone vs 57% in RAI + EBRT (effect size = 14%; 95% CI, −7% to 33%) RAI alone had increased LRF (effect size 32%)	Age, esophageal invasion predicted worse DFS Addition of EBRT to RAI improves disease control for locally advanced differentiated thyroid cancer
Anaplastic Thyroid Cancer			
MDACC (*Bhatia et al. Head Neck* 2010) RR *N* = 53 patients with anaplastic thyroid cancer	Mostly curative intent RT Median RT dose 55 Gy (4-70 Gy) 25% received IMRT median 60 Gy (39.9-69 Gy)	1-y OS for definitively irradiated patients: 29% Patients without distant metastases receiving ≥50 Gy had better survival	Use of IMRT vs 3DRT did not influence toxicity
RTOG 0912 (*Sherman et al. Lancet Oncol* 2022) Randomized phase II trial *N* = 71 patients with anaplastic thyroid cancer	Pazopanib + concurrent paclitaxel and RT (66 Gy in 33 fx) Placebo + concurrent paclitaxel and RT (66 Gy in 33 fx)	No difference in median survival (5.7 vs 7.3 mo) 1-y OS: 29% in paclitaxel and RT arm vs 37% in pazopanib arm (nonsignificant)	Pazopanib did not increase toxicity significantly. Most common toxicity events were radiation-related (dysphagia, dermatitis)

UNKNOWN HEAD AND NECK PRIMARY

ALAN SOSA • ADAM GARDEN

BACKGROUND

- **Definition:** Metastatic disease in the lymph nodes of the neck for which complete workup failed to determine primary tumor origin—diagnosis of exclusion. In some cases, the primary tumor can spontaneously regress leaving only the nodal disease; in others, the primary may evade detection due to small size.
- **Incidence/prevalence:** Accounts for 2-5% of all head and neck cancers. The incidence of cervical node from unknown primary (CUP) has diminished significantly with advances in diagnostic imaging and surgical techniques.
- **Outcomes:** With aggressive radiation approaches, the 5-year overall survival rate is between 80% and 90%; mucosal emergence occurs in <10%, and the most common site of recurrence is distant (20%).
- **Risk factors:** Risk factors include those common for head and neck cancer in general. Since CUP is often from undetected oropharyngeal cancer, HPV association is common.
- **Presentation:** Most commonly a painless neck mass, and most frequently in the upper neck.

TUMOR BIOLOGY AND CHARACTERISTICS

- **Pathology:** Derived from FNA or core biopsy. Open biopsy is discouraged because of risk of tumor spillage.
  - Most common histology is squamous cell carcinoma (75%), of which HPV (HPV-DNA via PCR and/or p16 on IHC) association is identified in up to 75% of patients. EBV association may also be detected. Skin cancers of the face and neck can present as CUP. It is important to obtain HPV-DNA, as p16 will not differentiate from a mucosal vs cutaneous probable site.
    - HPV+: Likely oropharynx or nasopharynx primary
    - EBV+: Likely nasopharynx primary
    - HPV−/EBV−: Head and neck primary including all head and neck subsites in addition to skin primary
- Adenocarcinoma histology is most likely associated with subclavicular primary origin (eg, esophageal or lung cancer), after salivary gland or thyroid primary tumors are excluded. Consider thyroglobulin, TTF1, calcitonin, and PAX8 IHC for undifferentiated carcinoma or adenocarcinoma.
- Other histologies include lymphoma, melanoma, and sarcoma.

ANATOMY

- Upper cervical nodes (levels II, III, and VA) are likely from HNC primary origin.
  - The presence of a level II cystic metastasis is a hallmark of HPV-related SCC. The tonsil and base of the tongue (lingual tonsil) are the most probable primary sites.
  - Level III metastasis without involvement of level II suggests larynx or hypopharynx primary origin, more so if viral markers are negative.
  - RP node involvement may suggest nasopharyngeal or oropharyngeal primary.
  - Parotid nodes (squamous cell) or external jugular nodes suggest a skin primary.
- Lower cervical nodes (levels IV and V) and supraclavicular nodes presentations are associated with a worse prognosis. Consider subclavicular primary origin (lung, gastrointestinal, breast) especially if there are no markers for thyroid cancer.
- See **Oral Cavity** chapter for discussion of LN levels.

WORKUP

- **History and physical:** CUP is a diagnosis of exclusion, so a directed history and exam is designed to find a primary. The history should include common symptoms of head and neck cancers, and a history of skin cancers. The oral cavity, pharynx, larynx, and skin should be carefully examined utilizing palpation and nasopharyngolaryngoscopy.
- **Labs:** CBC, CMP

- **Procedures/biopsy:** FNA (first-line) or core biopsy of enlarged LN(s). Ultrasound guidance is very useful for cystic nodes, as it is common for an FNA to sample a benign component in the absence of image guidance. Evaluation of histology with appropriate stains. For the most common histology (squamous), assess HPV status and EBV staining. Examination under anesthesia (EUA) with panendoscopy, biopsy of suspicious sites, directed mucosal biopsies of at-risk potential sites, ± palatine tonsillectomy (if no suspicious lesions are found). Consider bronchoscopy and EGD especially for low LNs (levels IV and V).
- **Imaging:**
  - FDG-PET/CT detects occult primary in 25% of cases and should be done before EUA with panendoscopy to potentially allow for EUA guidance. However, resolution limits detection size in tumors < 7 mm and in BOT.
  - CT and/or MRI of the head and neck, CT of the chest (>T0N2b). CT of the chest, abdomen, and pelvis for lower cervical nodes (levels IV-V)
- **Additional consultations:** Multidisciplinary evaluation with head and neck surgical oncology, radiation oncology, medical oncology, speech, nutrition, dental (fluoride/extractions)

Treatment Algorithm

T0N1[a]	1. Selective or comprehensive neck dissection, +/− postoperative RT if ≥2 LN or concurrent chemoRT if ENE on LN dissection pathology 2. Definitive RT[a]
T0N2-N3[a]	1. Definitive RT +/− neck dissection 2. Concurrent chemoRT[b] +/− neck dissection 3. Neck dissection[c] + adjuvant radiation +/− systemic therapy 4. Induction chemotherapy followed by RT +/− concurrent systemic therapy (uncommon, mainly if level IV disease)
Stage IVB (M+)	1. Systemic therapy or best supportive care 2. Surgery, RT, or systemic therapy/RT for selected cases with limited metastatic burden

[a]Favored in patients with open biopsy (violated neck)
[b]Concurrent chemotherapy preferred in the presence of large nodal volume or radiographic ENE
[c]May be favored for suspected skin primary or non–viral-mediated disease

Radiation Treatment Technique

- **Target:** As CUP is uncommon, there are no phase III trials to guide targets. The main controversy, which varies by the suspicion of where is the primary site, is the elective sites to cover, including the contralateral cN0 neck and putative mucosal sites. Review of the MDA practice and literature favors a more comprehensive approach.

Definitive Target Volumes	
CTV_{HD}	GTV nodal (or LN bed after excisional biopsy) + 1 cm
CTV_{ID}	LN levels 2 cm superior and inferior of CTV_{HD}
CTV_{ED}	Remainder LN not included in CTV_{ID} to encompass minimally: Ipsilateral* RP and levels IB-VI; contralateral RP, II-IV; select mucosa (based on HPV/EBV status) • HPV+ histology: Oropharynx and nasopharynx mucosa • HPV−/EBV− histology: Oropharynx mucosa, nasopharynx mucosa, and consider hypopharynx mucosa and larynx (controversial) • Skin primary suspected (pathology reveals squamous cell pathology and HPV−/EBV− especially if history of skin cancers): Consider definitive management of neck with radiation and/or surgery and close observation for the development of a primary
Postoperative Target Volumes	
CTV_{HD}	Tumor bed (determined by imaging and surgical/pathology findings) + 1 cm Consider boosting the resection bed if ECE is detected on pathology
CTV_{ID}	Operative bed covers the dissected neck

CTV_{ED}	Remaining LNs not included in CTV_{ID} in involved neck to encompass ipsilateral[a] levels I-V, bilateral RP nodes, and contralateral levels II-IV of uninvolved neck • HPV+ histology: Oropharynx and nasopharynx mucosa • HPV−/EBV− histology: Oropharynx mucosa, nasopharynx mucosa, and consider hypopharynx mucosa and larynx (controversial)
PTV	CTV + 3-mm margin

*Ipsilateral neck RT: Consider if histologic findings (eg, adenocarcinoma) or nodal location (eg, submental, submandibular, supraclavicular) suggest a primary outside of the pharyngeal axis without bilateral lymph node drainage. Examples of primary subsites with predominantly ipsilateral nodal drainage include well-lateralized gingival tumors, buccal tumors, and RMT.

- **Dose** (Fig. 29.1):

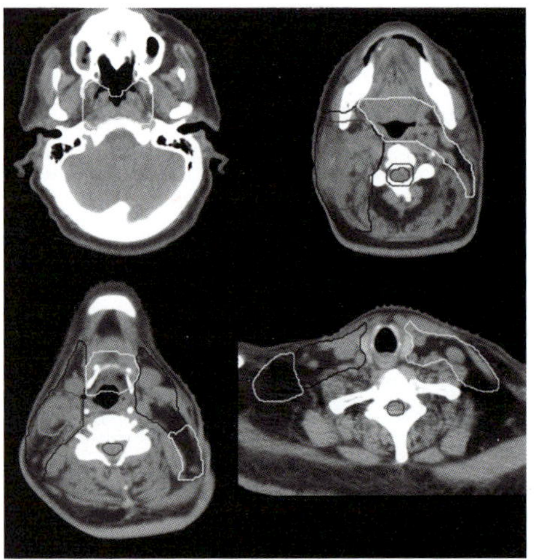

Figure 29.1 Target volumes for CUP with metastasis to right LN levels II-III, showing CTVHD (*red*), CTV_{ID} (*blue*), and CTV_{ED} (*yellow*). **See color insert.**

Definitive	
CTV_{HD}	70 Gy in 33 fractions
CTV_{ID}	60-63 Gy in 33 fractions
CTV_{ED}	56 Gy in 33 fractions

Consider boosting bulky adenopathy to 70 Gy.

Postoperative (After Neck Dissection)	
CTV_{HD}	60 Gy in 30 fractions
CTV_{ID}	57 Gy in 30 fractions
CTV_{ED}	54 Gy in 30 fractions
CTV_{boost}	63-66 Gy in 30 fractions (consider defining a smaller volume within CTV_{HD} if ECE)

- **Technique:** IMRT, IMPT
- **SIM:** Supine position, arms in shoulder straps to lower shoulders from treatment field, thermoplastic head and neck mask, wire and 3-mm bolus on surgical scar (if LN dissection or excisional biopsy)
- **IGRT:** Daily kV imaging +/− weekly 3D imaging
- **Planning directive:**
  Ensure each PTV coverage by prescription dose with the goal of V100% > 95%, V95% > 99%, V105% < 10%, D_{max} < 120%.

OAR dose should respect the following constraints, though goals can be considerably lower and attainable for these OARs:

Brainstem	D_{max} < 50 Gy
Spinal cord	D_{max} < 45 Gy
Mandible	D_{max} < CTV_{HD} prescription dose
Parotid	Mean < 26 Gy
Oral cavity	Mean < 30 Gy
Larynx	Mean < 30 Gy *(if larynx/hypopharynx not included in CTV_{ED})*
Cervical esophagus	Mean < 30 Gy
Submandibular gland	Mean < 39 Gy *(if level IB excluded in N0 neck)*
Brachial plexus	D_{max} < 63-66 Gy (lower dose if fraction to plexus > 2 Gy)

Chemotherapy

The chemotherapy regimen is extrapolated from data from head and neck cancers with detectable primary.

- **Concurrent:** Single-agent cisplatin, carboplatin, or cetuximab
- **Neoadjuvant:** Docetaxel, cisplatin, and 5-FU

Side Effect Management

See **Oral Cavity** chapter.

Follow-up

- CT of the neck at 8 weeks posttreatment +/− PET/CT at 12 weeks. Failure to achieve complete metabolic response mandates neck dissection.
- H&P exam with fiberoptic and skin examination q2-4mo for years 1-2, q6mo for years 3-5, and q12mo thereafter. Further follow-up imaging as clinically indicated.
- TSH q6-12mo. Annual low-dose chest CT or CXR for patients with smoking history; smoking cessation counseling as indicated

Notable Trials

Name/Inclusion	Arms	Outcomes	Notes
		Surgery alone	
Mayo Clinic (*Coster et al. IJROBP* 1992) Retrospective Unilateral CUP (*N* = 24)	**Unilateral CUP treated by dissection or excisional Bx** <u>Patient characteristics:</u> • 58% N1 disease • 33% ECE	Primary developed in 4% Neck recurrence in 25% (ECE in all neck recurrences but 1 patient) 5-y OS 66% **Conclusion:** Surgery alone may be sufficient in pN1 and no ECE; consider adjuvant RT if pN2+ or ECE	Both N1 patients who recurred had ECE
		Radiation	
Danish (*Grau et al. Radiother Oncol* 2000) Retrospective CUP treated with definitive therapy (*N* = 277)	**Comprehensive RT:** 81% bilateral neck RT + mucosal RT (OPX, NPX, larynx, hypopharynx) 10% ipsilateral RT 9% surgery alone	Mucosal primary emergence rate: 19% • 50% of emerging primaries were in lung/esophagus Emergence of primary higher w/ surgery alone vs RT (54% vs 15%) Relative risk of LRR • 1.9 for ipsilateral RT vs bilateral + mucosal RT	

Name/Inclusion	Arms	Outcomes	Notes
MD Anderson (*Kamal et al. Cancer* 2018) Retrospective CUP treated with IMRT (*N* = 260)	**IMRT to bilateral neck + mucosa** 30% presented after excisional Bx or neck dissection. Median CTVHD was 60 Gy 70% treated w/ definitive RT. Median CTVHD was 66 Gy Entire pharyngeal axis was irradiated in 30% **OPX/NPX** only in 63%	5-y OS: 84% 5-y LRC: 91% 5-y DMFS: 94% 7% had chronic RT-associated dysphagia No obvious benefit to adding chemotherapy	24% received induction chemotherapy 25% received concurrent chemoRT
Unilateral vs bilateral RT			
Princess Margaret (*Weir et al. Radiother Oncol* 1995) Retrospective CUP treated with RT (*N* = 144)	**RT to involved nodal region:** 59% **RT to bilateral neck + mucosal sites:** 41%	5-y actuarial regional failure: 49% Trend toward improved survival for treatment of both potential primary sites and nodes (*P* = .07) **No difference in both OS and CSS** after adjusting for extent of nodal disease RT of involved node alone may be adequate in select patients	Primary site occurrence was 2% for bilateral RT and 7% for unilateral RT
Loyola (*Reddy et al. IJROBP* 1997) Retrospective CUP treated with RT (*N* = 52)	**RT to unilateral neck:** 31% **RT to bilateral neck + mucosal sites:** 69%	Control of contralateral neck (*P* = .03) • 86% for bilateral RT • 56% for unilateral RT Mucosal primary emergence (*P* = .0005) • 8% for bilateral RT • 44% for unilateral RT Similar 5-y OS Bilateral RT + mucosal RT is superior for preventing contralateral and mucosal emergence	
Further De-escalation Efforts			
OPX-targeted RT (*Mourad et al. Anticancer Res* 2014) Retrospective CUP (*N* = 68)	**Targeted RT to OPX, RP nodes, and bilateral LNs** (no comprehensive mucosal RT) • 40% IMRT • 50% chemoRT Stage III: 9% Stage IVA: 75% Stage IVB: 16%	Actuarial LRC at median FU of 3.5 y: 95.5% Mucosal primary emergence: 1 patient Neck failures: 2 patients Median time to LRF: 18 mo OPX-targeted RT provides excellent oncologic and functional outcomes	Severe late complication (grade 3 or higher) was found in one patient with HIV (1.5%) with grade 4 dysphagia (ie, PEG tube dependent)

Name/Inclusion	Arms	Outcomes	Notes
Beth Israel (*Hu et al. Oral Oncol* 2017) Retrospective SCC of unknown primary (*N* = 60)	**RT to the OPX and bilateral necks** • 55% IMRT • 62% chemoRT N1: 18% N2: 75% N3: 7% 82% underwent neck dissection	5-y OS: 79% 5-y DM: 20% 5-y LRC: 90% 5-y primary emergence rate was 10% overall and 3% in non-OPX site No obvious benefit to adding chemotherapy	
TORS-assisted Workup (*Grewal et al. Laryngoscope* 2020) Retrospective Persistent CUP after TORS (pT0) (*N* = 172)	Persistent CUP (pT0) after TORS-assisted palatine and lingual tonsillectomy • 49% TORS → **PSRT** (pharyngeal-sparing radiation therapy) targeting only the at-risk neck and omitting treatment of the pharynx • 51% **PRT** (pharyngeal-targeted RT) based on institutional historical control subjects Adjuvant RT recommended for surgical pathology with ≥ 2 LNs, single node > 3 cm, or ENE Concurrent chemoRT for ENE	Median FU: 24 and 28 mo, respectively, for PSRT and PRT groups (*P* = .04) 2-y RFS and 2-y OS were similar between the arms • PSRT was associated with lower weight loss, feeding tube rates, opiate requirements, and unplanned hospitalizations	Many patients increasingly undergo TORS to facilitate identification of primary tumors Strong smoking history: pharynx and larynx included in CTV NPX included in patients with EBV-encoding RNA positivity

EARLY-STAGE NSCLC

YUFEI LIU • JOE CHANG

Background

- **Incidence/prevalence:** The second most common diagnosed cancer and leading cause of cancer death among men and women in the United States
- **Outcomes:** 5-Year survival estimated at 54% for localized disease, 26% for regional nodal involvement, and 4% for distant disease (SEER). NOTE: 5-Year survival often worse for patients treated with SABR compared with surgery; most patients treated with SABR are medically inoperable and expected to have shorter life expectancy due to greater comorbidities (selection bias). Recent pooled randomized data show that SABR yields equivalent or better OS compared with lobectomy and nodal dissection in medically operable patients (STARS/ROSEL trials).
- **Risk factors:** Smoking, radon, ionizing radiation, asbestos, chromium, male sex, family history, acquired lung disease (ie, interstitial pulmonary fibrosis), and other occupational exposures (silica, arsenic, beryllium, coal)
- **Prognostic factors:** Stage, performance status, weight loss, molecular mutations

Tumor Biology and Characteristics

- **Genetic markers:** Higher percentage of clinically relevant mutations that are targetable are found in adenocarcinomas. These include *EGFR* (~20% of adeno cases), *ALK* (~5%), *KRAS*, *ROS-1* (~2%), *BRAF*, *MET*, *RET*, and *PDL-1*.
- **Pathology:** Majority are adenocarcinomas (40% of lung malignancies), then squamous cell carcinomas (30%). Rarer histologies include large cell (15%), neuroendocrine, bronchoalveolar (arising from type II pneumocytes), and carcinoid.

Anatomy

- Right lung: 3 lobes (upper, middle, lower) and 2 fissures (major, minor)
- Left lung: 2 lobes (upper, lower) and 1 fissure (major). Lingula is an inferior project of left upper lobe and serves as the homologue of the right middle lobe
- Drainage most commonly to ipsi hilar/mediastinal nodes. Hematogenous spread common
- Lymph node names (numeric classifications) (Fig. 30.1):
  Supraclavicular: Low cervical, supraclavicular, and sternal notch (LN station 1)
  Superior mediastinal: Upper paratracheal (2R/L), prevascular (3a), retrotracheal (3p), and lower paratracheal (4R/L)
  Aortic: Subaortic (5) and para-aortic (6)

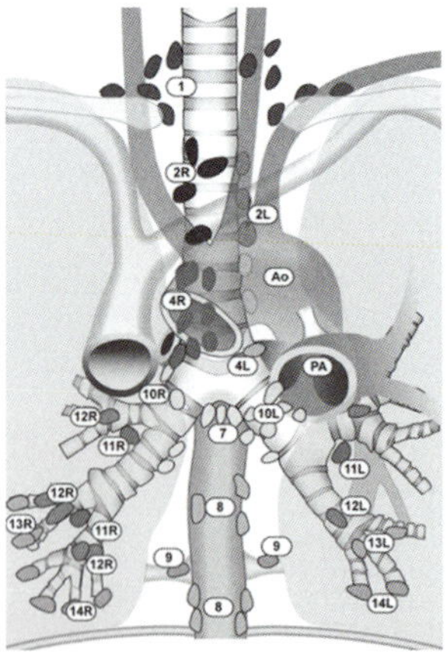

Figure 30.1 Diagram illustrating mediastinal and thoracic lymph node stations. (Used with permission of the American College of Surgeons, Chicago, Illinois. The original source for this information is the AJCC Cancer Staging System (2023))

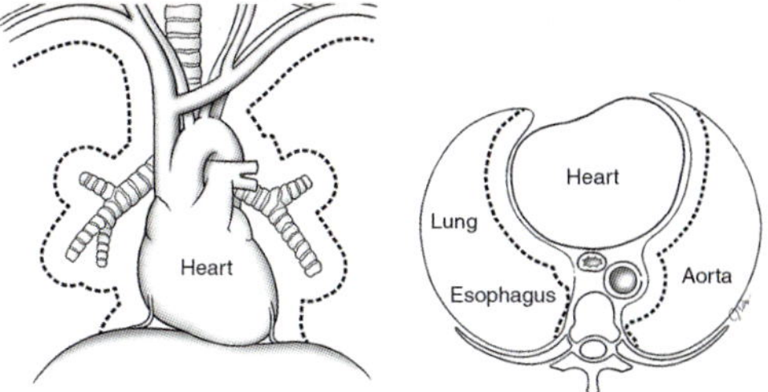

Figure 30.2 Central zone figure. (Reprinted from Chang JY, Bezjak A, Mornex F, et al. Stereotactic ablative radiotherapy for centrally located early stage non-small-cell lung cancer: what we have learned. *J Thorac Oncol.* 2015;10(4):577-585. Copyright © 2015 International Association for the Study of Lung Cancer. With permission.)

Inferior mediastinal: Subcarinal (7), paraesophageal (8), and pulmonary ligament (9)
N1: Hilar (10), interlobar (11), lobar (12), segmental (13), and subsegmental (14)

- Pancoast tumor (syndrome): Superior sulcus tumor associated with shoulder pain, Horner syndrome (ipsilateral ptosis, miosis, anhidrosis), and atrophy of hand muscles
- Early-stage (T1-3N0) tumors are divided into central and peripheral lesions. The central zone is defined as the region within 2 cm of the proximal bronchial tree (Fig. 30.2) (which extends from the trachea to the lobar bronchi and other central structures [esophagus, heart, pericardium, great vessels, vertebral body]). Peripheral lesions are beyond this 2-cm zone. Distinction is important for risk of lymph node spread and treatment planning.

Workup

- **History and physical:** Typically present with cough, shortness of breath, hemoptysis, weight loss, and/or incidental mass on chest x-ray/CT
- **Screening:** Annual low-dose CT scan recommended for patients aged 55-74 years with ≥30 pack-year smoking history and cessation <15 years ago *(NLST NEJM* 2011)
- **Labs:** CBC, CMP
- **Procedures/biopsy:** Consider CT-guided biopsy if able to obtain tissue of primary. Not necessary if pathology more easily obtained by sampling suspicious nodes during mediastinal staging. Selective sampling of hila/mediastinum (eg, mediastinoscopy, EBUS) is recommended for higher-risk characteristics including central tumors, radiographic suspicion of adenopathy, or ≥T2a tumors but should be considered for all tumors. Mutational testing recommended to assess for targetable mutations. Pulmonary function testing to evaluate surgical candidacy and to provide baseline
- **Imaging:** CT of the chest w/ contrast and PET/CT to rule out regional/distant disease for all patients. Brain MRI for all ≥T2a tumors (optional for T1b) or neurologic symptoms. Consider MRI of the shoulder for superior sulcus tumors and octreotide scans if with carcinoid histology.

NSCLC Staging (*AJCC 8th Edition*)

T Stage		**N Stage**	
T1	≤3 cm without main bronchus invasion	N1	Ipsi peribronchial/hilar LN
T1a	≤1 cm	N2	Ipsi mediastinal/subcarinal LN
T1b	>1-2 cm	N3	Scalene/supraclav LN or contra mediastinal/hilar LN
T1c	>2-3 cm	**M Stage**	
T2	>3-5 cm or involves main bronchus but not carina, invades visceral pleura, or associated atelectasis or obstructive PNA	M1a	Nodule in contra lobe, pleura, or pericardium, or malignant pleural or pericardial effusion
T2a	>3-4 cm	M1b	Single extrathoracic metastasis

T Stage		M Stage	
T2b	>4-5 cm	M1c	Multiple extrathoracic mets
T3	>5-7 cm or separate nodule in the same lobe or invades CW, phrenic nerve, parietal pericardium		
T4	>7 cm or separate nodule in different ipsi lobe or invades the diaphragm, mediastinum, heart, great vessels, trachea, recurrent laryngeal nerve, esophagus, vertebral body, carina		

Stage Grouping

	N0	N1	N2	N3	M1a-b	M1c
T1a-c	IA1-3	IIB	IIIA	IIIB	IVA	IVB
T2a	IB	IIB	IIIA	IIIB	IVA	IVB
T2b	IIA	IIB	IIIA	IIIB	IVA	IVB
T3	IIB	IIIA	IIIB	IIIC	IVA	IVB
T4	IIIA	IIIA	IIIB	IIIC	IVA	IVB

Locally Advanced NSCLC (stage III)

Used with permission of the American College of Surgeons, Chicago, Illinois. The original source for this information is the AJCC Cancer Staging System (2023).

Treatment Algorithm

Stages I-II (T1-3 satellite nodule, N0M0)	• Regional/distant disease ruled out during workup • Surgical candidate (usually postoperative predictive FEV1 > 40% and deemed surgical candidate by thoracic surgeon) → lobectomy plus mediastinal lymph node dissection • Nonsurgical candidate or decline surgery → SABR (aka SBRT) • For special circumstances in which patient tolerance and disease may be limiting, nonpreferred, alternative treatments include sublobar resection, radiofrequency ablation, cryotherapy, chemoradiation, and hypofractionated or conventional radiation

Radiation Treatment Technique (Stereotactic Ablative Radiotherapy, also Called Stereotactic Body Radiation Therapy)

- **SIM:** Supine with Vac-Lok device and arms above the head. Four-dimensional imaging required. If tumor moves more than 10 mm, consider breath-hold technique or gating if patient is able to hold breath. Scan from base of the skull to top of the kidneys to encompass lung volume across the entire respiratory cycle.
- **Dose:** Goal is BED > 100 (*Onishi Cancer* 2004 showed this is required for optimal local control).
  50 Gy to PTV with SIB GTV to 60 Gy in 4 fractions (peripheral)
  70 Gy to PTV with SIB GTV to 80 Gy in 10 fractions (central that cannot be safely treated with 50 Gy in 4 fractions, or peripheral lesion abutting the chest wall where 50 Gy in 4 fractions could lead to chest wall injury/pain)
  Note: For large-volume PTV in central regions, consider SIB (70 Gy to iGTV, 50-60 Gy to PTV in 10 fractions).
- **Target:** iGTV: Tumor across all phases of respiratory cycle (contour on maximum intensity projection [MIP]) or, when used, across all breath-hold trials (typically will have 5 breath-hold trials)
  PTV: iGTV + 5 mm
- **Technique:** 3DCRT, IMRT/VMAT. 6-10 MV photons with heterogeneity correction
- **IGRT:** Daily cone beam CT with respiratory management
- **Peripheral tumor planning directive (for 50 Gy in 4 fractions):**
  Chest wall: V30 ≤ 30 cc

Skin: V30 ≤ 50 cc
Vessels: V40 ≤ 1 cc, D_{max} ≤ 56 Gy
Trachea: V35 ≤ 1 cc, D_{max} ≤ 38 Gy
Bronchial tree: V35 ≤ 1 cc, D_{max} ≤ 38 Gy
Brachial plexus: V30 ≤ 0.2 cc, D_{max} ≤ 35 Gy
Esophagus: V30 ≤ 1 cc, D_{max} ≤ 35 Gy
Heart/pericardium: V40 ≤ 1 cc, V20 ≤ 5 cc, D_{max} ≤ 45 Gy
Spinal cord: V20 ≤ 1 cc, D_{max} ≤ 25 Gy
Ipsilateral lung: iMLD ≤ 10 Gy, iV10 ≤ 35%, iV20 ≤ 25%, iV30 ≤ 15%
Total lung: MLD ≤ 6 Gy, V5 ≤ 5%, V10 ≤ 17%, V20 ≤ 12%, V30 ≤ 7%

- **Central tumor planning directive (for 70 Gy in 10 fractions):**
  Chest wall/skin: V50 ≤ 60 cc, D_{max} ≤ 82 Gy
  Vessels: V50 ≤ 1 cc, D_{max} ≤ 75 Gy
  Trachea: V40 ≤ 1 cc, D_{max} ≤ 60 Gy
  Bronchial tree: V50 ≤ 1 cc, D_{max} ≤ 60 Gy
  Brachial plexus: V50 ≤ 0.2 cc, D_{max} ≤ 55 Gy
  Esophagus: V40 ≤ 1 cc, D_{max} ≤ 50 Gy
  Heart/pericardium: V45 ≤ 1 cc, D_{max} ≤ 60 Gy
  Spinal cord: V35 ≤ 1 cc, D_{max} ≤ 40 Gy
  Total lung: MLD ≤ 9 Gy, V40 ≤ 7%

Side Effect Management

- Esophagitis: Magic mouthwash (viscous lidocaine, Benadryl, nystatin), glutamine supplement (eg, Helios), aloe products, and narcotic elixir second line
- Chest wall pain: OTC analgesics (eg, Tylenol, NSAIDs) or neuropathic agents (select agent based on pain etiology—radicular/neurogenic, myositis/muscular), narcotics second line
- Pneumonitis: For symptomatic patients (shortness of breath, reduction in O_2 on pulse oxygenation), consider oral steroid taper (typically prednisone starting at 1 mg/kg daily for 2-3 weeks with taper). Bactrim prophylaxis for PCP pneumonia and antacid prophylaxis for gastric ulcers

Follow-up

- CT of the chest with contrast q3mo for years 1-2, q6mo for years 3-5, and annually thereafter
- PET for suspicious CT findings (establish postradiation changes vs recurrence)
- Biopsy for imaging findings consistent with recurrence

Notable Literature

Stereotactic body radiation therapy—single arm

Name/Inclusion	Arms	Outcomes	Notes
RTOG 0236 (*Timmerman et al. JAMA* 2010, Update *JAMA Oncol* 2018) 55 patients w/ peripheral inoperable stage I NSCLC	Phase II single arm 60 Gy/3 fx (54 Gy/3 fx with heterogeneity correction) over 1.5-2 wk	3-y LC 98%, LRC 87%, and OS 56%. 17% grade 3 or higher toxicity (4% grade 4 or higher) At 5 y, LC is 93%, LRC 75%, and OS 40%	EBUS not required Conclusion: Good local control and moderate toxicity with SBRT for medically inoperable stage I NSCLC
RTOG 0618 (*Timmerman et al. JAMA* 2018) 33 patients w/ peripheral operable stage T1-2N0 NSCLC	Phase II single arm 54 Gy/3 fx	4-y LRC 88%, DF 12%, DFS 57%, OS 56%. Median DFS and OS 55.2 mo	Conclusion: SBRT provides excellent local control in operable early-stage NSCLC

Name/Inclusion	Arms	Outcomes	Notes
RTOG 0813 (*Bezjak et al. JCO* 2019) 120 patients with central tumors (within 2 cm of tracheal-bronchial tree)	Phase I/II study of maximum tolerated dose (MTD) Dose started at 50 Gy/5 fx and escalated by 0.5 Gy/fx to 60 Gy/5 fx every other day	MTD 60 Gy/5 fx with DLT 7.2%. 2-y LC 88%, PFS 55%, OS 73% 55 Gy/5 fx or lower had no DLT	Conclusion: 60 Gy/5 fx for central tumors associated with excellent LC but significant DLT
RTOG 0915 (*Videtic et al. IJROBP 2015*, Update *IJROBP* 2019) 94 medically inoperable T1-2N0 peripheral NSCLC	34 Gy/1 fx	Grade 3+ AE 3% vs 11, LC 89% vs 93%, OS 30% vs 41%, PFS 19% vs 33%	Conclusion: Toxicity and LC similar in both arms. OS lower in single arm but underpowered. Needs prospective validation
	48 Gy/4 fx		

Comparison of SBRT vs surgery vs immunotherapy + SBRT (I-SABR)

Name/Inclusion	Arms	Outcomes	Notes
STARS/ROSEL (*Chang et al. Lancet Oncol* 2015) Pooled analysis of two randomized phase III trials. Total 58 medically operable patients	SBRT	3-y RFS 86% vs 80% Improved OS 95% vs 79% (HR 0.14, *P* = .037) Fewer grade 3+ events (10% vs 44%)	SBRT is a viable alternative to surgery in medically operable early-stage NSCLC patients
	Surgery		
Revised STARS (*Chang et al. Lancet Oncol* 2021) Single-arm prospective trial of 80 early-stage NSCLC patients treated with SBRT	SBRT only with protocol-specified propensity-matched analysis to prospective cohort of patients receiving video-assisted thoracoscopic surgical lobectomy with mediastinal lymph node dissection (VATS L-MLND)	3-y OS 91% for SBRT vs 91% in propensity-matched surgical cohort. 5-y OS 87% for SBRT vs 84% in propensity-matched surgical cohort. On MVA, no significant difference in OS. No grades 4-5 toxicity in SBRT cohort	SBRT is a viable and safe alternative to surgery in operable early-stage NSCLC patients with similar OS
I-SABR (***Chang et al. Lancet* 2023)** **156 stage treatment naive IA-IIB patients or isolated parenchymal recurrence <7 cm**	SABR (50 Gy in 4 fx or 70 Gy in 10 fx)	I-SABR significantly improved 4-y event-free survival from 53% with SABR to 77% (HR = 0.38, *P* = .0056)	No grade 3+ adverse events associated with SABR. In the I-SABR group, 10 participants (15%) had grade 3 immunological adverse events related to nivolumab
	4 cycles of nivolumab for 6 mo + SABR		

STAGE III NSCLC

YUFEI LIU • SAUMIL GANDHI

BACKGROUND

- **Incidence/prevalence:** Stage III NSCLC accounts for ~1/3 of all NSCLC cases.
- **Outcomes:** 5-Year OS for stage III is highly variable and dependent on numerous factors including performance status and comorbidities, estimated to be between 5% and 35% (IIIA, 35%; IIIB 25%, IIIC, 15%).
- **Demographics and risk factors:** See **Early-Stage NSCLC** chapter.

TUMOR BIOLOGY AND CHARACTERISTICS

See **Early-Stage NSCLC** chapter.

ANATOMY

See **Early-Stage NSCLC** chapter.

WORKUP

See **Early-Stage NSCLC** chapter.

TREATMENT ALGORITHM (STAGE III)

Resectable	**Neoadjuvant chemo/immunotherapy → surgery** • Allows for tailored RT based on surgical findings. Also selects for patients who do not metastasize after chemotherapy, therefore optimizing the benefits of local therapy • Checkmate 816 established benefit of adding nivolumab to neoadjuvant chemotherapy • PORT not routinely indicated (LungART) **Surgery → adjuvant chemo/immunotherapy** • IMpower010 established benefit of adding atezolizumab after adjuvant chemotherapy **Surgery → adjuvant chemo/TKI** • ADAURA established benefit of adjuvant osimertinib for completely resected patients who had EGFR mutations. **Neoadjuvant chemoRT → surgery** • May reduce tumor size to decrease extent of surgery • Not a preferred option in patients who would undergo pneumonectomy
Superior sulcus tumor	**Neoadjuvant chemoRT → surgery → completion chemoRT if unresectable** • Preferred approach for borderline resectable T3-4N0-1 tumors (SWOG 9416) **Surgery → chemoRT if unresectable** • Consideration for upfront resectable tumor especially for resectable tumors with significant symptoms (*Gomez et al. Cancer* 2012)
Unresectable criteria includes multiple N2 stations, N3, bulky/invasive LN, lobectomy not feasible, or medically inoperable	**Definitive chemoRT → adjuvant durvalumab** • Preferred approach given results of PACIFIC trial which showed improvement in overall survival • Consider RT alone in elderly patients or poor PS

Radiation Treatment Technique

- **Simulation:**
  - Supine, upper body cradle, arms above head, and wedge below knee. 4DCT preferred. Consider breath-hold if tumor moves >1 cm. Optional fusion with PET or CT with contrast
- **Dose:**
  - **Definitive (able to tolerate chemotherapy):** 60 Gy in 30 fractions with concurrent chemotherapy
    Consider simultaneous integrated boost to GTV to 66 Gy.
  - **PORT:** 50.4 Gy in 28 fractions or 50 Gy in 25 fractions
    Increase dose for areas of concern (60-66 Gy for positive margins).
    Add concurrent chemo for gross residual dx.
    Add sequential chemo for N2 disease.
  - **Neoadjuvant:** 45 Gy in 1.8 Gy/fx > surgery if operable or completion to 60-66 Gy radiation if inoperable
  - **RT alone (if unable to tolerate chemotherapy):** 60-66 Gy in 30 fractions or 45 Gy in 15 fractions to PTV and SIB to 52.5-60 Gy in 15 fractions to GTV
  - **Superior sulcus tumors:**
    Neoadjuvant: 45 Gy in 1.8 Gy/fx > surgery if operable or completion to 60-66 Gy radiation if inoperable
    Adjuvant: Consider Hyper FX regimen (60 Gy in 1.2 Gy/fx bid) to minimize late radiation effects and reduce risk of brachial plexopathy (Gomez et al. *Cancer* 2012)
- **Target:**
  - **Definitive/neoadjuvant:**
    CTV: GTV contoured on MIP + 8 mm, edited out of anatomical boundaries such as bone and heart, and includes involved nodal stations and, if dose constraints met, ipsilateral hilum (no other elective nodal irradiation except ipsilateral hilum if staging adequate)
    PTV: CTV + 5 mm if daily kV or CTV + 3 mm if daily CBCT
- **Technique:**
  IMRT/VMAT or protons
- **IGRT:**
  Daily kV imaging and weekly CBCT
- **Planning directive (for daily fractionation):**
  Spinal cord: D_{max} < 45 Gy
  Total lung: MLD < 20 Gy, V20 < 35%, V10 < 45%, and V5 < 60%
  Heart: V30 Gy < 45%, mean < 26 Gy
  Esophagus: D_{max} < 80 Gy, V70 < 20%, V50 < 40%, and mean < 34 Gy
  Kidney (bilateral): V20 Gy < 32%
  Liver: V30 Gy < 40%, mean liver <30 Gy
  Brachial plexus: D_{max} < 66 Gy

Surgery

- Surgical resection alone is not sufficient treatment for locally advanced NSCLC.
- Standard surgery is **lobectomy with mediastinal lymph node dissection**.
- Other options depending on the extent of disease include pneumonectomy, segmentectomy, and sleeve resection.

Systemic Therapy

- Most commonly given alone in the preoperative setting or concurrent with radiation
- **Concurrent chemo:**
  - Cisplatin and etoposide
  - Cisplatin and vinblastine
  - Carboplatin and pemetrexed
  - Cisplatin and pemetrexed
  - Carboplatin and paclitaxel
- **Neoadjuvant and adjuvant chemo:**
  - Multiple platinum-based combinations including cisplatin with etoposide, paclitaxel, pemetrexed, and vincristine
  - If patient can't tolerate cisplatin, consider carboplatin and paclitaxel.

- **Immunotherapy**
  - Adjuvant durvalumab for 1 year after definitive chemoradiation (if no progression of disease after definitive chemoradiation)
  - Nivolumab in conjunction with chemotherapy as neoadjuvant treatment for resectable patients planned for surgery
  - Atezolizumab or pembrolizumab after adjuvant chemotherapy for patients who underwent resection
- **Tyrosine kinase inhibitor**
  - Adjuvant osimertinib for patients who underwent surgical resection and have targetable EGFR mutations

Side Effect Management

See **Early-Stage NSCLC** chapter.

Follow-up

- History/physical and CT: Every 3 months for 2 years → annually for 3 years
- Postradiation toxicity

  Esophagitis peaks 1-2 weeks after radiation therapy and then resolves weeks-months

  Radiation pneumonitis: Occurs 6 weeks to 1 year following RT with symptoms of dyspnea, cough, and fatigue. Inflammatory changes within RT field on imaging. Treat with high-dose steroid taper.

  Esophageal stricture/fistula (months-years)

  Long-term dyspnea/fibrosis (months-years)

  Brachial plexopathy for apical tumors (years)

Notable Literature and Trials

Evidence supporting trimodality therapy

Name/Inclusion	Arms	Outcomes	Notes
INT 0139 (*Albain et al. Lancet* 2009) Phase III—429 operable stage IIIA (N2) patients receiving neoadj CRT randomized to surgery (pneumonectomy or lobectomy) vs no surgery. All patients received adj cisplatin/etoposide	Induction CRT 45 Gy/25 fx w/ cis/etop followed by surgery and 2 cycles adj cis/etop Induction CRT 45 Gy/25 fx w cis/etop followed by continued RT to 61 Gy and 2 cycles adj cis/etop	Median PFS improved in surgical arm (12.8 vs 10.5 mo, $P = .017$) but not 5-y OS (27% surgery vs 20% chemoRT, $P = .10$). Pneumonectomy associated with high mortality risk. Lobectomy associated with improved OS compared to no surgery	Conclusion: Definitive CRT is a viable alternative to induction CRT and surgery
SWOG 9416 (*Rusch et al. JCO* 2007) 111 T3-4N0-1 patients with superior sulcus tumors	Phase II single arm—45 Gy with concurrent cisplatin/etoposide → surgical resection if stable or response → adjuvant cisplatin/etoposide × 2 cycles	83 patients underwent complete resection and pathologic complete response seen in 61 patients. 5-y survival was 44% for all patients and 54% after complete resection	Conclusion: Established combined modality therapy as standard for superior sulcus tumors

Postoperative radiation (PORT)

Name/Inclusion	Arms	Outcomes	Notes
LungART (*Le Pechoux et al. Lancet Oncol* 2022) Phase III—501 NSCLC patients with N2 disease who had complete resection	PORT 54 Gy/27-30 fx No PORT	3-y DFS 47% vs 44% (NS), median DFS 30.5 mo vs 22.8 mo (NS), increased late grade 3-4 cardiopulmonary toxicity (11% vs 5%), 3 deaths in PORT group vs 0 in no PORT	Conclusion: PORT improved mediastinal relapse but did not lead to improvement in DFS and had increased toxicity. PORT not routinely indicated for N2 disease

Evidence supporting definitive chemoradiation approach

Name/Inclusion	Arms	Outcomes	Notes
EORTC 08941 (*Van Meerbeeck et al. JCNI* 2007) Phase III—579 patients w operable stage III NSCLC	Induction chemo + surgery Induction chemo + radiation (60-62.5 Gy)	5-y OS (15.5% vs 14%) and median survival (16.4 mo vs 17.5 mo) not significantly different between arms	PORT 56 Gy in surgery arm for positive margins (40% received in surgical arm) Conclusion: Sequential chemoRT is a viable alternative to induction chemo + surgery
RTOG 9410 (*Curran et al. JCNI* 2011) Phase III—610 patients w/ unresectable stage III NSCLC	Induction chemo (cisplatin/vinblastine) → radiation 63 Gy/34 fx Concurrent chemo-radiation (cisplatin/vinblastine) 63 Gy/34 fx Concurrent chemo-radiation (cisplatin/etoposide) 69.6 Gy/58 fx bid	5-y OS (10% vs 16% vs 13%) Median survival (14.6 mo vs 17 mo vs 15.6 mo) Grade 3-4 esophageal toxicity worse in bid chemoradiation arm	Conclusion: Concurrent chemoRT leads to improved survival compared to sequential chemo-radiation. BID chemoRT results in too much toxicity
NSCLC Collaborative Group Meta-Analysis (*Auperin et al. JCO* 2010) Combined data from 6 RCTs—total 1205 patients	Meta-analysis compared concurrent chemoRT to sequential chemoRT	Concurrent chemoRT led to a 4.5% absolute survival benefit at 5 y (P = .004)	Conclusion: Concurrent chemoRT leads to improved survival compared to sequential chemoRT

Benefit with adjuvant immunotherapy after chemoradiation

Name/Inclusion	Arms	Outcomes	Notes
PACIFIC (*Antonia et al. NEJM* 2017, *Update Spigel et al. JCO* 2022) Phase III—713 patients w/ unresectable stage III NSCLC	Chemoradiation + consolidation durvalumab (up to 1 y) Chemoradiation only	Significant improvement in median OS (47.5 mo vs 29.1 mo) and PFS (16.9 mo vs 5.6 mo) 5-y OS (42.9% vs 33.4%) 5-y PFS (33.1% vs 19.0%)	Conclusion: Consolidative durvalumab after definitive chemoradiation leads to improved freedom from progression and also overall survival

Dose escalation for definitive chemoradiation leads to worse outcomes

Name/Inclusion	Arms	Outcomes	Notes
RTOG 0617 (*Bradley et al. Lancet Oncol* 2015) Phase III—2 × 2 design w/ 544 patients w/ stage IIIA-B NSCLC comparing 60-74 Gy radiation along with adjuvant cetuximab	ChemoRT to 60 Gy/30 fx with carboplatin/ paclitaxel (+/− cetuximab) ChemoRT to 74 Gy/37 fx with carboplatin/ paclitaxel (+/− cetuximab)	Trial closed early due to futility OS worse in 74 Gy group (1 y: 80% vs 69.8%, $P = .004$) and adding cetuximab did not improve survival Increased grade 3+ esophagitis in 74 Gy arm	Conclusion: Dose escalation to 74 Gy does not improve outcomes Secondary analysis demonstrated correlation of increased heart V40 Gy with worse survival (*Chun et al. JCO* 2017)

SMALL CELL LUNG CANCER

YUFEI LIU • SAUMIL GANDHI

Background

- **Incidence/prevalence:** Approximately 30 000 cases of SCLC per year in the United States (15% of all lung cancer diagnoses). About 1/3 are diagnosed with limited stage disease.
- **Outcomes:** 5-Year survival for stage I, II, III, and IV disease is 31%, 19%, 8%, and 2%, respectively.
- **Demographics:** Average age of diagnosis is 70. Highest incidence in White male smokers
- **Risk factors:** Smoking is the biggest risk factor (>90% of patients are heavy smokers). Increasing age, asbestos, and radon gas exposure are also risk factors.

Tumor Biology and Characteristics

- **Genetics:** TCGA genomic profiling of 110 SCLCs identified loss of *TP53* and *RB1* in nearly all cases. 25% of patients exhibited inactivating NOTCH pathway mutations. Targetable mutations in *EGFR*, *ALK*, *K-RAS*, and *ROS-1* not seen in SCLC
- **Pathology:** Malignant epithelial tumor of small round blue cells of neuroendocrine origin (Fig. 32.1) and scant cytoplasm. Necrosis often extensively seen in pathologic specimens with high mitotic count. SCLC is grouped into two variants: small cell carcinoma and combined small cell carcinoma, which include SCLC cells and any histologic subtype of NSCLC. On pathology, positive staining seen for synaptophysin, chromogranin A, IGF-1, and CD56 and typically negative for TTF1 and keratin (which are positive in NSCLC)
- **Imaging:** Enhance significantly on contrasted CT and highly PET-avid as well (Fig. 32.1). Typically presents centrally as opposed to peripherally

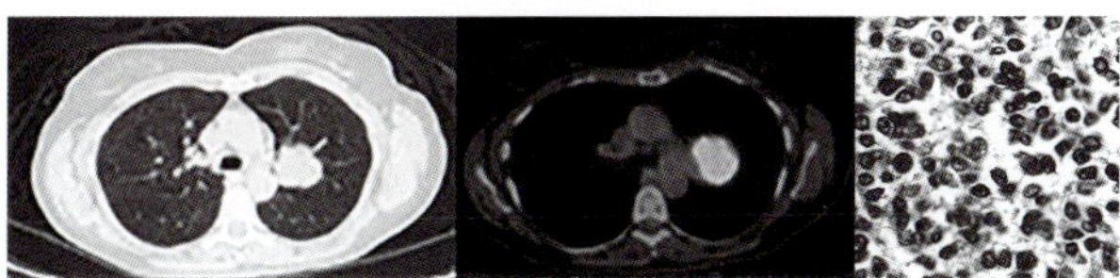

Figure 32.1 Representative CT (*left*) and PET (*middle*) images obtained from a patient presenting with cough/weight loss. The LUL mass and L hilar LNs were biopsied with pathology returning as SCLC. Note the small, round blue cells with scant cytoplasm and large nuclei, which is classic for SCLC (*right image*).

Workup

- **History and physical:** High frequency of bulky mediastinal lymphadenopathy leads to shortness of breath, hoarse voice, dysphagia, and/or superior vena cava syndrome. Evaluate for neurologic symptoms, paraneoplastic syndromes, and bone pain.
- **Labs:** CBC, CMP, LFTs, and LDH. SCLC is the most common solid malignancy associated with paraneoplastic syndromes: Syndrome of inappropriate antidiuretic hormone SIADH seen in 11-15% of patients. Ectopic Cushing syndrome (5%) and Lambert-Eaton syndrome (1-3%) are also observed.
- **Procedures/biopsy:** Bronchoscopy +/− FNA with biopsy if central, CT-guided, or thoracentesis for peripheral lesions. If cT1-T2N0 disease with no evidence of distant metastases, consider mediastinal staging.
- **Imaging:** CT of the chest with contrast and PET/CT done for staging (identifying distant metastases, distinguishing between limited stage and extensive stage). MRI of the brain w/ contrast performed on all patients as the brain is a sanctuary site with respect to chemotherapy and frequently the first site of failure in patients with SCLC

Anatomy

See Early-Stage NSCLC chapter.

Small Cell Lung Cancer Staging (*AJCC 8th edition*)

(Same as NSCLC; however, use of historical "limited" and "extensive" stage definitions is frequently made)

T Stage		**N Stage**	
T1	≤3 cm without main bronchus invasion	N1	Ipsi peribronchial/hilar LN
T1a	≤1 cm	N2	Ipsi mediastinal/subcarinal LN
T1b	>1-2 cm	N3	Scalene/supraclav LN or contra mediastinal/hilar LN
T1c	>2-3 cm	**M Stage**	
T2	>3-5 cm or involves the main bronchus but not carina, invades visceral pleura, or associated atelectasis or obstructive pneumonia	M1a	Nodule in contra lobe, pleura, or pericardium or malignant pleural or pericardial effusion
T2a	>3-4 cm	M1b	Single extrathoracic metastasis
T2b	>4-5 cm	M1c	Multiple extrathoracic mets
T3	>5-7 cm or separate nodule in the same lobe or invades CW, phrenic nerve, parietal pericardium		
T4	>7 cm or separate nodule in different ipsi lobe or invades the diaphragm, mediastinum, heart, great vessels, trachea, recurrent laryngeal nerve, esophagus, vertebral body, carina		

Stage Grouping

<table>
<tr><th></th><th>N0</th><th>N1</th><th>N2</th><th>N3</th><th>M1a-b</th><th>M1c</th></tr>
<tr><td>T1a-c</td><td>IA1-3</td><td rowspan="3">IIB</td><td rowspan="3">IIIA</td><td rowspan="3">IIIB</td><td rowspan="5">IVA</td><td rowspan="5">IVB</td></tr>
<tr><td>T2a</td><td>IB</td></tr>
<tr><td>T2b</td><td>IIA</td></tr>
<tr><td>T3</td><td>IIB</td><td rowspan="2">IIIA</td><td rowspan="2">IIIB</td><td rowspan="2">IIIC</td></tr>
<tr><td>T4</td><td>IIIA</td></tr>
</table>

VA Lung Cancer Study Group Staging

- Historical definitions:
  - **Limited stage:** Intrathoracic disease that can be encompassed within a reasonable radiation field, excluding those with pleural or pericardial effusions. However, applicability of these definitions to modern techniques is questionable. Overall, "limited" = localized; "extensive" = metastatic
  - **Extensive stage:** All others

Treatment Algorithm

Limited stage	• For solitary pulmonary nodule and medically operable based on PFTs → mediastinoscopy → proceed to surgery (lobectomy preferred) if negative lymph node involvement. Adjuvant platinum and etoposide 4-6 cycles followed by PCI. For positive nodes after resection, proceed to concurrent chemoRT followed by PCI • For locally advanced disease → chemoRT followed by PCI. If poor performance status, can consider chemotherapy alone or supportive care
Extensive stage	• Platinum and etoposide ×4-6 cycles with immunotherapy (atezolizumab or durvalumab) → for partial or complete response, consolidative chest RT. Weigh risks/benefits and consider PCI • Patients with symptomatic brain mets or cord compression, provide palliative RT +/− steroids and 4-6 cycles of platinum/etoposide → for partial or complete response, consolidative chest RT

Chemotherapy Treatment Guidelines

- **LS-SCLC:** Acceptable regimens for limited stage disease (maximum 4-6 cycles) Cisplatin or carboplatin with etoposide
  During concurrent chemoradiation, cisplatin/etoposide is recommended.
- **ES-SCLC:** Acceptable regimens for extensive stage disease (maximum 4-6 cycles) Cisplatin or carboplatin with etoposide along with atezolizumab (IMpower133 *NEJM* 2018) or durvalumab (CASPIAN *Lancet* 2019)

Radiation Treatment Technique

- **SIM:** 4DCT, supine, both arms overhead holding T-bar, upper Vac-Lok, wingboard, and knee wedge. Consider breath-hold technique if motion is >1 cm on 4DCT scan (Fig. 32.2).
- **Dose: Limited stage:** 45 Gy in 30 fractions twice a day (at least 6 hours apart) at 1.5 Gy/fx (preferred MDACC approach)
  If bid fractionation is not feasible, acceptable alternative is 1.8-2.0 Gy/d to a dose of 60-70 Gy. Radiation should be delivered concurrently with chemotherapy, ideally beginning during cycle 1.
  Extensive stage: 30 Gy in 10 fractions or 45 Gy in 15 fractions daily
- **Target:** Paradigm similar to NSCLC. GTV defined by most recent PET/CT. If chemo is given first, can limit GTV to postchemo tumor volume. Use prechemo PET/CT to define involved LN stations. Historically, elective nodal radiation was used, but it is omitted in current trials as rate of nodal failure is low when using PET/CT for staging.
  Margins: 5- to 10-mm CTV, 5-mm PTV expansion for daily CBCT
- **Technique:** IMRT/VMAT (Fig. 32.3)
- **IGRT:** For free breathing treatment setup, daily kV imaging, and weekly CBCT. For breath-hold treatment setup, CBCT before each fraction
- **Planning directive (either daily or bid fractionation)**
  Ensure coverage of PTV by >95% of prescription dose.
  Spinal cord: D_{max} < 36 Gy (bid), <45 Gy (daily)
  Mean lung dose <20 Gy, V20 < 35%, V10 < 45%, and V5 < 60%
  Heart: V30 < 45 Gy, mean heart dose < 26 Gy
  Esophagus: D_{max} < 80 Gy, V70 < 20%, V50 < 40%, mean dose < 34 Gy
  Kidney (bilateral): V20 < 32%
  Liver: V30 < 40%, mean liver dose < 30 Gy
  Brachial plexus: D_{max} < 50.6 Gy (bid), <3 cc, >44.5 Gy (bid), D_{max} < 66 Gy (daily)
  Chest wall: V40 < 150 cc (bid) (Figs. 32.2 and 32.3)

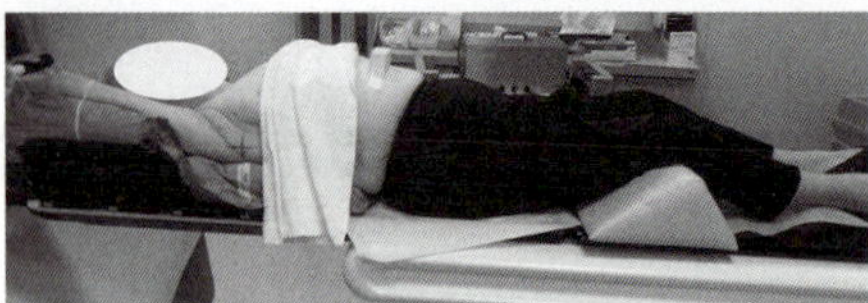

Figure 32.2 Typical SCLC/NSCLC simulation setup showing a patient positioned supine with a wingboard, upper Vac-Lok device, both hands overhead gripping a T-bar. Opaque markers mounted on a box are taped to the patient's abdomen to assess breathing.

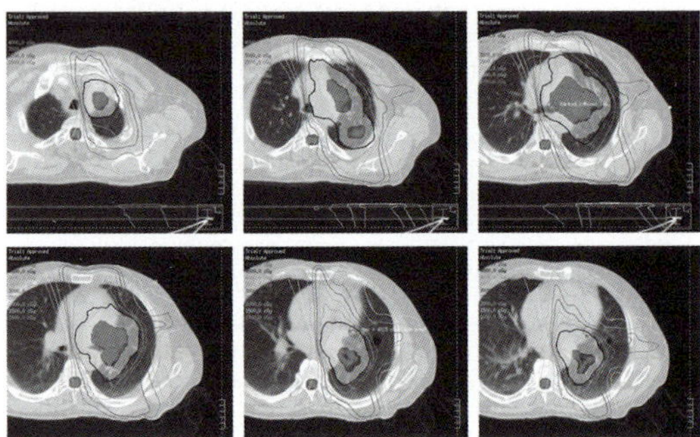

Figure 32.3 Limited stage SCLC IMRT plan. 45 Gy isodose line showed in *blue* surrounding PTV (*sky blue color wash*), CTV (*tan*), and GTV (*red*). Note sparing of contralateral lung. **See color insert**.

Prophylactic Cranial Irradiation (PCI)

- **Indication**
  - For limited stage, PCI should be discussed for patients with a partial or complete response following chemoRT, as it decreases the risk of developing brain metastasis by about 50% and improves OS based on clinical studies. Restage after completion of chemoRT and if no progression (local or distant), then consider starting PCI 6-12 weeks after chemoRT completion.
  - For extensive stage, a thorough discussion should take place in context of conflicting data (*Takahashi et al. Lancet Oncol* 2017; *Slotman et al. NEJM* 2007). Patients should be informed that it will reduce the risk of developing subsequent brain metastases with questionable OS benefit.
- **SIM:** Arms on chest holding A-bar, Aquaplast mask with isocenter placed at midbrain
- **Dose:** 25 Gy in 10 fractions
- **Target:** Whole brain, ensure coverage of cribriform plate and inferior edge should extend to C1/C2 vertebral bodies.
- **Technique:** 3DCRT. Beam arrangement typically opposed laterals or right and left anterior obliques (gantry angled to 85 and 275 degrees) to spare lens exposure due to beam divergence
- **IGRT:** Usually no image guidance, setup to marks only. Consider daily MV or kV imaging.

Surgery

- High local recurrence rates (35-50%) suggest that surgery may offer benefit in local control.
- Surgical resection generally only recommended for patients with a solitary pulmonary nodule, no evidence of local/regional lymphadenopathy, no distant metastatic disease, and no contraindications to surgery. Lobectomy preferred.

- The survival of patients undergoing surgery for pathologic stage I, II, and III disease was 48%, 39%, and 15%, respectively, at 5 years.
- No randomized trials exist for adjuvant therapy; however, most patients receive adjuvant chemotherapy and adjuvant radiation for those found to have pathologic N1 or N2 disease.

Side Effect Management

- Nausea: Zofran, Compazine, Reglan, low-dose dexamethasone, Haldol, IV fluids
- Pneumonitis: For symptomatic patients (eg, shortness of breath, drop in pO_2), consider oral steroid taper (typically prednisone starting at 1 mg/kg daily for 2-3 weeks, remember Bactrim prophylaxis for PCP pneumonia and antacid prophylaxis for ulcers).
- Esophagitis: Magic mouthwash (viscous lidocaine, Benadryl, nystatin), glutamine supplement (eg, Helios), aloe products, narcotic elixir second line
- Dermatitis: Aquaphor or other moisturizing cream, gel sheets
- Chest wall pain: Analgesics, physical therapy
- Neurocognitive side effects of PCI: Memantine 20 mg bid (start 20 mg daily ×1-2 weeks and then increase) to reduce risk of late neurocognitive side effects in patients with >6 months expected survival.

Side Effect Management

See **Early-Stage NSCLC** chapter.

Follow-up

- History/physical and CT: Every 3 months for 2 years → annually for 3 years

Notable Trials

Chemoradiation vs chemotherapy alone

Name/Inclusion	Arms	Outcomes	Notes
French Meta-Analysis (*Pignon et al. NEJM* 1992) Meta-analysis of 13 trials with 2140 patients w/ LS-SCLC	Meta-analysis comparing chemo alone to chemoRT	5% increase in 3-y overall survival with chemoRT (8.9 → 14.3%; *P* = .001). Local control improved from 16% to 34%. A trend was seen toward a larger reduction in mortality among younger patients (<55 y)	Conclusion: ChemoRT results in better local control and survival compared to chemo alone in patients with LS-SCLC Chemo was predominantly cyclophosphamide or doxorubicin-based as opposed to SOC cisplatin/etoposide

Daily vs twice daily thoracic radiation in limited stage disease

Name/Inclusion	Arms	Outcomes	Notes
INT 0096 (*Turrisi et al. NEJM* 1998) Phase III—417 patients with LS-SCLC	ChemoRT 45 Gy/25 fx QD w/ cisplatin/etoposide ChemoRT 45 Gy/30 fx bid w/ cisplatin/etoposide	Improved 5-y OS (16% vs 26%, *P* = .04) and median survival (19 vs 23 mo, *P* = .04) w/ bid along with decreased rate of local failure (52% vs 36%, *P* = .06) Increased incidence of grade 3 esophagitis (11% vs 27%, *P* < .001)	Conclusion: BID fractionation significantly improved overall survival over QD, but important to note that QD BED (assuming alpha/beta of 10) was lower

Name/Inclusion	Arms	Outcomes	Notes
CONVERT (*Faivre-Finn et al. Lancet Oncol* 2017) Phase III—547 patients with LS-SCLC	ChemoRT 45 Gy/30 fx bid w/ cisplatin/etoposide	2-y OS (56% vs 51%) and median OS (30 vs 25 mo) were not significantly different (P = .14). Grade 4 neutropenia increased with bid (49% vs 38%, P = .05). Similar grade 3 esophagitis rates (19% both arms)	Conclusion: Trial designed as superiority, so bid remains SOC as equivalence not demonstrated. However, in practice, this trial has been used to justify QD fractionation for patients who cannot tolerate bid
	ChemoRT 66 Gy/33 fx bid w/ cisplatin/etoposide		

Role of consolidative chemoRT in extensive stage disease

Name/Inclusion	Arms	Outcomes	Notes
Yugoslavia Trial (*Jeremic et al. JCO* 1999) Phase III—210 patients with ES-SCLC treated with EP × 3C and had distant CR and local CR or PR	54 Gy/36 fx bid with concurrent carboplatin/EP and then EP × 2C	Improved MS (17 vs 11 mo, P = .041) with radiation	Conclusion: Consolidative RT improved survival compared to further chemo for ES-SCLC patients with good response to initial chemo Patients with distant CR had PCI
	EP × 4C		
Netherlands Trial (*Slotman et al. Lancet* 2015) Phase III—498 patients with ES-SCLC with ECOG 0-2, initial response to chemo, and received PCI	Thoracic RT (30 Gy/10 fx)	Primary end point of 1-y OS not different (33% vs 28%, P = .066), but on secondary analysis, 2-y OS improved (13% vs 3%, P = .004) along with 6-mo PFS (24% vs 7%, P = .001)	Conclusion: Consolidative thoracic radiation results in improved disease control and survival in ES-SCLC patients who respond to chemo and have good performance status and PCI
	Observation		

Prophylactic cranial irradiation in SCLC

Name/Inclusion	Arms	Outcomes	Notes
French Meta-Analysis (*Auperin et al. NEJM* 1999) Meta-analysis of 7 trials with 987 patients w/ SCLC (85% LS-SCLC)	Meta-analysis comparing PCI to no PCI. Various doses and fractionations for PCI	Improved 3-y OS (20.7% vs 15.3%, P = .01) and 3-y LC (33.3% vs 58.6%, P < .001) for PCI. Larger RT doses (8, 24-25, 30, 36-40 Gy) led to greater decrease in risk of mets, but no impact on survival	Conclusion: Meta-analysis of mostly LS-SCLC patients showed survival and local control benefit of PCI

SCLC 6-15

Name/Inclusion	Arms	Outcomes	Notes
EORTC 08993-22993 (*Slotman et al. NEJM 2007*) Phase III—286 patients with ES-SCLC, ECOG 0-2, response to chemo, and no evidence of brain mets (imaging not required)	PCI (20-30 Gy/10 fx)	Improved 1-y OS (27.1% vs 13.3%, *P* = .003), MS (6.7 vs 5.4 mo, *P* = .03) and incidence of symptomatic brain mets (14.6% vs 40.4%, *P* < .001) with PCI	Conclusion: PCI improved survival and reduced the incidence of symptomatic brain mets in ES-SCLC patients with response to chemo Caveat: Brain imaging was not required prior to randomization
	No PCI		
Japanese Trial (*Takahashi et al. Lancet 2017*) Phase III RCT of PCI vs no PCI in ES-SCLC patients with any response chemo. Brain MRI required within 4 wk of randomization.	PCI (25 Gy/10 fx)	Reduced incidence of brain mets at 1 y with PCI (32.9% vs 59.0%, *P* < .001), but no difference in survival (median: 11.6 vs 13.7 mo, *P* = .094)	Conclusion: PCI should be considered on a case-by-case basis for eligible patients with ES-SCLC as there was no survival benefit shown in this trial
	Observation		

THYMOMA AND THYMIC CARCINOMA

VINCENT BERNARD • ZHONGXING LIAO

BACKGROUND

- **Incidence/prevalence:** Rare, ~0.15/100 000, the most common neoplasm of the anterior mediastinum
- **Outcomes:** 5-Year OS by Masaoka stage: stage I, 95%; stage II, 90%; stage III, 60%; and stage IV, 11-50%. Thymic carcinoma, 20-30%
- **Demographics:** Median age 40-60 years; equal in males and females
- **Risk factors:** May be related to autoimmune disorders including myasthenia gravis. No other known etiologic risk factors

TUMOR BIOLOGY AND CHARACTERISTICS

- **Pathology:** Histologic subtypes include benign, medullary, and spindle cell, mixed; moderately malignant, lymphocyte-rich, lymphocytic, predominantly cortical, organoid, cortical, epithelial, atypical, squamoid, and well-differentiated thymic carcinoma; and highly malignant, thymic carcinoma (<1% of thymic tumors).

ANATOMY

Thymus originates from thymic *epithelial* cells (third pharyngeal pouch); involved in processing and maturation of T lymphocytes to recognize foreign Ag from self-Ag

- Thymomas: 1-2% lymph node metastasis rate and 1% distant metastasis (mostly to the lung)
- **Thymic** carcinomas: 30% lymph node metastasis rate and 12% distant metastasis (lung, bone, liver)
- Lymph node drainage to the lower cervical, internal mammary, and hilar nodes
- **Differential of mediastinal mass**

  Anterior: Thymoma, thymic carcinoma, carcinoid, germ cell tumor, lymphoma, and goiter

Middle: Cysts > lymphomas, teratomas > sarcomas, and granuloma
Posterior: Neurogenic tumors (PNET, schwannomas, neurofibroma, neuroblastoma, ganglioneuroma) and pheochromocytoma

Workup and Staging

- **History and physical:** 1/3 asymptomatic (incidental), 1/3 myasthenia gravis, and 1/3 thoracic symptoms (cough, SOB, CP, SVC). Ask for B symptoms (rule out lymphoma). Thymoma diagnosed clinically if mediastinal mass + symptoms of myasthenia, red cell aplasia, or hypogammaglobulinemia
- **Labs:** LDH, ESR, and AFP/HCG (rule out germ cell tumor). Paraneoplastic syndromes include myasthenia gravis (35-50%), due to autoAb to postsynaptic AChR; **symptoms**, easy fatigability, double vision, and ptosis; **diagnosis**, Tensilon test (edrophonium); **treatment**, AChE inhibitors (pyridostigmine) or thymectomy. May also present with red cell aplasia (5%), immune deficiency syndromes (ie, hypogammaglobulinemia, 5%), autoimmune disorders (collagen vascular, dermatologic, endocrine), and other malignancies (lymphomas, GI/breast carcinoma, Kaposi sarcoma)
- **Imaging/procedures:** CT of the chest with contrast preferred. MRI optional. PET/CT if lymphoma or thymic carcinoma suspected, PFTs. If thymoma is suspected, straight to surgery (avoid biopsy if resectable to avoid seeding)

New Thymoma and Thymic Carcinoma Staging

Masaoka Stage	
	Completely encapsulated (micro and macro)
IIA	Microscopic transcapsular invasion
IIB	Macroscopic invasion into fatty tissue or adherent to pleura/pericardium
III	Macroscopic invasion into other organs (ie, pericardium, vessels, lung)
IVA	Mets to pleura/pericardium

Treatment Algorithm*

- Prognosis: associated with completeness of resection
- If myasthenia gravis, signs and symptoms should be controlled medically before surgery

WHO Designations	
Type A-AB	Benign thymoma
Type B1-B3	Malignant thymoma
Type C	Thymic carcinoma

Masaoka Stage	Recommended Treatment
Stage I	Surgical resection
Stage II	Surgical resection Consider PORT particularly for high-risk factors (close/positive margins, high grade, pleural adhesion)
Stage III	Surgical resection → consider PORT
Stage IV	Induction chemo → surgery → consider PORT
Thymic carcinoma	**Operable:** Max surgery → consider chemoRT for cases of limited disease **Inoperable:** Consider induction chemo, RT, or chemoRT

*With new AJCC staging, these recommendations may change.

Radiation Treatment Technique

- **SIM:** 4DCT, supine, upper Vac-Lok device. Consider breath-hold if tumor moves >1 cm.
- **Dose:** Unresectable: 60-70 Gy (45-50 Gy to PTV and 60-70 Gy SIB to GTV)
  PORT: R0 resection = 45-50 Gy; R1 resection = 54 Gy; R2 resection = 60-70 Gy
- **Target:** GTV: grossly visible tumor/tumor bed (clips can be useful if placed)
  CTV: Entire pretreatment superior-inferior extent of disease, posttreatment lateral extent (respect anatomic boundaries and follow pleural spaces)
  PTV: 0.5-1 cm based on IGRT
- **Technique:** IMRT or VMAT

- **Planning directive (for conventional fractionation):**

RT Alone	ChemoRT	Neoadjuvant ChemoRT
Lung: V20 ≤ 40% Heart: V30 ≤ 45% mean < 26 Gy Spinal cord: D_{max} < 45 Gy Esophagus: V50 < 50%	Lung: V20 ≤ 35%, V10 ≤ 45% V5 ≤ 65% Heart: V30 ≤ 45% mean < 26 Gy Spinal cord: D_{max} < 45 Gy Esophagus: V50 < 40%	Lung: V20 ≤ 30%, V10 ≤ 40% V5 ≤ 55% Heart: V30 ≤ 45% mean < 26 Gy Spinal cord: D_{max} < 45 Gy Esophagus: V50 < 40%

Chemotherapy

- **Induction:** Can downstage if unresectable
  First line: Cytoxan/Adriamycin/cisplatin (CAP) +/− prednisone
- **Adjuvant:** Thymoma with gross residual disease or thymic carcinoma with R1-R2 resection
  Possible chemotherapy regimens include
  VP-16/ifosfamide/cisplatin (VIP)
  Cisplatin/VP-16 (EP)
  Carboplatin/paclitaxel
  Cisplatin/Adriamycin/vincristine/Cytoxan (ADOC)

Side Effects

See **Early-Stage NSCLC** chapter.

Follow-up

- History/physical q3-12mo + annual CT of the chest for life (late recurrences can occur for >10 years)

Notable Literature

Adjuvant radiation therapy after surgical resection

Name	Arms	Outcomes	Notes
Peking 1999 (*Zhang Chin Med J (Engl)* 1999) Prospective randomized trial of 12 patients with stage I thymoma	1. Surgery 2. Surgery followed by adjuvant RT (lymphocytic predominant, 50 Gy/25 fx; epithelial/mixed, 60 Gy/30 fx)	10-y OS: 92% (surgery) vs 88% (surgery + RT), not significant	Adjuvant RT is not necessary for stage I thymoma
ITMIG 2016 (*Rimner et al. JTO* 2016) Retrospective database review of 1263 patients with stage II-III thymoma and R0 resection	1. R0 resection without PORT 2. R0 resection with PORT	10-y OS: 79% (no PORT) vs 86% (PORT), *P* = .002 Recurrence-free survival: not affected by PORT	PORT improves 10-y OS in stage II-III completely resected thymoma, but selection bias must be considered

MESOTHELIOMA

VINCENT BERNARD • ZHONGXING LIAO

Background

- **Incidence/prevalence:** Approximately 3000 cases diagnosed annually in the United States. Overall incidence is decline in the United States due to less asbestos exposure.
- **Outcomes:** Median survival is ~12 months (range 4-20 months). MS 8 months sarcomatoid, 19 months epithelioid, and 13 months mixed subtype. Stage I

MS = 20 months, stage II MS = 19 months, stage III MS = 16 months, stage IV MS = 11 months (*Rusch et al. J Thorac Oncol* 2012)

- **Demographics:** Peak incidence in fifth to seventh decades
- **Risk factors:** 70-80% related to asbestos exposure (commonly found in insulation, ship building, construction work, and brake pads, 90% male predominance). Rod/needle (amphibole) greater risk factor than serpentine (chrysotile). Latency is 20-40 years due to chronic pleural irritation leading to malignant transformation. Smoking + asbestos increases risk.

Tumor Biology and Characteristics

- **Genetics:** Four distinct molecular subtypes: sarcomatoid, epithelioid, biphasic-epithelioid (biphasic-E), and biphasic-sarcomatoid (biphasic-S) based on RNA-seq. Mutations in *BAP1, NF2, TP53, SETD2, DDX3X, ULK2, RYR2, CFAP45, SETDB1, and DDX51.* Loss of tumor suppressor genes p14, p16, and NF-2. Alterations in Hippo, mTOR, histone methylation, RNA helicase, and p53 signaling pathways
- **Pathology:** Sarcomatoid (15-25%), epithelioid (40-60%, best prognosis), and mixed subtypes (25-35%). May be confused with adenocarcinoma (IHC or electron micro required to differentiate)
- **Imaging:** Appears as a pleural thickening, possibly with pleural plaques, calcifications, involvement of interlobar fissures often associated with pleural effusion on x-ray and CT imaging

Anatomy

- Mesothelium is a membrane composed of simple squamous epithelium, which forms the lining of pleura (thoracic cavity), mediastinum, pericardium, peritoneum, tunica vaginalis testis, and tunica serosa uteri.
- The inner lining of the pleura is the visceral pleura and outer lining is the parietal pleura. Parietal pleura includes the mediastinal and diaphragmatic pleura.
- Pleura extends from SCV fossa (thoracic inlet) superiorly to the insertion of the diaphragm inferiorly.
- Mesothelioma spreads by direct extension and seeding into the pleural space, through the chest wall, into the mediastinum, to the peritoneum, and to the lymph nodes. It has a tendency to grow along tracks of biopsies or chest tubes. Lymph node drainage:
  - Peribronchial, internal mammary nodes (IMN), hilar, and ipsi and contralateral mediastinum
  - Spreads to level 8 (lower paraesophageal), level 9 (pulmonary ligament), and diaphragmatic nodes more frequently than NSCLC
  - Axillary and/or supraclav (SCV) nodes at risk if with chest wall involvement

Workup

- **History and physical:** Cough and shortness of breath are the most common presenting symptoms. Ask about asbestos exposure. Evaluate performance status. Typically present with weight loss and respiratory symptoms
- **Labs:** CBC, CMP, and PFTs
- **Procedures/biopsy:** Historically, biopsy is done via thoracentesis, but if VATS is being done, obtain biopsy at that time. Perform pulmonary function tests to evaluate operability. VATS to r/o c/l or peritoneal dz. Mediastinoscopy to r/o N2/N3 disease. Renal scan prior to RT
- **Imaging:** CT of the chest/abdomen with contrast for pleural effusions or calcified pleural plaques. Chest MRI with contrast and PET/CT scan optional and typically done to determine chest wall/diaphragm invasion.

Treatment Algorithm

Stages I-III and epithelioid (medically operable)	Surgical resection (EPP) → chemotherapy → RT Surgical resection (P/D) → chemotherapy → RT (on protocol) Chemotherapy → surgical resection (EPP) → RT Chemotherapy → surgical resection (P/D) → observation vs RT (on protocol)
Sarcomatoid, mixed histology, medically inoperable, stage IV	Chemotherapy (PS 0-2) vs best supportive care (PS 3-4)

Surgery

- Surgical resection possible in only a minority of patients with T1-3N0-1
- Extrapleural pneumonectomy (EPP) provides the greatest cytoreduction and includes the en bloc resection of the parietal and visceral pleura, lung, pericardium, and ipsilateral diaphragm. Mediastinal lymph node sampling of at least three stations is recommended. Graft is placed in the region of the diaphragm.
- Pleurectomy and decortication (P/D) is the complete removal of the pleura, and all gross tumor +/− en bloc resection of the pericardium and/or diaphragm with reconstruction, P/D can be considered for patients with more extensive disease (greater nodal burden, more invasive disease) or medically high risk. Allows expansion of the ipsi lung and reduces recurrent pleural effusions
- Pleurodesis with talc can be palliative.

Radiation Treatment Technique

- **SIM:** Supine, arms up, with a wingboard, upper body Vac-Lok device, and T-bar. 4DCT scan. Wire scar/drain sites. Consider 5-mm bolus (3 cm) around the scar/drain sites. Scan from thoracic inlet (starts at ribs around T1) through below the ribs (at least L2 or as inferiorly as possible). If PD or biopsy only, get quantitative perfusion scan to assess lung function (FEV1 [% contribution contralateral lung] should be >30% predicted).
- **Dose:** 45-50.4 Gy in 28 fractions at 1.8 Gy/fx, consider SIB to gross disease, positive margin, and PET-avid regions to 60 Gy (2.4 Gy/fx) to increase the likelihood of local control.

  Palliation: Several possible regimens, including 45 Gy in 15 fractions, 30 Gy in 10 fractions, or 20 Gy in 5 fractions. ≥4 Gy for skin nodules/pain from chest wall invasion

  Prophylactic: 7 Gy × 3 to drain sites (*Boutin et al. Chest* 1995), although may not reduce rate of seeding (*Clive et al. Lancet Oncol* 2016), so not done routinely at MDACC
- **Target:** Ipsilateral hemithoracic pleural surfaces, including the parietal/visceral pleura, diaphragm, and involved nodal stations (Fig. 34.1). Modify contours to include scars and drains with ~2.5-cm margin. Approach center of the sternum anteromedially and approach/abut the spinal canal posteromedially. Include the diaphragm crus/insertion (~L2) inferiorly. Utilize surgical clips, scars, and drain sites. High-risk areas for contouring misses: costophrenic, costodiaphragmatic, anteromedial pleural reflection, and cardiophrenic angles. If treatment after P/D or biopsy alone, consider 1-cm outside chest wall, 0.6 cm into lung parenchyma (+/− inclusion of fissures) with "donut" technique.

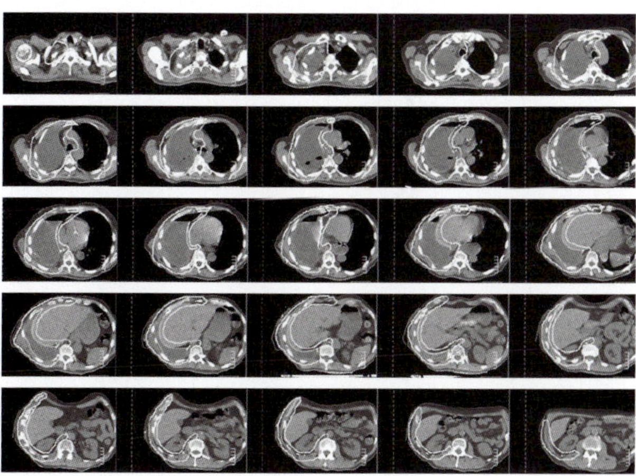

Figure 34.1 IMRT/VMAT contours for right-sided mesothelioma.

- **Technique:** IMRT/VMAT (Fig. 34.2)

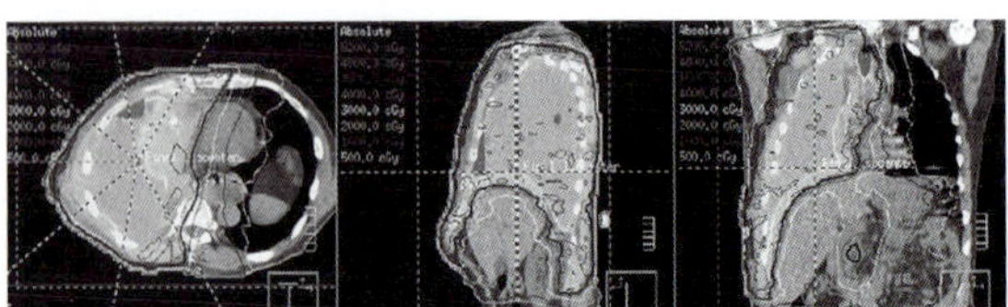

Figure 34.2 IMRT/VMAT plan for right-sided mesothelioma.

- **IGRT:** Daily kV imaging with once or twice weekly CBCT up to daily CBCT (depending on setup stability)
- **Planning directive (for 45 Gy in 25 fractions sp EPP and with optional boost to 54-60 Gy for R1/R2 resection AND hemithoracic RT on protocol sp P/D):**
  Target: V95% or D95% of the PTV is 45 Gy; D99-100% of CTV gets 45 Gy
  Contralateral lung: MLD < 8 Gy, V20 < 7%
  Liver: V30 < 50%, mean < 30 Gy
  Contralateral kidney: V15 < 20%
  Ipsilateral kidney: V20 < 33% (compromise coverage, if necessary, based on renal scan results)
  Stomach: Mean < 30 Gy
  Esophagus: V55 Gy < 70%, V60 Gy < 30%,
  Mean < 34 Gy
  Heart: V40 Gy < 70%, V45 Gy < 30, V30 Gy < 45%, Mean < 26 Gy%
  Spinal cord: D_{max} < 50 Gy, V45 Gy < 10%
  Major vessels: 5 cc < 70 Gy, 10 cc < 60 Gy
  Brachial plexus: D_{max} < 60 Gy, 1 cc < 50 Gy, 10 cc < 40 Gy
  For palliative cases, utilize standard lung constraints (see "NSCLC").

CHEMOTHERAPY

- **Agents:** Cisplatin and pemetrexed +/− bevacizumab, or nivolumab and ipilimumab

SIDE EFFECT MANAGEMENT

- Nausea: Zofran, Compazine, Reglan, low-dose dexamethasone, Haldol, IV fluids
- Pneumonitis: For symptomatic patients (eg, shortness of breath, drop in pO_2), consider oral steroid taper (typically prednisone starting at 1 mg/kg daily).
- Esophagitis: Magic mouthwash (viscous lidocaine, Benadryl, nystatin), glutamine supplement (eg, Helios), aloe products, narcotic elixir second line
- Dermatitis: Aquaphor or other moisturizing cream, gel sheets
- Chest wall pain: Analgesics, physical therapy

FOLLOW-UP

- CT of the chest/abdomen/pelvis: at 6 weeks, then q3mo for 2 years, and then q6-12mo thereafter. PET/CT scan can also be used at 3 months and then PRN for suspicious findings on CT imaging.

Notable Literature

EPP +/− hemithoracic RT

Name	Arms	Outcomes	Notes
SAKK 17/04 Trial (Stahel *Lancet Oncol* 2015) Randomized phase II trial of 54 patients after neoadjuvant cisplatin and pemetrexed > EPP	Hemithoracic RT Observation	No LRR benefit, OS benefit, or QOL improvement with RT	Role of radiation in EPP setting should be discussed with patients and evaluated in further protocols. The rationale for continued use of RT in the EPP setting comes from retrospective studies showing reasonable outcomes with multi-disciplinary management

Intensity-modulated radiation therapy s/p EPP

Name	Arms	Outcomes	Notes
Harvard (*Allen et al. IJROBP* 2006) Retrospective review of 13 patients treated with IMRT to 54 Gy	IMRT to 54 Gy with most patients receiving heated intraoperative cisplatin	46% fatal pneumonitis, pulmonary death	MLD 15.2 Gy, V20 17.6% No pulmonary death: MLD 12.9 Gy, V20 10.9%
MD Anderson (*Rice et al. IJROBP* 2007) Retrospective review of 63 patients s/p EPP, stages III-IV	IMRT to 45-50 Gy after EPP	MS: 14.2 mo, LRR 13%, DM 54%, pulmonary death: 9.5%	Pulmonary death: MLD 10.2 Gy, V20 9.8%. No pulmonary death: MLD 7.6 Gy, V20 3.6%. Recommended constraints: MLD < 8.5 Gy, V20 < 7%
MD Anderson (*Gomez et al. J Thorac Oncol* 2013) Retrospective review of 86 patients	IMRT to 45-50 Gy after EPP	Median OS 14.7 mo, grade 5 pulmonary toxicity (*n* = 5), LRR 16%, DM 59%, grade 3+ toxicity: skin 17%, lung 12%, heart 2.3%, GI 16%	

Intensity-modulated radiation therapy s/p P/D

Name	Arms	Outcomes	Notes
MD Anderson (*Chance et al. IJROBP* 2015) Retrospective study of 48 patients	1. Hemithoracic IMRT post P/D 2. Hemithoracic IMRT post EPP	P/D IMRT associated with OS 28.4 vs 14.2 mo, PFS 16.4 vs 8.2 mo	Nearly all had neoadjuvant chemotherapy
MSKCC (*Gupta et al. IJROBP* 2005) Retrospective study of 125 patients	RT after P/D, median dose 42.5 Gy	MS 13.5 mo, 2-y OS 23%, LC 42%	RT dose <40 Gy, nonepithelioid, left-sided disease, and use of implant worse. 12 patients with pneumonitis, 8 patients with pericarditis, 2 patients died from grade 5 toxicity

Chemotherapy

Name	Arms	Outcomes	Notes
University of Chicago (*Vogelzang et al. JCO* 2003) 456 patients not eligible for curative surgery. Phase III randomized	Pemetrexed + cisplatin Cisplatin	Response rate: for pemetrexed + cisplatin 41% vs cisplatin 17% (*P* = .001), TTP 6 vs 4 mo, OS 12 vs 9 mo (*P* = .02)	Treatment with pemetrexed plus cisplatin resulted in superior survival time, time to progression, and response rates compared with treatment with cisplatin alone in patients with malignant pleural mesothelioma

ESOPHAGEAL CANCER

VINCENT BERNARD • STEVEN LIN

Background

- **Incidence/prevalence:** The seventh leading cause of cancer death in men in the United States; 21 560 cases diagnosed each year (16 120 estimated deaths); lifetime risk 0.5%
- **Outcomes:** 5-Year survival for local, regional, and distant disease 42.9%, 23.4%, and 4.6%, respectively (SEER)
- **Demographics:** More common in men; squamous cell carcinoma prevalent in developing nations (>90%). Adenocarcinoma more common in developed countries including the United States (~70% cases). Typically diagnosed between ages 50 and 70. Men account for 80% of the diagnoses.
- **Risk factors:** Squamous cell carcinoma risks include tobacco, smoking, alcohol, and asbestos. Adenocarcinoma risks include obesity, hiatal hernia, elevated BMI, and Barrett esophagus/GERD.

Tumor Biology and Characteristics

- **Genetics:** HER-2 (25% of adenocarcinomas+), COX-2, EGFR overexpression; *TP53* mutations common
- **Pathology:** Squamous cell carcinoma or adenocarcinoma; Barrett esophagus is the replacement of squamous with columnar epithelium and is associated with progression to adenocarcinoma.

Anatomy

- The esophagus extends from the pharynx to the stomach, the trachea anteriorly.
- Total length of the esophagus estimated to be 25 cm
- Cardia marks the junction of the stomach and esophagus.
- Locations of esophageal tumors and lymph node drainage summarized below

Name		Location (Landmarks)	Elective Nodal Coverage
Cervical		15-18 cm from upper incisors (C6 is distal hypopharynx)	Periesophageal, mediastinal, supraclavicular
Upper thoracic		18-24 cm from incisors (carina at ~24 cm)	
Mid thoracic		24-32 cm from incisors	Periesophageal, mediastinal
Lower thoracic/GEJ		32-40 cm from incisors	Periesophageal, mediastinal, perigastric, celiac
GEJ Tumor Classifications	Siewert type 1	1-5 cm superior to cardia	Recommend covering LN stations described in *Matzinger et al. Radiother Oncol* 2009
	Siewert type 2	At cardia or up to 1 cm superior, 2 cm inferior	
	Siewert type 3	2-5 cm inferior to cardia	

WORKUP

- **History and physical:** Typically present with progressive dysphagia, weight loss, and/or worsening heartburn
- **Screening:** Indicated for patients with documented Barrett esophagus (usually via biannual EGDs) (Fig. 35.1). Risk of development to esophageal cancer is 0.1-0.4% per year.
- **Labs:** CBC and CMP. Consider HER-2 tested for adenocarcinoma if metastatic.
- **Procedures/biopsy:** EGD and EUS +/− FNA (most sensitive for nodal staging). Consider bronchoscopy to rule out tracheal invasion of tumors located above the carina.
- **Imaging:** CT of the chest/abdomen/pelvis with contrast and PET/CT to rule out regional/distant disease for all patients

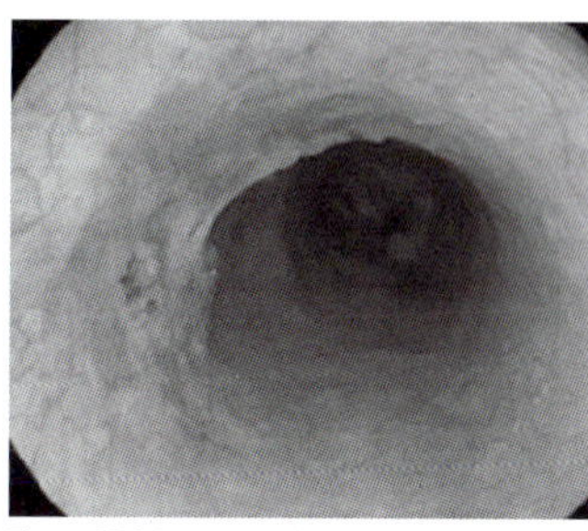

Figure 35.1 Image taken from surveillance upper endoscopy of a 63-year-old male with long-standing history of Barrett esophagus. Note the ulcerated mucosal lesion, which was biopsied and consistent with superficially invasive esophageal adenocarcinoma.

TREATMENT ALGORITHM

cTis-T2[a], N0	Esophagectomy, endoscopic resection or ablation if patient can tolerate and extent of disease permits
cT1bN1[b] and higher, operable	Preoperative chemoradiation and then surgery (or definitive chemoradiation) Perioperative chemotherapy and then surgery Surgery upfront (uncommon) with postoperative chemoRT if LN+[c], ≥pN1+, +margins
cT1bN1 and higher, cervical location squamous histology	Definitive chemoradiation preferred. Surgery can be very morbid in this location
cT1bN1 and higher, inoperable	Definitive chemoradiation
M1	Palliative RT, chemotherapy, or best supportive care

[a]Low-risk cT1b-cT2 lesions: <3 cm, no LVI, well differentiated
[b]Including high-risk lesions: ≥3 cm, LVI, poorly differentiated
[c]Postoperative chemoradiation only recommended for ≥pN1+ if adenocarcinoma histology, observation recommended for ≥pN1+ squamous cell histology

RADIATION TREATMENT TECHNIQUE

- **SIM:** NPO ×3 hours. Supine, arms up if tumor below carina (arms down if tumor above carina), immobilization device, iso at carina; scan from the mandible through stomach and celiac axis. Consider oral contrast to delineate tumor and head and neck mask for cervical primaries. 4DCT for GEJ tumors to account for movement
- **Dose:** 50.4 Gy in 1.8 Gy/fx with concurrent chemotherapy
- **Target:** GTV = PET/CT + primary and nodal disease at EGD/EUS
  CTV = 3- to 4-cm mucosal margin superiorly/inferiorly and 1-cm radial margin, trimmed from surrounding structures (Fig. 35.2)
  PTV = 5-mm margin with daily kV imaging
- **Technique:** 3D, IMRT, and proton therapy (under investigation)
- **IGRT:** Daily kV imaging, consider weekly CBCT
- Planning directive (for conventional fractionation):
  PTV: 50.4 Gy in 28 fractions
  Esophagus minus GTV: D_{max} < 70 Gy, V50 < 50%
  Heart: V30 < 45%, mean < 26 Gy

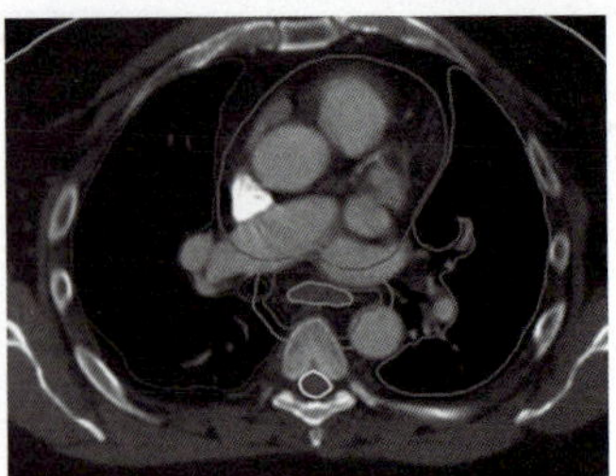

Figure 35.2 Representative cross-sectional image illustrating typical contours for an esophageal adenocarcinoma patient. GTV, CTV, and PTV contours showed in *orange*, *red*, and *pink*, respectively. **See color insert.**

Total lung: mean dose <20 Gy; V5 < 65%, V10 < 45%, V20 < 25%
Liver minus GTV: Mean dose <32 Gy, V20 < 50%, V30 < 30%
Kidney: V20 < 33% each kidney
Spinal cord: D_{max} < 45 Gy
Stomach: D_{max} < 54 Gy

Surgery

- **Approaches to esophagectomy:**
  - Transhiatal esophagectomy: Upper midline laparotomy and L neck incision; often uses gastric pull-through approach for cervical anastomosis; usually avoids thoracotomy
  - Transthoracic esophagectomy, Ivor-Lewis approach: R thoracotomy of the abdomen and upper abdominal laparotomy incisions allow for direct visualization of thoracic esophagus but limit length of proximal esophagus that can be removed.
  - Transthoracic esophagectomy, modified Ivor-Lewis approach: L thoracoabdominal incision only with anastomosis in L chest
- **Conduits:** Following esophagectomy. Connection between the remaining esophagus and stomach, colon, or jejunum
- **Lymph node dissection**: Should include at least 15 LNs if no preoperative chemoRT

Chemotherapy

- **Concurrent with RT, preoperative or definitive:** Paclitaxel/carboplatin or 5-FU/cisplatin, or 5-FU/oxaliplatin
- **Adjuvant:** Nivolumab after CRT with R0 and residual disease (per CheckMate 577)
- **Perioperative (thoracic adenocarcinoma or GEJ):** Fluorouracil/leucovorin/oxaliplatin/docetaxel (FLOT), 5-FU/cisplatin

RT Side Effect Management

- Nausea: Zofran, Compazine, Reglan, low-dose dexamethasone, Haldol, and IV fluids
- Esophagitis: Magic mouthwash (viscous lidocaine, Benadryl, nystatin), glutamine supplement (eg, Helios), aloe products, and narcotic elixir second line
- Thrush: Nystatin swish/swallow, fluconazole
- Weight loss: Nutrition consult/diet modifications, opiates if needed; may require feeding tube
- Leukopenias due to chemotherapy: Weekly labs with transfusion/Neupogen PRN
- Pneumonitis: Approximately 6 weeks to 1 year after RT and may present with cough, dyspnea, and fever. Prescribe steroid taper (60 mg for 2-3 weeks with taper) and/or NSAIDs. Patient may even require O_2.
- Late effects: Tracheoesophageal fistula (5-10%) if esophageal tumor invades trachea; presents as choking with PO intake, coughing, or recurrent pneumonias; treatment may involve stent or surgery (Ke et al. *J Thorac Dis* 2015). RT-induced pericarditis and coronary artery disease in long-term survivors

Follow-up

- History/physical: Every 3-6 months for 1-2 years → every 6-12 months for 3-5 years
- CT of the chest/abdomen with contrast: Every 4-6 months for the first year and every 6-9 months for the next 2 years
- EGD: Every 3-6 months × 2 years and then 6-12 months in definitive chemoRT or early-stage surgical patients

Notable Literature

Outcomes with definitive chemoradiation

Name	Arms	Outcomes	Notes
RTOG 85-01 (*Cooper et al. JAMA* 1999; *Herskovic et al. NEJM* 1992) Phase III randomized trial of 129 patients with cT1-3, N0-N1, M0 esophageal cancer	RT alone (50 Gy + 14 Gy boost) ChemoRT (30 Gy + 20 Gy boost with) with 5-FU and cisplatin	5-y OS: 0% (RT alone) 5-y OS: 27% (chemoRT)	ChemoRT improves survival in locally advanced esophageal cancer Acute toxicity worse in chemoRT arm No significant differences in late effects
INT-0123/RTOG 94-05 (*Minsky et al. JCO* 2002) Phase III randomized trial of 50 patients. Stopped early during interim analysis	50 Gy chemoRT with concurrent 5-FU and cisplatin High-dose (65 Gy) chemoRT with concurrent 5-FU and cisplatin	2-y OS and LR: equivalent (*P* value not provided) Treatment-related death: 2% (standard), 10% (high dose)	High-dose chemoRT does not improve outcomes OS or LR
ARTDECO (*Hulshof et al. JCO* 2021) 260 patients with medically inoperable and/or irresectable esophageal carcinoma	Standard-dose chemoRT (50.4 Gy) High-dose chemoRT (61.6 Gy)	3-y LPFS: 70% (SD) vs 73% (HD), not significant LPFS for SCC: 75% (SD) vs 79% (HD), not significant	Radiation dose escalation up to 61.6 Gy to the primary tumor did not significantly improve local control over 50.4 Gy No significant difference in LPFS for both AC and SCC
Xu et al. CCR 2022 Multicenter phase III trial of 319 patients with inoperable squamous cell carcinoma	Standard-dose chemoRT (50 Gy) High-dose chemoRT (60 Gy)	3-y locoregional PFS: 49.5% (60 Gy), 48.4% (50 Gy), not significant 3-y overall survival rates: 53.1% (60 Gy), 52.7% (50 Gy), not significant.	The 60 Gy arm had similar survival end points, but a higher severe pneumonitis rate compared with the 50 Gy arm

Neoadjuvant chemoradiation improves overall survival

Name	Arms	Outcomes	Notes
CROSS Trial (*Shapiro et al. Lancet Oncol* 2015; *van Hagen et al. NEJM* 2012) Phase III randomized trial of 368 patients with cT1N1 or T2-3N0-1	Surgery alone Preoperative chemoRT (41.4 Gy/23 fx with carboplatin/paclitaxel) followed by surgery	Median OS: 24 mo (surgery alone), 49.4 mo (preoperative chemoRT), $P = .003$ R0 resection rates: 69% (surgery alone), 92% (preoperative chemoRT), $P < .001$ pCR rate: 29% overall, 49% (SCC), 23% (adenocarcinoma)	Preoperative chemoRT improves OS, R0 resection rates, and pCR in resectable esophageal cancer patients

Adjuvant systemic therapy

Study Name	Arms	Outcomes	Notes
CheckMate 577 (*Kelly et al. NEJM* 2021) Phase III, double-blind, placebo controlled randomized trial of 794 patients with resected stage II-III disease 2:1 Randomization	Nivolumab (532 patients) Placebo (262 patients)	Nivolumab median DFS: 22.4 mo (95% CI, 16.6-34.0), improved compared to placebo median DFS: 11.0 mo (95% CI, 8.3-14.3) HR for DFS: 0.69 (96.4% CI, 0.56-0.86; $P < .001$)	Adjuvant nivolumab after resection improved DFS in patients with esophagela and gastroesophageal junction cancers who received neoadjuvant CRT

COLORECTAL CANCER

CHIKE ABANA • EMMA HOLLIDAY • PRAJNAN DAS

Background

- **Incidence/prevalence:** The fourth most commonly diagnosed cancer and the second leading cause of death among men and women in the United States. Approximately >43 000 cases are diagnosed annually in the United States.
- **Outcomes:** 5-Year survival across all stages estimated at 67% (SEER data)
- **Demographics:** Lifetime risk 1 in 20 (5%). Highest incidence in Western countries
- **Risk factors:** Increasing age, familial syndromes (FAP, HNPCC [Lynch syndrome], Peutz-Jeghers syndrome, juvenile polyposis), inflammatory bowel disease, personal or family history of polyps, obesity, sedentary lifestyle, EtOH consumption, tobacco use, low-fiber diet, and Western diet

Tumor Biology and Characteristics

- **Genetics:** TCGA genomic profiling identified ~16% of colorectal cancers hypermutated. Frequent mutations in *APC* (FAP), *MLH1/MSH2/MSH6/PMS2* (HNPCC), TP53, *SMAD4* (juvenile polyposis), *PIK3CA*, and *KRAS* (*Cancer Genome Atlas Network Nature* 2012)
- **Pathology:** Majority adenocarcinomas (>90%). Minority neuroendocrine, mesenchymal tumors, or lymphomas. IHC testing for mismatch repair proteins (MLH1, PMS2, MSH2, and MSH6) commonly conducted and predictive of response to immunotherapy (*Le et al. Science* 2017). Consider testing for *BRAF* and *KRAS* mutations.
- **Imaging:** MRI accurate tool for local staging and for assessment of pelvic lymphadenopathy. Tumors typically visualized on high-resolution T2-weighted sequences, with increased signal on DWI sequence. Endorectal US can help to distinguish between T1 and T2 tumors.

Anatomy

- Rectum: Begins at the rectosigmoid junction at the level of S3. Total length of the rectum estimated to be between 12 and 15 cm. Squamous mucosa ends at the dentate line (~2 cm from anal verge). Internal anal sphincter ends 2 cm superior to dentate line (~4 cm from anal verge).
- Colon: Cecum is the junction between the small and large intestines (intraperitoneal) → ascending colon (retroperitoneal) → transverse colon (intraperitoneal) → descending colon (retroperitoneal) → sigmoid colon (intraperitoneal).
- Lymph node drainage:
  - Upper half rectum: Superior hemorrhoidal → IMA → para-aortic
  - Lower half rectum: Inferior + middle hemorrhoidal → internal iliac, obturator presacral nodes
  - Involvement of anal canal: Superficial inguinal nodes
  - Invading anterior structures (prostate, bladder, vagina) → external iliac

Workup

- **History and physical:** DRE for all patients and pelvic exam in women
- **Labs:** CBC, CMP, CEA, MMR/MSI testing
- **Procedures/biopsy:** Colonoscopy with biopsy of primary(ies). Proctoscopy/flexible sigmoidoscopy for precise location for surgery/RT planning; diverting ostomy if obstructed or <1 cm luminal diameter
- **Imaging:** Contrast-enhanced CTs of the chest/abdomen/pelvis (important to image the liver) for all patients. "Rectal protocol" MRI of the pelvis (perpendicular to axis of rectum). Contrast-enhanced PET/CT is not routinely indicated. EUS for T1 vs T2 differentiation

Treatment Algorithm for Rectal Cancer

Stage I	• Transanal excision (TAE, see criteria below) → observation (if pT1N0M0 with R0 resection) or adjuvant tx if pT2/+margin/LVI/G3 on path • Total mesorectal excision (TME; LAR if ≥5 cm from AV or APR if <5 cm from AV) → observation (if pT1-2N0M0 with R0 resection) or adjuvant tx (if +margin/T3-4N0/T1-4N+)

Stage II-III	• Preoperative short-course RT (SC-RT) or long-course chemoRT (LC-CRT) → TME • **TNT:** Induction chemo → LC-CRT → TME, or preoperative SC-RT or LC-CRT → consolidation chemo → TME
Stage IV (oligometastatic)	• Oligometastatic: Chemotherapy → +/− LC-CRT or SC-RT → TME and definitive local treatment of metastatic disease (in either order) → chemotherapy • Widespread metastasis: Chemotherapy or best supportive care

Treatment for colon cancer is surgical + adjuvant chemo without routine use of adjuvant RT. Local control benefit of adjuvant RT was seen in T4 tumors invading adjoining structures, associated with perforation or fistula, or in the setting of residual disease (*Willett et al. Cancer J Sci Am* 1999). However, this was not confirmed when tested in the phase III Int 0130 trial comparing adjuvant chemo to chemo+RT (*Martenson et al. JCO* 2004) in T4 or T3N+ patients. Consider RT to metastatic sites if oligometastatic with good PS.

Radiation Treatment Technique for Rectal Cancer

- **SIM:** Prone on a bellyboard, Vac-Lok device, comfortably full bladder, and marker on anal verge (wire perineal scars if postoperative). Scan from midlumbar spine to middle femur, isocenter midline at top of femoral heads. Consider supine with a vaginal dilator in younger women with low-lying rectal tumor to reduce the dose to the anterior vagina.
- **Dose:**
  LC-CRT: 45 Gy in 25 fractions at 1.8 Gy/fx → cone-down boost to 50.4 Gy in 1.8 Gy/fx
  SC-RT: 25 Gy at 5 Gy/fx
  Recurrent after prior RT: 39 Gy in 1.5 Gy/fx bid
- **Target:** Preoperative: GTV, mesorectum, internal iliac, obturator, presacral nodes
  Postoperative: Tumor bed, anastomosis, mesorectum, internal iliac, obturator, presacral nodes

Considerations: If T4 disease (invasion into anterior structures including the bladder, vagina, prostate), cover external iliac nodes. If primary tumor extends beyond dentate line, consider covering inguinal nodes. If locally advanced or recurrent, consider intraoperative radiation therapy (10-15 Gy, electrons, or HDR brachytherapy).

- **Technique:** 3DCRT (3-field PA and opposed laterals) for LC-CRT or SC-RT (Fig. 36.1), or IMRT for SC-RT or when inguinal nodes are included

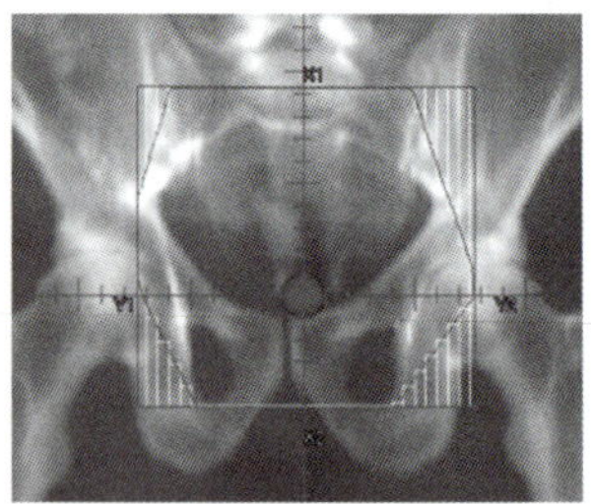

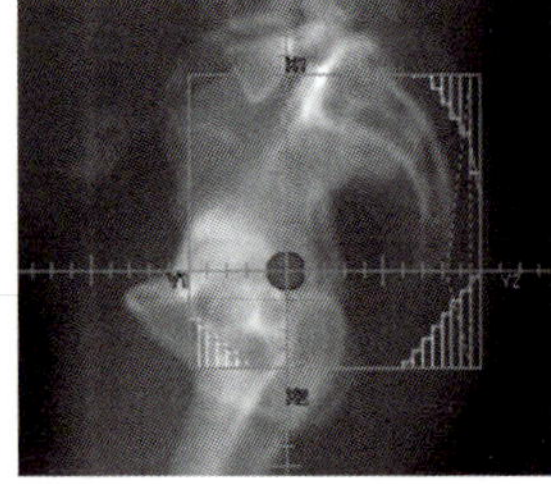

Figure 36.1 Standard PA and lateral fields.

- **IGRT:** Weekly kV imaging for LC-CRT align to bone or daily CBCT imaging for SC-RT to verify full bladder, no pelvic tilt/gas bubbles
- **Planning directive**
  LC-CRT, that is, conventional fractionation (*Park et al. Pract Radiat Oncol* 2022):
  PTV D95% ≥ 95%; D0.03 cc ≤ 110%
  Spinal cord D_{max} < 45 Gy

CC 7-2

Bowel "bag" V45 < 195 cc
Small bowel V35 < 150 cc; V50 < 10 cc; V45 < 10%; V20 < 50%; D120 cc ≤ 35 Gy; D35 cc ≤ 45 Gy; D0.03 cc ≤ 54 Gy
Bladder V45 ≤ 15%; D_{mean} ≤ 40 Gy
Femoral heads V30 < 50%; V45 < 5%
Bone marrow V10 < 90%
Genitalia: V20 < 50% and V30 < 35%

SC-RT:

PTV D95% ≥ 95%; D0.03 cc ≤ 115%
Small bowel D_{max} < 27.8 Gy; V25 < 65 cc; V22.2 < 100 cc
Bladder D_{max} < 27.8 Gy; V25 < 15%; V22.2 < 40%
Femoral heads D_{max} < 27.8 Gy; V25 < 25%; V22.2 < 40%

Surgery

- Transanal excision (TAE): Sphincter-preserving, full-thickness local excision with adequate margin. Consider for low-lying (<10 cm) T1N0 lesions <30% circumferential involvement, <3 cm in size, ≥3-mm margins, low-intermediate grade (no G3), and no LVI. Consider postoperative chemoRT or radical surgery if path shows high-risk features, staging is upgraded, or there are inadequate margins.
- Total mesorectal excision (TME):
  - Low anterior resection (LAR): Sphincter-preserving TME if ≥5 cm from AV. Sharp dissection outside the mesorectal fascia, temporary diverting loop ileostomy for anastomosis healing, and ligation of superior and middle hemorrhoidal arteries. Adequate LN dissection removes ≥12 LNs.
  - Abdominoperineal resection (APR): TME if <5 cm from AV, with complete removal of the rectum and anal canal and permanent colostomy. Adequate LN dissection removes ≥12 LNs.

Chemotherapy

- **Concurrent:** Capecitabine (825 mg/m² bid, 5 days a week) or continuous infusion 5-FU (225 mg/m²/d)
- **Adjuvant/neoadjuvant:** FOLFOX (folinic acid + 5-FU + oxaliplatin), or capecitabine, or CAPOX (capecitabine + oxaliplatin)

Side Effect Management

- Nausea: First-line Zofran (8 mg q8h PRN) → second-line Compazine (10 mg q6h prn) → ABH (lorazepam 0.34 mg, diphenhydramine 25 mg, and haloperidol 1.5 mg) 1 capsule q6h
- Diarrhea: First-line Imodium titrating to a max of 8 pills/day → second-line alternating Lomotil 2 pills and Imodium 2 pills every 3 hours
- Cystitis: *Urgency/frequency and dysuria*. UA to r/o UTI. Treat if positive.
- Skin care: First-line sitz baths, Aquaphor, and Domeboro powder → second-line Silvadene cream and hydrogel dressings (Cool Magic)
- Proctitis: *Diarrhea/abdominal pain*. First-line alternating Lomotil and Imodium (as above) → second-line steroid enemas
- Hand and foot syndrome: Redness, swelling, and pain in the hand and foot. Consult with medical oncology about reducing concurrent capecitabine dose.

Follow-up

- History/physical and CEA: Every 3-4 months for 3 years → every 6 months for 2 years
- CT of the chest/abdomen/pelvis: Every year
- Colonoscopy: At years 1 and 3 and every 5 years thereafter
- Vaginal dilators for women

Notable Trials

Name/Inclusion	Arms	Outcomes	Notes
Neoadjuvant Chemoradiation			
German rectal trial (*Sauer et al. NEJM* 2004; *Sauer et al. JCO* 2012) T3/4 or N+ 421 patients total	Preoperative LC-CRT (5-FU, 50.4 Gy/28 fx) → surgery → 5-FU Surgery → post-operative LC-CRT (5-FU, 50.4 Gy/28 fx) + 5.4 Gy boost → 5-FU	10-y OS 59.6% vs 59.9%, *P* = .85 10-y LR 7.1% vs 10.1%, *P* = .048 G3-4 acute tox 27% vs 40%, *P* = .001 G3-4 late tox 14% vs 24%, *P* = .01 Sphincter preservation in unfavorable patients 39% vs 19%, *P* = .004	Preoperative LC-CRT improves local control and reduces toxicity compared to post-operative LC-CRT
Short-Course Radiation Therapy (SC-RT)			
Dutch Trial (*Kapiteijn et al. NEJM* 2001; *van Gijn et al. Lancet Oncol* 2011) Resectable cancers 1861 patients	Preoperative SC-RT (25 Gy/5 fx) → TME surgery TME surgery (APR, LAR, or Hartmann procedure)	10-y LR 5% vs 11%, *P* < .0001	Preoperative SC-RT reduces LR over surgery alone
TROG 01.04 (*Ansari et al. Ann Surg* 2017; *Ngan et al. JCO* 2012) T3N0-2M0 Powered to detect 3-y LR of 15% for SC-RT and 5% for LC-CRT 326 patients	Preoperative SC-RT (25 Gy/5 fx) → surgery → adjuvant 5-FU Preoperative LC-CRT (5-FU, 50.4 Gy/28 fx) → surgery → adjuvant 5-FU	5-y LR 7.5% vs 5.7%, *P* = .51 5-y DR 27% vs 30%, *P* = .92 5-y OS 74% vs 70%, *P* = .62 G3-4 acute tox 1.9% vs 27.1%, *P* < .001 G3-4 late tox 6% vs 8%, *P* = .53	No difference in outcomes and late toxicity between preoperative SC-RT and LC-CRT
Stockholm III (*Erlandsson et al. Lancet* 2017; *Pettersson et al. Br J Surg* 2015) Noninferiority trial SC-RT: 25 Gy/5 fx LC-CRT: 385 patients	SC-RT → surgery 1 wk later SC-RT → surgery 4-8 wk later LC-CRT → surgery 4-8 wk later	pCR SC-RT + wk 1 surgery vs SC-RT + wk 4-8 surgery: 2% vs 12%, *P* = .001 and postoperative complications 53% vs 41%, *P* = .001 No difference in postoperative comp or late toxicity, OS, DM, LR, or RFS among all 3 arms	SC-RT + delayed surgery at 4-8 wk post-RT yields better pCR and fewer postoperative complications than immediate surgery or LC-CRT
Total Neoadjuvant Treatment (TNT)			
RAPIDO (*Bahadoer et al. Lancet Oncol* 2021; *Dijkstra et al. Ann Surg* 2023) High risk 920 patients	TNT w/ SC-RT (25 Gy/5 fx) → CAPOX/FOLFOX4 → TME LC-CRT (50.4 Gy/28 fx or 50 Gy/25 fx, + capecitabine) → TME → optional CAPOX/FOLFOX	pCR 28% vs 14%, *P* < .0001 3-y disease-related treatment failure (DrTF) 23.7% vs 30.4%, *P* = .019 3-y DM 20.0% vs 26.8%, *P* = .005 No difference in, OS, postoperative complications or quality of life at 3 y 5-y LRR 10% vs 6%, *P* = .027	TNT w/ SC-RT had better pCR, DrTF, and DM, but worse LRR TNT w/ SC-RT, large lateral Ns, +CRM, tumor deposits, and pN+ were predictors of LRR

Name/Inclusion	Arms	Outcomes	Notes
PRODIGE-23 (*Conroy et al. Lancet Oncol* 2021) T3/T4 LC-CRT: capecitabine + 50 Gy/25 fx 461 patients	TNT w/ mFOLFIRINOX → LC-CRT → TME → capecitabine/ mFOLFOX6 LC-CRT → TME → capecitabine/ mFOLFOX6	pCR 27.8% vs 12.1%, $P < .001$ 3-y DFS 76% vs 69%, $P = .034$ 3-y MFS 79% vs 72%, $P = .017$ G3+ toxicity 45% vs 76%, $P \leq .0001$ No difference in 3-y OS	TNT with LC-CRT led to better pCR, DFS, MFS, and toxicity at 3 y
TNT for Organ Preservation			
OPRA (*Garcia-Aguilar et al. J Clin Oncol* 2022) Stage II and III distal rectal cancer 360 patients Goal was to determine what sequence of TNT more likely to achieve pCR and organ preservation with "watch-and-wait" (DRE + flex sig q4mo for 2 y then q6mo for 3 y) LC-CRT: 50 Gy/25 fx + 4-6 Gy optional boost with concurrent capecitabine or 5-FU	Induction FOLFOX/ CAPEOX → LC-CRT → TME if no CR, or "watch-and-wait" if complete or near CR LC-CRT → consolidation FOLFOX/ CAPEOX → TME if no CR, or "watch-and-wait" if complete or near CR	3-y TME-free survival 41% vs 53%, $P = .01$ No difference in 3-y LRFS, DMFS, or OS No difference in 3-y DFS in both arms (76%) vs historical controls treated with CRT, TME, and adjuvant chemo (75%)	LC-CRT f/b consolidation chemo f/b selective "watch-and-wait" increased the rate of organ preservation compared to induction chemo f/b LC-CRT
Omission of Radiation Therapy in Select Patients			
MERCURY (*Taylor et al. J Clin Oncol* 2014) Low-risk criteria included clear (>1 mm) CRM, T2/ T3a/T3b (<5 mm beyond muscularis propria), no EMVI and clear intersphincteric plane for low-lying tumors < 5 cm from AV 374 patients	MRI-identified low-risk patients for TME-only tx	*5-y OS was 68%, DFS was 85%, and LR was 3%*	High-resolution MRI preoperative assessment of CRM involvement identified low-risk patients for whom RT could be safely omitted with 97% LC rate after good quality TME

ANAL CANCER

CHIKE ABANA • EMMA HOLLIDAY

BACKGROUND

- **Incidence/prevalence:** Very rare; makes up only 3% of all GI malignancies, but the incidence is increasing. Estimated 9760 new cases in 2023 leading to an estimated 1870 deaths
- **Outcomes:** 5-year overall survival for T2-T4; M0 was 76% (RTOG 0529; *Kachnic et al. IJROBP* 2022).
  By stage (*Gunderson et al. IJROBP* 2013 after RTOG 9811):

T2N0 5-y OS 87%, LRF 17%	T2N+ 5-y OS 70%, LRF 26%
T3N0 5-y OS 74%, LRF 18%	T3N+ 5-y OS 57%, LRF 44%
T4N0 5-y OS 57%, LRF 40%	T4N+ 5-y OS 42%, LRF 60%

- **Risk factors:** HPV, HIV/AIDS, smoking, increased number of sexual partners, receptive anal intercourse, smoking, immunosuppression, female gender, older age (most 50-60+), and chronic anal/perianal wounds

TUMOR BIOLOGY AND CHARACTERISTICS

- **HPV association:** 80-90% of anal cancers are HPV+; HPV16 is present in 70% of tumors. HPV+ anal cancers have a better prognosis. HPV vaccination has been shown to decrease the incidence of premalignant anal lesions in men who have sex with men (*Lawton et al. Sex Transm Infect* 2013), but there has been no evidence of benefit for widespread cancer/premalignancy screening programs (*Leeds et al. World J Gastrointest Surg* 2016).
- **Pathology:** ~90% squamous cell carcinoma and ~10% adenocarcinoma (have a much worse prognosis and typically treated with rectal cancer paradigm of neoadjuvant chemoRT → APR TME)
- **Imaging:** Primary anal tumors are not typically well visualized on cross-sectional imaging. So physical exam and anoscopy is very important.

ANATOMY

- The anal region includes the anal canal (~3-5 cm from the anal verge) and the anal margin (5-6 cm radius of perianal skin around the anal verge). Dentate line represents a histologic boundary separating squamous from columnar/glandular epithelium and occurs ~2 cm into the anus.
- Lymph node drainage:
  - Anal margin: Superficial inguinal nodes
  - Anal canal below the dentate line: Superficial inguinal nodes
  - Anal canal above the dentate line: Anorectal, perirectal, paravertebral nodes → internal iliac nodes
  - Invasion into anterior structures (prostate, bladder, vagina): External iliac nodes

WORKUP

- **History and physical:** DRE and inguinal nodal exams for all patients, last colonoscopy
- **Labs:** CBC, CMP, LFTs, HIV testing (CD4 count and VL if positive), Pap smear/cervical screening for all females if they are not up to date. PSA and prostate cancer screening for all males
- **Procedures/biopsy:** Anoscopy or flexible sigmoidoscopy for biopsy of primary and documentation of largest measurement for T staging; colonoscopy if ≥45 years
- **Imaging:** Contrast-enhanced CTs of the chest and abdomen for systemic staging and a CT or an MRI recommended for pelvis. The authors favor a contrast-enhanced PET/CT for both locoregional and systemic staging, and pelvic MRI reserved for patients with bulky T3 or T4 disease for whom better visualization of the tissue planes is desired.

Treatment Algorithm

M1 anal canal or anal margin cancer	Systemic chemotherapy (5-FU/cisplatin) +/– local RT vs clinical trials
T1N0, well-differentiated anal margin cancer	Local excision → observation if adequate margins. If inadequate margins, re-excision preferred or can consider local RT +/– concurrent chemotherapy
T1N0, poorly differentiated or T2-T4, N0 or any T, N+ anal margin cancer	Definitive chemoradiation

Radiation Treatment Technique

- **SIM:** Supine, frog-legged position, and custom immobilization device for the lower body. Place radiopaque BB at the anal verge to help delineate tumor during treatment planning, place wire around any perianal extension, and consider bolus. Consider full bladder to displace small bowel. Use vaginal dilator for women to displace the anterior vaginal wall. Use scrotal shelf for men to minimize skin toxicity. Position and immobilize penis midline and pointed down.
- **RTOG0529 dose:**

	Dose/Fractions (dose per fraction)	
	Primary Tumor Involved Nodes	**Elective Nodal Volume**
Primary Tumor Stage		
T2	50.4 Gy/28 fx (1.8 Gy/fx)	42 Gy/28 fx (1.5 Gy/fx)
T3/T4	54 Gy/30 fx (1.8 Gy/fx)	45 Gy/30 fx (1.5 Gy/fx)
Nodal Size		
≤3 cm	50.4 Gy/30 fx (1.68 Gy/fx)	
>3 cm	54 Gy/30 fx (1.8 Gy/fx)	

- **MDACC dose:**

	Dose/Fractions (dose per fraction)	
	Primary Tumor Involved Nodes	**Elective Nodal Volume**
Primary Tumor Stage		
T1	50 Gy/25 fx (2 Gy/fx)	43 Gy/25 fx (1.72 Gy/fx)
T2	54 Gy/27 fx (2 Gy/fx)	45 Gy/27 fx (1.67 Gy/fx)
T3/T4	58 Gy/29 fx (2 Gy/fx)	47 Gy/29 fx (1.62 Gy/fx)
Nodal Size		
<2 cm	50 Gy/25 fx* (2 Gy/fx)	
2-5 cm	54 Gy/27 fx* (2 Gy/fx)	
>5 cm	58 Gy/29 fx* (2 Gy/fx)	

*The tumor, involved LNs, and elective nodal volume are treated using one IMRT plan with a simultaneous integrated boost technique. The number of fractions should be determined by the largest of either the primary tumor or the involved LN. For example, a T2 tumor with a 1.5-cm inguinal node would be treated in 27 fractions. The primary tumor would receive 54 Gy, the inguinal node would receive 50 Gy, and the elective nodal volume would receive 45 Gy.

- **Target:** CTVp (primary) = anal GTV + 1 cm
  CTVn (involved nodes) = nodal GTV + 5 mm
  CTVe (elective nodal volume) = Should extend at least 2 cm inferior to anal GTV and include the entire mesorectum to the pelvic floor. Nodal areas include inguinal, perirectal, presacral, internal, and external iliacs to the level of the bifurcation of the common iliacs (~L5/S1)
  PTV margin with daily kV or CBCT to bone is 5 mm from CTV.
- **Technique:** IMRT/VMAT
- **Target delineation:**
  Primary and nodes:
  Utilize information from physical exam, CT, PET/CT or MRI, and endoscopy reports to delineate the GTVp and GTVn.

CTVp = GTVp + 1 cm	CTVn = GTVn + 5 mm
PTVp = CTVp + 5 mm	PTVn = CTVn + 5 mm

Elective nodal volume:

Should include the entire mesorectum to the pelvic floor.

+/– extension into ischiorectal fossa (RTOG and ECOG atlases states only extend a few mm beyond levators if no ischiorectal fossa involvement; Australasian atlas includes the entire ischiorectal fossa.)

The inguinal nodal area should be covered from the inguinal ligament superiorly to the lesser trochanter inferiorly. The lateral border is the iliopsoas (I), the medial border is the adductor longus (AL) and pectineus (P), the posterior border is the I and P, and the anterior border is the sartorius (S).

In the **mid pelvis**, the CTVe should extend to the lateral pelvic sidewall (muscle or bone). There should be an extension of ~1 cm into the bladder and cover the posterior internal obturator vessels.

In the **high pelvis**, the perirectal coverage should extend to the rectosigmoid junction. The superior border of CTVe should extend to where the common iliacs bifurcate into internal and external iliacs (~L5/S1). The internal, external, and presacral nodal basins should be covered. A margin of ~7 mm in soft tissue around the external iliac vessels should be added excluding muscle and bone.

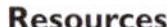

Resources:

RTOG Atlas (used for RTOG 0529): https://www.rtog.org/CoreLab/ContouringAtlases/Anorectal.aspx

Australasian GI Trials Group Atlas: *Ng et al. Int J Radiat Oncol Biol Phys* 2012

Inguinal Nodal Atlas: *Kim et al. Pract Radiat Oncol* 2012

ECOG-ACRIN EA2182 (DECREASE) Atlas: *Damico et al. Pract Radiat Oncol* 2022

- **IGRT:** daily kV imaging and/or daily CBCT aligning to the pelvic bones, but reviewing daily also to ensure consistent bladder filling, bowel loop position, and soft tissue alignment
- **Planning directive:**

  Ensure coverage of GTV by prescription Gy isodose line.

  Femoral heads V45 < 20%

  Small bowel V20 < 50%, V45 < 10%, V50 < 5%, V30 < 200 cc, V35 < 150 cc, V45 < 20 cc, V50 < 10 cc

  Bowel bag V45 < 195 cc (*Kavanaugh et al. Int J Radiat Oncol Biol Phys* 2010)

  Bladder V50 < 30%

  Genitalia V30 < 20%, V20 < 67%

  Pelvic bone marrow V10 < 90%

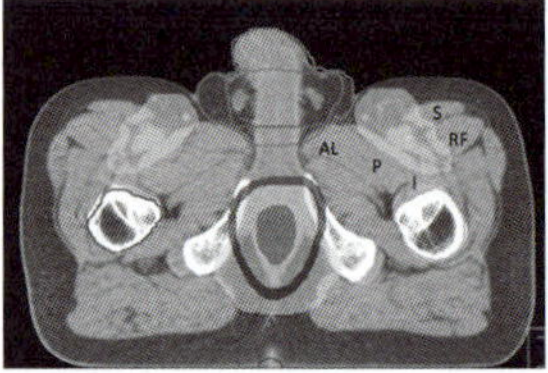

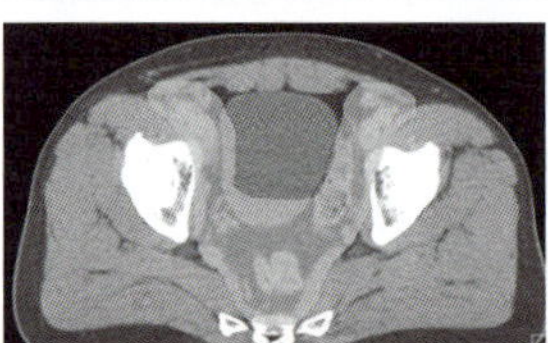

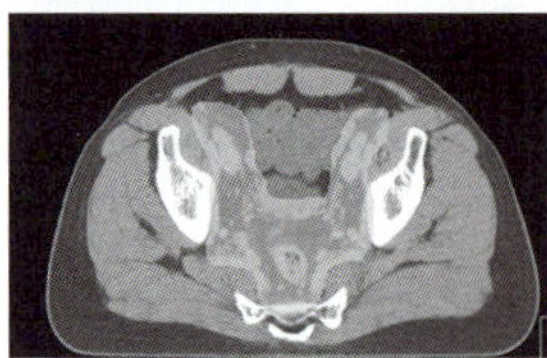

Figure 37.1 RTOG Atlas (used for RTOG 0529): https://www.rtog.org/CoreLab/ContouringAtlases/Anorectal.aspx. **See color insert.** (Australasian GI Trials Group Atlas: *Ng et al. Int J Radiat Oncol Biol Phys* 2012; Inguinal Nodal Atlas: *Kim et al. Pract Radiat Oncol* 2012.)

Chemotherapy

- **Concurrent:**
  - **Most widely accepted regimen:** Continuous infusion 5-FU 1000 mg/m^2/d IV days 1-4 and 29-32. Mitomycin C 10 mg/m^2 IV bolus days 1 and 29 or mitomycin C 12 mg/m^2 (capped at 20 mg) on day 1
  - **MDACC preferred regimen:** Weekly bolus cisplatin 20 mg/m^2 and continuous infusion 5-FU 300 mg/m^2 administered Monday to Friday on the days of radiation

- **Other consensus-listed regimens:** Capecitabine 825 mg/m² PO bid, Monday to Friday on the days of radiation. Mitomycin C 10 mg/m² days 1 and 29 or mitomycin C 12 mg/m² IV bolus on day 1

Side Effect Management

- Nausea: First-line Zofran (8 mg q8h prn) → second-line Compazine (10 mg q6h prn) → ABH (lorazepam 0.34 mg, diphenhydramine 25 mg, and haloperidol 1.5 mg) 1 capsule q6h
- Diarrhea: First-line Imodium titrating to a max of 8 pills/day → second-line alternating Lomotil 2 pills and Imodium 2 pills every 3 hours to a max of 8 pills/day → third-line tincture of opium 1 g anhydrous morphine/100 cc, 0.6 mL orally four times daily. Late toxicity: nightly Metamucil (regular dose + ½ volume of water and consume no water for the rest of the night); pelvic floor PT
- Cystitis/urethritis: *Urgency/frequency and dysuria.* UA to r/o UTI, exam to r/o vaginal mucositis or candidiasis in women. Treat if positive. If negative, consider Pyridium OTC or prescription for urethritis; ibuprofen/oxybutynin for cystitis/bladder spasm; and tamsulosin for weak stream in men.
- Dermatitis: Grade 1: sitz baths and Aquaphor → Grade 2: NDX (nystatin, desitin, xylocaine), topical corticosteroids/mometasone (0.1%), or OTC lantiseptic cream → Grade 3: Silvadene cream 1% tid, perineal cool pads, and hydrogel dressings (Cool Magic) → Grade 4: treatment break and surgical consult
- Proctitis/anal mucositis: sitz baths → topical lidocaine (combine with nifedipine for hemorrhoids/fissures) → gabapentin 600 mg/d wk 2 and titrate to 2700 mg/d by wk 3. Most patients require opiate pain medications.
- Tenesmus/bowel spasms w/o productive diarrhea: dicycloverine qid
- Consider dihydropyrimidine dehydrogenase deficiency for early onset (week 1-2), severe diarrhea/mucositis/cytopenia
- Hematologic toxicity:
  - When is chemotherapy held?
    - If platelets <75K, hold. If <50K, hold then dose reduce. Consider transfusion if bleeding.
    - If Hbg < 8, hold. Give PRBC transfusion, then dose reduce.
    - If ANC < 1, hold. If <0.5, hold then dose reduce. If reoccurs, hold permanently.
  - When is RT held?
    - If platelets <25K or ANC < 0.5
  - When is GCSF given?
    - >24 hours after/before chemo and on Friday/Saturday after RT
    - Weigh the risks of concurrent G-CSF w/ neutropenic fever and needing/prolonging tx breaks

Follow-up

- Skin and toxicity check at 6 weeks posttreatment with a DRE
- First restaging at 12 weeks posttreatment includes DRE, anoscopy, and CT of the chest/abdomen/pelvis. If disease is persistent, reevaluate in 4 weeks and continue monitoring until complete clinical response (CR). If no complete CR by 6 months, consider biopsy.
  **It is important not to biopsy prematurely as only 52% of patients on ACT II achieved a complete CR (cCR) by 11 weeks from the start of treatment, but 72% of the patients who didn't achieve a complete CR by 11 weeks had achieved a complete CR by 26 weeks.*
- Once complete CR achieved, DRE q3mo, anoscopy q6mo, and CT of the chest/abdomen/pelvis annually if initially T3, T4, or N+ disease
- If biopsy-proven locally recurrent disease, perform systemic restaging and proceed to salvage abdominoperineal resection +/– inguinal nodal dissection. If metastatic disease is found, treat with cisplatin/5-FU systemic therapy or enroll on a clinical trial.

Notable Trials

Name/Inclusion	Arms	Outcomes	Notes
Concurrent ChemoRT vs RT Alone			
UKCCCR ACT I (*Northover et al. Br J Cancer* 2010) T2-T4M0 patients 577 patients total	5-FU/MMC chemoRT (45 Gy/20-25 fx; 15 Gy or 25 Gy Ir-192 boost if >50% response) RT	12-y OS 33% vs 28%, *P* = .12 12-y LC 66% vs 41%, *P* < .0001 12-y CFS 30% vs 20%, *P* = .004 12-y DFS 30% vs 18%, *P* = .004	Established long-term outcome benefits of 5-FU/MMC chemoRT over RT only
EORTC 22861 (*Bartelink et al. JCO* 1997) T3-T4 and N1-N3 patients 110 patients total Patients were taken off trial and given APR if no response	5-FU/MMC chemoRT (45 Gy/25 fx; boost 15 Gy if CR or 20 Gy if <CR) RT	5-y LC 68% vs 50%, *P* = .02 5-y CFS 68% vs 40%, *P* = .002 No difference in 5-year OS or DFS	Established long-term outcome benefits of 5-FU/MMC chemoRT over RT only
Optimal Concurrent ChemoRT Regimen			
RTOG 9811 (*Gunderson et al. JCO* 2012) T2-T4 and M0 patients 682 patients 10-14 Gy boost for T3/T4 or N+ disease or residual T2 disease after the first 45 Gy	5-FU/MMC chemoRT (3D-CRT 45 Gy/25 fx → 10-14 Gy boost) Induction cis/5-FU ×2 → cis/5-FU chemoRT	5-y DFS 68% vs 58%, *P* = .006 5-y OS 78% vs 71%, *P* = .026 No difference in LC or CFS	Superiority study Established improved long-term outcomes with concurrent MMC over cisplatin for chemoRT
UKCCCR ACT II (*James et al. Lancet Oncol* 2013) 940 patients 3D-CRT: 50.4 Gy/28 fx Only 44% of patients randomized to maintenance chemo completed it	5-FU/MMC chemoRT→ Cis/5-FU Cis/5-FU chemoRT→ Cis/5-FU 5-FU/MMC chemoRT Cis/5-FU chemoRT	26-wk LC, 3-yr CFS, PFS, and OS were all no different. G3 hematologic toxicity: cis/5-FU 16% vs 5-FU/MMC 26%	5-FU-MMC remains SoC w/o need for maint. chemo. 26 wk after start of chemoRT is the earliest time to assess cCR unless obvious disease progression
Induction Chemotherapy and Additional RT Boost			
ACCORD 03 (*Peiffert et al. JCO* 2012) >4 cm or N+ M0 307 patients Patients with no response were taken off trial and given APR	Induction cis/5-FU→ chemoRT (45 Gy/25 fx) → 15 Gy boost Induction cis/5-FU→ chemoRT→ 20-25 Gy boost ChemoRT→15 Gy boost ChemoRT→ 20-25 Gy boost	No difference in 5-year LC, OS, CFS (primary endpoint), or DFS among all arms	Demonstrated no benefit for induction chemo or RT boost

Name/Inclusion	Arms	Outcomes	Notes
IMRT for Toxicity Reduction			
RTOG 0529 (*Kachnic et al. IJROBP* 2013; *Kachnic et al. IJROBP* 2022) T2-T4 and M0 63 patients Goal: reduction in G2+ acute GI/GU toxicity by ≥15% with IMRT compared to RTOG 98-11's 2D/3D RT 49% required treatment break	RT doses: T2N0 or ≤3 cm nodes = 50.4 Gy/28 fx T3-T4 or >3 cm nodes = 54 Gy/30 fx	No difference in G2+ acute GI/GU toxicity G3+ GI/GU tox 21% vs 37%, $P = .0052$ G3+ skin tox 23% vs 49%, $P \leq .0001$ G2+ heme tox 73% vs 85%, $P = .032$	Comparable rates of LRF, CFS, DFS, OS, and DM to RTOG 98-11's 2D/3D RT Established IMRT as preferred modality for CRT

PANCREATIC CANCER

BRIAN DE • ETHAN LUDMIR • EUGENE KOAY

BACKGROUND

- **Incidence/prevalence:** The 12th most commonly diagnosed cancer and the 4th most common cause of cancer death in the United States. Estimated ~64 000 new cases diagnosed per year in the United States
- **Outcomes:** The 5-year survival is 12%.
- **Demographics:** Lifetime risk is 1 in 64. Slightly higher incidence in males vs females (1.1:1). More common in developed nations. Typically diagnosed between ages 50 and 70 years
- **Risk factors:** Increasing age, familial-associated genetic changes (p16 and BRCA2), obesity, ETOH consumption, chronic pancreatitis, diabetes, periodontal disease, red meat, tobacco use, exposure to 2-naphthylamine, and benzidine

TUMOR BIOLOGY AND CHARACTERISTICS

- **Genetics:** Familial component in 10% of cases. The most common mutated oncogenes in PCA include *KRAS*, *CDKN2A*, *TP53*, and *SMAD4*.
- **Pathology:** Majority are ductal adenocarcinomas (80%). Other less common subtypes include mucinous cystadenocarcinoma, acinar cell carcinoma, and adenosquamous carcinoma.
- **Imaging:** Predominately hypointense compared with normal pancreatic tissue on CT scans with contrast. Hypointense on T1-weighted MRI. Associated imaging findings include pancreatic duct dilatation, abrupt changes in duct caliber, and parenchymal atrophy distal to the lesion.

ANATOMY

- The pancreas is divided into the head, neck, body, and tail.
- Retroperitoneal structure, with pancreatic duct merging with the common bile duct to drain into the second portion of the duodenum at the ampulla of Vater
- The pancreas is next to numerous critical GI structures including the duodenum, jejunum, stomach, spleen, liver/gallbladder, and both the celiac and SMA axes, which makes treatment challenging.
- Lymphatic drainage is to peripancreatic, celiac, SMA, porta hepatis, and para-aortic lymph nodes.
- Bony landmarks: Celiac artery at the level of **T12**, SMA at the level of **L1**, pancreas is seen at the level of **L1-L2**.

Workup

- **History and physical:** Examination focusing on abdominal symptoms including bloating, abdominal pain, and history of pancreatitis. Evaluation of systemic symptoms including jaundice, weight loss, and back pain.
- **Labs:** CBC, CMP, LFTs, and CA19-9
- **Procedures/biopsy:** Endoscopic ultrasound with biopsy if able. Consider endoscopic evaluation with endoscopic retrograde cholangiopancreatography (ERCP) or percutaneous transhepatic cholangiography (PTC) for evaluation and biopsy. If jaundice, consider stent placement. If resectable, consider staging laparoscopy in high-risk patients.
- **Imaging:** CT of the chest and abdomen with contrast, pancreas protocol (early arterial, pancreatic, and portal venous phase) within 4 weeks of surgery and following neoadjuvant treatment; ideally performed prior to stenting
- **Multidisciplinary discussion:** Prospective discussion facilitated by high-quality imaging is vital. Resections are ideally performed at high-volume centers (at least 15-20 pancreatic per year).

Definitions of Resectability (*Katz J Am Coll Surg* 2008)

	Potentially Resectable	Borderline Resectable	Locally Advanced
Portal vein/SMV	TVI < 180 degrees	TVI ≥ 180 degrees and/or reconstructable occlusion	Unable to reconstruct
Hepatic artery	No TVI	Reconstructable short-segment TVI of any degree	Unable to reconstruct
Superior mesenteric artery	No TVI	TVI < 180 degrees	TVI ≥ 180 degrees
Celiac trunk	No TVI	TVI < 180 degrees	TVI ≥ 180 degrees

TVI, tumor-vessel interface.

Treatment Schema

PCA Stage	Treatment
Resectable PCA	*Preoperative approach:* chemo → chemoRT → surgery *Adjuvant approach:* Surgery → chemo → restage → consider postoperative chemoRT in selected cases
Borderline PCA	Chemo → chemoRT or SBRT → assess for resectability → surgery
Locally advanced PCA	Chemo → restage → consider dose-escalated RT/SBRT*

*Stereotactic body radiation therapy (SBRT) is contraindicated when there is significant bowel (duodenum) invasion.

Radiation Treatment Technique

Conventional RT

- **SIM:** Supine, wingboard, T-bar, Vac-Lok, and Iso at T12 right of midline. Scan from carina to iliac crest. IV contrast
- **Dose:** Preoperative: capecitabine + 50-50.4 Gy, 1.8-2 Gy/fx
  Postoperative: capecitabine + 50-50.4 Gy, 1.8-2 Gy/fx
- **Target:** Preoperative: tumor, involved nodes, celiac, SMA, +/– porta hepatis (for pancreatic head only)
  Postoperative: tumor bed, celiac, SMA, porta hepatis (for pancreatic head only), para-aortics (*Goodman et al. IJROBP* 2012)
  Locally advanced: tumor, involved nodes, celiac, SMA
- **Technique:** 3D or IMRT

Dose-escalated regimens/SBRT

- **SIM:** Arms extended overhead, upper Vac-Lok, T-bar, and wingboard. IV contrast, breath-hold scans. Patient is NPO 3 hours prior to SIM and treatment. Fiducials
- **Dose:** Dose-escalated: 60-67.5 Gy/15 fx; SBRT: 33-36 Gy/5 fx (Fig. 38.1)

- **Target:** GTV and tumor-vessel interface (TVI), consider elective nodal irradiation
- **Technique:** 6 MV photons delivered by VMAT

Contouring and Target Delineation for Pancreatic SBRT[a]	
GTV	Primary tumor
TVI	The circumferential extent of major vessels in direct contact with GTV
PRV	Stomach/duodenum/small bowel + 3 mm
PTV1	GTV + TVI + 3 mm
PTV2	PTV1 – PRV
PTV3	(TVI + 3 mm) – PRV
Treatment Planning	
36 Gy delivered to the interface of the tumor and vessel, PTV3	
33 Gy delivered to the main target, PTV2	
25 Gy delivered to the areas of overlap of 3 mm of critical structures, PTV1[b]	

[a]Adapted from Alliance trial A021501 contouring guidelines.
[b]Elective nodal irradiation may be considered; single institution data suggest improved LRC with ENI

- **IGRT:** Daily cone beam CT and kV. Consider CT-on-rails for dose-escalated regimens.
  Respiratory motion management, for example, breath hold
  We strongly recommend implanting fiducials for SBRT cases.

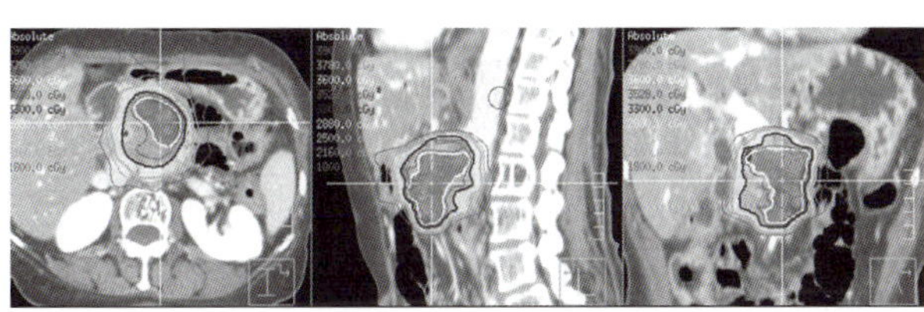

Figure 38.1 Representative cross-sectional axial, sagittal, and coronal images (L→R) from a SBRT treatment plan for locally advanced pancreatic cancer. The *white* isodose line represents 36 Gy encompassing the *red color* wash, which delineates PTV3 (tumor-vessel interface minus PRV). The *sky-blue* isodose line represents 25 Gy, which is encompassing the *yellow contour* that represents PTV1 (gross tumor + TVI + 3 mm). This patient had fiducials placed, which was used daily for image guidance along with CBCT. **See color insert.**

- **Planning Directive (for SBRT) and Conventional RT:**

	SBRT	Conventional RT
Spinal cord	V20 < 1 cc	≤45 Gy
Duodenum	Max dose < 40 Gy	Max dose 54 Gy (consider V54 ≤ 1 cc if needed)
Liver	V12 < 50%	Mean < 28 Gy; V20 < 50%; V30 < 33%
Stomach	Max dose < 40 Gy	Max dose < 54 Gy
Kidneys	V12 < 25%	V20 < 33% for each kidney, mean < 18 Gy

Surgery

- Pancreaticoduodenectomy (Whipple procedure): En bloc removal of the distal stomach, 1st and 2nd position of the duodenum, head of the pancreas, common bile duct, and gallbladder. Anastomoses: pancreas/jejunum, gallbladder/jejunum, stomach/jejunum

Chemotherapy

- **Concurrent with standard dose RT:** capecitabine
- **Neoadjuvant:** FOLFIRINOX (5-fluorouracil, leucovorin, irinotecan, and oxaliplatin) or gemcitabine and nab-paclitaxel
- **Metastatic:** FOLFIRINOX or gemcitabine and nab-paclitaxel

Side Effect Management

- Nausea: First-line ondansetron (8 mg q8h prn) → second-line prochlorperazine (10 mg q6h prn) → ABH (lorazepam 0.34 mg, diphenhydramine 25 mg, and haloperidol 1.5 mg) 1 capsule q6h
- Diarrhea: First-line loperamide titrating to a max of 8 pills/day → second-line alternating diphenoxylate/atropine 2 pills and loperamide 2 pills every 3 hours. Patients will be evaluated and receive CREON (lipase replacement) prior to initiation of therapy.
- Fatigue: Supportive care
- Chronic side effects: Ulcer formation, bowel perforation, and bowel stenosis. Refer to GI specialists.

Follow-up

- History/physical, CT of the chest, abdomen, and pelvis, CA 19-9 level: Every 3 months

Notable Trials

Name/Inclusion	Arms	Outcomes	Notes
Resected Pancreatic Cancer			
ESPAC 1 (*Neoptolemos et al. NEJM* 2004) 2 × 2 randomization 289 patients with resectable cancer	Surgery → obs Surgery → chemo alone (5-FU) Surgery → split course chemoRT (40 Gy + 5-FU) Surgery → split course chemoRT → chemo (5-FU)	5-y OS 10% chemoRT vs 20% without 5-y OS 21% chemo vs 8% without	Chemo improved OS whereas chemoRT worsened OS. Many criticisms: lack of central QA, selection bias RTOG 0848 (results pending) will address the role of adjuvant chemoRT
PRODIGE 24/ CCTG PA.6 (*Conroy et al. NEJM* 2018; *JAMA Onc* 2022) 493 patients R0-1 resection	Surgery → gem x6 Surgery → mFOLFIRINOX x12	Median DFS (21.4 vs 12.8 mo), DMFS (29.4 vs 17.7 mo), and OS (53.5 vs 35.5 mo) improved with adjuvant mFOLFIRINOX	Adjuvant mFOLFIRINOX improved DFS, DMFS, and OS vs gem
PREOPANC (*Versteijine et al. JCO* 2020, 2022) 246 Resectable and borderline resectable patients	Surgery → gem x6 Gem x3 + RT (36 Gy/15 fx during cycle 3) → surgery → gem x4	Preoperative chemoRT ↑ R0 resection (71% vs 40%), median OS (15.7 vs 14.3 mo)	ChemoRT associated with higher R0 rate and improved OS. Supports neo-adjuvant chemoRT for both resectable and borderline tumors
Alliance A021501 (*Katz et al. JAMA* 2022) 126 Borderline resectable patients	Induction mFOLFIRINOX x8 → surgery → FOLFOX x4 Induction mFOLFIRINOX x7 → SBRT (33-40 Gy/5 fx) or hypofrac IGRT (25 Gy/5 fx) → surgery → FOLFOX x4	RT arm reached futility due to low R0 (33% RT vs 57% chemo alone) Survival numerically favored chemo alone arm, but not significant: 18 mo OS (67% vs 47%), median OS (30 vs 17 mo), and median EFS (15 vs 10 mo)	Unclear if designed and powered appropriately; no *P* values reported, as outcomes cannot be statistically compared. More metastatic patients in RT arm at time of surgery

Name/Inclusion	Arms	Outcomes	Notes
Locally Advanced Pancreatic Cancer			
LAP 07 (*Hammel et al. JAMA* 2016) 449 stage III locally advanced Two-step randomization first induction regime then adjuvant chemoRT if disease controlled	Induction gem x4 > gem x2 Induction gem/erlotinib x4 > gem/erlotinib x2 > maintenance erlotinib Induction gem x4 > chemoRT (54 Gy + concurrent cape) Induction gem/erlotinib x4 > chemoRT > maintenance erlotinib	No difference in OS: median 16.5 mo for chemo vs 15.2 mo for chemoRT RT improved LC, 68% vs 54% (*P* = .04)	Improvement in LC was seen with addition of RT, but no difference in OS
Phase II SBRT (*Herman et al. Cancer* 2015) 49 patients	Gemcitabine → SBRT (6.6 Gy x5)	Median OS 13.9, 1-y LC 78%	Favorable results seen with SBRT

GASTRIC CANCER

BRIAN DE • PRAJNAN DAS

GC 7-15

Background

- **Incidence/prevalence:** 26 500 new cases in the United States annually. More common in East Asia (Japan, China, Korea) relative to the United States
- **Outcomes:** 5-Year survival across all stages estimated at 33% (SEER data)
- **Demographics:** 35% gastric cardia/fundus, 25% body, 40% distal/antrum
- **Risk factors:** Lynch syndrome, E-cadherin alteration (*CDH1*), Juvenile polyposis syndrome (*SMAD4*), Peutz-Jeghers syndrome (*STK11*), familial adenomatous polyposis (*APC*), Li-Fraumeni (*TP53*), *BRCA1/BRCA2*, xeroderma pigmentosum, Cowden (*PTEN*), GERD/gastritis/Barrett esophagus, pernicious anemia, diet high in salted meats and nitrates and low in fruits and vegetables, smoking, obesity

Tumor Biology and Characteristics

- **Genetics:** 60% have p53 loss; HER2 overexpression seen in ~20% of patients (*Bang et al. Lancet* 2010); other subtypes include EBV+ (10%) and microsatellite instability (MSI; 20%) (*TCGA* 2014). Many are associated with *Helicobacter pylori* and EBV; others have *CDH1* mutation or mismatch repair w/ *MLH1* silencing (CIMP phenotype).
- **Pathology (Lauren histologic classification):**
  - **Intestinal subtype:** Male predominant; arises from precursor lesions; better prognosis, more often localized; EBV- and MSI-associated; arises in GEJ/cardia
  - **Diffuse subtype:** Female predominant; no precursor lesions; worse prognosis, more invasive and more common intraperitoneal spread; locations diffuse

Anatomy

- From cranial to caudal: Esophagus → GE junction → cardia → fundus → body → antrum/pyloric antrum → pylorus → duodenum (Fig. 39.1)
- Siewert classification: Type I—5-1 cm proximal to GEJ, type II—epicenter of tumor located between 1 cm proximal and 2 cm distal to GEJ, type III—2-5 cm distal to GEJ

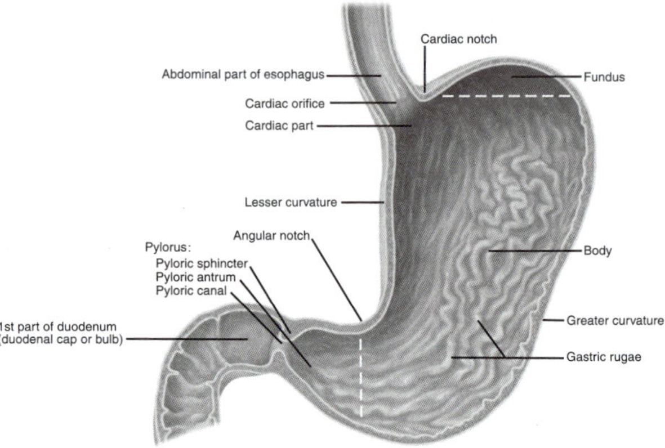

Figure 39.1 Anatomy of the stomach. (Reproduced with permission from Gest TR. Lippincott Atlas of Anatomy. 2nd ed. Philadelphia, PA: Wolters Kluwer; 2019.)

- Lymph node drainage:
  - Fundus/cardia → perigastric, celiac, left gastric, splenic, hepatic
  - Body → perigastric, celiac, left gastric, splenic, hepatic, sub/suprapyloric, pancreaticoduodenal
  - Antrum/pylorus → perigastric, celiac, left gastric, hepatic, sub/suprapyloric, pancreaticoduodenal
- Vascular supply (from celiac artery)
  - Left gastric: Lesser curvature
  - Right gastric: Lesser curvature/inferior stomach
  - Right gastroepiploic: Greater curvature
  - Left gastroepiploic: Upper greater curvature
  - Short gastric arteries: Fundus/proximal stomach

Workup

- **History and physical:** Standard H&P beginning with assessment of hemodynamic stability; dysphagia, indigestion, early satiety, loss of appetite, nausea, abdominal pain, weight loss, obstruction, anemia, hematemesis, melena; examine for adenopathy
- **Labs:** CBC, CMP, CEA, *H pylori*
- **Procedures/biopsy:** Esophagogastroduodenoscopy (EGD) with biopsies along with endoscopic ultrasound (EUS) (depth of tumor + LN involvement; ~85-90% accurate; nodal Sn/Sp are ~83%/67%). Nutritional assessment/counseling. Consider Her2-neu, MSI/MMR, PD-L1, and *NTRK* testing if M1 disease is suspected. **Need laparoscopic evaluation** particularly if T4 or undergoing neoadjuvant therapy (20-30% of patients with >T1 tumors and negative imaging: + peritoneal involvement)
- **Imaging:** CT of the chest, abdomen, and pelvis with IV and oral contrast. Guidelines recommend PET/CT if there is no evidence of M1 disease (false negative ~40% of the time, particularly in diffuse subtype).

Treatment Algorithm

T1N0	Surgery (gastrectomy vs endoscopic mucosal resection)
T2+ or N+ (combined modality)	Surgery → chemo → chemoRT → chemo—**INT 0116** Surgery → chemo (cape/ox ×6)—**CLASSIC** Perioperative chemo (chemo → surgery → chemo)—**MAGIC, FLOT-4** Induction chemo → preoperative chemoRT → surgery—**MDACC**
Stage IV	Chemotherapy Palliative chemoRT

Radiation Treatment Technique

Preoperative

- **SIM: Supine, arms up, upper body cradle, 3 hours NPO**, 4DCT, scan carina to pelvic brim, isocenter midline @T12; no IV or oral contrast
- **Dose:** 45-50.4 Gy in 25-28 fractions at 1.8 Gy/fx
- **Target: GTV:** based on EGD/CT/PET + 3 cm mucosal expansion = mucosal target volume (MTV) (Fig. 39.2)
  CTV = MTV + involved nodes + elective nodes* + 1 cm
  PTV = CTV + 0.5 cm
  *Elective nodes may be omitted in select cases; institutional practices vary.

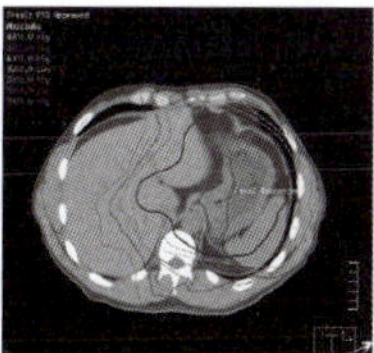
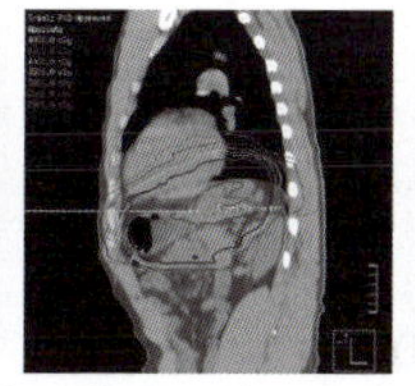
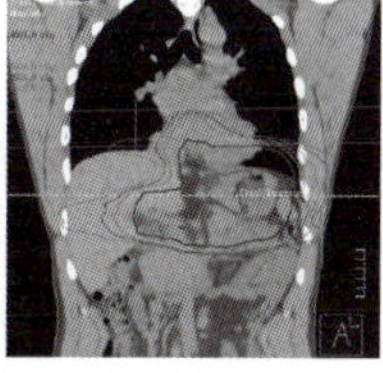

Figure 39.2 Representative axial, sagittal, and coronal cross-sectional images (L → R) illustrating a typical IMRT treatment plan for preoperative radiation for gastric adenocarcinoma. The 45-Gy isodose line is shown in *blue*, which encompasses the MTV (*red line*), involved and elective nodes, with a 1-cm expansion. This patient's primary tumor was located at the GEJ extending 4 cm into the cardia. **See color insert.**

- **Elective Nodes**

GEJ/fundus/cardia	Perigastric, celiac, left gastric artery, splenic artery, splenic hilar, hepatic artery, porta hepatis
Body	Perigastric, celiac, left gastric artery, splenic artery, splenic hilar, hepatic artery, porta hepatis, sub/suprapyloric, pancreaticoduodenal
Antrum/pylorus	Perigastric, celiac, left gastric artery, hepatic artery, porta hepatis, sub/suprapyloric, pancreaticoduodenal

- **Technique:** IMRT
- **IGRT:** Daily kV or CBCT

Adjuvant/postoperative

- **Dose:** 45-50.4 Gy in 25-28 fractions at 1.8 Gy/fx, consider boost if R1/R2 resection
- **Target:** Draw tumor bed using preoperative imaging, op note, clips, and path. Same elective regions as preoperative, cover anastomosis (may be high in the thorax) and gastric remnant.
- **Technique:** IMRT
- **IGRT:** Daily kV or CBCT
- **Planning directive (for conventional fractionation):**
  Cord Max < 45 Gy
  Lung: V20 < 30%, V10 < 45%, V5 < 65%, MLD < 20 Gy
  Heart: V30 < 10%, mean < 10 Gy, ALARA
  Kidney: Each kidney V20 < 33%, mean < 18 Gy
  Liver: V30 < 30%, V20 < 50%, mean < 25 Gy
  Bowel bag: V45 < 195 cc

Surgery

- For distal tumors (body/antrum) → subtotal gastrectomy; proximal tumors → total gastrectomy
- D1 dissection: removes involved proximal or distal or entire stomach + perigastric LNs
- D2 dissection: D1 + celiac, L gastric, hepatic, splenic, splenic hilum (celiac + branches); **recommended procedure at experienced centers**

- D3 dissection—D2 + PA +/− porta hepatis
- Billroth I anastomosis (end-to-end gastrojejunal w/ gastric resection margin) or Billroth II (end-to-side anastomosis, gastric resection margin NOT used)
- Aim for removal of at least 16 nodes, but assessment of >30 nodes is desirable.

Chemotherapy

- **Concurrent preoperative:** Fluoropyrimidine (+/− oxaliplatin) OR paclitaxel/carboplatin
- **Concurrent postoperative:** 5-FU alone (infusional or capecitabine)
- **Perioperative:** 5-FU + leucovorin + oxaliplatin + docetaxel
- **Postoperative:** Capecitabine + oxaliplatin OR 5-FU-oxaliplatin

Side Effect Management

- Nausea: Use PPI, first-line Zofran (8 mg q8h prn) → second-line Compazine (10 mg q6h prn) → ABH (lorazepam 0.34 mg, diphenhydramine 25 mg, and haloperidol 1.5 mg) 1 capsule q6h
- Anorexia: Maintain hydration, IVF if necessary, dietary counseling including protein heavy intake, consider J-tube placement if persistently inadequate intake
- Skin care: Aquaphor
- Hand and foot syndrome: *Redness, swelling, and pain in hand and foot.* Consult with medical oncology about reducing concurrent capecitabine dose.

Follow-up

- History/physical: Every 3-6 months for 2 years → every 6-12 months for 5 years
- EGD: As clinically indicated
- CT C/A/P w/ contrast (or PET/CT): Every 6-12 months for 2 years and then annually

Notable Trials

Name/Inclusion	Arms	Outcomes	Notes
	Postoperative ChemoRT		
Intergroup 0116 *(Macdonald et al. NEJM 2001; Smalley et al. JCO 2012)* 559 stage IB-IV gastric, R0 resection, PS ≤ 2, and maintaining 1500 kcal/d diet Mostly D0 and D1 dissections (10% D2)	Surgery alone Surgery → postoperative chemoRT (5-FU/LV ×1 before, 2 during, 2 after)	ChemoRT improved median OS (39 vs 27 mo), 3-y OS (50% vs 41%), RFS (48% vs 31%), LR (19% vs 29%), RR (65% vs 72%), and DM (33% vs 18%)	Adjuvant chemoRT improves OS, RFS, LR, and DM in resected gastric cancer. Subgroup analysis showed no benefit in women and patients with diffuse subtype
CRITICS *(Cats et al. Lancet Oncol 2018)* 788 stage IB-IV gastric All received neoadjuvant ECC/EOC ×3 + gastrectomy with planned D1-D3 dissection	ECC/EOC ×3 → surgery → ECC/EOC ×3 ECC/EOC ×3 → Surgery → chemoRT (45 Gy/25 fx + cape/cis)	5-y OS similar (~41% both arms), no difference in EFS or LRC, heme toxicity higher in chemo alone arm (postoperative nonfebrile neutropenia 34% vs 4%)	No difference in OS with perioperative chemo compared with adjuvant RT Poor completion rates in both groups (~60% in each arm started postoperative therapy)
ARTIST *(Lee et al. JCO 2012; Park and Sohn et al. JCO 2015)* 458 stage IB-IVA gastric All received D2 dissection	Surgery → cape/cis ×6 Surgery → chemoRT (45 Gy/25 fx + cape) → cape/cis ×2	5-y OS ~75% in both arms Subgroup analysis: Improved DFS among N+ patients with chemoRT (76% vs 72%) and intestinal subtype (94% vs 83%)	No significant difference in OS between adjuvant chemo and chemoRT, but DFS benefit for N+ and intestinal subtype

Name/Inclusion	Arms	Outcomes	Notes
ARTIST-2 (*Park et al. ASCO 2019*) 546 stages II-III gastric, D2 dissection, node positive	Surgery → chemo (S-1) Surgery → chemo (S-1 + oxali; SOX) Surgery → chemo (S-1 + oxali) + 45 Gy/25 fx (SOXRT)	Stopped early due to futility 3-y DFS 65% vs 78% vs 73%; S-1 DFS lower than SOX or SOXRT	SOX and SOXRT both resulted in improved DFS over S-1, but no benefit seen to adding RT to SOX
Preoperative ChemoRT			
CROSS (*Eyck et al. JCO; 2021; Shapiro et al. Lancet Oncol 2015; van Hagen et al. NEJM 2012*) 368 patients esophageal + GE junction T1-T3, N0-N1	Surgery alone ChemoRT (41.4 Gy/23 fx + carbo/ taxol) → surgery	With chemoRT, improved 5-y OS (47% vs 34%), 10-y OS (38% vs 25%), and median OS (49 vs 24 mo); higher for SCC vs adeno but both benefit	Adding concurrent carbo/taxol to preoperative RT improves OS vs surgery alone R0 resection 92% vs 69%
RTOG 9904 (*Ajani et al. JCO 2006*) 43 patients localized gastric adenocarcinoma, confirmed by negative laparoscopic evaluation—49 patients D2 dissection in 50%	Chemo (cis/5-FU ×2) → chemoRT (45 Gy/25 fx + 5-FU + weekly taxol) → surgery	pCR 26%, R0 resection 77%, 1-y OS 72%, median OS 23 mo 1-y OS higher among those achieving pCR (82% vs 69%)	Favorable pCR and OS associated with preoperative chemoRT were observed
Perioperative Chemotherapy			
MAGIC (*Cunningham et al. NEJM 2006; Smyth et al. JAMA Oncol 2017*) 503 patients gastric/ GE junction ≥ stage II At least D1 dissection in 85%	Surgery alone Surgery + peri-operative ECF ×3	Perioperative chemo resulted in longer 5-y OS (36% vs 23%) and lower LR (15% vs 21%) pCR 0%	Perioperative ECF improves PFS and OS MSI/MMR negative prognostic factors with chemo, but positive without
FLOT-4 (*Al-Batran et al. Lancet 2019*) 716 patients gastric or GEJ adenocarcinoma stage ≥cT2 or N+ Treated with D2 dissection	Surgery + perioperative ECF/ ECX ×3 Surgery + perioperative FLOT ×4	FLOT improved median OS (50 vs 35 mo), 5-y OS (45% vs 36%), DFS (30 vs 18 mo)	Perioperative FLOT improved DFS and OS over ECF/ECX Both regimens poorly tolerated (ECF/ECX 37% and FLOT 46% completed all cycles)

HEPATOBILIARY CANCER

BRIAN DE • ETHAN LUDMIR • EUGENE KOAY

Hepatocellular Carcinoma (HCC)

- **Incidence/prevalence:** Sixth most common cancer worldwide, third leading cause of cancer mortality. Screening programs are effective—those with risk factors should be screened with US and AFP q3-6 months.
- **Risk factors:** Cirrhosis from any cause, including hepatitis (B > C; accounts for 75% of cases; B can occur without cirrhosis), alcoholic, autoimmune, NASH-related, A1AT deficiency, primary biliary cholangitis, and hemochromatosis

- **Evaluation/workup:** Calculate Child-Pugh score (albumin, total bili, INR, ascites, encephalopathy); imaging w/ triphasic CT or MRI; hepatitis serologies; CBC (platelets), AFP, LFTs, bilirubin, alk phos, albumin, PT/INR. Consider SPECT.

Treatment Algorithm for HCC

Resectable, operable candidate	Child-Pugh A (occasionally B) → surgical resection; 5-y OS 40-80%
Liver transplant candidate	Child-Pugh B-C okay; Based on **UNOS criteria** (AFP level ≤ 1000 ng/mL + solitary lesion 2-5 cm, or 2-3 lesions each 1-3 cm, no macrovascular invasion, no extrahepatic disease) → transplant list. Can use SBRT, EBRT, or other local therapies as bridge to transplant
Unresectable/ not transplant candidate	Transcatheter arterial chemoembolization (TACE), radiofrequency ablation (RFA), Sir-Spheres Y-90, SBRT/EBRT, atezolizumab + bevacizumab for CP A only (*Finn et al. NEJM* 2020); tremelimumab-actl + durvalumab (*Abou-Alfa et al. NEJM Evid* 2022)

Selecting Local Therapy

RFA	Tumor ≤4 cm, CP A/B, >1 cm from the liver capsule, vessels, diaphragm, dome of the liver
TACE/TARE	NO portal vein thrombosis (need vascular access)
Radiation	Portal vein thrombosis okay, large tumors okay (as long as adequate preserved functional liver)

Cholangiocarcinoma

- **Incidence/prevalence:** 10% intrahepatic, 60% perihilar, 30% distal. Extrahepatic includes perihilar and distal. The second most common primary hepatobiliary malignancy after HCC. Estimated 8000 cases per year in the United States
- **Risk factors:** Chronic inflammation of the gallbladder or gallbladder tracts: primary sclerosing cholangitis, liver flukes, chronic calculi, chronic typhoid
- **Evaluation/workup:** Triphasic CT or MRI with contrast. MRCP or ERCP (particularly if obstruction, need stenting), EGD/colonoscopy, hepatitis serologies, CA 19-9, AFP, CEA, and LFTs. Biopsy with MSI/MMR, TMB, and molecular testing. Evaluate for resectability (hepatic duct involvement, encasement of portal vein, stage III-IV disease, late-stage cirrhosis, medically unfit for surgery → pursue alternate treatment options).

Treatment Algorithm for Cholangiocarcinoma

Distal	More likely to be resectable → requires pancreaticoduodenectomy → adjuvant chemo or chemoRT if R1 or N+ (*Horgan et al. JCO* 2012)
Intrahepatic	Surgery when feasible. If unresectable, OS improved with ablative RT (BED > 80.5; *Tao et al. JCO* 2016)
Perihilar	If resectable requires hepatic lobectomy + involved bile ducts + nodal dissection → adjuvant chemo or chemoRT if R1 or N+. Often unresectable. Definitive RT if unresectable

Anatomy

- The liver has eight independent segments.
- The middle hepatic vein divides the liver into right and left lobes.
- The portal vein divides the liver into upper and lower segments.
- Dual blood supply by portal vein and hepatic artery

Radiation Treatment Technique for HCC/ Cholangiocarcinoma

- **SIM:** NPO for 3 hours, with IV contrast, 5-6 deep inspiration breath-hold scans for reproducibility; begin scans 30 seconds after contrast administration for variable phases
- **Dose:** Depends on tumor location, size, and anatomy; BED > 80 if possible. SBRT (50 Gy in 4-5 fractions), hypofractionated IMRT (60-67.5 Gy in 15 fractions) or standard fractionation (54-50.4 Gy in 28 fractions). Consider lower doses for postoperative cases with R0 resection. Need >5 mm from GI mucosa. Preserve >700-800 cc functional liver
- **Target:** Tumor defined on liver protocol CT/MRI and breath-hold scans from simulation to accommodate respiratory movement; contour GI mucosal avoidance structure based on anatomic movement + 5 mm
  If extrahepatic cholangiocarcinoma, consider elective treatment of portal and celiac vein LN basins to 45 Gy in 25 fractions.
- **Technique:** IMRT, SBRT, or protons; use daily CT on rails or fiducials with CBCT for cases with escalated dose/SBRT
- **Constraints:**

Structure	4 or 5 fractions (50 Gy)	15 fractions (60-67.5 Gy)	25 or 28 fractions (50-50.4 Gy)
Spinal cord	D_{max} < 18 Gy; 10 cc < 15 Gy	D_{max} < 36 Gy	D_{max} < 45 Gy
Liver (minus GTV)	700 cc < 15 Gy; mean < 16 Gy	Child-Pugh A 700 cc < 24 Gy; mean < 24 Gy Child-Pugh B 700 cc < 18 Gy; mean < 18 Gy	Child-Pugh A 700 cc < 28 Gy; mean < 28 Gy Child-Pugh B 700 cc < 24 Gy; mean < 24 Gy
Kidneys	V15 < 67% for contralateral, V15 < 35% for both	V20 < 33% for each	V20 < 33% for each
Stomach	D_{max} < 28 Gy	D_{max} < 45 Gy	D_{max} < 55 Gy
Duodenum	D_{max} < 28 Gy	D_{max} < 45 Gy	D_{max} < 55 Gy
Small bowel	D_{max} < 28 Gy	D_{max} < 45 Gy	D_{max} < 55 Gy
Large bowel	D_{max} < 30 Gy	D_{max} < 50 Gy	D_{max} < 60 Gy
Heart	V40 < 10%	V40 < 10%	V40 < 10%
Common bile duct	D_{max} < 55 Gy	D_{max} < 70 Gy	D_{max} < 80 Gy

Notable Trials

Name/Inclusion	Arms	Outcomes	Notes
Hepatocellular Carcinoma			
RTOG 1112 (*Dawson et al. ASTRO* 2022) 193 patients >1 cm, unsuitable or refractory to TACE or drug eluting beads, unsuitable for surgery, transplant or RFA	Sorafenib SBRT (27.5-50 Gy in 5 fractions) + sorafenib	Favored SBRT, including longer median OS (15.8 vs 12.3 mo, 1-sided *P* = .0554), median PFS (9.2 vs 5.5 mo), and TTP	Addition of SBRT → longer OS vs sorafenib alone Large tumors (up to 20 cm) permitted on this study

Name/Inclusion	Arms	Outcomes	Notes
Phase II hypofrac proton (*Hong et al. JCO* 2016) 80 patients with unresectable HCC or ICC, Child-Pugh A/B	Definitive RT (maximum dose 67.5 Gy [RBE] in 15 fractions for peripheral, 58.05 Gy [RBE] for central	2-y LC 95% for HCC and 94% for ICC 2-y OS 63% for HCC and 47% for ICC	High-dose hypofrac proton therapy confers excellent LC and OS
Extrahepatic Cholangiocarcinoma			
SWOG 0809 (*Ben-Josef et al. JCO* 2015) 79 patient with ECC or GBC, pT2-4 or N+ or R1 resection	Surgery → cape/gem ×4 → chemoRT (52.5-59.4 Gy to tumor bed, 45 Gy to regional nodes + concurrent cape)	2-y OS 65% (67% for R0 and 60% for R1 patients), median OS 35 mo LR in 14 patients, DM in 24 patients, combined in 9 patients Toxicities: G3 52%, G4 11%	Use of adjuvant chemoRT led to favorable outcomes
Palliation			
CCTG HE1 (*Dawson et al. ASCO GI* 2022; abstract) 66 patients with HCC or liver mets Pain score ≥4 (out of 10)	Best supportive care (BSC) BSC + palliative RT (8 Gy in 1 fraction)	Greater improvement (≥2 points on pain scale) with RT vs BSC alone (67% vs 10%) Trend toward improved OS at 3 mo with RT (51% vs 22%)	Palliative RT delivered in a single fraction → favorable pain control and possibly longer OS. Full results pending

GENERAL BREAST CANCER

KELSEY CORRIGAN • WENDY WOODWARD

Background

- **Incidence/prevalence:** See other breast cancer chapters.
- **Outcomes:** See other breast cancer chapters.
- **Risk factors:** Increasing age, personal or family history of breast cancer, genetic mutations (BRCA1/2, p53 [Li-Fraumeni], PTEN [Cowden], STK11 [Peutz-Jeghers], ATM [ataxia-telangiectasia]), prior chest radiotherapy, prior anthracycline/alkylating agent exposure, estrogen exposure (obesity, hormone therapy/contraceptive use, early menarche, late menopause, nulliparity), alcohol consumption

Breast Cancer Screening Guidelines

- **Average-risk patients:**
  - **American Cancer Society:** Annual mammogram (MMG) for patients age 40-54 (optional for age 40-44), biennial MMG beginning at age 55
  - **U.S. Preventive Task Force:** Biennial screening MMG from age 50 to 74 *Recommends against breast self-examination
  - **Breast MRI:** Not required for screening, useful for women with dense breasts
- **High-risk patients** (defined as BRCA carriers, untested women with 1-degree relatives with BRCA, p53, or PTEN mutations, women with 1-degree relative with premenopausal BrCa, women with prior chest RT between 10 and 30 years of age, or women with lifetime risk of BrCa ≥ 20%):
- **American Cancer Society:** Annual MMG and MRI for patients starting at age 30 or 10 years earlier than affected 1-degree relative

Tumor Biology and Characteristics

- **Genetics:**
  BRCA1: 60-80% lifetime risk of breast cancer and 40% risk for ovarian cancer
  BRCA2: 40-50% lifetime risk of BrCa and 10-20% risk for ovarian cancer. Genetic counseling recommended if high-risk features present for hereditary breast cancer
- **Pathology:** See other breast cancers.
- **Imaging:** See other breast cancers.

BI-RADS Categories for MMGs			
1	Negative	4	New suspicious abnormality (biopsy)
2	Stable benign findings	5	New finding highly suggestive of malignancy (biopsy and treat)
3	New finding, likely benign (recommend biopsy or repeat MMG in 6 mo)	6	Known biopsy, proven malignancy

Anatomy

Field borders are not to rigidly supersede volume-based target definitions edited for patient- and tumor-specific factors. Breast contouring should include all of the glandular breast tissue and the clinically apparent breast mound.

- **Breast anatomic breast borders:**
  - Superior: Inferior border of clavicular head or 2nd anterior rib
  - Inferior: Loss of apparent breast parenchyma or 6th anterior rib
  - Lateral: Midaxillary line
  - Medial: Sternum-rib junction
- **Regional nodal borders** *(nodal volumes are described in the RTOG atlas and should be edited for clinical risk; nodes should always be contoured if targeted)*:
  - Axillary: Level 1 (inferior and lateral to pectoralis minor), level 2 (subpectoral and constrained by pectoralis minor, includes Rotter nodes), and level 3 (medial and superior to pectoralis minor; should be entirely within the SCV field)
  - Internal mammary: Superior aspect of medial 1st rib (superior) to superior aspect of 4th rib (inferior)

- Supraclavicular: Cricoid (superior), inferior border of clavicular head (inferior). Medial border should cover the volume even if it includes the trachea. Contour and block the esophagus unless N3c targets would be compromised.

Breast Cancer Staging (AJCC 8th edition)

T Stage		N Stage	Clinical	Pathologic
Tis	Ductal carcinoma in situ	N0	No regional LN(s) involved	pN0: None pN0(i+): ITCs only pN0(mol+): Positive by RT-PCR only
T1mi	TS ≤ 1 mm	N1mi	Micromets (~200 cells, >0.2 mm but ≤2 mm)	
T1a	TS > 1 mm but ≤5 mm	N1	Mobile ipsi level I-II axillary LN(s)	pN1a: 1-3 axilla LN(s) pN1b: Ipsi IM LN(s) pN1c: pN1a + pN1b
T1b	TS > 5 mm but ≤10 mm	N2a	Matted/fixed ipsi level I-II axillary LN(s)	4-9 axillary LN(s)
T1c	TS > 10 mm but ≤20 mm	N2b	Only ipsi IM LN(s) involved	
T2	TS > 20 mm but ≤50 mm	N3a	Ipsi infraclavicular LN(s)	≥10 axillary LN(s) or infraclavicular LN(s)
T3	TS > 50 mm	N3b	Ipsi IM and axillary LN(s)	
T4a	Extension to chest wall (invasion of pectoralis in the absence of chest wall invasion does not qualify)	N3c	Ipsi supraclavicular LN(s)	
T4b	Ulceration and/or ipsilateral satellite nodules and/or edema without meeting criteria for T4b	**M stage**		
		M0	No distant metastases cM0(i+): tumor cell deposits ≤2 cm detected only by microscopic or molecular techniques	
T4c	Both T4a and T4b present			
T4d	Inflammatory carcinoma (see **IBC** chapter)	M1	Distant metastases present	

Summative Stage: Prognostic Stage Groups should now be used in countries that routinely test for receptors and grade, see AJCC 8th edition

<table>
<tr><th></th><th>N0</th><th>N1mi</th><th>N1</th><th>N2</th><th>N3</th><th>M1</th></tr>
<tr><th>T0</th><td>0</td><td rowspan="2">IB</td><td rowspan="2">IIA</td><td rowspan="4">IIIA</td><td rowspan="5">IIIC</td><td rowspan="5">IV</td></tr>
<tr><th>T1</th><td>IA</td></tr>
<tr><th>T2</th><td>IIA</td><td colspan="2">IIB</td></tr>
<tr><th>T3</th><td>IIB</td><td colspan="2"></td></tr>
<tr><th>T4</th><td colspan="4">IIIB</td></tr>
</table>

Abbreviations: TS, tumor size; Ipsi, ipsilateral; IM, internal mammary; ITCs, isolated tumor cells.

Systemic Therapy

Preference at MDACC is for neoadjuvant chemotherapy (NAC) if the decision to give chemotherapy is known. NAC is the first option in a patient who wants BCS but cannot proceed due to tumor size. Below are common regimens based on FDA approval as of 1/2023. Care should be taken to review subsequent changes.

	ER/PR+HER2−	ER/PR +/−HER2+	ER/PR−HER2−
DCIS	+ Hormone therapy	+/− Hormone therapy (for ER+ only)	Observation
T1mi/T1a, N0	+/− Hormone therapy[a]	+/− HER2-targeted systemic therapy[a] +/− Hormone therapy (ER+ only)[a]	+/− Chemotherapy[a]
T1b/1c/2, N0	+/− Chemotherapy (Oncotype DX[b] or other genomic study) + Hormone therapy	+ HER2-targeted systemic therapy +/− Hormone therapy (ER+ only)	+ Chemotherapy with pembrolizumab[c]
≥T3 and/or ≥N1mi[d]	+ Chemotherapy + Hormone therapy + CDK 4/6 inhibitor[d]	+ HER2-targeted systemic therapy +/− Hormone therapy (ER+ only)	+ Chemotherapy with pembrolizumab[c]

[a]Choice of hormone therapy, chemotherapy, or HER2-targeted systemic therapy is unclear and depends on discussion of factors including patient preference, age, and pathology factors (size, grade, margin, etc.).
[b]For postmenopausal patients, if Oncotype DX score <26, then no chemotherapy; score ≥26, then addition of chemotherapy to endocrine therapy is recommended. For premenopausal patients with pN0, if Oncotype DX score <15, then no chemotherapy; score 16-25, unclear, consider addition of chemotherapy; score ≥26, then addition of chemotherapy to endocrine therapy is recommended. For premenopausal patients with 1-3 positive LNs, if Oncotype DX score <26, unclear, consider addition of chemotherapy; score ≥26, then addition of chemotherapy to endocrine therapy is recommended.
[c]Pembro is preferred regardless of PD-L1 status (*Schmid et al. Keynote 522, NEJM* 2020); however, capecitabine should be given adjuvantly (6-8 cycles) for patients who received NAC without pembro and had residual invasive disease.
[d]For N1mic or greater patients with ER/PR+HER2− BrCa who received NAC, abemaciclib should be given adjuvantly with hormone therapy for 2 years (*Martin et al. monarchE, JAMA Onc* 2022).

- Chemotherapy (for HER2−): AC (Adriamycin, cyclophosphamide) ×4, ddAC (dose-dense AC, administered twice for every 4-week cycle) ×4, or FAC (fluorouracil, Adriamycin, and cyclophosphamide) ×4 → paclitaxel q1wk ×12
- HER2-targeted systemic therapy (for HER2+): THP (paclitaxel, Herceptin, pertuzumab) ×6, then consider ddAC q2wk ×4 pre/postoperative → maintenance Herceptin q3wk (total 1 year)
  - Alternate Her2+ regimen: TCHP (paclitaxel, carboplatin, Herceptin, pertuzumab) ×6 → maintenance trastuzumab q3wk (total 1 year)
  - Ado-trastuzumab should be given adjuvantly (14 cycles) for patients who received NAC and had residual invasive disease.
- Hormone therapy: Tamoxifen or aromatase inhibitor for 5-10 years
- PARP inhibitors (Olaparib) should be given adjuvantly (total 1 year) for patients with germline BRCA1/2 mutation who received NAC and had residual invasive disease.

DUCTAL CARCINOMA IN SITU (DCIS)

KELSEY CORRIGAN • WENDY WOODWARD

BACKGROUND

- **Incidence/prevalence:** Approximately 70 000 cases diagnosed annually in the United States. DCIS accounts for 15-30% of all detected breast cancer.
- **Outcomes:** Mortality from DCIS is very low. 20-Year breast cancer–specific mortality is 3.3% (*Narod et al. JAMA Oncol* 2015).
- **Risk factors:** See **General Breast Cancer** chapter.

Tumor Biology and Characteristics

- Genetics: See **General Breast Cancer** chapter.
- Pathology: Subtypes of DCIS include comedonecrosis and noncomedo (cribriform, papillary, medullary, and solid type).
- Imaging: On mammogram, characteristically appears as linear or granular calcifications. May underestimate size by 1-2 cm. On *ultrasound*, typically presents as hypoechoic mass with ductal extension. On *MRI*, regional branching or linear enhancement is seen on T1.

Workup

- **History and physical, labs:** Including bilateral breast examination and axilla palpation. Consider genetics evaluation. β-HCG (if premenopausal)
- **Procedures/biopsy:** Core needle biopsy of suspicious breast lesions, pathology staining of biopsy for ER/PR status. Two commercially available genomic tests may further refine risk of recurrence estimates: DCISionRT and Oncotype DX. Neither has prospectively demonstrated prediction of radiation therapy benefit (*Woodward, IJORBP* 2023).
- **Imaging:** Bilateral diagnostic mammogram (MMG), breast ± regional LN basin ultrasound, consider MRI for dense breasts.

Treatment Algorithms

Low-risk:	**BCS → observation or RT and/or hormone therapy**[a]
Non–low-risk:[b]	**BCS → APBI/WBI → RT boost → hormone therapy**[a] **OR total mastectomy +/− SLNB → observation or hormone therapy**[a]

[a]If ER/PR+

[b]Non–low-risk defined as one or more of the following: <50 years old, symptomatic presentation, palpable tumor, tumor size ≥ 1.5 cm, multifocal, intermediate or high grade, central necrosis, comedo histology, or radial margin < 1 cm

Radiation Treatment Technique for WBI

- **SIM:** Supine, upper Vac-Lok device, ipsilateral arm abducted/externally rotated over the head. Use slant board (5-15 degrees) to make breasts fall downward but balance with degree of inframammary fold (can worsen skin reactions). Consider wiring surgical scar and treatment borders, deep inspiration breath-hold for left-sided tumors to reduce heart/lung doses, and prone simulation for larger BMI and/or pendulous breasts.
- **Dose:** 40.05 Gy in 15 fx or 26 Gy in 5 fx (given daily over 1 week or weekly over 5 weeks) → boost to 10-16 Gy in 2 Gy/fx (9 Gy in 3 Gy/fx is reasonable if the volume is small).

Considerations:

- Boost patients with non–low-risk DCIS (BIG 3-07/TROG 07.01, *Chua et al. Lancet* 2022)
- Boost doses: 10 Gy for negative SM, 14 Gy for close SM, and 16 Gy for positive SM (reexcision preferred but if not possible [ie, positive SM at fascia] give higher boost dose)
- Consider simultaneous integrated boost for patients receiving HF-WBI and are eligible for a boost: 48 Gy in 15 fx at 3.2 Gy/fx (*Vicini et al. ASTRO* 2022)
- Consider 42.5 Gy in 16 fx if a boost was intended but not feasible (eg, complicated surgical bed)

- **Target:** Clinical breast mound including all glandular breast tissue (Fig. 42.1)
- **WBI technique:** Opposed lateral tangents and appositional electron field for boost
    - For APBI, see **ESBC** chapter.

Initial WBI Field Treatment Borders Finalize Using RTOG Consensus Guidelines and CT/Volume-Based Contouring	
Superior	Typically, 2 cm below humeral head if not using high tangents
Inferior	2 cm below inframammary fold
Anterior	Flash ipsilateral breast
Posterior	≤2 cm of ipsilateral lung

Medial	Sternum (avoid treating contralateral breast)
Lateral	Midaxilla (cover entire ipsilateral breast)
Cone-Down Tumor Bed Boost	
2-cm expansion around tumor bed to block edge if using an appositional electron field. Resimulate during treatment with breast compression device if needed to flatten tumor bed and improve setup reproducibility	

- **IGRT:** Weekly MV imaging once setup is stable
- Planning directive for WBI:
  - Breast: V98 ≥ 100%, V100 > 90%
  - Entire breast/CW covered by 98% isodose line (IDL)
  - Entire tumor bed covered by 100% IDL
  - Boost target covered by 90% IDL
  - Heart: V5 ≤ 40% (≤50% for left-sided tumors)
  - *Expected mean heart dose for left intact breast with no IMC < 1 Gy*
  - Total lung: V20 < 35%, V40 < 20%
  - Evaluate each beam separately for adequate coverage.
  - Avoid 106% hot spots, consider using wedges or field-in-fields.

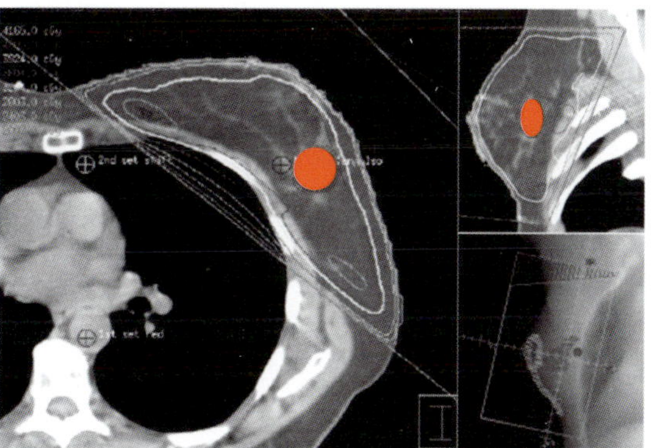

Figure 42.1 CT-based XRT planning images and DRR of the left lateral tangent beam. Contours: *Maroon*, tumor bed. Isodose lines on CT images: *White*, 98% IDL.

Systemic Therapy

- Chemotherapy not part of management for DCIS
- Consider endocrine therapy for 5 years for estrogen receptor (ER)-positive DCIS.
  - **Tamoxifen** 20 mg PO daily for premenopausal women
  - **Aromatase inhibitors (anastrozole, letrozole)** for pre- or postmenopausal women

    *Give ovarian suppression or ablation for premenopausal women receiving aromatase inhibitors.

Surgical Definitions and Pathology Information

- **Breast-conserving surgery (BCS) or lumpectomy:** Removal of tumor and surrounding area of breast tissue to ensure negative margins
- **Total or skin-sparing mastectomy:** Complete removal of the breast ± overlying skin
- **Sentinel lymph node biopsy (SLNB):** Not indicated in DCIS. May be offered if high risk for occult invasive disease and if mastectomy is planned. Blue dye and/or radioactive tracer is injected into the ipsilateral breast to help locate typically 1-3 sentinel nodes for removal.

- **Pathology report:** Review ER/PR status, tumor grade, tumor size, extent (multifocal?), surgical margin status (either positive, close [0-1.9 mm], or negative [≥2 mm]).

Side Effect Management

- **Skin care:** Aquaphor → Cool Magic → Mepilex dressings → Silvadene

Follow-up

- History and physical: Every 6-12 months ×5 years, then annually
- Bilateral diagnostic mammogram: Every year

Notable Trials

*For APBI and HF-WBI trials, see **ESBC** chapter.

WBI after lumpectomy results in ~50% reduction in ipsilateral breast recurrence

Name/Inclusion	Arms	Outcomes	Notes
NSABP B17/B24 (*Wapnir et al. JNCI* 2011) 2612 patients with DCIS or invasive Randomization shown is from B17 trial	BCS BCS + WBI (50 Gy in 25 fx)	15-y IBTR 19% vs 9% (HR 0.48, *P* < .001) No difference in OS or CSS	9% of patients received boost as part of WBI Conclusion: Ipsilateral breast tumor recurrence reduced with BCS + WBI
EORTC 10853 (*Donker et al. JCO* 2013) 1010 women with DCIS only	BCS BCS + WBI (50 Gy in 25 fx)	15-y IBTR 30% vs 17% (HR 0.52, *P* < .001) No difference in OS or CSS	5% of patients received boost Conclusion: Ipsilateral breast tumor recurrence reduced with BCS + WBI
SweDCIS (Warnberg et al. *JCO* 2014) 1046 women with DCIS only	BCS BCS + WBI (48-50 Gy in 24-25 fx)	20-y IBTR 32% vs 20% (*P* < .001) No difference in OS or CSS	Boost not recommended Conclusion: Ipsilateral breast tumor recurrence reduced with BCS + WBI
EBCTCG DCIS meta-analysis (*Correa et al. JNCI* 2010) 3729 women with DCIS only Meta-analysis of four randomized trials	BCS BCS + WBI	10-y IBTR 28% vs 13% (*P* < .001)* *Regardless of patient age, extent of BCS, use of TAM, margin status, tumor grade, or size	Proportional reduction in IBTR greater in older vs younger women (≥50 vs <50) Conclusion: RT after BCS decreases any IBTR by ~50%

Tamoxifen after lumpectomy further reduces breast recurrence

Name/Inclusion	Arms	Outcomes	Notes
UK/ANZ (*Cuzick et al. Lancet Oncol* 2011) 1701 women with DCIS only	2 × 2 comparing BCS ± WBI ± tamoxifen (TAM) (20 mg po daily ×5 y)	10-y IBTR ± WBI 19% vs 7% (HR 0.32, *P* < .001) 10-y IBTR ± TAM 20% vs 16% (HR 0.68, *P* = .04)	Conclusion: Ipsilateral breast tumor recurrence reduced with both WBI and TAM

Name/Inclusion	Arms	Outcomes	Notes
NSABP B17/B24 (*Wapnir et al. JNCI* 2011) 2612 patients with DCIS or invasive Randomization shown is from B24 trial	BCS + WBI (50 Gy in 25 fx) BCS + WBI + TAM	15-y contralateral breast tumor occurrence 11% vs 7% (HR 0.68, $P = .023$) No difference in OS or CSS	9% of patients received boost Conclusion: Contralateral breast tumor occurrence reduced with TAM

Omission of RT after BCS for low-risk DCIS

Name/Inclusion	Arms	Outcomes	Notes
ECOG 5194 (*Solin et al. JCO* 2015) 665 patients with "low-risk" DCIS: grades 1-2, ≤2.5 cm **OR** grade 3, ≤1 cm *All had normal postoperative MMG and margins ≥3 mm	BCS BCS + WBI	12-y IBTR in grades 1-2 patients: 14% (8% invasive) 12-y IBTR in grade 3 patients: 25% (13% invasive)	31% of patients received TAM Conclusion: High-grade patients had unacceptable IBTR, thus high-grade DCIS is a poor prognostic factor for RT omission
RTOG 9804 (*McCormick et al. JCO* 2015) 636 patients with "low-risk" DCIS: grades 1-2, ≤2.5 cm, margins ≥3 mm	BCS BCS + WBI	7-y IBTR 0.9% vs 6.7% (HR 0.11, $P < .001$) Grades 1-2 toxicities: 30% vs 76%	TAM 20 mg po daily given in both arms (69% compliance) Conclusion: Ipsilateral breast tumor recurrence reduced with BCS + WBI, but acceptable risk
RTOG 9804 15-year update (*McCormick et al. JCO* 2021) 636 patients with "low-risk" DCIS: grades 1-2, ≤2.5 cm, margins ≥3 mm	BCS BCS + WBI	15-y risk of local failure ~1%/y vs ~0.5%/y Excellent OS and DFS in both groups	Conclusion: Ipsilateral breast tumor recurrence reduced with BCS + WBI, but acceptable risk

Hypofractionated whole breast radiation is safe for DCIS

Name/Inclusion	Arms	Outcomes	Notes
MDACC RCT (*Shaitelman et al. JAMA Oncol* 2015) 287 women ≥40 yo with stages 0-II BrCa (22% DCIS) who received BCS	CF-WBI (50 Gy/25 fx + boost) HF-WBI (42.56 Gy/16 fx + boost)	Acute grade 2 toxicity 78% vs 47% ($P < .001$) Better QOL and less fatigue with HF-WBI vs CF-WBI	Conclusion: Less acute toxicities and improved QOL in patients who received HF-WBI

Boost for non–low-risk DCIS

Name/Inclusion	Arms	Outcomes	Notes
BIG 3-07/TROG 07.01 (*Chua et al. Lancet* 2022) 1608 women with "non–low-risk" DCIS (at least one of the following): <50 y old, symptomatic, palpable tumor, tumor ≥1.5 cm, multifocal, grades 2-3, central necrosis, comedo histology, or radial margin <1 cm	WBI without boost WBI + boost (16 Gy/8 fx)	5-y LC 93% vs 97% ($P < .001$) Acute grade 2+ breast pain 10% vs 14% ($P < .01$) and induration 6% vs 14% ($P < .001$)	48% received HF-WBI (42.56 Gy/16 fx) and 52% received CF-WBI (50 Gy/25 fx) Conclusion: Local control improved with worse acute toxicities in patients who received WBI + boost

EARLY-STAGE BREAST CANCER (ESBC)

KELSEY CORRIGAN • WENDY WOODWARD

Background

- **Definition:** Stage I/II patients (T1/2 N0/1mic/1); T3N0 (stage IIB) is included in **LABC** chapter.
- **Incidence/prevalence:** Most commonly diagnosed cancer among women and second leading cause of death in the United States. Approximately 250 000 new cases of invasive breast cancer (BrCa) annually and 40 000 deaths annually. Lifetime risk is 1 in 8 (12%).
- **Outcomes:** 5-Year survival ~90%
- **Risk factors:** See **General Breast Cancer** chapter.
- **Screening guidelines:** See **General Breast Cancer** chapter.

Tumor Biology and Characteristics

- **Pathology:** Majority invasive ductal carcinoma (~90%). Remaining 10% is invasive lobular carcinoma, which is bilateral in up to 30% of cases. Pathologic evaluation for tumor grade, size, extent (multifocal?), and surgical margin (SM) status (either positive, close [0-1.9 mm], or negative [≥2 mm]). IHC testing for ER (≥1% threshold), PR, Her2 (IHC: 3+ on ≥10% breast tissue threshold, if Her2+ utilize FISH testing and test if ratio > 2.0), and Ki-67
- **Molecular subtypes (incidence and receptor-based surrogates):**
  - Luminal A–like (70%): grades 1-2, high ER+/PR+, Her2−, low Ki-67
  - Luminal B–like (10%): grade 3, low ER+/PR+, +/−Her2+, high Ki-67
  - Her2-like (10%): grade 3, ER/PR−/+, Her2+, high Ki-67
  - Basal-like (10%): grade 3, triple negative (TNBC), BRCA1 associated

Note: gene expression and receptor subtypes are not perfectly correlated.

- **Multigene panels and signature scores:** Routinely utilize recurrence scores including Oncotype DX DCIS recurrence score. Retrospective analyses of the NSABP data suggest that recurrence score is prognostic for LRR in node-negative and node-positive ER+ patients (*Paik et al. NEJM* 2004).
- **Imaging:** *MMG*: linear or granular microcalcifications, masses, skin thickening, nipple retraction, or distortions. *Ultrasound*: hypoechoic mass with irregular margins and ductal extension ± infiltration of surrounding tissue. *MRI*: regional branching, mass, or linear enhancement on T1
- **Anatomy:** See **General Breast Cancer** chapter.

Workup

- **History and physical:** Including bilateral breast examination and axilla palpation. Consider genetics evaluation.
- **Labs:** β-HCG (if premenopausal), CBC, LFTs
- **Procedures/biopsy:** Core needle biopsy of suspicious breast lesions, pathologic staining of biopsy for ER/PR status, and Her2 expression. Consider obtaining Oncotype DX score if indicated.
- **Imaging:** Bilateral diagnostic MMG, breast, and regional LN basin ultrasound. Consider MRI for dense breasts, suspected multicentric/multifocal disease, occult primary, or chest wall invasion. If abnormal LFTs, or symptoms, bone scan and/or CT of the chest, abdomen, and pelvis

Treatment Algorithms

- **Overall treatment:** Both adjuvant and neoadjuvant chemotherapy are equally valid, consider neoadjuvant for cN+ or if patient desires BCS but cannot due to size of primary disease. Institutional preference is for neoadjuvant approach.
- **Adjuvant systemic therapy approach:** Mastectomy/BCS + SLNB ± ALND → systemic therapy (if any) → RT → completion hormone/HER2-targeted systemic therapy (if any)
- **Neoadjuvant systemic therapy approach:** Systemic therapy (if any) → mastectomy/BCS + SLNB ± ALN procedure (TAD or ALND) → RT → completion hormone/HER2-targeted systemic therapy (if any)

	Surgery	LN Status	Radiation
No neoadjuvant systemic	**BCS + SLNB/ALND**	pN0/(i+)[a]	• No radiation
		pN0/(i+)/mic	• APBI • WBI • WBI + RNI[c]
		1-2 LN+	• WBI[b] • WBI + RNI[c]
		≥3 LN+	• WBI + RNI
	Mastectomy + SLNB/ALND	0-2 LNs	• No radiation • PMRT[c]
		≥3 LN+	• PMRT
Neoadjuvant systemic	**BCS + SLNB/ALND**	ypN0	• WBI • WBI + RNI[d,e]
	Mastectomy + SLNB/ALND	yp ≥1 LN+	• WBI + RNI
		ypN0	• No radiation • PMRT[d,e]
		yp ≥1 LN+	• PMRT

[a]Consider radiation omission (CALGB9343): age ≥70, tumor size ≤3 cm, N0, margin >2 mm, ER+, and willing to undergo hormone therapy.

[b]Patients with LN+ SLNB and no ALND w/ significant risk factors (http://www3.mdanderson.org/app/medcalc/bc_nomogram2), consider modifying tangents to include level 1 and 2 LNs (high tangents).

[c]Consider WBI + RNI/PMRT in patients meeting the following criteria:

- pN1 and ≥**1** of the following: Age ≤40 and upfront surgery, ≥3 LN+ and upfront surgery, cT3N1, ER− and upfront surgery, age <50 and Oncotype DX RS >18, ER− and upfront surgery, and ypN+
- p1-2 LN+, age >40, ER+ and ≥**2** of the following: Luminal B (Ki-67 >20% or Her 2+), grade 3, LVSI, Oncotype DX RS > 18
- pN0/pN0(i+)/mic and ≥**3** of the following: Age ≤40, >1 LN with micromet (0.21-2 mm), T3, central/medial tumor, ER−, grade 3, LVSI, Ki-67 >20% Oncotype DX RS > 18

[d]Consider WBI + RNI/PMRT in patients with ≥cT3N1 or <cT3N1 and ≥1 of the following: premenopausal, TNBC, greater initial clinical tumor burden, residual tumor in the breast.

[e]Consider omission of RNI/PMRT in patients who are ypT0N0 as part of a clinical trial.

Radiation options

- **Whole breast irradiation (WBI):** See **DCIS** chapter. In a patient with cN0 but involvement of 1-2 LNs identified on SLNB and who did not have an ALND, consider contouring level I-II LNs and modifying WBI tangents to encompass (high tangents).
- **WBI + regional nodal irradiation (RNI):** See **LABC** chapter.
- **Postmastectomy radiation therapy (PMRT):** Chest wall radiation and RNI, see **LABC** chapter.

- Accelerated partial breast irradiation (APBI): If patient meets eligibility criteria:

APBI Suitability Criteria (N0(i+/i−) Tumors Only)

	Age	Margins	T Stage	DCIS
Suitable (if all criteria match)	≥50	≥2 mm	Tis or T1	• Screen-detected • Low to intermediate grade • ≤2.5 cm • Margin ≥3 mm
Cautionary	• 40-49 if all other criteria for "suitable" are met • ≥50 if ≥1 unsuitable pathology factors exist* and otherwise all other criteria for "suitable" are met	<2 mm		≤3 cm and does not meet criteria for "suitable"
Unsuitable* (if any criteria match)	• <40 • 40-49 and do not meet criteria for cautionary	Positive		>3 cm

*Unsuitable pathology factors: Size 2.1-3 cm, T2, margins <2 mm, limited/focal LVSI, ER−, clinically unifocal with size 2.1-3 cm, invasive lobular histology, pure DCIS ≤ 3 cm if criteria for "suitable" not fully met, extensive invasive component ≤3 cm

ASTRO Consensus Guidelines, Adapted from *Correa et al. Pract Radiat Oncol* 2017.

Radiation Treatment Technique

For WBI, see **DCIS** chapter. For chest wall + RNI, see **LABC** chapter.

Radiation Treatment Technique for APBI

- Dose:
  - 10-year data options: 40 Gy in 15 fx, 30 Gy in 5 fx QOD
  - 5-year data options: 26 Gy in 5 fx QD, 38.5 Gy in 10 fx bid (Fig. 43.1, uncommonly used)
- Target:
  - CTV: Surgical cavity + 15-20 mm; but limited to 5 mm from skin and excludes chest wall/pectoralis muscles

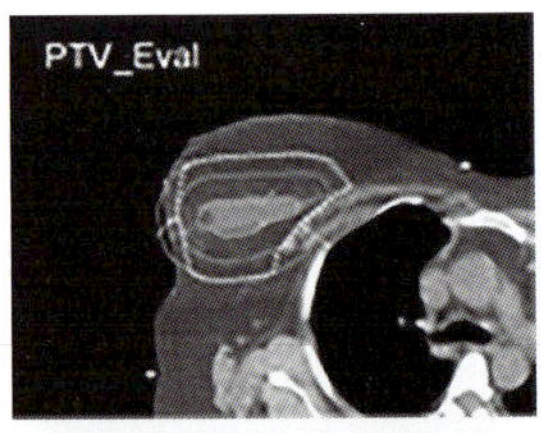

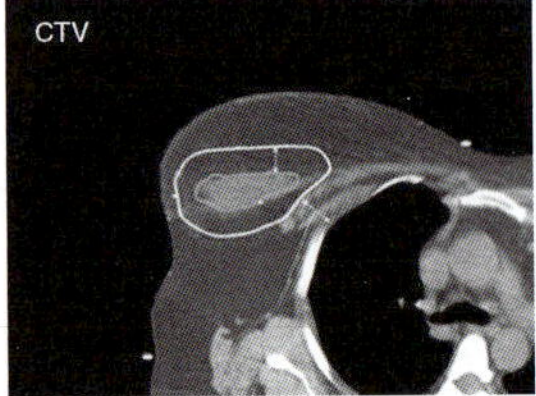

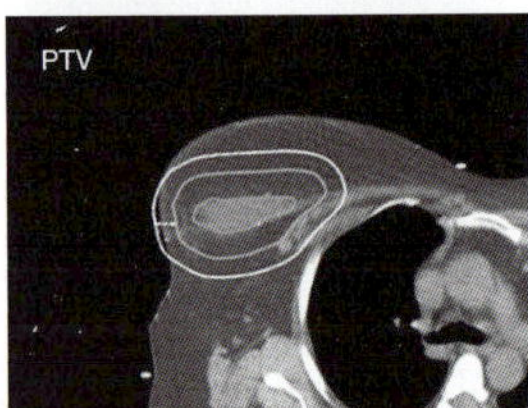

Figure 43.1 External beam APBI volumes. (From NSABP B-39.)

- PTV: CTV + 5-8 mm (5 mm if tumor bed clips are visible on kV x-rays or using CBCT for daily IGRT)
- PTV_Eval: PTV but limited to 5 mm from skin and excludes chest wall/pectoralis muscles

- **Technique:** 3DCRT (multiple noncoplanar beams) or VMAT
  - **VMAT:** Contour and dose constraints according to dosing protocol chosen
- **SIM:** Supine, upper Vac-Lok device, ipsilateral arm abducted/externally rotated over the head, head turned slightly away (open neck). Use 5- to 15-degree slant board if breast intact or to minimize SCV lung dose. Wire surgical scar. Deep inspiration breath-hold for left-sided tumors to reduce heart/lung doses

Planning Directive for APBI

Planning directives are different based on dose regimen and fractionation scheme. We recommend using the dose constraints published in the clinical trial supporting the dose regimen that is chosen.

IGRT (EBRT APBI)

- kV every treatment, align to clips and soft tissue; weekly CBCT for VMAT

Side Effect Management/Follow-up

- **Skin care:** Aquaphor → topical steroids → Cool Magic/Mepilex dressings → Silvadene
- **Fatigue:** Encourage exercise and adequate daily protein intake, good sleep hygiene → referral to fatigue clinic
- **Lymphedema:** Referral to physical therapy for education and sleeve fitting → plastic surgery options include LN transfer and lymphatic bypass

Systemic Therapy

See **LABC** chapter.

Surgical Definitions

- **Breast-conserving surgery (BCS) or lumpectomy:** Removal of tumor and surrounding area of breast tissue to ensure negative margins
- **Total or skin-sparing mastectomy:** Complete removal of the breast ± overlying skin
- **Sentinel lymph node biopsy (SLNB):** Conducted in all cN0 patients. Blue dye and/or radioactive tracer injected into the ipsilateral breast to locate one to three sentinel nodes for removal
- **Targeted axillary dissection (TAD):** Removes SLNs and a biopsy-proven involved clipped LN. Consider for patients with cN+ disease who receive NAC for improved axillary staging to help with the decision for ALND.
- **Axillary lymph node dissection (ALND):** Omitted for cN0 and SLNB+ if T1-2 and 1-2 positive LNs when doing lumpectomy and no neoadjuvant therapy (*Guiliano et al. JAMA* 2011).

Notable Trials

Radiation after BCS improves local control and breast cancer deaths

Name/Inclusion	Arms	Outcomes	Notes
EBCTCG meta-analysis (*Lancet* 2011) Patients from 86 randomized trials	BCS BCS + WBI	10-y tumor recurrence 35% vs 19% ($P < .001$) 15-y risk of BrCa death 25% to 21% ($P < .001$)	Conclusion: RT after BCS improves recurrence rates and cancer-specific mortality

Lumpectomy boost after whole breast radiation:

Name/Inclusion	Arms	Outcomes	Notes
EORTC Boost Trial (*Bartelink et al. Lancet Oncol* 2015)$ 5318 patients with DCIS or invasive	BCS + WBI (50 Gy in 25 fx) BCS + WBI + boost (16 Gy in 8 fx)	17-y IBTR 16% vs 12% ($P < .001$) No difference in OS or DMFS	Conclusion: Addition of boost with WBI improves local control

Omission of RT after BCS is acceptable in low-risk breast cancer patients

Name/Inclusion	Arms	Outcomes	Notes
CALGB 9343 (*Hughes et al. JCO* 2013) 636 women with low-risk ESBC (age ≥70 y, T1 N0, ER+)	BCS BCS + WBI (45 Gy/25 fx + 14 Gy boost) → tamoxifen (TAM) ≥5 y	10-y LRFS 98% vs 90% ($P < .001$)	Conclusion: WBI reduces recurrence risk, but LRF risk still acceptable with observation
PRIME II (*Kunkler et al. Lancet Oncol* 2015) 636 women with low-risk ESBC (age ≥65 y, HR+, T1/2 N0, grade 3 or LVSI, margins ≥1 mm)	BCS BCS + WBI (40-50 Gy in 15-25 fx) → hormone ≥5 y	5-y IBTR 4% vs 1% ($P < .001$) No difference in OS	Conclusion: WBI reduces recurrence risk, but risk still acceptable with observation in some patients
PRIME II 10-y update (*Kunkler et al. NEJM* 2023) 658 women with low-risk ESBC as above	BCS BCS + WBI (40-50 Gy in 15-25 fx) → hormone ≥5 y	LF 10% vs 1% ($P < .001$) No difference in OS Low-ER+ had greater LF: 19% vs 0% ($P < .001$)	Conclusion: WBI reduces recurrence risk, especially in low-ER+ ESBC patients

Hypofractionation has equivalent efficacy and at least as good cosmesis as conventional fractionated radiation

Name/Inclusion	Arms	Outcomes	Notes
Canada (*Whelan et al. NEJM* 2010) 1234 women with T1/2 N0, margin-negative	CF-WBI (50 Gy in 25 fx) HF-WBI (42.56 Gy in 16 fx)	10-y LR 7% vs 6% (NS) No difference in OS or DFS Excellent/good cosmesis in 70% vs 71% (NS)	No boost allowed Conclusion: HF-WBI is noninferior to CF-WBI
UK Start (START A + START B) (*Haviland et al. Lancet Oncol* 2013) 2236 women (START A) and 2215 women (START B) with pT1-3a N0-1, margin-negative	CF-WBI (50 Gy in 25 fx) HF-WBI (multiple regimens: 40 Gy in 15 fx, 41.6 Gy in 13 fx, and 39 Gy in 13 fx)	10-y LR 4-6% vs 5-7% (NS) No difference in OS or DFS Better long-term cosmesis in 40 Gy vs 50 Gy arm (START B)	61% of patients received 10 Gy boost Conclusion: HF-WBI is safe and effective with better cosmesis
MDACC (*Shaitelman et al. JAMA Oncol* 2015; *Weng et al. IJORBP* 2021) 287 women with Tis-2 N0-1a	CF-WBI (50 Gy in 25 fx + 10-14 Gy/5-7 in fx boost) HF-WBI (42.56 Gy in 16 fx + 10-12.5 Gy in 4-5 fx boost)	Less toxicity in HF-WBI: dermatitis, 36% vs 69%; pruritus, 54% vs 81%; pain, 55% vs 74%; hyperpigmentation, 9% vs 20%; fatigue, 9% vs 17%	Conclusion: Lower toxicity rates with HF-WBI

Simultaneous integrated boost with HF-WBI has equivalent efficacy and cosmesis as sequential boost with HF- or CF-WBI

Name/Inclusion	Arms	Outcomes	Notes
RTOG 1005 (*Vicini et al. ASTRO* 2022) 2262 women with high-risk ESBC (Tis + high-grade + age <50 **OR** stage I/II + high-risk factor [cN1, LVSI+, close/ positive SM, ER/ PR-negative, high-grade, Oncotype ≥26, age <50])	HF- or CF-WBI with sequential boost (42.7 Gy/16 fx or 50 Gy/25 fx + 12-14 Gy/6-7 fx)	7-y LR 2.6% vs 2.2% (NS) Grade 3+ AEs in 3.5% vs 3.3% (NS) No difference in physician- or patient-reported cosmesis	Conclusion: HF-WBI with concurrent boost is equivalent to HF- or CF-WBI with sequential boost
	HF-WBI with concurrent boost (48 Gy/15 fx at 3.2 Gy/fx)		

Ultra-hypofractionation has equivalent efficacy and at least as good cosmesis as hypofractionated and conventional fractionated radiation

Name/Inclusion	Arms	Outcomes	Notes
UK Fast (*Brunt et al. JCO* 2020) 915 women with T1/2 N0, margin-negative	CF-WBI (50 Gy in 25 fx)	10-y LR 1.3% vs 1% (NS) No difference in OS or DFS Similar normal tissue effects (NTEs) in 28.5 Gy vs 50 Gy (OR 1.22, $P = .25$) but worse NTEs in 30 Gy vs 50 Gy (OR 2.12, $P < .001$)	No boost allowed Conclusion: Ultra-HF-WBI using 28.5 Gy is equivalent to CF-WBI
	Ultra-HF-WBI (28.5-30 Gy in 5 fx once weekly)		
UK Fast Forward (*Brunt et al. Lancet Oncol* 2020) 4096 patients with T1-3 N0, margin-negative	HF-WBI (40 Gy in 5 fx)	5-y LR 2.1% vs 1.8% (27 Gy) vs 1.4 % (26 Gy) (NS) No difference in OS or DFS Similar NTEs in 26 Gy vs 40 Gy (OR 1.12, $P = .20$) but worse NTEs in 27 Gy vs 40 Gy (OR 1.55, $P < .0001$)	No boost allowed Conclusion: Ultra-HF-WBI using 26 Gy is noninferior to HF-WBI
	Ultra-HF-WBI (26 Gy in 5 fx or 27 Gy in 5 fx given daily)		

Partial breast irradiation is associated with good efficacy and cosmesis

Name/Inclusion	Arms	Outcomes	Notes
GEC-ESTRO (*Strnad et al. Lancet* 2016) 1184 patients T1/2 (≤3 cm) N0, margin-negative	CF-WBI (50-50.4 Gy in 25-28 fx + 10 Gy in 5 fx boost)	5-y IBTR 1.4% vs 0.9% (NS)	Conclusion: APBI using brachytherapy is noninferior to CF-WBI
	Interstitial brachytherapy (32 Gy in 8 fx or 30.3 Gy in 7 fs bid)		
RAPID (*Olivotto et al. JCO* 2013) 2315 women with T1/2 (≤3 cm) N0	WBI (50 Gy in 25 fx or 42.56 Gy in 16 fx)	Increased fibrosis and worse cosmesis in APBI arm at 3 y	10 Gy boost allowed for WBI arm Conclusion: Increased toxicity with APBI
	External APBI (38.5 Gy in 10 fx bid)		

Name/Inclusion	Arms	Outcomes	Notes
IMPORT LOW (*Coles et al. Lancet* 2017) 2016 women with pT1-2 (≤3 cm) N0-1, margin ≥ 2 mm disease	WBI (40 Gy in 15 fx) PBI (40 Gy in 15 fx) Reduced dose WBI (36 Gy in 15 fx with 40 Gy to partial breast)	5-y LR: 1.1% (WBI) 0.5% (PBI) vs 0.2% (reduced dose) (NS) Similar to improved cosmesis with PBI and reduced dose	Conclusion: PBI and reduced dose WBI are noninferior to WBI
FLORENCE (*Meattini et al. JCO* 2020) 520 patients >40 yo with ESBC and primary tumor size ≤2.5 cm	CF-WBI (50 Gy in 25 fx + 10 Gy in 5 fx boost) APBI (30 Gy in 5 fx QOD using IMRT technique)	10-y IBTR 2.5% (WBI) vs 3.7% (APBI) (NS) No difference in BCSS and OS Improved toxicity and cosmesis in APBI ($P < .001$)	Conclusion: Equivalent survival outcomes and better toxicity/ cosmesis in APBI vs CF-WBI

Axillary LN dissection can be omitted in select patients with positive SLNB

Name/Inclusion	Arms	Outcomes	Notes
ACOSOG Z11 (*Guiliano et al. JAMA* 2017) 856 women with T1/2, cN0, 1 or 2 SLN+	BCS with SLNB (→ +/− WBI) BCS with SLNB + ALND (→ +/− WBI)	10-y OS 86% vs 85% (NS) 10-y DFS 80% vs 78% (NS) 46% of SLN+ were micromets 27% of patients treated with ALND had additional positive nodes beyond SLN+	Post hoc analysis (*Jagsi et al. JCO* 2014): 50% of patients received high tangents and 20% had separate regional nodal fields Conclusion: SLNB noninferior to SLNB + ALND; consider adj WBI with high tangents
TAD (*Caudle et al. JCO* 2016) 191 patients with cN+ who received neoadjuvant therapy → BCS or mastectomy	Surgery with SLND +/− targeted axillary dissection (TAD) +/− ALND	False-negative rate (FNR) with SLND alone: 10.1% FNR with TAD alone: 4.2% FNR with SLND+TAD: 2%	Conclusion: TAD improves evaluation of residual nodal mets after neoadjuvant chemotherapy

Regional nodal irradiation (RNI) associated with similar axillary control compared with LN dissection in low-risk patients

Name/Inclusion	Arms	Outcomes	Notes
AMAROS (*Donker et al. Lancet Oncol* 2014) 4806 patients with T1/2	BCS → SLND. If SLN+ → axillary RT BCS → SLND. If SLN+ → ALND	5-y axillary recurrence 1.2% vs 0.4% (NS) 5-y OS 94% vs 94% (NS) 5-y DFS 87% vs 83% (NS)	Conclusion: ALND and axillary RT have noninferior survival outcomes. Less morbidity with axillary RT

Regional nodal irradiation (RNI) associated with improved efficacy in high-risk patients

Name/Inclusion	Arms	Outcomes	Notes
NCIC MA.20 (*Whelan et al. NEJM* 2015) 1832 patients with high-risk (T3 **OR** tumor size >2 cm and <10 ALNs removed and either grade 3, ER−, or LVIS) pN0 or pN1-3 s/p BCS + adjuvant chemo	WBI WBI + RNI	10-y DFS 77% vs 82% (*P* = .01) No difference in OS Increased acute grade 2+ pneumonitis (1.2% vs 0.2%, *P* = .01) and lymphedema (8.4% vs 4.5%, *P* = .001) in RNI group	RNI included IMC, SCV, and axillary coverage Conclusion: RNI reduced rates of breast cancer recurrence in N+ or high-risk N0 patients

Inclusion of IM nodes in comprehensive RT fields may improve efficacy

Name/Inclusion	Arms	Outcomes	Notes
EORTC 22922/10925 (*Poortmans et al. NEJM* 2015) 4004 patients with axillary N+ (~55%) or medial tumors s/p BCS or MRM	Adjuvant PMRT to CW alone Adjuvant PMRT + IMC/medial SCV RT (RNI)	10-y DFS 69% vs 72% (*P* = .04) 10-y DMFS 75% vs 78% (*P* = .02) Trend toward higher 10-y OS 80.7% vs 82.3% (*P* = .056) No increased toxicities in RNI	Conclusion: Addition of RNI (IMC and SCV) to PMRT improved outcomes without increase in toxicity
KROG 08-06 (*Kim et al. JAMA Onc* 2022) 735 patients with pN+ s/p BCS or mastectomy with ALND followed by adjuvant breast/CW RT	RNI without internal mammary node irradiation (IMNI) RNI + IMNI	7-y DFS 85% vs 82% (NS) in all patients In patients with medial/central tumors who received IMNI: DFS 92% vs 82% (*P* < .01) BCSM 5% vs 10% (*P* = .04) No difference in toxicities	Conclusion: Patients with medial/central tumors may benefit from including IMNI in RNI

LOCALLY ADVANCED BREAST CANCER (LABC)

KELSEY CORRIGAN • WENDY WOODWARD

BACKGROUND

- **Definition:** ≥T3 or ≥N1 (stage IIB/III) patients. IBC patients are a subset of LABC (see separate **Inflammatory/Recurrent Breast Cancer** chapter). Stage IV patients are not included.
- **Incidence/prevalence:** 8-15% of all detected breast cancers in the United States, with decreased rates in regions of increased screening. Impoverished or minority communities can experience higher rates of LABC and increased mortality.
- **Outcomes:** 5-year survival rates for stage IIIA and IIIB breast cancers are 52% and 48%, with median survival for stage III at 4.9 years (SEER data).
- **Risk factors:** See **General Breast Cancer** chapter.

Tumor Biology and Characteristics

- **Pathology:** See **ESBC** chapter. Predominant histologies include infiltrating ductal and lobular carcinoma. More favorable histologies, such as tubular or medullary carcinoma, are less common in LABC.
- **Genetics and molecular subtypes:** See **ESBC** and **General Breast Cancer** chapters.

Anatomy/Workup/Staging/Treatment Algorithm

See **ESBC** and **DCIS** chapters.

Radiation Treatment Technique for Comprehensive Breast/Chest Wall Irradiation

- **SIM:** Supine, upper Vac-Lok device, ipsilateral arm abducted/externally rotated over the head, head turned slightly away (open neck). Use 5- to 15-degree slant board if breast intact or to minimize SCV lung dose. Wire surgical scar and treatment borders (optional). Deep inspiration breath-hold for left-sided tumors to reduce heart/lung doses. Aquaplast masks are appropriate for patients who need supraclavicular nodal boosts or who will be treated with IMRT/VMAT or proton therapy.
- **Dose:** 50 Gy in 25 fractions → boost to 10-16 Gy in 2 Gy/fx; 40.05 Gy in 15 fx + boost may be increasingly considered as additional data showing equivalence report out.
- **Target:** Entire breast/chest wall and regional nodes (SCV, IMC, undissected cN+; Figs. 44.1 and 44.2)

Comprehensive Breast/CW Treatment Borders for Locally Advanced Breast Cancer: Multi-isocenter Technique *(example fields may be found at the back of the book insert)*

A general starting point for 3D treatment fields/borders is detailed below. This technique must also include volume-based planning with contouring of target nodal CTVs (regional nodal volumes including undissected axillary levels, supraclavicular nodes, internal mammary nodes).

- Utilize upfront and cross-sectional imaging for CTV delineation.
- **Field borders are then modified accordingly to encompass these CTVs.**
- When using IMRT/VMAT or proton therapy, the breast/CW and nodal regions should be contoured as CTV. The CTV should be expanded by a 0.5-cm margin to generate the PTV (exclude 3 mm from skin and 3 mm at the lung interface).
- Please see the RTOG and ESTRO Breast Cancer Atlas for contouring guidelines for most cases (https://www.rtog.org/LinkClick.aspx?fileticket=vzJFhPaBipE=>). Consider the radcomp atlas for T4d and N3a or c disease.

Tangents	***Medial and lateral photon tangents***
Superior	Nondivergent field border ~2 cm below humeral head (sagittal) and just below clavicular head (coronal) if not using high tangents
Inferior	2 cm below inframammary fold
Anterior	Flash ipsilateral breast/CW
Posterior	≤2 cm of ipsilateral lung, include pectoralis muscles, chest wall muscles, and ribs
Medial	Sternum (avoid treating contralateral breast, allow IMC field width of at least 4 cm)
Lateral	Midaxilla (cover entire ipsilateral breast/CW)
IMC and medial CW:	***Typically a 15- to 25-degree angled electron field with a mid IMC isocenter. May use upper and lower IMC fields with different electron energies to reduce heart dose***
Superior	Matched to nondivergent superior border of tangent fields
Inferior	Matched on skin rendering to inferior border of medial tangent
Medial	Allow for at least 2 cm on IMC and CW scar, width of at least 4 cm
Lateral	
Posterior	Electron energy chosen such that 90% isodose line covers IMC

SCV/ICV:	***Typically a 15- to 20-degree angled photon field with an SCV isocenter and half beam block***
Superior	At cricoid (if ICV LN+, raise to arytenoids; if SCV LN+, raise to mastoid)
Inferior	Matched to nondivergent superior border of tangent fields
Medial	Angled off spinal cord, pedicles of vertebrae
Lateral	To cover lateral edge of pectoralis muscle. Contour the undissected axilla (including level III) to ensure coverage while also blocking humeral head

Boost Volumes: Tumor Bed/CW and Involved Node
BCS boost: At least 2-cm expansion around tumor bed and involved nodes
CW boost: Determined clinically using visual inspection and CT imaging of the surgical bed to determine and cover the surgical laps
Boosts are usually conducted with appositional electron field(s).
Resimulate with breast compression device if needed for boost RT planning.

- **Considerations:** Boost doses: 10 Gy for negative SM; 14 Gy for <2 mm SM; 16 Gy for positive SM (ie, positive SM at fascia; though, reexcision preferred). If gross or residual nodes, consider 16 Gy boost with a 2-cm CTV margin. Use 3-mm bolus postmastectomy (every other day for 2 weeks and then PRN to achieve brisk skin reaction), but avoid for intact breast due to cosmetic concerns.
- **Technique:** Multi-isocenter technique utilizing photon-based tangent fields matched to AP oblique SCV field and appositional electron IMC field. Consider VMAT or proton therapy for patients with extensive disease, implants/expanders, depth of IMC nodes >4 cm, mid-tangent separation >25.5 cm, and re-RT. Consider using the Radcomp atlas for VMAT contouring for advanced disease. Dose constraints are modified as clinically indicated per the MDACC IBC Algorithm on page 10: https://www.mdanderson.org/content/dam/mdanderson/documents/for-physicians/algorithms/cancer-treatment/ca-%20treatment-breast-inflammatory-web-algorithm.pdf

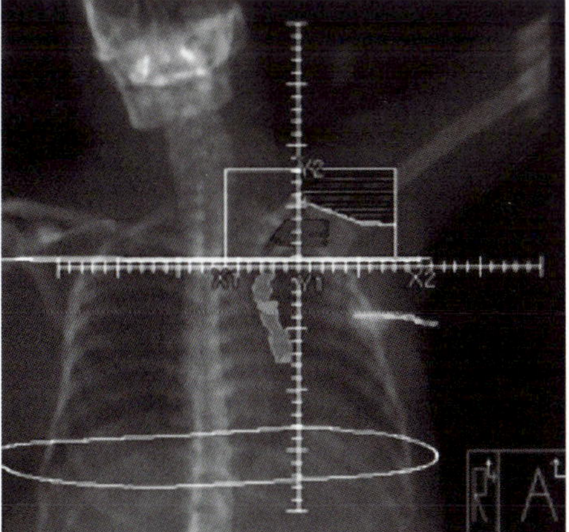

Figure 44.1 Supraclavicular/infraclavicular field design: DRR matched to nondivergent tangent fields. Contours: blue, level III axilla on DRR; green, IM nodes in 1st 3 interspaces; orange, mastectomy scar. Lines: yellow, superior and inferior borders of tangent fields. Blocks: purple, humeral head block. **See color insert.**

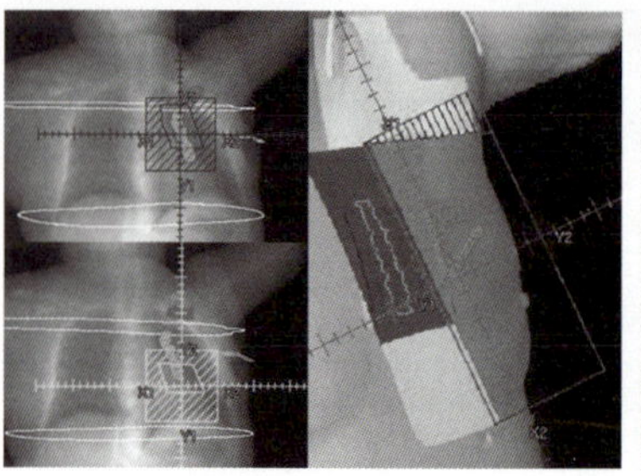

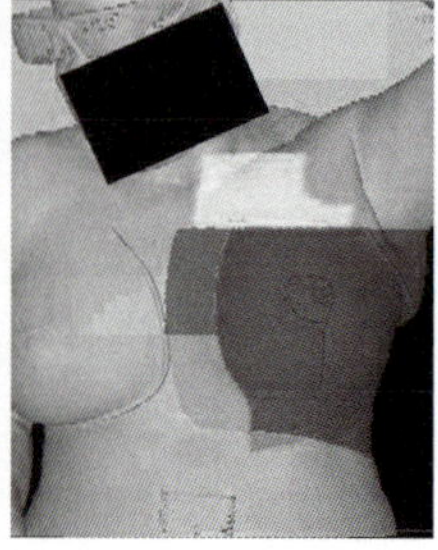

A B

Figure 44.2 **A.** IMC Field Design: DRRs and skin rendering matched to nondivergent tangent fields and SCV field. Contours: Blue, Level III axilla on DRR; Green, IM nodes in 1st 3 interspaces; Orange, Mastectomy scar. Lines: Yellow, Superior and inferior borders of tangent fields. Fields: Yellow, AP oblique SCV field; Purple/Aqua, appositional upper and lower IMC fields; Red, Medial tangent field. **B**. Composite Skin Rendering of Comprehensive Treatment Fields (w/o Boost). Fields: Yellow, AP oblique SCV field; Purple/Orange, appositional upper and lower IMC fields; Red/Aqua, Medial and lateral tangent fields. **See color insert.**

IGRT/Planning Directive

- **IGRT:** Weekly MV for 3D photon therapy once setup is stable. Daily kV with weekly CBCT for IMRT/VMAT or proton therapy.

Planning directive considerations for comprehensive breast/chest wall

- Evaluate each beam separately for adequate coverage.
- Entire breast/CW covered by 98% isodose line (IDL)
- All nodal CTV covered by >90% IDL
- Evaluate cold triangle between IMC and tangents.
- Continuous coverage of 35 Gy line, most notably at IMC and tangent interface
- Boost target covered by 90% IDL

Dose constraints

• Total lung:	D_{mean} < 20 Gy V20 < 35% V40 < 20%
• Heart:	ALARA; D_{mean} < 1-4 Gy, V20 < 4%
• Brachial plexus:	$D_{max} \leq 66$ Gy
• Contralateral breast (VMAT):	$D_{mean} \leq 5$ Gy

Side Effect Management/Follow-up

- Same as **ESBC** chapter

Systemic Therapy

- See **General Breast Cancer** chapter.

Notable Trials

Neoadjuvant chemotherapy improves outcomes in LABC:

Name/Inclusion	Arms	Outcomes	Notes
NSABP B18 (*Fisher et al., JCO*, 1997) 1523 operable patients	Preoperative AC Postoperative AC	Tumor size reduced in 80% (26% pCR) and nodal reduction in 89% (44% pCR) in preoperative AC group 12% more lumpectomies performed in preoperative AC group No difference in OS or DFS, but trend favored preoperative AC in women <50 years old (*P* = .06, *P* = .09)	Conclusion: preoperative AC reduced size of breast and nodal tumor sizes; should be considered for tumors too large for BCS
NSABP B27 (*Rastogi et al., JCO*, 2008) 1567 operable patients	Preoperative AC Preoperative AC + Taxotere Preoperative AC with postoperative Taxotere	Preoperative AC + Taxotere showed increased pCR (26% vs 13%, *P* < .001) No difference in DFS or OS	Conclusion: preoperative chemo is equivalent to postoperative chemo. Addition of taxanes to AC improves response

Improved outcomes with PMRT:

Name/Inclusion	Arms	Outcomes	Notes
Premenopausal Danish Trial (DBCG 82b) (*Overgaard et al., NEJM*, 1997) 1708 premenopausal patients with T3/T4 or axillary N+ s/p MRM + ALND	CMF (chemo) CMF + PMRT (50 Gy/25 fx or 48 Gy/22 fx)	PMRT improved 10-y DFS from 34% to 48%, 10-y OS from 45% to 54%, and LRR 9% vs 32% (all *P* < .001)	PMRT included CW, scar, and regional LN (SCV/ICV/IMC) Conclusion: improved outcomes with PMRT
Postmenopausal Danish Trial (DBCG 82c) (*Overgaard et al., Lancet*, 1999) 1375 postmenopausal women <70 y old with T3/T4 or axillary N+ disease s/p MRM + ALND	Tamoxifen alone Tamoxifen + PMRT (50 Gy/25 fx or 48 Gy/22 fx)	PMRT improved 10-y DFS from 24% to 36% (*P* < .001) and 10-y OS 36% to 45% (*P* = .03)	Conclusion: improved outcomes with PMRT
Danish Trial 30-year update (*Overgaard et al., Radiother Oncol*, 2022)	Systemic therapy alone Systemic therapy + PMRT	RT improved LRR (9% vs 37%), DFS (56% vs 67%), and OS (81% vs 86%), *P* < .0001	Conclusion: improved long-term outcomes with PMRT

Name/Inclusion	Arms	Outcomes	Notes
Early Breast Cancer Trialists' Collaborative Group (EBCTCG meta-analysis) (*Clarke et al., Lancet,* 2005; update *McGale et al., Lancet,* 2014) 78 randomized trials of 42 000 women	Several subgroups analyzed: **N0 s/p BCS:** adj RT reduced 5-y LR (22.9% → 6.7%) and 15-y breast cancer mortality (BCM) (31.2% → 26.1%) **N+ s/p BCS:** adj RT reduced 5-y LR (41.1% → 11%) and 15-y BCM (55% → 47.9%) **N0 s/p MRM:** PMRT reduced 5-y LR (6.3% → 2.3%) but increased 15-y BCM (27.7% → 31.3%) *2014 update: no benefit to PMRT in N0 MRM patients **N+ s/p MRM:** PMRT reduced 5-y LR (22.8% → 5.8%) and 15-y BCM (60.1% → 54.7%) *2014 update: significant reduction in LR and BCM in N+ MRM patients **ER+ vs ER−:** Tamoxifen use for 5 y reduced LR risk by ~50% in ER+ patients		Conclusion: improved outcomes with adjuvant PMRT and tamoxifen

Hypofractionation emerging as an option in LABC:

Name/Inclusion	Arms	Outcomes	Notes
Chinese RCT (*Wang et al., Lancet Onc,* 2019) 820 patients s/p mastectomy with path showing T3/4 or 4 +LNs	HF-WBI (43.5 Gy/15 fx) CF-WBI (50 Gy/25 fx)	5-y LRR 8.3% vs 8.1% (NS) Decreased rates of grade 3 acute skin toxicity in HF-WBI vs CF-WBI (3% vs 8%, $P < .0001$)	Noninferiority study Conclusion: decreased toxicity with no difference in tumor recurrence in HF-WBI
DBCG RCT (*Offersen et al., ESTRO,* 2022) 2879 patients s/p mastectomy or BCS with path showing pN+	HF-WBI (40 Gy/15 fx) CF-WBI (50 Gy/25 fx)	3-y LRR 1.8% vs 1.8% (NS) No difference in rates of lymphedema (11.8% vs 11.6%)	Noninferiority study Conclusion: no difference in toxicity or tumor recurrence in HF-WBI

INFLAMMATORY/RECURRENT BREAST CANCER

KELSEY CORRIGAN • WENDY WOODWARD

Background

- **Definition:** Inflammatory breast cancer (IBC) is primarily a clinical diagnosis requiring (1) rapid onset of breast erythema, edema, and/or peau d'orange with or without a palpable mass or skin thickening, (2) <6-month duration of symptoms, (3) erythema occupying at least 1/3 of the breast, and (4) pathologic confirmation of invasive carcinoma. Note: Erythema not classically "red" in all skin tones, and pathologic evidence of lymphatic involvement not required.
- **Incidence/prevalence:** IBC accounts for 1-4% of all detected breast cancer with ~70% presenting with regional disease and 30% with metastatic disease.
- **Outcomes:** Lower than non-IBC. Best reported outcomes with trimodality treatment. Retrospective series suggest presence of dermal lymphatic invasion, lack of breast-feeding, obesity, and triple-negative subtype are negative prognostic indicators.
- **Risk factors:** Bimodal incidence by age. IBC tends to be diagnosed at younger ages with increased prevalence in African American/Hispanic vs white women and is associated with obesity. Pregnancy is not protective. No difference in BRCA status or family history compared to non-IBC.

Tumor Biology and Characteristics

- **Pathology:** Although all subtypes present, there is higher incidence of ER/PR− and Her2 +/− than non-IBC. Luminal A not associated with clearly favorable prognosis. Commonly, dermal lymphatic invasion or tumor emboli are noted in the involved skin but are not required for diagnosis. Emboli-clogged dermal lymphatics are purported cause of erythema and swelling.
- **Molecular/biologic features:** 90% express RhoC (*van Golen et al. Cancer Res* 2000). All E-cadherin positive. IBC tumors can demonstrate increased angiogenic properties such as increased mRNA expression of VEGF and VEGFR, as well as several cytokines (IFN-γ, IL-1, IL-12, bFGF, FGF-2, IL-6, and IL-8). Role for tumor-promoting stromal macrophages is demonstrated.

Workup

See **General Breast Cancer** chapter.

- **Imaging modifications:** Bilateral breast and bilateral nodal imaging required (*contralateral nodes involved in 10%*). CT of the chest/abdomen/pelvis/neck or PET/CT. Prechemo cross-sectional imaging of involved regional nodes and including the neck helpful in RT planning. Upfront medical photography. Mammogram can be negative except for skin thickening. Consider MRI with and without contrast.

Treatment Algorithm

An aggressive trimodality approach is optimal. M1 patients are routinely offered total mastectomy for optimal local control.

- **Algorithm:** Neoadjuvant chemotherapy ± Her2-targeted therapy (HER2+) or pembrolizumab (TNBC) → non–skin-sparing MRM → PMRT → maintenance pembro (TNBC), abemaciclib/completion hormone therapy (ER+) × 5-10 years and/or completion Her2-targeted therapy × 1 year (HER2+). TDM-1 should be given if residual HER2+ disease. Adjuvant olaparib should be given in patients with BRCA mutations.

Radiation Treatment Technique for Comprehensive Chest Wall (CW) Irradiation

- **Dose:** If pCR to NAC and age > 45 years old: 50 Gy/25 fx + 16 Gy/8 fx boost (qd) If <pCR to NAC or age ≤ 45 years old: 51 Gy/34 fx + 15 Gy/10 fx boost (bid)
  - Ensure 98% of the prescription doses are given to the CW, and 90% of the prescription doses are given to the undissected ax/ICV nodes and SCV/IMC nodes.
- **Target/technique/SIM:** Same as PMRT techniques listed in **LABC** chapter. Critical to use upfront imaging and photographics to increase field size and cover all disease prior to neoadjuvant chemotherapy. For VMAT, use Radcomp contours.

Comprehensive CW Treatment Borders for Inflammatory Breast Cancer: Multi-isocenter Technique
*See **LABC** chapter for PMRT field design and details.*

Special Considerations: Treatment + Field Design Modifications	
Inflammatory Breast Cancer/T4 Disease/Recurrent	
Radiation fields	• Wider medial margin needed on scar and surgical bed. Cover scar + 3 cm minimum. Compromise contralateral breast if needed for coverage. • Double treat all junctions (~2- to 3-mm field overlap) to ensure skin is fully treated unless upfront images suggest skin disease does not encroach on the junction (SCV/tangents) and constraints are not met. • Boost fields should include the CW + involved undissected unfront cN+.

Special Considerations: Treatment + Field Design Modifications	
Bolus	• Daily treatment: 3-mm bolus qod × 2 wk, then prn • Twice daily treatment: 3-mm bolus bid ×1 wk, qAM ×1 wk, then prn • Skin is a target. Goal is to achieve brisk erythema/moist desquamation. • Bolus over ICV in the SCV field to increase skin dose since close proximity to the chest wall

Systemic Therapy

- See **General Breast Cancer** chapter for systemic therapy regimens. IBC patients are treated primarily with neoadjuvant systemic therapy.
- Minimal response or progressive disease with neoadjuvant systemic therapy → follow closely and perform MRM before the window of operability is lost given morbidity of local failure. Consider preoperative radiotherapy if margin-negative surgery is unlikely.

Surgical Options and Pathology

- **Non–skin-sparing modified radical mastectomy (MRM):** Complete removal of the breast, overlying skin, and axillary levels I-II. SLNB not effective in IBC. Cannot place tissue expander due to non–skin-sparing procedure.
- **Delayed reconstruction recommended to avoid potential delay in adjuvant treatment and to optimize radiation.**
- **Pathology report:** Review ER/PR/Her2 status, tumor grade, tumor size, extent (multifocal?), surgical margin status (either positive, close [0-1.9 mm], or negative [≥2 mm]), extent of response to chemotherapy, presence of dermal lymphatic invasion/tumor emboli.

Notable Studies (All Retrospective Single Institution)

Dose and local control in IBC (Adapted from *Woodward et al. IJORBP,* 2014):

Name/Inclusion	Dose	Outcomes	Notes
MDACC (*Bristol et al. Int J Radiat Oncol Biol Phys* 2008) Nonmetastatic IBC, *N* = 256, 1977-2004	60-66 Gy, prn bolus (66 Gy bid)	For those that completed all treatment vs did not complete tx: 5-year LRC 84% vs 51%, 5-year DMFS 47% vs 20%, and 5-year OS 51% vs 24% (all *P* < .001)	192 patients completed treatment Conclusion: Treatment completion associated with better outcomes
MDACC (*Stecklein et al. Pract Radiat Oncol* 2019) Nonmetastatic IBC, *N* = 103, 2007-2015	60 Gy qd 66 Gy bid	5-year LRC: 95% vs 100% No difference in toxicity between qd vs bid	Conclusion: good outcomes with acceptable toxicity in PMRT for nonmetastatic IBC
Cleveland (*Rehman et al. Int J Radiat Oncol Biol Phys* 2012) Nonmetastatic IBC, *N* = 104, 2000-2009	45-66 Gy, with bolus NS	5-year LRC in all patients: 83% 5-year LRC in patients who received ≥60.4 Gy: 100%	Conclusion: Improved outcomes with dose-escalated PMRT
Florida (*Liauw et al. Cancer* 2004) Nonmetastatic IBC, *N* = 61, 1982-2001	42-60 Gy, qd with bolus	5-year LRC: 78% Trend toward better LRC with ≥60 Gy (*P* = .06)	Conclusion: Improved outcomes with dose-escalated PMRT

Name/Inclusion	Dose	Outcomes	Notes
MSKCC (*Damast et al. Int J Radiat Oncol Biol Phys* 2010) *N* = 107, 1995-2006	50 Gy, qd with bolus	5-year LRC: 87% 100% LC with ≥ 60 Gy	Conclusion: Excellent outcomes with dose-escalated PMRT
Mayo (*Brown et al. IJORBP* 2014) Nonmetastatic IBC, *N* = 49, 2000-2010	60-66 Gy, qd with bolus	5-year LRC: 81% pCR associated with better LRC	Conclusion: Daily RT with aggressive bolus has similar outcomes
Penn (*Abramowitz et al., Am J Clin Oncol*, 2009) *N* = 19, 1986-2006	46-50 Gy, qod with bolus	5-year LRC: 88% Only patients with dermal lymphatic invasion (DLI) had LRR	Conclusion: DLI and IBC associated with worse outcomes following PMRT
British Columbia Cancer Agency (*Panades et al. JCO* 2005) *N* = 148, 1980-2000	42.4 Gy (hypofx), with bolus NS	5-year LRC: 63% pCR associated with better LRC	Conclusion: Trimodality therapy improves pCR and LRC

Dose escalation/patient selection in IBC:

Name/Inclusion	Dose	Outcomes	Notes
MDACC (*Bristol et al. Int J Radiat Oncol Biol Phys* 2008) 256 nonmetastatic IBC patients treated with trimodality therapy	60-66 Gy, prn bolus (66 Gy bid)	Patients with unknown/close/+ margins, <pCR to NAC, or age < 45 benefited from dose escalation of PMRT from 60 to 66 Gy	Conclusion: Improved outcomes with dose-escalated PMRT
MDACC (*Rosso et al. Ann Surg Oncol* 2017) Prospective study with 114 nonmetastatic IBC patients receiving trimodality treatment	AC ± carboplatin (for TNBC) ± Her2-directed therapy (for HER2+) → Taxol → MRM → PMRT to >60 Gy → ± hormone therapy	2-y LRR: 3.2% 5-y OS: 69.1% Improved DFS in Her2+, clinical stage IIIB, complete or partial response to NAC, pCR, and lower initial nodal burden	Conclusion: Improved outcomes with dose-escalation and completion of trimodality therapy

Aggressive local therapy in metastatic IBC:

Name/Inclusion	Dose	Outcomes	Notes
MDACC (*Akay et al. Cancer* 2014) 172 stage IV IBC patients	46% underwent curative primary tumor resection → PMRT (51 Gy in 34 fx bid + 15 Gy in 10 fx CW boost)	5-y OS: 29% 5-y DPFS: 17% MVA showed improved OS with response to chemotherapy (HR 0.49, *P* = .005) and surgery + PMRT (HR 0.9, *P* = .0001)	55% of patients had oligomet IBC Conclusion: Aggressive multimodality therapy improves outcomes for metastatic IBC

Recurrent Breast Cancer

Background

- **Definition:** Recurrences can be local (ipsilateral breast/tumor bed), regional (in nearby lymph nodes), or distant. Contralateral breast disease is not considered recurrent.
- **Outcomes:** Dependent on type/timing, 5-year OS 50% (any recurrence) vs 70% (CW only)

- **Workup:** Similar workup to IBC workup, note previous therapies received. Depending on site and timing of recurrence, repeat biopsy. Multidisciplinary evaluation is essential.

Surgical options and systemic therapy

- Dependent on multidisciplinary evaluation and prior therapies received
- Trimodality treatment preferred when possible (Aebi et al. *Lancet Oncol* 2014)

Treatment algorithm

Locoregional recurrence after mastectomy, no prior RT	Evaluation for chemotherapy → surgery → comprehensive RT
Ipsilateral breast recurrence after BCS and prior RT	Mastectomy → no RT*
Ipsilateral breast/node recurrence after BCS and prior RT	Mastectomy ± nodal dissection → consideration of nodal irradiation*

*Careful review of prior records, consideration of reirradiation in extenuating circumstances in which safety may not be compromised.

Considerations for prior RT

General principles: Prior dose recall is 50% at 10 years; flap placement can reduce volume of previously irradiated tissue. If adequate dose for tumor control cannot be given safely, the risk-benefit ratio favors no treatment.

If indications for local recurrence are high and other therapies not feasible, reirradiation may be considered. Greater consideration for radiation techniques that limit reirradiation of ribs and other normal structures (eg, electrons/protons).

Radiation treatment technique for recurrent breast cancer

- **Rationale:** Recurrent disease in the setting of prior therapy as opposed to persistent or inadequately treated disease has had time and pressure to increase resistance. As such, an empiric 10% dose escalation is recommended.
- **Dose:** 54 Gy in 27 fractions → boost of 12 Gy/6 fx (empiric 10% dose escalation)
- **Target/technique/SIM** for locoregional recurrence is similar to PMRT techniques in **LABC** chapter.

PROSTATE CANCER (DEFINITIVE)

KEVIN DIAO • CHAD TANG

BACKGROUND

- **Incidence/prevalence:** Most common nonskin cancer in men with 268 000 new cases of prostate cancer per year and 34 000 deaths in the United States in 2022. Lifetime risk is estimated to be ~12.5% (1 in 8 men).
- **Outcomes:** Prostate cancer–specific survival at 10 years with treatment is 99% for low risk (*Hamdy et al. NEJM* 2016), 95% for intermediate risk (*Pisansky et al. JCO* 2015), and 84% for high risk (*Nguyen et al. Cancer* 2013).
- **Demographics:** Average age of diagnosis is 66. Rare under age 40. African American men have higher rates of prostate cancer, present with more advanced disease at a younger age, and have shorter progression-free survival than White men. Asian American men have lower rates of prostate cancer than White men.
- **Risk factors:** Older age, African American race, family history, smoking

TUMOR BIOLOGY AND CHARACTERISTICS

- **Genetics:** 5-10% familial (*Bratt et al. J Urol* 2002). RR of 2.5 and 3.5 in patients with 1 and 2 first-degree relative(s), respectively (*Johns and Houlston BJU Int* 2003). Associated with *BRCA2*, *ATM* mutations, and increased risk in patients with Lynch syndrome and Fanconi anemia. Over 100 single-nucleotide polymorphisms associated with increased risk of prostate cancer (*Allemailem et al. Am J Transl Res* 2021)
- **Pathology:** Majority acinar adenocarcinoma (~95%), but more high-risk variants include sarcomatoid, ductal, squamous, small cell, urothelial (*Humphrey Histopathology* 2011)
- **Imaging:** 1.5 T (with endorectal coil) or 3 T (with/without endorectal coil) multiparametric MRI with contrast: T2 hypointense (Fig. 46.1), contrast enhancing, and DWI restricted

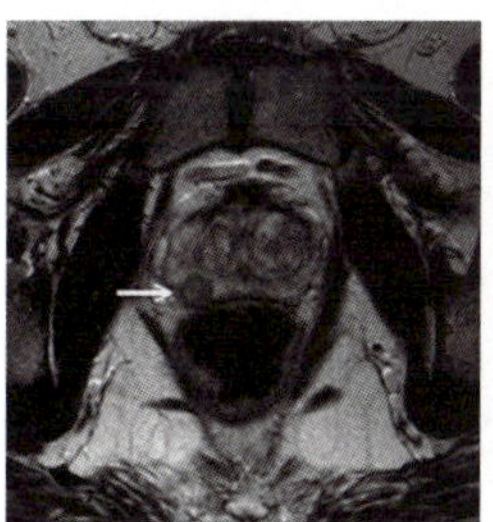
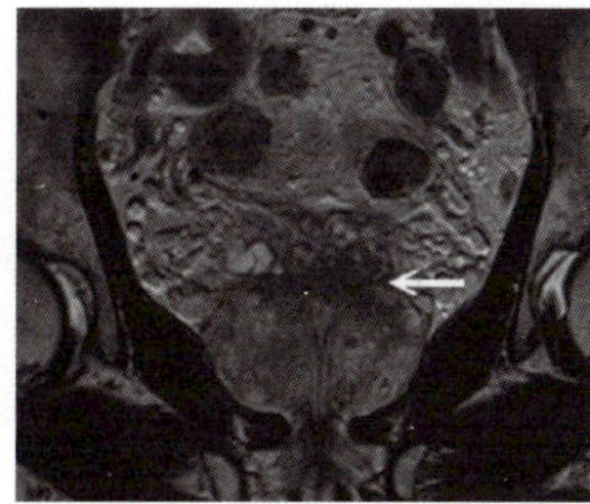

Figure 46.1 Representative MRI T2 sequence identifies dominant lesion appearing as T2 hypointense on axial **(left)** and coronal **(right)** cross-sectional images (*white arrows*). (Reproduced with permission from Abdellaoui A, Iyengar S, Freeman S. Imaging in Prostate Cancer. Future Oncol. 2011;7(5):679-691.)

- **Anatomy:** Prostate bordered by bladder/bladder neck (superiorly), fascia of urogenital diaphragm (inferiorly), attached to pubic symphysis by puboprostatic ligament (anteriorly), separated from rectum by Denonvilliers' fascia and attached to the rectum near the prostate apex via the rectourethralis muscle (posteriorly), and levator ani muscles (laterally)
  - Prostatic lymph node drainage
    - First echelon: Periprostatic, obturator
    - Second echelon: External iliac, internal iliac, presacral, presciatic
    - Third echelon (M1a): Common iliac, inguinal, retroperitoneal

Workup

- **History and physical:** Specific attention to PSA screening history, history of urologic procedures including TURPs, AUA score, SHIM score, history of IBD (ulcerative colitis and Crohn's), collagen vascular disease, and colonoscopy within last 3 years (avoid colonoscopy within 2 years after RT). Digital rectal exam (DRE)
- **Labs**: PSA, testosterone. If treating with hormone therapy: CBC, LFTs
- **Procedures/biopsy:** 10-12 core US-guided biopsy. MRI-guided fusion biopsy if discordant finding between MRI, DRE, and/or US-guided biopsy
- **Imaging**
  - MRI of the pelvis/prostate >6 weeks after biopsy
  - Tc-99m bone scan and abdominopelvic soft tissue imaging for ≥unfavorable intermediate risk
  - Consider PSMA PET, which has superior sensitivity/specificity to conventional imaging (40% sensitivity, 95% specificity for pelvic LN metastases and 85% sensitivity, 98% specificity for distant metastases), especially in high or very high risk.
  - Consider DEXA scan prior to long-term ADT.

Prostate Cancer Staging *(AJCC 8th Edition)*

T Stage (c = clinical, p = pathologic)[a]		
T1	Clinically inapparent tumor that is not palpable	
T1a	Incidental histologic finding in ≤5% tissue resected	
T1b	Incidental histologic finding in >5% tissue resected	
T1c	Identified by needle biopsy in one or both sides, but not palpable	
T2	Palpable and confined within prostate	
cT2a	Involves ½ of one side	pT2: organ confined disease
cT2b	Involves >½ of one side but not both sides	
cT2c	Involves both sides	

T Stage	
T3	Extraprostatic tumor, no fixation or adjacent structure invasion
T3a	Extraprostate extension (unilateral or bilateral)
T3b	Invades seminal vesicle(s)
T4	Fixed or invades other adjacent structures
N Stage	
N0	No regional lymph nodes
N1	Involves regional lymph nodes
M Stage	
M0	No distant metastases
M1	Distant metastasis
M1a	Nonregional lymph node(s)[b]
M1b	Bone(s)
M1c	Other site(s) +/− bone disease

Gleason Score	Grade Group	NCCN Risk Group	
6 (3 + 3)	1	Low or very low	cT1-T2a, GG1, and PSA < 10 (*very low* if all of: cT1c, <3 biopsy cores positive, ≤50% each core, and PSA density <0.15 ng/mL/g)
7 (3 + 4)	2	Favorable intermediate	GG1-2, only 1 intermediate-risk factor (GG2, cT2b-c, 10 ≤ PSA < 20), and <50% biopsy cores positive
7 (4 + 3)	3	Unfavorable intermediate	GG3, ≥2 intermediate-risk factors, or ≥50% biopsy cores positive
8	4	High or very high	≥cT3a, GG4-5, or PSA ≥ 20 (*very high* if any of: cT3b-4, primary Gleason 5, ≥2 high-risk factors, or >4 cores GG4-5)
9-10	5		

<table>
<tr><th colspan="8">Summative Stage</th></tr>
<tr><th>T stage</th><th>GG1</th><th>GG2</th><th>GG3</th><th>GG4</th><th>GG5</th><th>N1</th><th>M1</th></tr>
<tr><td>cT1-2a, pT2 (PSA < 10)</td><td>I</td><td rowspan="3">IIB</td><td colspan="2" rowspan="3">IIC</td><td rowspan="5">IIIC</td><td rowspan="5">IVA</td><td rowspan="5">IVB</td></tr>
<tr><td>cT1-2a, pT2 (10 ≤ PSA < 20)</td><td rowspan="2">IIA</td></tr>
<tr><td>cT2b-c (PSA < 20)</td></tr>
<tr><td>cT1-T2 (PSA ≥ 20)</td><td colspan="4">IIIA</td></tr>
<tr><td>cT3-4</td><td colspan="4">IIIB</td></tr>
</table>

[a]Unless noted, pathologic stage is the same as clinical stage. Imaging (MRI, CT scan, etc.) can only be used to determine N stage and not T stage.
[b]Nonregional LNs refer to common iliacs and superior and inguinals and inferior.
Used with permission of the American College of Surgeons, Chicago, Illinois. The original source for this information is the AJCC Cancer Staging System (2023).

Treatment Algorithm

Low or very low risk	• **Active surveillance**
	  • Biopsy, PSA, prostate MRI at baseline
	  • PSA every 6 mo
	  • DRE and prostate MRI every 12 mo
	  • Repeat prostate biopsy 12 mo after diagnosis and no more often than every 12 mo thereafter
	  • Consider definitive treatment if >10 y life expectancy and GS increases, ≥50% cores positive, or patient preference
	• **EBRT**
	  • No ADT unless needed for prostate shrinkage
	• **Brachytherapy monotherapy** (see **Brachytherapy** chapter)
	  • AUA < 15 on LUTS medication, no TURP or prostate surgery, no large median lobe, no pubic arch interference (based on axial CT or MRI), able to tolerate anesthesia
	  • No ADT unless needed for prostate shrinkage to allow brachy eligibility in which case 3-6 mo ADT given prior to brachy reassessment
	• **Radical prostatectomy +/− bilateral pelvic lymph node dissection**

Favorable intermediate risk	• **EBRT**
	  • No ADT unless needed for prostate shrinkage
	• **Brachytherapy monotherapy**
	  • Typically only in patients with favorable intermediate-risk disease. See low-risk brachytherapy for other criteria
	• **Radical prostatectomy +/− bilateral pelvic lymph node dissection**
	• **Active surveillance**
	  • May consider in patients with life expectancy <5 y. See low risk active surveillance for monitoring approach

Unfavorable intermediate risk	• **EBRT with ADT**
	  • Total 6 mo of neoadjuvant/concurrent/adjuvant ADT
	• **EBRT + brachytherapy boost +/− ADT**
	  • Consider 6 months ADT for young patients and/or bulky disease
	  • Treat prostate +/− SVs only with EBRT
	• **Radical prostatectomy + bilateral pelvic lymph node dissection**

High or very high risk	• **EBRT with ADT ± abiraterone** • Total 18-24 mo of neoadjuvant/concurrent/adjuvant ADT • Treat pelvic LNs if high risk of involvement or imaging suspicious • Consider abiraterone if LN+ or ≥2 of: cT3-4, GG4-5, PSA ≥ 40
	• **EBRT with ADT + brachytherapy boost** • Total 12 months of neoadjuvant/concurrent/adjuvant ADT • Treat pelvic LNs if high risk of involvement or imaging suspicious • Consider brachytherapy boost 2-4 wk after EBRT • **Radical prostatectomy + bilateral pelvic lymph node dissection**
LN+ disease	• **EBRT with ADT ± abiraterone** • Total 24 mo of neoadjuvant/concurrent/adjuvant ADT • Consider abiraterone • Treat pelvic LNs

RADIATION TREATMENT TECHNIQUE

- **SIM:** Fiducial marker placement (2 carbon for proton; 3 gold for photon) and consider rectal spacer hydrogel prior to simulation; head first, supine, lower extremity immobilization (Fig. 46.2), bladder full, empty rectum (milk of magnesia day before and enema day of SIM). Endorectal balloon if proton simulation or if sigmoid/small bowel close to radiation field. Isocenter in middle of the prostate.
- **Dose:** 78 Gy in 39 fractions, 72 Gy in 30 fractions, 70 Gy in 28 fractions, 60 Gy in 20 fractions, 36.25/40 Gy in 5 fractions PTV/CTV (SBRT)
  50.4 Gy in 28 fractions pelvis, SIB involved LN to 58.8-61.6 Gy and prostate to 70 Gy
  46 Gy in 23 fractions pelvis, boost involved LN to 54-60 Gy and prostate to 78 Gy
- **Target:** Prostate only (low risk)
  Prostate, proximal 1.5-2 cm of seminal vesicles (intermediate risk)
  Prostate, full seminal vesicles, ± pelvic lymph nodes (high risk)
- **Technique:** IMRT/VMAT; SBRT; consider protons

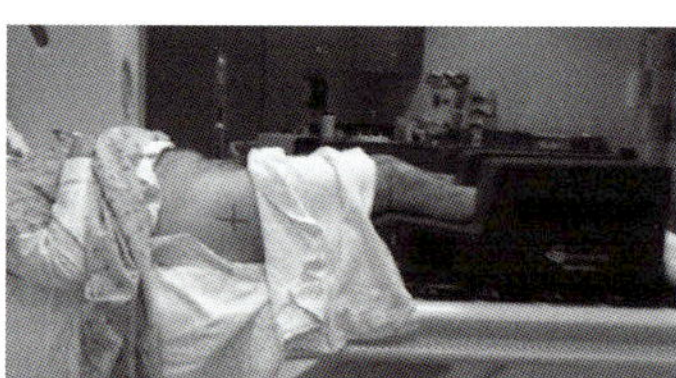

Figure 46.2 Standard setup at simulation for definitive EBRT for prostate cancer. The lower extremities are typically immobilized with a Medtec© device. Hands holding an A-bar.

CTV for Intact Prostate/Seminal Vesicles	
Low risk	Prostate
Intermediate risk	Prostate + proximal 1.5-2 cm of seminal vesicles (SVs)
High risk	Prostate + entire SV. Consider treating distal SVs to lower dose if no MRI evidence of involvement
IMRT PTV = CTV + 0.4 cm posterior, 0.6 cm elsewhere	
Proton PTV = CTV + 0.4 cm posterior, 0.6 cm anterior, 0.6 cm superior/inferior, 1.1 cm lateral	
SBRT PTV = CTV + 0.3 cm in all dimensions	
CTV for Pelvic Lymph Nodes	
Start at the bifurcation of the aorta (typically L4/L5) or vertebral body above any radiographically involved LNs.	
Include presacral, prevertebral, posterior mesorectal nodes to bottom S3.	
Stop external iliac nodes as the external iliac vessels cross the medial portion of the acetabulum or enter the inguinal canal.	
Stop internal iliac nodes as the seminal vesicles join the top of the prostate gland.	

- Bladder volume scan prior to each treatment, treat if +/− 20% of simulation
- **Conventional/hypofractionated image guidance:**
  Daily kV imaging with alignment to intraprostatic fiducials
  Consider weekly or daily CBCT if fiducial is not available, LN field, or if anticipated problems with setup.
- **SBRT image guidance:**
  Daily CBCT align soft tissue and intrafractional ExacTrac to intraprostatic fiducials, apply shifts >1 mm discrepancy, daily enema prior to treatment

Dose Constraints by Fractionation				
	78 Gy 39 fx	**70 Gy 28 fx**	**60 Gy 20 fx**	**SBRT (5 fx)**
PTV	V100 ≥ 98%	V100 ≥ 98%	V100 ≥ 98%	V100 ≥ 98%
Rectum	V80 ≤ 3% V70 ≤ 15% V60 ≤ 40% V40 ≤ 60%	V65 ≤ 10 cc V65 ≤ 15% V55 ≤ 25% V45 ≤ 45%	V60 ≤ 1% V50 ≤ 22% V40 ≤ 38% V30 ≤ 57% V20 ≤ 85%	V38.1 < 1 cc V34.4 < 3 cc V32.6 < 10% V29 < 20% V18.1 < 50%
Bladder	V70 ≤ 15% V60 ≤ 40% V40 ≤ 60%	V65 ≤ 15% V55 ≤ 25% V45 ≤ 45%	V60 ≤ 3% V56.8 ≤ 5% V48 ≤ 25% V40 ≤ 50%	V38.1 < 1 cc V32.6 < 10% V18.1 < 50%
Small bowel	D_{max} <55 Gy	D_{max} <52 Gy V46.5 ≤2 cc	D_{max} < 40 Gy V37 ≤ 90 cc V33 ≤ 130 cc	V30 < 1 cc V18.1 < 5 cc
Sigmoid	D_{max} <60 Gy	D_{max} <55 Gy	D_{max} < 50 Gy	V25 ≤ 20 cc
Femoral heads	D_{max} <55 Gy V50 ≤5% V45 ≤10%	D_{max} <52.5 Gy V50 ≤1%	D_{max} < 37 Gy V35 ≤ 5%	V14.5 < 5%
Urethra (if visualized)	N/A	N/A	N/A	V44 < 20%

Surgery

- Radical prostatectomy either open or minimally invasive, generally robotic. Robotic surgery associated with lower blood loss and decreased hospital stays. Oftentimes combined with pelvic lymph node dissection, especially for intermediate/high-risk patients.

Chemotherapy/hormone therapy

- **Androgen deprivation therapy:** Neoadjuvant/concurrent/adjuvant ADT using GnRH agonist (leuprolide +/− 14-30 days bicalutamide) or antagonist (degarelix, relugolix). GnRH antagonists have faster testosterone suppression and recovery, fewer cardiovascular events. Total 6 months ADT for unfavorable intermediate-risk patients receiving EBRT, 24 months in high-risk patients with EBRT, and 12 months with EBRT + brachytherapy boost. ADT duration may vary based on response, tolerance, and patient factors.
- **Abiraterone:** Consider treatment intensification with addition of abiraterone to ADT for a subset of very high-risk patients (≥2 of cT3/4, GG4-5, PSA ≥ 40) or LN+ (*Attard et al. Lancet* 2022). Given with prednisone 5 mg daily.
- **Second-generation antiandrogens:** Enzalutamide, apalutamide, and darolutamide are FDA approved for nonmetastatic castrate-resistant prostate cancer (*Hussain et al. NEJM* 2018, *Smith et al. NEJM* 2018, *Fizazi et al. NEJM* 2019). Can consider in place of abiraterone if abiraterone/prednisone is contraindicated. Darolutamide may be associated with less CNS toxicity. No benefit to addition of either apalutamide or enzalutamide to abiraterone and ADT with RT for localized therapy.

Side Effect Management

- Obstruction: *Decreased flow/hesitancy/frequency*. 1st-line tamsulosin (0.4 mg 30 minutes after dinner up to 2 tablets per evening) → 2nd-line terazosin (1 mg 30 minutes after dinner, can titrate up to 10 mg as tolerated)
- Overactivity: *Urgency/frequency*. 1st-line ibuprofen (200 mg 2-3 tablets bid prn; avoid in kidney disease) → oxybutynin (5 mg 2-4 times per day)

- Cystitis: *Urgency/frequency + dysuria.* UA + urine culture to r/o UTI. Treat UTI if positive. If negative, 1st-line over the counter phenazopyridine (AZO) +/− cranberry tablets (100-200 mg tid after meals; short course, turns urine orange; avoid in kidney disease) → 2nd-line ibuprofen (200 mg 2-3 tablets bid prn; avoid in kidney disease)
- Diarrhea: 1st-line diet modification (low residue, lower fiber, and low dairy) → 2nd-line Imodium titrating to a max of 8 pills/day → 3rd-line alternating Lomotil 2 pills and Imodium 2 pills every 3 hours
- Proctitis: *Rectal pain.* 1st-line cortisone suppository → 2nd-line steroid enemas
- Rectal bleeding: Consider steroid enemas, hyperbaric oxygen, GI referral for argon plasma coagulation
- Hematuria: Urology referral for cystoscopy, consider hyperbaric oxygen

Follow-up

- History and PSA (measure testosterone if on ADT until full recovery): Every 6 months for 2 years then every 6-12 months until year 5, annually thereafter.
- Consider DRE every 12 months.
- Minimize instrumentation (eg, colonoscopy, cystoscopy) in first 2 years

Randomized Evidence

Name/Inclusion	Arms	Outcomes*	Notes
		Low Risk	
ProtecT (*Hamdy et al. NEJM* 2016) **QOL** (*Donovan et al. NEJM* 2016) Age 50-69 Early stage (mostly GG1, cT1c, PSA <10)	Active monitoring Radical prostatectomy RT (74 Gy) + 3-6 mo ADT	Improved 10-y DMFS with RP (2.4%) or RT (2.7%) vs AS (5.6%) but similar PCSS (99%) and OS (88%)	RP associated w/ worse sexual fx and urinary incontinence, RT w/ worse urinary and bowel bother. 53% of AS patients rec'd definitive treatment
		Intermediate Risk	
RTOG 0815 (*Krauss et al. ASTRO* 2021) At least 1 of: cT2b-c, GG2, >10 PSA ≤ 20 Excluded if all 3 and ≥50% biopsy cores positive	RT alone (79.2 Gy or 45 Gy w/ brachy boost) RT + 6 mo ADT	ADT improved 5-y bPFS (14% vs 8%), DMFS (3% vs 0.6%), PCSM (1% vs 0%). Similar OS (90 vs 91%)	ADT beneficial for intermediate-risk prostate cancer even w/ dose-escalated RT. Pending subset analysis for favorable intermediate. Pelvic RT not allowed
RTOG 9408 (*Jones et al. NEJM* 2011) cT1-T2b, PSA < 20, GG1-2	EBRT alone (66.6 Gy prostate, 46.8 Gy pelvis) EBRT + 4 mo ADT	ADT improved 10-y OS (62% vs 57%) and PCSM (4% vs 8%)	Established role of neoadjuvant ADT in intermediate-risk prostate cancer
Harvard (*D'Amico et al. JAMA* 2008) cT1-T2b, ≥1 of GG ≥ 2, PSA > 10, or T3 on MRI	EBRT alone (70 Gy, prostate only) EBRT + 6 mo ADT	ADT improved 8-y OS (74% vs 61%) and PCSM (4% vs 13%)	Established role of adjuvant ADT in intermediate-risk prostate cancer
		High Risk	
POP-RT (*Murthy et al. JCO* 2021) N0 prostate cancer with LN risk ≥20% using Roach formula	Prostate only RT (68 Gy 25 fx) Whole pelvic RT (50 Gy 25 fx)	Pelvic RT improved 5-y bPFS (95% vs 81%) and DMFS (96% vs 89%). Similar OS (93% vs 91%)	All patients received ≥2 y ADT. 80% of patients were staged/restaged with PSMA-PET

Name/Inclusion	Arms	Outcomes*	Notes
ASCENDE-RT (*Morris et al. IJROBP* 2017, *Rodda et al. IJROBP* 2017) Intermediate and high risk Excluded if PSA > 40, ≥cT3b, prior TURP, pre-ADT prostate volume > 75 cc	EBRT (46 Gy pelvic, 78 Gy prostate) + 12 mos ADT EBRT (46 Gy pelvic) + LDR brachytherapy boost (I-125 115 Gy) + 12 mo ADT	Brachy boost improved 9-y bPFS (83% vs 62%) but not DMFS (89% vs 85%), PCSS (95% vs 92%), or OS (91% vs 89%)	Approx. 69% high risk. Brachy boost associated w/ worse 5-y grade ≥3 GU toxicity (18% vs 5%) w/ half of events being urethral strictures requiring dilatation
RTOG 9202 (*Horwitz et al. JCO* 2008) cT2c-4N0, PSA < 150, pelvic LN+ allowed	EBRT + 4 mo neoadjuvant ADT EBRT + 4 mo neoadjuvant ADT + 24 mo adjuvant ADT	Long-term ADT improved 10-y DFS (22.5% vs 13.2%), DM (15% vs 23%), biochemical failure (52% vs 68%) but not OS (54% vs 52%)	RT was 65-70 Gy (45 Gy to whole pelvis). ADT was goserelin. Subset analysis of GG3-5 demonstrated OS benefit
STAMPEDE meta-analysis (*Attard et al. Lancet* 2022) LN+ or ≥2 of: cT3/4, GG 4-5, or PSA ≥ 40	ADT alone +/− RT (74 Gy) ADT + abiraterone +/− RT (74 Gy) ADT + abiraterone + enzalutamide +/− RT (74 Gy)	Addition of abiraterone to ADT +/− RT improved 6-y DMFS (82% vs 69%) as well as OS, PCSS, bPFS, and PFS. More G3+ toxicities in first 2 years (37% vs 29%)	RT mandated for node negative and encouraged for node positive. 85% had planned RT. Addition of enzalutamide to abiraterone and ADT did not improve outcomes
Miscellaneous (hypofractionation, dose escalation, SBRT)			
RTOG 0415 (*Lee et al. JCO* 2016) Low-risk prostate cancer (cT1b-T2c, GG1, PSA < 10)	73.8 Gy in 41 fractions 70 Gy in 28 fractions	5-y DFS (86% vs 85%) with 70 Gy noninferior to 73.8 Gy	Late grade ≥2 and ≥3 GI and GU toxicities increased with hypofx but standard arm not dose escalated
PROFIT (*Cotton et al. JCO* 2017) NCCN intermediate-risk prostate cancer	78 Gy in 39 fractions 60 Gy in 20 fractions	5-y bPFS (85% in both arms) with 60 Gy noninferior to 78 Gy	ADT not permitted. No difference in late grade ≥3 GI or GU toxicity
MDACC dose escalation (*Pasalic et al. IJROBP* 2019) cT1-T3, N0, PSA ≤ 30 Included mix of low-, intermediate-, and high-risk patients	Standard dose RT (70 Gy in 35 fractions) Dose escalated (DE) RT (78 Gy in 39 fractions)	DE-RT reduced 15-y failure rate (12% vs 19%), DM (1% vs 3%), and PCSM (3% vs 6%)	ADT not allowed. Only dose escalation study to demonstrate improvement in DM and PCSM
PACE-B (*Tree et al. Lancet Oncol* 2022) Low- or intermediate-risk prostate cancer	Standard RT (78 Gy in 39 fractions or 62 Gy in 30 fractions) SBRT (40 Gy in 5 fractions to CTV, 36.25 Gy in 5 fractions to PTV over 1-2 weeks)	At 2 years, RTOG grade ≥2 GU (3% vs 2%) and GI toxicity (2% vs 3%) were similar for SBRT and standard RT, respectively. Awaiting biochemical outcomes	Worse CTCAE grade ≥2 GU toxicity with SBRT (12% vs 7%). PTV margin 5-9 mm and 3-7 mm posterior, SBRT 4-5 mm and 3-5 mm posterior. No rectal spacers used

Name/Inclusion	Arms	Outcomes*	Notes
HYPO-RT-PC (*Widmark et al. Lancet Oncol* 2019) **QOL** (*Fransson et al. Lancet Oncol* 2022) Intermediate- or high-risk prostate cancer	Conventional RT (78 Gy in 39 fractions)	5-y FFS was 84% in both groups. SBRT is noninferior to conventional RT	Higher grade ≥2 GU toxicity with SBRT at 1 y (6% vs 2%). Patient-reported acute QOL worse but long-term QOL similar
	SBRT (42.7 Gy in 7 fractions qod)		

*Primary study end point underlined.

PROSTATE CANCER (ADJUVANT/ SALVAGE)

KEVIN DIAO • UGUR SELEK • SEUNGTAEK CHOI

Background, Tumor Biology, and Characteristics

See Definitive Prostate Cancer chapter.

Workup for PSA Recurrence

- **History and physical:** AUA score, SHIM score, IBD (ulcerative colitis and Crohn's), collagen vascular disease, and colonoscopy (within 3-5 years). Initial stage. Type and date of surgery, PSA measurements after surgery. Digital rectal exam. Delay postoperative RT until urinary function is maximized/stabilized to ≤1 pad/day (typically ≥3 months from the date of surgery).
- **Labs:** PSA, testosterone. If treating with hormone therapy: CBC
- **Procedures/biopsy:** Consider image-guided biopsy if nodule is palpated or visible on imaging.
- **Imaging:** MRI of the pelvis/prostate and PSMA-PET preferred (33% yield for PSA < 0.2, 45% for PSA < 0.5 *Perera et al. Eur Urol* 2020). If unavailable, Tc-99m bone scan and CT of abdomen and pelvis with contrast.
- **Anatomy:**
  - Prostate fossa: Top of pubic symphysis (superiorly), 1 cm below vesicourethral anastomosis (inferiorly), bladder wall or posterior edge of pubic bone (anteriorly), anterior rectal wall (posteriorly), and pelvic floor muscles/fascia (laterally)
  - SV fossa: Top of the prostate fossa (inferiorly), posterior wall of the bladder (anteriorly) to the anterior rectum wall (posteriorly) up to the remnants of the vas deferens (superiorly)
  - Prostatic lymph node drainage
    - First echelon: Periprostatic, obturator
    - Second echelon: External iliac, internal iliac, presacral, presciatic
    - Third echelon (M1a): Common iliac, inguinal, retroperitoneal

PC 9-8

Prostate Cancer Staging (AJCC 8th Edition)

See Definitive Prostate Cancer chapter.

Treatment Algorithm

Adjuvant (PSA undetectable)	• EBRT
	  • Not routinely indicated, consider for multiple risk factors: pGS 8-10, positive margins, SV involvement, ECE, pN1, high genomic risk classifier score, unable to have follow-up
	  • PSA undetectable to be considered adjuvant
	  • ADT not typically given for adjuvant pN0

Salvage (PSA detectable)	• EBRT +/− ADT • Salvage RT for ultrasensitive PSA < 0.2 controversial • 0.2 ≤ PSA ≤ 0.5 consider 4-6 mo ADT* • PSA > 0.5 consider pelvic RT + 6 mo ADT • 6-12 mo ADT for clinical/radiologic recurrence • If cN1 consider 12-24 mo ADT +/− abiraterone
Pathologic lymph node involvement	• EBRT + ADT • ≥12 mo ADT for pN1 • If PSA undetectable treat fossa as per adjuvant • If PSA detectable treat fossa as per salvage

*Factors favoring ADT use include negative margins, Gleason ≥ 8, and short time to PSA recurrence.

Radiation Treatment Technique

- **SIM:** Lower extremity immobilization, bladder full, empty rectum (milk of magnesia day before and enema day of SIM), +/− endorectal balloon. Isocenter middle of fossa
- **Dose:** 66 Gy in 33 fractions to the prostate fossa (postoperative adjuvant). Consider 59.4 Gy in 33 fractions to SV fossa (if pSV−).
  66-70 Gy in 33-35 fractions to the prostate fossa (postoperative salvage). Consider 59.4-63 Gy in 33-35 fractions to SV fossa (if pSV−).
  Pelvic LN radiation to 46 Gy in 23 fractions. Sequential boost to gross LNs to 54-60 Gy
  Consider SIB to gross disease in the fossa to 72-74 Gy in 35 fractions (Fig. 47.1).
- **Target:** Prostate fossa and SV fossa ± pelvic lymph nodes
- **Technique:** IMRT/VMAT

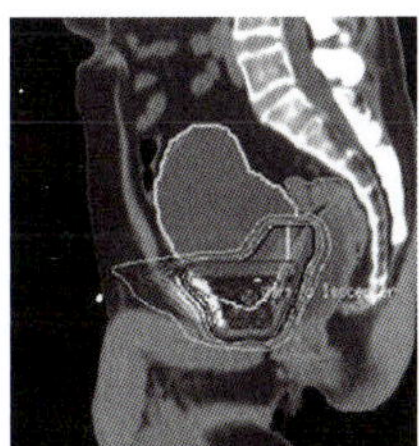
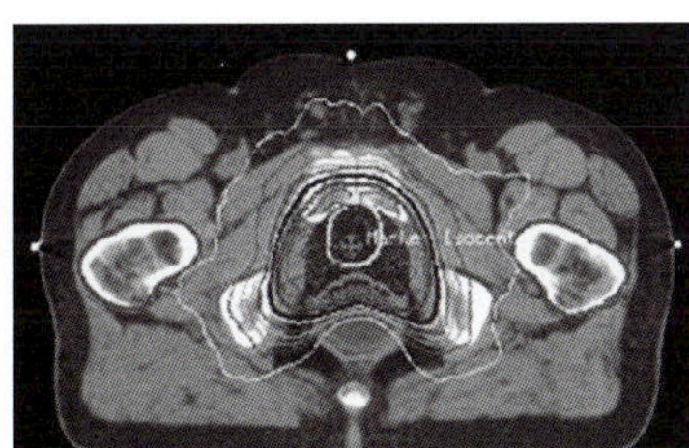

Figure 47.1 Sagittal and axial views showing an RT plan treating the prostate fossa to 70 Gy (*blue color wash*) and SV fossa (*yellow color wash*) to 63 Gy. **See color insert**.

CTV for Postoperative Prostate/Seminal Vesicle Fossa	
Superior	Level of cut of vas deferens or 3-4 cm above superior symphysis
Inferior	1 cm below vesicourethral anastomosis
Anterior	Pubic symphysis, can reduce cover to top 1/3 of symphysis to spare bladder dose
Posterior	Anterior rectal wall, mesorectal fascia
Lateral	Levator ani muscles, sacrorectogenitopubic fascia
IMRT PTV = CTV + 0.5 cm posterior, 0.7 cm elsewhere	
CTV for Pelvic Lymph Nodes	
Start at the bifurcation of the aorta (typically L4/L5) or vertebral body above any radiographically involved LNs.	
Include presacral, prevertebral, posterior mesorectal nodes to bottom S3, excluding bone, bowel, bladder, and muscle.	
Stop external iliac nodes as the external iliac vessels cross the medial portion of the acetabulum or enter the inguinal canal.	
Stop internal iliac nodes as the seminal vesicles join the top of the prostate gland.	

- **IGRT:** Daily kV imaging with alignment to bone. Consider CBCT if anticipated problems with setup.
- **Planning directive (for conventional fractionation):**
  PTV:V100 ≥ 98%
  Rectum:V70 Gy ≤ 15%,V60 Gy ≤ 40%,V40 Gy ≤ 60%, respectively (do not have V30 line encompass the entire rectum on a single axial slice)
  Bladder:V70 Gy ≤ 15%
  Femoral heads:V45 Gy ≤ 10%;V50 Gy ≤ 5%; D_{max} < 55 Gy
  Small bowel: D_{max} < 50-54 Gy
  Sigmoid: D_{max} < 60 Gy

Chemotherapy/Hormone Therapy

- **Androgen deprivation therapy:** Neoadjuvant/concurrent/adjuvant leuprolide. Consider 4-6 months for early salvage (0.2 ≥ PSA ≥ 0.5), 6 months for salvage (PSA ≥ 0.5), and ≥12 months for pLN+ disease. If ≥2 of: ≥pT3b, ≥GS 8, PSA ≥0.5, consider 12 months ADT. If cN1 consider 12-24 months ADT +/− abiraterone. May omit ADT for early salvage PSA < 0.5 especially if positive surgical margin, GS 6-7.

Side Effect Management

See Definitive Prostate chapter.

Follow-up

- History and PSA (get testosterone if on ADT): Every 3-6 months for 2 years, then every 6-12 months until year 5, annually thereafter
- Consider DRE every 12 months.
- Minimize instrumentation (eg, colonoscopy, cystoscopy) in first 2 years.

Randomized Evidence

Name/Inclusion	Arms	Outcomes	Notes
EORTC 22911 (*Bolla et al. Lancet* 2012) pT3 (ECE or SVI) or + surgical margins after radical prostatectomy	Adjuvant RT (60 Gy, 50 Gy followed by 10 Gy cone-down boost) Observation	Adjuvant RT improved 10-y bPFS (61% vs 41%, *P* < .001). MFS and OS not different. More late toxicity with adjuvant RT at 10 years (71% vs 60%)	Enrolled patients were 70% adjuvant (PSA undetectable) and 30% salvage (PSA detectable)
ARTISTIC Meta-Analysis (*Vale et al. Lancet* 2020) See specific trials for individual inclusion criteria Postoperative PSA ≤ 0.2, ≥1 high-risk feature: pT3/4, Gleason 7-10, preoperative PSA ≥ 10 ng/mL, +margins, assigned between 4 to 22 weeks after RP	Adjuvant RT (64-66 Gy in 2 Gy fractions or 52.5 Gy in 20 fractions +/− pelvic RT +/− ADT) Early salvage RT triggered by PSA ≥0.2 (64-66 Gy in 2 Gy fractions or 52.5 Gy in 20 fractions +/− pelvic RT +/− ADT)	No difference in 5-y EFS (89% vs 88%, HR 0.95, *P* = .70). 39% of patients in the early salvage arm received RT with a median follow-up time of 60-78 months. Increased toxicity with adjuvant RT in all 3 trials	Prospectively planned meta-analysis of RADICALS, RAVES, and GETUG-AFU 17. EFS defined as rising PSA ≥ 0.4 after RT, PSA ≥2.0 at any point, clinical or radiographic progression, nontrial treatment, death from PCA
RTOG 9601 (*Shipley et al. NEJM* 2017) T2 with +margins or T3, pN0, postoperative PSA between 0.2 and 4.0 ng/mL. Pelvic lymph node dissection required	Salvage RT alone (64.8 Gy in 36 fractions) Salvage RT + 24 mo ADT (bicalutamide 150 mg qd)	Long-term ADT improved 12-y OS (76% vs 71%, *P* = .04), PCA death (6% vs 13%, *P* < .001), and DM (15% vs 23%, *P* = .005)	High rate of gynecomastia with ADT (70% vs 11%, *P* < .001) due to use of bicalutamide. Pelvic RT not allowed

Name/Inclusion	Arms	Outcomes	Notes
GETUG-AFU 16 (*Carrie et al. Lancet Oncol* 2016, *Lancet Oncol 2019*) pT2-T4a, pN0, postoperative PSA between 0.2 and 2.0 ng/mL	Salvage RT alone (66 Gy in 33 fractions) Salvage RT + 6 months ADT (goserelin)	Short-term ADT improved 10-y PFS (664% vs 49%, P < .001) and MFS (HR = 0.73) but not OS (10 y: 86% vs 85%)	Pelvic RT allowed in patients without node dissection and risk >15% according to Partin table
RTOG 0534/ SPPORT (*Pollack et al. Lancet* 2022) pT2-3 disease, pGS of ≤9, postoperative PSA between 0.1 and 2.0 ng/mL	Prostate bed RT (PBRT) alone (64.8-70.2 Gy in 1.8 Gy fractions) PBRT + 4-6 months ADT PBRT + pelvic LN RT (45 Gy in 1.8 Gy fractions) + 4-6 months ADT	5-y PFS 87% vs 81% vs 71%, (group 3 > 2 > 1). Acute ≥G2/3 toxicity worse in group 3 > 2 > 1 (44%, 36%, and 18%, respectively) but late toxicity similar	PFS included BCF (Phoenix definition), clinical failure, or death from any cause

BLADDER CANCER

KEVIN DIAO • SEUNGTAEK CHOI

Background

- **Incidence/prevalence:** Fourth most common diagnosed cancer in men and 11th in women in the United States. Approximately 81 000 cases will be diagnosed in 2022 in the United States, with 17 000 deaths predicted. Approximately 25% of cases are muscle invasive.
- **Risk factors:** Tobacco use (urothelial type), industrial exposures (aromatic amines, hair dyes, arsenic), *Schistosoma* infection (squamous cell histology), chronic cystitis (recurrence infections, indwelling catheter use), cyclophosphamide

Tumor Biology and Characteristics

- **Genetics:** Papillary tumors are frequently seen to have mutations in *FGFR3*, and nonpapillary tumors often have mutated *TP53* and *RB1*.
- **Pathology:** Majority urothelial carcinomas (>90%). Minority squamous cell carcinomas and small cell carcinomas. Common presentation with a synchronous primary in the upper urinary tract (ureter and renal pelvis).
- **Imaging:** Direct visualization with cystoscopy and exam under anesthesia is required to assess location and stage. CT urogram can demonstrate three-dimensional lesions and LN involvement. Bladder MRI appearance is T1 hypointense and T2 intense.
- **Anatomy:**
  - Situated anterior to the rectum; in men superior to the prostate and in women both superior and anterior to the vagina/uterus
  - Urothelial lining is in the bladder, upper GU tract up to the renal pelvis, and inferiorly to the urethra. This contributes to the risk of "field cancerization effect" in which the entire GU tract may be subject to the same neoplastic effect seen in the bladder, requiring assessment of the entire GU epithelium when bladder cancer is identified.
  - Lymph node drainage: Perivesical, presacral, internal iliac, external iliac, and obturator nodes

Workup

- **History and physical:** History of exposure including aniline dyes, smoking, and bladder parasites. Symptoms including hematuria, bladder cramping, and dysuria
- **Labs:** CBC and basic chemistry panel including alkaline phosphatase

- **Procedures/biopsy:** Bimanual exam under anesthesia for staging and transurethral resection of bladder tumor (TURBT) to assess depth of invasion
- **Imaging:** Direct visualization using cystoscopy with TURBT is required. CT urogram (triple phase CT of upper GU tract, abdomen, and pelvis) or MR urogram. Chest x-ray or CT chest in patients with muscle-invasive disease. Bone scan, PET scan, and/or MRI brain (especially small cell) can be considered for locally advanced or node-positive patients or for those with symptoms concerning for metastatic disease (Fig. 48.1).

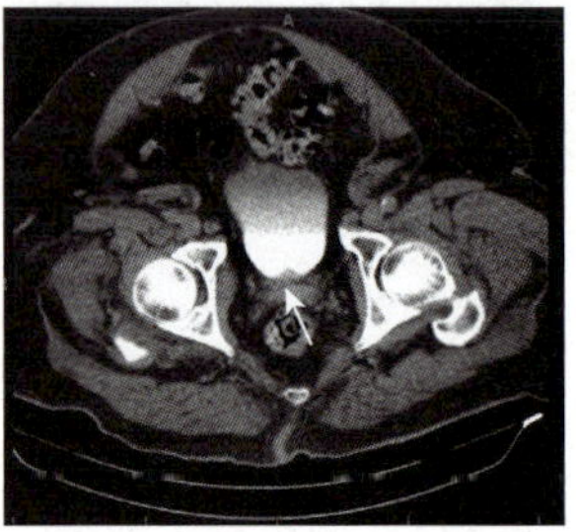

Figure 48.1 Representative CT urogram cross-sectional image from a bladder cancer patient. Mild thickening at the posterior wall of the bladder (*arrow*) represents the primary tumor.

TREATMENT ALGORITHM

Stage 0	• Transurethral resection of bladder tumor (TURBT) alone
Stage I	• TURBT + intravesical BCG or chemotherapy × 6 weeks +/− maintenance for 1-3 years • Radical cystectomy or bladder preservation (chemoradiation) for BCG-unresponsive, recurrent disease
Stage II	• Neoadjuvant chemotherapy → radical cystectomy with prostatectomy (in men) • Partial cystectomy if only involving bladder dome and 2 cm of margin can be achieved • Bladder preservation (chemoradiation)
Stage III	• Neoadjuvant chemotherapy → radical cystectomy with prostatectomy (in men) • Bladder preservation (chemoradiation)
Stage IV	• Systemic therapy, palliative radiation, or best supportive care

RADIATION TREATMENT TECHNIQUE

- **SIM:** Supine, arms on chest. When treating with a bladder boost, two simulations are needed—whole pelvic and whole bladder fields are treated with an empty bladder, and boost fields utilize a full bladder (Fig. 48.2). Empty rectum
  - Whole pelvis to 45-50.4 Gy in 25-28 fractions at 1.8 Gy/fx → Bladder tumor boost to 60-65 Gy in 1.8-2.0 Gy/fx
  - Consider treating boost field before whole bladder due to difficulty maintaining full bladder at end of treatment.
  - 64 Gy in 32 fractions to whole bladder
  - 55 Gy in 20 fractions to whole bladder
- **Boost target:** Initial TURBT area or known bladder tumor with 2-cm mucosal margin
- **Technique:** 3DCRT or IMRT; IMRT may help reduce small bowel dose.

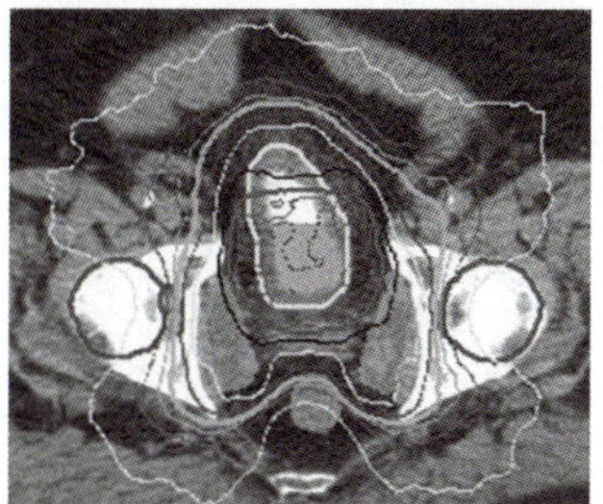

Figure 48.2 IMRT bladder conservation radiation plan treating to 45 Gy (*blue isodose line*) in 25 fractions to LNs and whole bladder followed by a sequential boost to the bladder resection cavity to 64.8 Gy (*red isodose line*) in 36 fractions. **See color insert.**

Initial fields (whole pelvis): 45-50.4 Gy in 25-28 fractions	
GTV	Visible tumor using multimodality evaluation (cystoscopy with bladder mapping + imaging)
CTV	Entire bladder, extravesical tumor, prostate, prostatic urethra (males), and draining nodes (presacral, obturator, internal iliac, and external iliac) up to L5-S1
PTV	1 cm margin on bladder, extravesical tumor with 5-mm margin on nodal fields with CT planning, organ/nodal contouring, and daily imaging
Tumor/tumor bed boost (whole pelvis): 18-20 Gy in 10-11 fractions	
Cover tumor/tumor bed as identified by bladder mapping, if 3DCRT, then tumor + 1.5-2 cm margin	

- **IGRT:** Daily US bladder + daily kV aligned to bone + CBCT at least weekly, consider more frequent CBCT if difficulty with bladder filling or performing partial bladder boost
- **Planning directive (for 1.8-2 Gy/day fractionation):**
  Spinal cord D_{max} < 45 Gy
  Femoral heads V45 < 20%
  Small bowel V50 < 10 cc, D_{max} < 54 Gy
  Bowel "bag" V45 < 195 cc

Surgery

- **Transurethral resection of bladder tumor (TURBT):** Cystoscopically guided tumor resection with the goal of resecting all visible tumors with negative margins. Random biopsies should be performed to identify multifocal disease or carcinoma in situ. A thorough mapping of the bladder assists in radiation boost planning.
- **Cystectomy:** Resection of the bladder and prostate (in males). If ileal conduit (neobladder) is created, surgeon should ensure that urethral margin is negative.
- **Lymphadenectomy:** Surgeons should perform bilateral pelvic lymphadenectomy at the same as surgery with the goal of disease cure. Completion of a pelvic lymphadenectomy (specifically external iliac, internal iliac, and obturator lymph nodes) has demonstrated improvements in disease-specific survival and pelvic recurrence risk.

Chemotherapy

- **Concurrent:** Cisplatin weekly (30-40 mg/m^2) or every 3 weeks (100 mg/m^2). Alternatively, combination 5-FU and MMC can be utilized. Acceptable single agents include 5-FU, docetaxel, or gemcitabine.
- **Adjuvant/neoadjuvant:** Multiagent cisplatin-based chemotherapy is most frequently utilized, such as gemcitabine and cisplatin or ddMVAC.

Side Effect Management

- **Nausea:** 1st-line Zofran (8 mg q8h prn) → 2nd-line Compazine (10 mg q6h prn) → ABH (lorazepam 0.34 mg, diphenhydramine 25 mg, and haloperidol 1.5 mg) 1 capsule q6h

- **Diarrhea:** 1st-line Imodium titrating to a max of 8 pills/day → 2nd-line alternating Lomotil 2 pills and Imodium 2 pills every 3 hours
- **Cystitis:** *Urgency/frequency and dysuria*. UA/UCx to rule out UTI. Treat if positive. Hyoscyamine (0.125 mg q4-6h prn, do not take more than 12 pills in a day)
- **Obstruction:** *Decreased flow/hesitancy/frequency*. 1st-line tamsulosin (0.4 mg 30 minutes after dinner up to 2 tablets per evening) → 2nd-line terazosin (1 mg 30 minutes after dinner, can titrate up to 10 mg as tolerated)
- **Bladder Spasm:** *Abdominal cramping or pain/urine leakage*. Mirabegron (25 → 50 mg daily) or tolterodine (ER 2 → 4 mg daily) or Hyoscyamine (ER 0.375 → 0.75 mg daily).

Follow-Up

- History/physical, alternating cystoscopy with urine cytology and CT abdomen/pelvis +/− CT chest/CXR every 3 months × 2 years, then every 6 months × 2 years, then annually
- Vaginal dilators for women

Evidence

Name/Inclusion	Arms	Outcomes	Notes
SWOG 8710 (Grossman et al. *NEJM* 2003) Muscle-invasive bladder cancer (T2-T4a)	Radical cystectomy alone Neoadjuvant chemotherapy + radical cystectomy	Neoadjuvant chemo trend to improved median OS (77 mo vs 46 mo, $P = .06$) and higher rate of no residual disease (38% vs 15%, $P < .001$)	Chemotherapy was 3 cycles of MVAC (methotrexate, vinblastine, doxorubicin, cisplatin)
BC2001 (James et al. *NEJM* 2012, Huddart et al. *IJROBP* 2013) Muscle-invasive bladder cancer (T2-T4a), N0, M0 *2 × 2 factorial design (chemoradiotherapy vs radiotherapy alone and whole bladder vs reduced high-dose volume radiotherapy [RHDVRT])*	Radiotherapy alone (55 Gy in 20 fractions or 64 Gy in 32 fractions) Radiotherapy with concurrent chemotherapy (5-FU and MMC) Standard whole bladder radiotherapy (sRT) Reduced high-dose volume radiotherapy (RHDVRT)	Concurrent chemotherapy improved 2-y locoregional DFS (67% vs 54%, $P = .03$) but not 5-y OS (48% vs 35%, $P = .16$) No difference in 5-y OS (38% vs 44%), 2-y LRC (61% vs 64%), or grade 3-4 toxicities between sRT or RHDVRT, respectively	Grades 3-4 toxicities more common with chemoRT during treatment (36% vs 27.5%, $P = .07$) but not during follow-up For sRT, bladder + 1.5 cm = 100% dose. For RHDVRT, GTV + 1.5 cm = 100% dose, bladder + 1.5 cm = 80% dose Pelvic lymph nodes not treated
BC2001/BCON meta-analysis (Choudhury et al. *Lancet Oncol* 2021) Locally advanced bladder cancer (high grade T1 or T2-T4, N0, M0)	Conventional radiotherapy (64 Gy in 32 fractions) Hypofx radiotherapy (55 Gy in 20 fractions)	Hypofx was noninferior to conventional RT in terms of LRR and late bladder/rectal toxicity. Lower risk of invasive LRR with hypofx RT (HR 0.71, 95% CI 0.52-0.96)	Fractionation schedule chosen according to local standard practice (nonrandomized). Approximately half of patients received each. Bladder-only treatment
RTOG Pooled Analysis (Mak et al. *J Clin Oncol* 2014) Muscle-invasive bladder cancer from RTOG 8802, 8903, 9506, 9706, 9906, and 0233	Bladder preservation with combined modality therapy (variable chemo and RT dosing and technique)	5- and 10-y OS of 57% and 36%, respectively, and 5- and 10-y DSS of 71% and 65%, respectively	Long-term DSS with combined modality therapy comparable to results from modern radical cystectomy studies

TESTICULAR CANCER

KEVIN DIAO • SEUNGTAEK CHOI

BACKGROUND

- **Incidence/prevalence:** Approximately 9900 new cases of testicular cancer in 2022. Incidence of testicular germ cell tumors increasing in the past two decades. Overall represents 1% of new cancers in males
- **Outcomes:** 5-Year survival in patients with testicular cancer is 95%.
- **Demographics**: Most common solid malignancy in males between ages 15 and 35
- **Risk factors:** Family history, cryptorchidism, testicular dysgenesis, Klinefelter syndrome, previous history of testicular cancer
- **Pathology:** 95% of testicular tumors are germ cell tumors (GCTs), classified as seminoma or nonseminoma. Nonseminomatous tumors consist of varied histologies including embryonal, choriocarcinoma, yolk sac, tumor, and teratomas. Non-GCTs include lymphoma and sex cord-stromal tumors.
- **Serum markers:**
  - **Seminomas:** Mild elevation of β-HCG can be observed (~100 IU/L). Alpha-fetoprotein rarely elevated. LDH may be elevated and is associated with prognosis but is a nonspecific marker.
  - **Nonseminomatous tumors:** Moderate to extreme elevation of β-HCG observed (>10 000 IU/L) in 10-20% of early-stage tumors and 40% of late-stage tumors. Moderate to extreme elevation of alpha-fetoprotein (>10 000 ng/mL), often associated with a yolk sac component. LDH may be elevated and is associated with prognosis but is a nonspecific marker.
- **Imaging:** Hypoechoic mass on testicular transscrotal ultrasound

WORKUP

- **History and physical:** History and examination including testicular. Discussion of sperm banking.
- **Labs:** AFP, β-HCG, LDH, chemistry panel, and CBC. Repeat AFP, β-HCG, and LDH after orchiectomy for staging purposes
- **Procedures/biopsy:** Radical inguinal orchiectomy, consider inguinal biopsy of contralateral testes if indicated. **Note:** Avoid transscrotal procedures as this may alter lymphatic drainage.
- **Imaging:** Testicular ultrasound, CT abdomen/pelvis, chest imaging (chest x-ray or CT of chest)
- **Anatomy:**
  - Testicle surrounded by fibrous tunica layer (tunica vaginalis: outer layer, tunica albuginea: inner layer). Each testicle divided into lobules with multiple seminiferous tubules. Seminiferous tubules drain into the rete testis, which is attached to the spermatic cord via epididymis, which empties into the vas deferens and then the urethra at the prostate. Blood-testis barrier established by tight junctions between Sertoli cells
  - Testicle/scrotum lymph node drainage
    - Testes: Retroperitoneal/para-aortic nodes
    - Scrotum: Inguinal lymph nodes

TREATMENT ALGORITHM—PURE SEMINOMA

All algorithms describe treatment after an initial radical inguinal orchiectomy, preferably a high ligation of the spermatic cord.

Stage IA-IB	• Surveillance (preferred for pT1-T3) • Single-agent carboplatin (AUC = 7 × 1-2 cycles) • EBRT (para-aortic nodes only)
Stage IIA	• EBRT to include para-aortic and ipsilateral iliac nodes • BEP chemotherapy ×3 cycles or EP ×4 cycles
Stage IIB	• BEP ×3 cycles or EP ×4 cycles (primary chemotherapy preferred) • EBRT to include para-aortic and ipsilateral iliac nodes
Stage IIC, III	• BEP ×3-4 cycles or EP ×4 cycles

TREATMENT ALGORITHM—NONSEMINOMA

All algorithms describe treatment after an initial radical inguinal orchiectomy, preferably a high ligation of the spermatic cord.

Stage IA	• Surveillance (preferred) • Nerve sparing retroperitoneal lymph node dissection (RPLND) → postoperative chemotherapy (BEP/EP) for pN2/N3 otherwise surveillance • BEP ×1 cycle
Stage IB	• Surveillance • Nerve-sparing RPLND → postoperative chemotherapy (BEP/EP) for pN2/N3 otherwise surveillance • BEP ×1 cycle

Stage IIA	• Markers negative
	  • Nerve-sparing RPLND → postoperative chemotherapy (BEP/EP) for pN2/N3 otherwise surveillance
	  • BEP ×3 cycles or EP ×4 cycles → RPLND if negative markers and ≥1 cm residual mass otherwise surveillance after chemo
	• Persistent marker elevation
	  • BEP ×3 cycles or EP ×4 cycles → RPLND if negative markers and ≥1 cm residual mass otherwise surveillance after chemo

Stage IIB-III	• BEP ×3 cycles or EP/VIP ×4 cycles → surgical resection of significant masses otherwise surveillance after chemo

RADIATION TREATMENT TECHNIQUE—SEMINOMA

- **SIM:** Headfirst, supine, Med-Tec lower extremities, clamshell contralateral testis
- **Dose:** 20 Gy in 10 fractions to at-risk lymphatics (para-aortic, ipsilateral iliacs) in stages I-II seminoma
  Boost grossly positive lymph nodes ≤3 cm to 26 Gy in 13 fractions and >3 cm to 30 Gy in 15 fractions
- **Target:** Para-aortic lymph nodes in all patients being treated (Fig. 49.1)
  Add ipsilateral iliac lymph nodes (common, internal, external) for "dogleg" field in stage II
  Boost gross nodes with 2-cm margin to block edge for stage II (Fig. 49.2)
- **Technique:** AP/PA with photons or single PA beam with protons
- **IGRT:** Daily kV aligned to bone

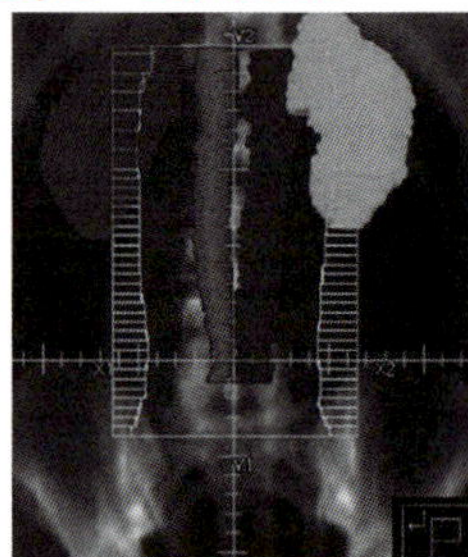

Figure 49.1 Example para-aortic radiation plan utilized to treat stage I patients. (*Wilder et al. IJROBP* 2012).

Field Borders—Dogleg (ie, Para-Aortic and Ipsilateral Iliacs)	
Superior	Bottom of T11
Inferior	Para-aortic—bottom of L5 Ipsilateral iliac—superior acetabulum
Medial	Tip of contralateral transverse process
Lateral	Tip of ipsilateral transverse process Consider covering ipsilateral renal hilum for left-sided tumors

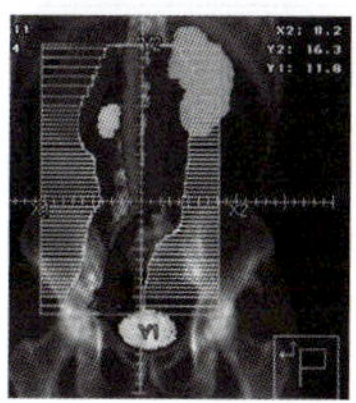

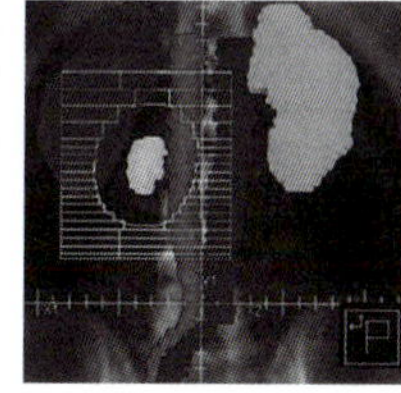

Figure 49.2 Example para-aortic and ipsilateral iliac LN field for a stage II seminoma showing the initial field **(left panel)** and subsequent sequential nodal boost **(right panel)**. (*Wilder et al. IJROBP* 2012).

- **Planning directive:**
  Kidney V20 < 20%

SURGERY

- Radical inguinal orchiectomy with high ligation of spermatic cord is therapeutic, establishes diagnosis, and establishes T stage.
- Nerve-sparing retroperitoneal lymph node dissection used in treatment of some stage IIB or higher seminoma patients and in select nonseminoma tumors.

CHEMOTHERAPY

- **BEP:** Bleomycin 30 units every 21 days, etoposide 100 mg/m^2, cisplatin 20 mg/m^2
- **EP:** Etoposide 100 mg/m^2, cisplatin 20 mg/m^2 every 21 days
- **VIP:** Vincristine 75 mg/m^2, ifosfamide 1200 mg/m^2 every 21 days with mesna 240 mg/m^2 prior to ifosfamide, cisplatin 20 mg/m^2

SIDE EFFECT MANAGEMENT

- Nausea: For prophylaxis, 4-8 mg po 1-2 hours prior to each fraction of RT. For treatment, 8 mg po q8h until 1-2 days after RT completion

FOLLOW-UP

After definitive treatment with adjuvant radiation, chemotherapy, and/or LN dissection

- History and physical, testosterone: Every 6 months for years 1-2, then yearly
- CT of chest/abdomen/pelvis with contrast yearly for 1-3 years after treatment, then as indicated. Can substitute CT chest with chest x-ray
- For nonseminoma, obtain serum markers on the same schedule as history/physical exams.

Active surveillance after orchiectomy without adjuvant therapy

- History and physical, testosterone: Every 2 months for year 1, every 3 months for year 2, and every 4-6 months for years 3-5. Annually after year 5
- CT of chest/abdomen/pelvis with contrast every 4-6 months for years 1-2 and every 6-12 months for years 3-4. Annually thereafter. Can substitute CT chest with chest x-ray
- For nonseminoma, obtain serum markers on the same schedule as history/physical exams.

RELEVANT EVIDENCE

Name/Inclusion	Arms	Outcomes	Notes
MRC TE19/EORTC 30982 (*Oliver et al. J Clin Oncol* 2011) Stage I, pT1-T3, pure seminoma patients with normal postoperative AFP/beta-hCG	Single agent carboplatin (AUC = 7 ×1 cycle) External beam radiotherapy (20 Gy in 10 fx or 30 Gy in 15 fx)	5-y relapse-free survival was not different at 95-96%. Contralateral seminoma was more common in RT arm (5-y incidence: 1.2% vs 0.2%, P = .03)	Most patients (87%) received para-aortic field only. Established the noninferiority of adjuvant carboplatin compared to adjuvant radiotherapy in stage I seminoma

Name/Inclusion	Arms	Outcomes	Notes
MRC TE10 (*Fossa et al. J Clin Oncol* 1999) Stage I, pT1-T3, pure seminoma patients with normal postoperative AFP/beta-hCG	Dogleg field (para-aortic and ipsilateral iliac)—30 Gy in 15 fractions Para-aortic field only—30 Gy in 15 fractions	No difference in 3-y recurrence-free survival (96% in both arms). Four pelvic relapses in para-aortic only arm, no pelvic relapses in dogleg arm	Para-aortic field associated with less acute toxicity and higher sperm counts. Established para-aortic only field as standard treatment for stage I seminoma
MRC TE18 (*Jones et al. J Clin Oncol* 2005) Stage I, pT1-T3, pure seminoma patients with normal postoperative AFP/beta-hCG	Standard dose RT (30 Gy in 15 fractions) Reduced dose RT (20 Gy in 10 fractions)	No difference in 5-y recurrence-free survival (for 20 and 30 Gy: 95% and 97%). All but one relapse occurred within 3 y of treatment	Para-aortic fields were standard, dogleg for prior inguinopelvic or scrotal surgery. Established the dose of radiation in stage I seminoma
Active Surveillance Retrospective Review (*Kollmannsberger et al. J Clin Oncol* 2015) Retrospective review of 2483 stage I seminoma or nonseminoma testicular cancer patients	Active surveillance following orchiectomy	13% of seminoma patients experienced a relapse with vast majority within 3 y. 5-y DSS was 99.7%	Salvage options for recurrent testicular cancer after active surveillance of stage I disease are highly effective and leads to excellent outcomes
SAKK 01/10 (*Papachristofilou et al. Lancet Oncol* 2022) Single-arm, multicenter, phase II trial. Stage IIA or IIB classic seminoma	Single-agent carboplatin (AUC = 7 ×1 cycle) followed by involved-node RT (30 Gy in 15 fractions for stage IIA and 36 Gy in 18 fractions for stage IIB)	3-y PFS was 93.7% which did not meet prespecified target of 95%. Serious adverse events were rare	De-escalated combination therapy with single-agent carboplatin and INRT did not meet primary end point but warrants further study given the favorable side effect profile and high PFS

PENILE CANCER

KEVIN DIAO • SEUNGTAEK CHOI • KAREN E. HOFFMAN

Background

- **Incidence/prevalence:** Rare cancer, approximately 2050 new cases diagnosed in 2023 accounting for 0.4-0.6% of all malignant neoplasms in men.
- **Outcomes:** 5-Year survival is 65%.
- **Demographics:** Higher incidence in Asia, Africa, and South America. Most commonly seen in ages between 50 and 70 years
- **Risk factors:** Increasing age, phimosis, balanitis, chronic inflammation, penile trauma, lack of neonatal circumcision, lichen sclerosus, STDs (particularly HPV types 16 and 18 and HIV), and tobacco use

Tumor Biology and Characteristics

- **Genetics:** Overall about 50% associated with HPV infection, but this varies with histology; oncogenic HPV types (ie, 16, 18, others) result in E6 and E7 suppression of p53 and Rb, respectively.
- **Pathology:** Majority are squamous cell carcinomas (95%).

- **Anatomy:**
  - **Penile shaft:** Consists of skin, subepithelial tissues, corpus cavernosum, and corpora spongiosum, which surrounds the urethra
  - **Head of penis (glans penis):** Primarily consists of an expansion of the corpora spongiosum. Urethral meatus located at the tip. The corona is the proximal rounded surface, which is the junction between the penile shaft and glans.
  - **Lymph node drainage:** Superficial inguinal nodes → deep inguinal nodes → external/internal iliac nodes

Workup

- **History and physical:** Exposure history and examination of the penis and inguinal LNs
- **Labs:** CBC and chemistry panel including calcium
- **Procedures/biopsy:** Punch, excisional, or incisional biopsy of primary lesion. Percutaneous LN biopsy of palpated LNs. If planning for definitive radiation (eg, brachytherapy or external beam), circumcision should always precede RT to prevent radiation-related complications.
- **Imaging:** If palpable inguinal adenopathy then CT or MRI of abdomen and pelvis to evaluate pelvic/inguinal LNs. If no palpable adenopathy routinely CT or MRI utilized for ≥T1b primary tumor, obese patients, and those with prior inguinal surgery

Treatment of the Primary

Most patients are treated with partial or complete penectomy. Limited excisions and laser ablation are appropriate for lower-stage lesions to accomplish organ preservation.

Surgery

- Penile organ-sparing approaches:
- Wide local excision (WLE): Consider for Tis, Ta, T1, and select T2 lesions involving the distal glans penis only
- Mohs surgery: An alternative to WLE in some select patient cases
- Glansectomy: Consider in patients with glans-only tumors; clinical Ta, T1, and select T2 tumors
- Penectomy: Partial or total penectomy. Partial penectomy is sufficient for most distal tumors. Consider total penectomy for large tumors when the remaining phallus would not provide enough length to stand and void.

Radiation therapy for the primary penile tumor may also permit organ preservation.

Interstitial brachytherapy

- **Indication:** Tumor ≤ 4 cm, no deep shaft invasion (<1 cm), ideally confined to the glans, but minor extension across the coronal sulcus is acceptable.
- **Dose:** c/LDR: 60 Gy over 5 days, ~50 cGy/h
  HDR: 3 Gy bid ×5 days
- **Toxicity:** Meatal stenosis (8-25%; especially >50 Gy); tissue necrosis (<20%)

Definitive external beam RT

- **Indication:** T1-2N0
- **Dose:** Shaft: 45-50 Gy
  10-20 Gy boost to primary disease + 2 cm margin
  Consider concurrent cisplatin-containing regime.
- **Target:** GTV, penile shaft
- **Technique:** VMAT. Electrons can be considered for superficial lesions
- **SIM:** Arms on chest holding a bar, frog leg, lower Vac-Lok, rice, wax, or lucite block technique to provide full bolus to penile skin surface (Fig. 50.1). Reproducible setup can be challenging.

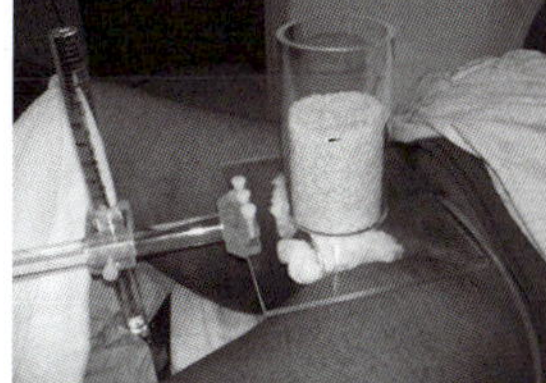

Figure 50.1 Simulation setup for a man receiving primary external beam radiation therapy for penile cancer. Setup shows Vac-Lok device immobilization into a frog-leg position. Rice bolus utilized to ensure dose coverage to the penis surface.

Regional Lymph Node Management

- No palpable or visible nodes pT stage ≥T1b: Dynamic sentinel LN biopsy or superficial inguinal dissection
- Biopsy-proven nodal disease (mobile <4 cm): Complete ipsilateral inguinal LN dissection and modified contralateral dissection → pelvic LN dissection for extranodal metastasis, >2 inguinal LN metastases, or bilateral inguinal LN metastases.
- Among patients with bulky inguinal metastases, inguinal and pelvic LN dissection, chemotherapy, and radiotherapy may be indicated. External beam RT can be used as neoadjuvant treatment to downsize unresectable LNs, definitive treatment instead of LN dissection, as adjuvant treatment after LN dissection for patients at high risk of recurrence, or as palliative treatment. The optimal integration of chemotherapy, chemoradiation, and surgery is being studied in the ongoing International Penile Advanced Cancer Trial (InPACT; NCT02305654).

External beam RT for LN management

- **SIM:** Arms on chest holding a bar, frog leg, and lower Vac-Lok. Consider bolus for superficial LN coverage in thin men.
- **Indication:** Adjuvant radiation considered for N3 disease, ≥3 LNs involved, bilateral positive nodes or ECE
- **Dose:** 60-70 Gy to gross nodes or sites of ECE
  45-50.4 Gy to at-risk inguinal/pelvic node basins and the prepubic fat (Fig. 50.2)
  Concurrent chemotherapy preferred utilizing a cisplatin-containing regime
- **Technique:** VMAT

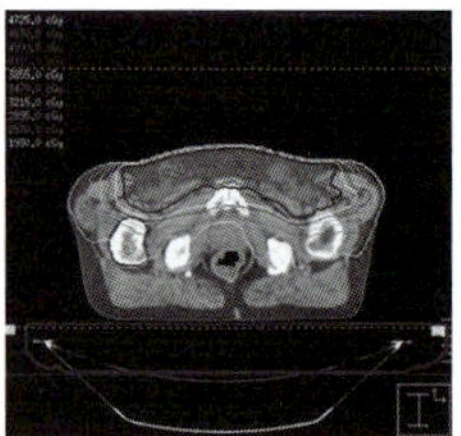

Figure 50.2 Example of neoadjuvant treatment of inguinal LNs and prepubic fat.

Follow-up

- History/physical: Every 3 months for years 1-2, every 6-12 months for years 3-5, and yearly after year 5. CT or MRI of the abdomen/pelvis for LN+ and CT or x-ray chest for N2-3 disease.

Relevant Evidence

Name/Inclusion	Arms (All Nonrandomized)	Outcomes	Notes
Outcomes after definitive organ preservation surgery for invasive penile cancer (*Philippou et al. J Urol* 2012) Retrospective review of 179 patients with invasive penile cancer.	Organ-sparing surgery (including glansectomy, excisions, and distal corporectomy)	With a mean follow-up of 43 mo, the incidence of local, regional, or distant recurrence was 9%, 11%, and 5%, respectively	5-y DSS after recurrence was 55% but for those with isolated local recurrence 5-y DSS was 92%. Surgical margins of <5 mm is adequate

Name/Inclusion	Arms (All Nonrandomized)	Outcomes	Notes
Outcomes after definitive external beam radiation (*Ozsahin et al. IJROBP* 2006) Retrospective review of 60 patients treated with surgery ± postoperative RT or definitive RT	Surgery (*n* = 27) +/− postoperative RT (*n* = 22) Organ sparing treatment, including definitive RT (*n* = 29) and excisional biopsy with refusal of RT (*n* = 4)	Rate of local failure was 13% with surgery vs 56% with organ-sparing (*P* < .001). 73% of local failures salvaged with surgery. 5-y intact penis survival was 43%. No difference in OS w/ surgery or definitive RT (56% vs 53%, *P* = .16).	Local control with primary surgery is superior but this does not translate to a survival difference. Approximately 50% rate of successful organ preservation with definitive RT
Outcomes after definitive brachytherapy (*Crook et al. World J Urol* 2009) Retrospective review of 67 patients with T1-T3 penile cancer	Definitive brachytherapy (PDR or manually-loaded LDR with Iridium-192) with 60 Gy delivered over 4-5 days	5-y local control was 87% and 5-y penile preservation was 88%. 10-y OS 59%, and 10-y CSS was 84%	Late soft tissue necrosis and urethral stenosis rates were 12% and 9%, respectively. Definitive brachytherapy is effective for T1-2 and select T3 penile cancers
Risk factors for regional recurrence (*Reddy et al. BJU Int* 2017) Single-institution, retrospective review of 182 patients	Men who underwent lymph node dissection for penile squamous cell carcinoma	On multivariate analysis, cN3 (HR = 3.53, *P* = .001), ≥3 pathologically involved lymph nodes (HR = 3.78, *P* < .001) and ENE (HR = 3.32, *P* < .001) were associated with worse RFS	Patients with these pathologic features may benefit from adjuvant therapies including chemoRT. This is being prospectively evaluated in the ongoing InPACT Trial (NCT02305654)

KIDNEY CANCER

KEVIN DIAO • CHAD TANG

Background

- **Incidence/prevalence:** Eighth most common cancer in the United States with 79 000 new cases and 13 920 deaths in 2022. Incidence has been steadily increasing (10.2 per 100 000 persons in 1990, 15.8 per 100 000 persons in 2019).
- **Outcomes:** 5-Year overall survival of 76.5% (93% localized, 72% regional metastases, 15% distant metastases)
- **Demographics:** Approximately twice more common in males than females. Median age of diagnosis is 65. Although notable pediatric tumors exist, rare under age 40. Less common among Asian American and Pacific Islanders and more common among American Indian and Alaskan Natives.
- **Risk factors:** Smoking, hypertension, obesity, chronic kidney disease, occupational exposure, chronic analgesic use.

Tumor Biology and Characteristics

- **Genetics:** Less than 5% of all cases due to hereditary syndrome. RCC is associated with pathogenic *VHL*, *BRCA1*, *MET*, *FH*, *FLCN*, and *TSC* mutations, as well as autosomal dominant polycystic kidney disease.

- **Pathology:** Majority renal cell carcinoma (85%) or transitional cell carcinoma (8%). Less common histologies include oncocytomas, collecting duct tumors, and renal sarcomas. Distinct subtypes of RCC include clear cell (80%), papillary (10%), chromophobe (5%), and oncocytic (3%).
- **Anatomy:** The kidneys are in the retroperitoneum with the right kidney displaced inferior and medial compared to the left (T12 to L3) due to presence of the liver. The kidney is covered by the renal capsule, and together with the adrenal gland are surrounded by perirenal fat, renal fascia (Gerota fascia is the anterior renal fascia), and pararenal fat. The renal artery, vein, and ureter attach at the concave medial border of the kidney known as the renal hilum. The kidney consists of an outer cortex and inner medulla formed by nephrons eventually draining into minor calyces, major calyces, the renal pelvis, and ureter.
- Kidney lymph node drainage can be unpredictable, however, most commonly:
  - Right kidney: Renal hilum, paracaval, retrocaval, interaortocaval nodes
  - Left kidney: Renal hilum, para-aortic, preaortic, interaortocaval nodes
- **Imaging:** Typically solid, homogeneous or with areas of necrosis, cystic changes, and/or hemorrhage. Soft tissue density (20-70 HU) on noncontrast CT scan with variable contrast enhancement less than that of the normal renal cortex.

Workup

- **History and physical:** History of kidney function impairment including due to partial or radical nephrectomies. Signs or symptoms of distant metastases (headache, nausea/vomiting, vision changes, cough, dyspnea, bone pain). Palpation of flank and abdomen
- **Labs**: CBC, CMP with creatinine and GFR, LDH, urinalysis. Split function renal perfusion scan
- **Procedures/biopsy:** Most patients with localized disease proceed directly to surgery without biopsy. For those with suspected metastatic disease, biopsy of a metastasis is preferred. Consider biopsy of primary lesion prior to definitive SBRT.
- **Imaging:** Abdominal/pelvic CT scan with and without contrast. CT urography if visualization of the renal pelvis and collecting system is required. Ultrasound may be useful to distinguish a simple cyst from complex cyst or solid tumor. MRI can be considered if CT and ultrasound are inconclusive or the patient is unable to tolerate contrast. Bone scan, CT chest, PET-CT, and/or brain MRI if clinical suspicion for distant metastases

Treatment Algorithm

Stage I (T1a)	• Partial nephrectomy (preferred) • Radical nephrectomy • Ablative therapy (cryotherapy, RFA) • Active surveillance
Stage I (T1b)	• Partial nephrectomy • Radical nephrectomy • Active surveillance (if limited life expectancy)
Stages II-III	• Partial nephrectomy (if solitary kidney, multiple tumors, chronic kidney disease) • Radical nephrectomy (if central tumor, suspected lymph node involvement, or renal vein, IVC, or adrenal gland invasion) • Consider 1 y of adjuvant pembrolizumab for high risk (pT2 + grade 4 or sarcomatoid features, pT3-4, or pN1)
Unresectable or poor surgical candidate	• Ablative therapy, ie, cryotherapy or radiofrequency ablation for smaller masses <3 cm • Definitive stereotactic body radiotherapy (SBRT)
Stage IV	• If oligometastatic (1-5 sites), consider nephrectomy and local therapy to all sites of disease +/− 1 y of adjuvant pembrolizumab • If oligoprogressive (1-3 growing sites) on systemic therapy, consider maintenance on current systemic therapy and definitive radiation to oligoprogressive sites • For polymetastatic patients with favorable risk factors, good performance status, and resectable primary, consider initial cytoreductive nephrectomy followed by systemic therapy • For all other patients, upfront systemic therapy

Radiation Treatment Technique

- **SIM:** Supine, long stereotactic Vac-Lok. Qfix for legs. NPO 3 hours. Arms above head. 4DCT +/− breath hold for >1 cm tumor motion
- **Dose:** 42 Gy in 3 fractions delivered every other day.
- **Target:** Internal gross tumor volume (iGTV) defined on CT sim without contrast fused with diagnostic CT, MR sim, or CT sim with IV contrast + 5 mm planning target volume (PTV)
  - Consider creating multiple PTV substructures each excluding critical OARs that would exceed respective tolerance doses with a 5- to 7-mm PRV margin.
  - iGTV_42 (iGTV minus 7 mm PRV around small bowel, duodenum, stomach, and large bowel)
  - PTV_42 (5 mm iGTV expansion minus 7 mm PRV around small bowel, duodenum, and stomach, and large bowel)
  - PTV_36 (5 mm iGTV expansion minus 5 mm PRV around small bowel, duodenum, and stomach)
  - PTV_26 (uniform 5 mm iGTV expansion)
- **Technique:** SBRT
- **Image guidance:** Daily CT on rails, MR linac, or CBCT align to soft tissue. Ensure critical structures (stomach, duodenum, small bowel, large bowel) are out of high-dose isodose lines.
- **Dose constraints:**
  - Kidney (ipsilateral): V10 < 50% (33% ideal, 10% ideal if solitary kidney)
  - Kidney (contralateral): D_{max} < 10 Gy
  - Small bowel, duodenum, stomach: D_{max} < 28 Gy
  - Large bowel: D_{max} < 40 Gy
  - Abdominal wall/muscle: V25 < 25 cc
  - Spinal cord: D_{max} < 22 Gy
- **Target coverage goals:**
  - Prioritize OAR constraints over target coverage.
  - For PTV_42, PTV_36, and PTV_26, goal V100% > 95%
  - For edited iGTV_42, goal V100% > 98%
  - No specific target goal for unedited iGTV—V100% coverage of 70-80% is not uncommon

Surgery

- **Radical nephrectomy**: Complete removal of the kidney and Gerota fascia with or without the adrenal gland. Involves ligation of the renal artery and vein. Laparoscopic approach is associated with less blood loss and faster recovery time. Radical nephrectomy leads to high rates of long-term CKD (65% with new-onset GFR < 60 mL/min and 36% with GFR < 45 mL/min).
- **Partial nephrectomy**: Preferred approach for smaller (≤7 cm) tumors when technically feasible, especially for patients with preexisting CKD. Robot-assisted laparoscopic approach has longer operative time but less blood loss, shorter hospitalization, and less complications. Partial nephrectomy has lower rates of long-term CKD compared to radical nephrectomy (20% with new-onset GFR < 60 mL/min and 5% with GFR < 45 mL/min).

Systemic Therapy

- **Immunotherapy:** Consider 1 year of adjuvant pembrolizumab in patients with high-risk locoregional disease or oligometastatic disease after metastasectomy occurring within 1 year of nephrectomy. Multiple effective immunotherapy and small molecule TKI combinations exist for advanced or metastatic RCC (pembrolizumab and axitinib or lenvatinib, nivolumab and cabozantinib). Dual checkpoint inhibitor therapy with ipilimumab and nivolumab followed by maintenance nivolumab may also be used. IL-2 no longer commonly used due to high rates of toxicity. mTOR inhibitors (everolimus, temsirolimus) are less effective than other agents but can be considered as a later-line option. Very limited role for conventional chemotherapy for most RCC histologies.

Side Effect Management

- New-onset/worsening chronic kidney disease: Expected reduction in eGFR of 5-15 mL/min depending on dosimetry and time elapsed since RT. Rare to require dialysis after SBRT but possible (<5%, typically with those with baseline eGFR ~30 mL/min).

- Duodenal or peptic ulcer: If suspected, refer to GI for upper endoscopy. When target is close to duodenum or stomach, consider prophylactic proton pump inhibitor (ie, pantoprazole 40 mg po daily) starting with first day of RT and continuing for 6 months afterward.
- Diarrhea: Imodium 2 mg titrating up to a max of 8 pills (16 mg) per day PRN
- Nausea: Zofran 8 mg 1 hour prior to RT fraction for prophylaxis or q8hrs PRN

Follow-up

- Abdominal/pelvic CT with and without contrast every 6 months after SBRT for 3 years and then annually thereafter for 5 years. In patients who cannot tolerate CT contrast, use abdominal/pelvic MRI with and without contrast. H&P, labs, and CT chest annually for 5 years. Individualized follow-up after 5 years but consider abdominal and chest imaging with longer intervals in patients with good performance status.

Relevant Evidence

Name/Inclusion	Arms	Outcomes*	Notes
Single Arm, Nonrandomized Data			
IROCK (*Siva et al. Lancet Oncol* 2022) Nonrandomized individual patient meta-analysis from 12 institutions in 5 countries Localized, de novo primary RCC treated with SBRT, at least 2-y follow-up	Single or multifraction SBRT Single fraction most commonly 25 in 1 fraction and multifraction most commonly 35-48 Gy in 3-5 fractions	Local failure rate of 5.5% at 5 y. Single fraction fewer local failures than multifraction (*P* = .02). Median decrease in eGFR of 14.2 mL/min at 5 y post-SBRT	Biopsy confirmation in 83%. 75% were surgically inoperable, 29% had solitary kidney. 4% required dialysis post-SBRT. Most common failure pattern was distant (5-y FFDM 87.3%)
Definitive radiotherapy in lieu of systemic therapy for oligometastatic RCC (*Tang et al. Lancet Oncol* 2021) Single arm, single institution, phase II trial Metastatic RCC with ≤5 metastatic sites, ≤1 prior line of systemic therapy	SBRT (≤5 fx and ≥7 Gy/fx) or hypofx IMRT (60-70 Gy in 10 fx or 52.5-67.5 Gy in 15 fx) to all sites of metastatic disease without systemic therapy	Median PFS was 22.7 mo and 1-y PFS of 64%. 1-y systemic therapy-free survival of 82%. 20% G2+ and 10% G3+ toxicity rate	All patients received nephrectomy before enrollment. 90% had pretreatment biopsy of a metastatic lesion
SBRT for oligoprogressive metastatic RCC (*Hannan et al. Eur Urol Oncol* 2021) Single arm, single institution, phase II trial Metastatic RCC with ≤3 sites of progression involving ≤30% of all sites, on 1st to 4th line systemic therapy	SBRT to oligoprogressive metastases upfront and longitudinally as long as irradiated sites controlled and overall disease remained oligoprogressive	At median f/u of 10.4 mo, SBRT extended duration of ongoing systemic therapy by >6 mo in 14 (70%) patients. Local control rate was 100%. Median OS not reached	One G3 (5%) GI toxicity. No significant decline in QOL. SBRT can safely extend the duration of systemic therapy in patients with oligoprogressive metastatic RCC

Name/Inclusion	Arms	Outcomes*	Notes
Randomized Data			
KEYNOTE-564 (*Choueiri et al. NEJM* 2021) Phase III, randomized, placebo-controlled trial Locoregional RCC with clear cell component and high risk of recurrence (pT2 + grade 4 or sarcomatoid features, pT3/4, pN1, or M1 with no evidence of disease)	Surgery with negative margins followed by placebo	Pembro significantly improved 2-y DFS (77.3% vs 68.1%, P = .002). Rate of G3+ toxicity was 32.4% with pembro or 17.7% with placebo	6% of patients included were M1 with NED. All subgroups appeared to benefit, though some were too small to draw definitive conclusions
	Surgery with negative margins followed by pembrolizumab q3wk for up to 17 cycles (1 y)		

*Primary study end point underlined

CERVICAL CANCER

LAUREN ANDRING • SHANE STECKLEIN • ANUJA JHINGRAN

Background

- **Incidence/prevalence:** Uncommon in developed countries and incidence continues to decrease. Third most common gynecologic cancer in the United States (14 100 diagnoses, 4280 deaths per year [ACS 2022]). Majority of cases occur in developing countries; 4th most common cancer and cause of cancer-related death in women worldwide [GLOBOCAN 2020].
- **Outcomes:** 5-Year survival across all stages is estimated at 67% (SEER data).
- **Demographics:** Lifetime risk 1 in 142 (0.7%). In the United States, incidence in Hispanic and African-American women are higher than that in non-Hispanic white women.
- **Risk factors:** Infection with high-risk human papillomavirus (HPV; virotypes 16, 18, 31, 33), immunosuppression, smoking, multiparity, early age at coitarche, multiple sexual partners

Tumor Biology and Characteristics

- **Pathology:** 80% are squamous carcinomas and 20% are adenocarcinomas; rare subtypes include neuroendocrine (small cell, large cell, low-grade carcinoidlike). Nearly all squamous and adenocarcinomas are positive for HPV DNA and p16 staining; neuroendocrine cancers are positive for CD56, chromogranin A, and synaptophysin.
- **Imaging:** PET-CT is most accurate for detection of nodal metastasis. MRI pelvis is useful for establishing extent of primary cervical disease; tumor is best visualized on T2-weighted images with intravaginal gel (Fig. 52.1). Lung and liver are the most common sites of metastatic disease.

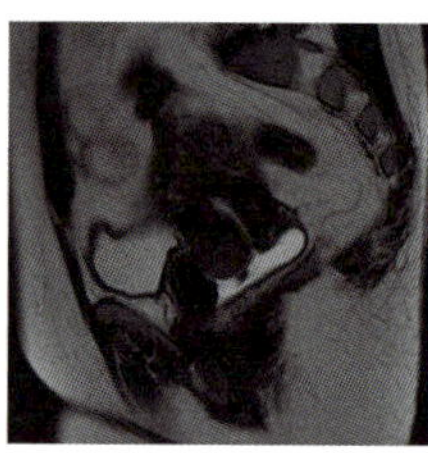

Figure 52.1 MRI T2 sequence in sagittal axis for a patient with a newly diagnosed 3-cm cervical adenocarcinoma of the anterior lip. Note the hyperintense signal in the vagina indicating presence of intravaginal gel, which allows for improved contrast and detection of cervical tissue.

Anatomy

- Cervix is located at the caudal portion of the uterus. Composed of muscle covered by stratified squamous epithelium (ectocervix) or simple columnar epithelium (endocervix)
- Length of endocervical canal is ~2 cm.
- Lymph node drainage:
  - External iliac → common iliac → para-aortic
  - Obturator and internal iliac → common iliac → para-aortic
  - Presacral → para-aortic
  - Tumors that involve the uterine fundus can spread directly to the para-aortic lymph nodes via lymphatics along the gonadal veins.
  - Tumors that involving distal 1/3 of vagina can spread to Inguinal lymph nodes.
  - Tumors invading rectovaginal septum, cul-de-sac, or rectum can spread to perirectal lymph nodes

Workup

- **History and physical:** Presentation may include postcoital bleeding, irregular or heavy vaginal bleeding, vaginal discharge, and lower back or pelvic pain. May be asymptomatic and detected during routine gynecologic examination. Conduct complete pelvic examination including external visualization, digital, speculum, bimanual, and recto-vaginal examination. Fiducial markers should be placed at caudal extent of vaginal disease.
- **Screening:** Women aged 21-65 years should be screened with (Papanicolaou ["Pap"] smear) every 3 years. Consider lengthening screening interval to every 5 years with combination Pap smear and HPV testing for women aged 25-65 years.
- **Labs:** CBC, CMP, and LFTs. Consider HIV testing and pregnancy test.
- **Procedures/biopsy:** Cervical biopsy and cone biopsy as indicated. For advanced stages (stage ≥ IB3), consider examination under anesthesia, cystoscopy, and/or proctoscopy as indicated.
- **Imaging:** PET/CT. Pelvic MRI with intravaginal water-based gel. Chest imaging with chest x-ray or CT chest
- **Referral:** Oncofertility, smoking cessation

Cervical Cancer Staging (*FIGO* 2018)

Note: FIGO cervical cancer staging is based on clinical examination, imaging, and pathology. Pathologic findings supersede imaging and clinical findings.

T Stage	
IA1	Microscopic tumor, confined to cervix, ≤3 mm depth
IA2	Microscopic tumor, confined to cervix, 3-5 mm depth
IB1	Microscopic tumor >IA2, or clinically visible lesion ≤2 cm
IB2	Clinically visible lesion >2 cm ≤4 cm
IB3	Clinically visible lesion >4 cm
IIA1	Involvement of upper 2/3 of the vagina ≤4 cm
IIA2	Involvement of upper 2/3 of the vagina >4 cm
IIB	Involvement of parametria
IIIA	Involvement of distal 1/3 of the vagina
IIIB	Extension to the pelvic sidewall, hydronephrosis, or nonfunctioning kidney
IIIC1	Pelvic lymph node metastasis
IIIC2	Para-aortic lymph node metastasis
IVA	Spread of tumor to adjacent pelvic organs
IVB	Spread of tumor to distant organs

Treatment Algorithm

Stage IA1	Simple (type I) hysterectomy*
Stage IA2-IB2	Modified radical (type II) hysterectomy with pelvic lymphadenectomy*
Stage IB3-IVA	Definitive chemoradiation
Stage IVB	Chemotherapy or best supportive care. Consider definitive therapy for patients with oligometastatic disease

*Motivated women with tumors ≤2 cm may be a candidate for fertility-sparing approaches, which include cone biopsy (stages IA1 and IA2) ± LN dissection or radical trachelectomy (stage IB1) ± LN dissection.

- Indications for postoperative radiotherapy (SedLIS criteria [GOG 92]):
  - At least two of three: LVSI, deep (>1/3) cervical stromal invasion, tumor size >4 cm
- Beyond sedLIS (*Levinson et al. Gyn Onc* 2021)
  - For SCC: LVSI (HR 1.58), size >4 cm (HR 2.67), and DOI (HR 4.31)—DOI most predictive for recurrence
  - For adenocarcinoma: only size >4 cm associated with recurrence (HR 4.69)
- Indications for postoperative chemoradiotherapy (Peters criteria [GOG 109]):
  - Positive margin, positive nodes, positive parametria

Radiation Treatment Technique

- **SIM:** Supine, lower Vac-Lok (add upper Vac-Lok if treating extended fields), arms on chest (above head if treating extended fields), full and empty bladder. Scan from midlumbar spine to midfemur (extend scan superiorly to T10 if treating extended fields). Place isocenter midline, midplane, ~2 cm superior to femoral heads.
- **Dose:**
  - Overall goal is HR-CTV D90 to ≥87 Gy (EQD_2) (EMBRACE), gross lymph nodes to ≥60 Gy (EQD_2), and subclinical nodal volumes to 43-45 Gy (EQD_2).
  - External beam: 45 Gy in 25 fractions at 1.8 Gy/fx (consider 43.2 Gy in 24 fractions at 1.8 Gy/fx for clinically node-negative patients). Boost grossly involved lymph nodes with simultaneous integrated boost to 50 Gy in 25 fractions at 2 Gy/fx, followed by sequential boost to 60-66 Gy. A 5-10 Gy boost to bulky parametrial disease can be considered. If node is 2 cm or less consider SIB to 56 Gy at 2.2 Gy/d (EMBRACE).
  - Initial brachytherapy (BT) dose to the HR-CTV:
    - HDR: 5.5-6 Gy × 5 fractions or 7Gy × 4 fractions ($EQD_{2,\alpha/\beta=10}$ = 40 Gy)
    - LDR/PDR: Generally, ~18-22 Gy × 2 fractions
    - Goal for combined EBRT and BT HR-CTV D90 > 87 Gy (EQD2)
    - Details regarding brachytherapy doses and volumes. See **Brachytherapy** chapter.
    - Consider a hybrid applicator or interstitial needles to shape dose distribution to improve target coverage and decrease dose to OARs (Fig. 52.2).
- **Targets:**

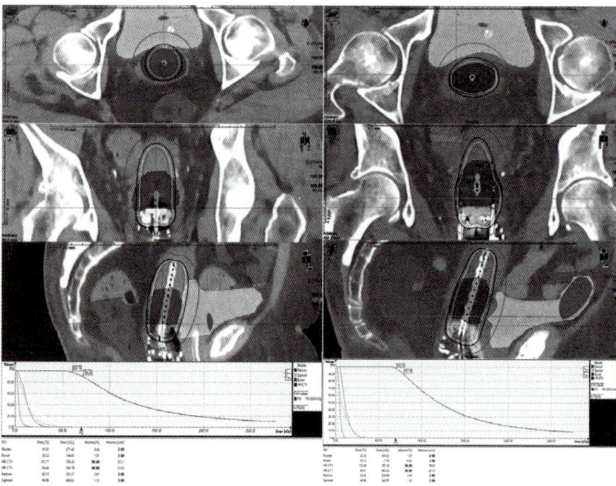

Figure 52.2 Plan comparison: fraction 1 utilizes a fixed intracavitary system with tandem and ovoids, fraction 2 utilizes a hybrid applicator with interstitial needles. **See color insert.**

Definitive Radiotherapy	
External Beam	
Uterocervix ITV	Uterus/cervix (use full/empty bladder scans) + parametria + uterosacral/cardinal ligaments
Pelvic LN CTV	Start at the bifurcation of the aorta (typically L4/L5) or vertebral body above any radiographically involved LNs. Include: obturator, internal/external iliac, presacral, common iliac, +/− para-aortic
PTV = uterocervix ITV + LN CTV + 0.7 cm	
Brachytherapy	
HR-CTV	Entire cervix and any gross residual disease at time of applicator placement

Postoperative Radiotherapy	
External Beam	
Vaginal cuff ITV	Vaginal cuff (full/empty) + parametria remnants
Pelvic LN CTV	Include: obturator, internal/external iliac, presacral, common iliac, +/− para-aortic (Fig. 52.2)
Brachytherapy	Proximal 2-3 cm of vaginal cuff

Considerations: If tumor involves distal 1/3 of the vagina, cover inguinal lymph nodes. If disease invades posteriorly into the rectovaginal septum, cul-de-sac, or rectum, cover the perirectal lymph nodes.

- **IGRT:** Daily kV with weekly CBCT
- **Dose constraints (external beam only)**
  Bladder V45 Gy < 50%
  Rectum V45 Gy < 80%
  Femoral heads V40 < 15%
  Kidney (each) V20 < 33%, mean < 18 Gy
  Small bowel V40 < 30%
  Duodenum V55 < 15 cc, V60 < 2 cc
  Spinal cord < 45 Gy max
- **Dose constraints (brachytherapy; doses include external beam contribution)**
  HR CTV D90% > 87 Gy
  Bladder D2cc < 80 Gy
  Sigmoid D2cc < 75 Gy
  Rectum D2cc < 70 Gy

Chemotherapy

- **Concurrent:** Cisplatin (40 mg/m^2 once weekly) for 5-6 cycles

Side Effect Management

- Diarrhea: Imodium titrating to a maximum of 8 pills/day; schedule Imodium if diarrhea persists on prn dosing → consider alternating Lomotil and Imodium or recommending 1-2 pills before meals and at bedtime → 3rd-line tincture of opium. Rule out other causes of diarrhea, especially if presentation is early during radiation (eg, *Clostridium difficile*).
- Cystitis: UA with culture and sensitivity to rule out UTI. Treat if positive. Pyridium for noninfectious radiation cystitis
- Nausea: 1st-line Zofran (8 mg q8h prn) → 2nd-line Compazine (10 mg q6h prn, can alternate with Zofran) → 3rd-line Emend (aprepitant) → 4th-line ABH (lorazepam 0.34 mg, diphenhydramine 25 mg, and haloperidol 1.5 mg) 1 capsule q6h.

Follow-up

- H&P 1 month after completing radiotherapy, PET-CT 3 months thereafter. Interval H&P every 3-6 months for 2 years, every 6-12 months for 3-5 years, and then annually
- Cervical/vaginal cytology as recommended for detection of lower genital tract neoplasia
- Imaging of para-aortic nodes for patients with positive pelvic nodes who were treated with pelvic RT may be performed to detect salvageable para-aortic recurrences. Additional imaging can be performed based on symptoms or examination findings suggestive of recurrence.
- Vaginal dilators or intercourse 2-3 times per week starting 2-3 weeks after completing radiotherapy to mitigate vaginal stenosis.

NOTABLE TRIALS AND PAPERS

Name/Inclusion	Arms	Outcomes*	Notes
	The Role of Surgery		
Milan (*Landoni et al. Lancet* 1997) 343 patients w/ stage IB-IIA	Radical hysterectomy Definitive RT	5-y PFS and OS better after surgery for adeno (66% vs 47%, $P = .02$) and (70% vs 59%, $P = .05$) No diff for SCC histology	Established role of surgery for early-stage disease, especially adenocarcinoma histology Toxicity > after surgery (28% vs 12%)
ConCerv (*Schmeler et al. Int J Gyncol Canc* 2021) Phase 2 single arm, 100 patients w/ IA2-IB1, DOI < 10 mm, no LVSI, < 2 cm, −margin	44 patients: conization + LN assess 56 patients: simple hyst w/ LN assess	2-y LR 3.5% +LN 5%	Established role for conservative surgery (and potentially fertility sparing) in early stage, low-risk cervical cancer
	Adjuvant Therapy After Surgery		
GOG 92 (*Sedlis et al. Gynecol Oncol* 1999) 277 patients w/ IB and 2 of 3 risk factors: LVSI, >1/3 stromal invasion, and size >4 cm	137 patients: pelvic RT 140 patients: no further treatment (NFT)	LR higher in NFT (28% vs 15%, RR 0.53) Grades 3-4 adverse event 6% in RT vs 2.1% NFT	Established role for postoperative RT if **SedLIS criteria** met
Beyond Sedlis (*Levinson et al. Gyn Onc* 2021) Analysis of GOG 49, 92, 141. Stage I, surgically managed	715 patients w/ SCC, 105 patients w/ adeno	SCC: LVSI (HR 1.58), size >4 cm (HR 2.67), and DOI (HR 4.31) Adeno: size >4 cm (HR 4.69)	Risk factors for recurrence depend on histology. Established nomograms for recurrence
GOG 109 (*Peters et al. JCO* 2000) 268 patients w/ IA-IIA (+LN, +margin, or +PM) post hyst. w/ PLND	127 patients: chemoRT + RT 116 RT alone	PFS and OS improved in chemoRT + RT (HR ~2)	Established role of postoperative CRT if **Peters criteria** met
STARS (*Huang et al. JAMA Oncol* 2021) 1048 patients IB-IIA s/p hyst. w/ risk factors: +LN, +margin, +PM, LVSI, pr >1/3 depth of invasion	350 patients: RT alone 345 patients: concurrent chemoRT (CCRT) w/ cis 353 patients sequential chemoRT (SCRT): (CHT ×2 → RT → CHT ×2)	SCRT associated with best DFS (HR 0.52 vs RT alone, HR 0.65 vs CCRT)	SCRT may provide better DFS compared to CCRT postoperatively
	Concurrent Chemoradiation		
RTOG 9001 (*Eifel et al. JCO* 2004) 386 stage IIB-IVA patients	Extended field radiation Pelvic RT + concurrent cis/5-FU	50% decrease in recurrence w/ CRT. 8-y OS (67% CRT vs 41% RT, $P < .001$)	Established role of definitive chemoRT for advanced disease
Additional chemoRT Trials: *GOG-120, GOG-123, GOG-85, SWOG 8797, NCIC*			Defined role of definitive chemoRT

Name/Inclusion	Arms	Outcomes*	Notes
OUTBACK Trial (*Mileshkin et al. JCO* 2021) Postoperative RT: 919 patients with locally advanced disease	463 patients: chemoRT → adjuvant carbo/taxol ×4	No SS diff in OS or PFS 1-y AE g3-5 higher in adj CHT (81% vs 62%)	No role for adjuvant chemotherapy after chemoRT for locally advanced disease
	456 patients: chemoRT		
CALLA Trial (*Mayadev et al. ASTRO* 2022) Postoperative RT: 770 patients with locally advanced disease	385 patients: chemoRT + durvalumab	No SS diff in PFS (HR = 0.84, *P* = .174)	chemoRT alone remains SOC for locally advanced disease
	385 patients: chemoRT + placebo		
Role of IMRT Postoperative			
NRG-RTOG 1203/ TIME-C (*Klopp et al. JCO* 2018; *Yeung et al. JCO* 2020) Postoperative RT: 234 patients w/ cervical or endometrial ca postoperative requiring RT	RT with 4-field	Less GU and GI patient reported AEs w/ IMRT 18% less diarrhea, 8% less fecal incontinence, 8.5% less interference from fecal intolerance	Established role of IMRT for postoperative RT
	RT with IMRT		
Image-Guided Adaptive Brachytherapy			
EMBRACE-I (*Potter et al. Lancet Oncol* 2021) Prospective, observational, multicenter of patients w/ IB-IVA cerv ca. receiving definitive chemoRT	1341 patients receiving definitive chemoRT w/ MR-guided BT	D90 EQD2 90 Gy 5-y LC: 92% 5-y G3-5 GU events: 6.8%; GI: 8.5%; vaginal: 5.7%	Established the role for MR-guided BT
EMBRACE-II (*Potter et al. ctRO* 2018) Prospective dose and volume prescription protocol			Provides uniform dose, target, technique, and constraint recommendation for MR-guided BT

ENDOMETRIAL CANCER

WENDY MCGINNIS • ANN KLOPP

Background

- **Incidence/prevalence:** Most common gynecologic cancer in high-income countries (65 950 diagnoses and 12 550 deaths in the United States in 2022 [SEER]), second most common gynecologic cancer in low- and middle-income countries, and second most common cause of gynecologic cancer deaths; overall incidence is increasing.
- **Outcomes:** 5-Year survival across all endometrial histologies and stages is estimated at 91% localized, 71% regional, 20% distant, 84% overall (SEER).
- **Demographics:** Lifetime risk 3.1%. Generally, postmenopausal women of 55-85 years old, Caucasian > African American disease prevalence, but African American women have higher mortality rates than other racial groups and are more likely to be diagnosed with high-risk histologies including serous and carcinosarcomas.
- **Risk factors:** Unopposed estrogen (obesity, PCOS, nulliparity, early menarche, late menopause, tamoxifen), DM, Lynch/Cowden syndromes (consider genetic testing if <50 years old with family history of colorectal cancer +/− endometrial cancer)

Tumor Biology and Characteristics

- Histomorphologic classification (historic):
  - Classic histologic subtypes:
    - Type 1: Endometrioid (75-80%), mucinous (1-5%); genomic perturbations in *PTEN*, *KRAS*, *PIK3CA*, *PAX2*, and *CTNNB1* (β-catenin). May be associated with microsatellite instability (MSI)
    - Type 2: Nonendometrioid (10-15%); serous, clear cell, carcinosarcoma (previously malignant mixed müllerian tumor [MMMT]), squamous cell, and undifferentiated); genomic perturbations in *TP53*, *ERBB2* (HER2), *CDKN2A* (p16), and *CDH1* (E-cadherin) and may overexpress EGFR or HER2
  - Uterine sarcoma (5%): Leiomyosarcoma, endometrial stromal sarcoma, and adenosarcoma
- Molecular subtypes: The Cancer Genome Atlas (TCGA) categorization:
  - DNA polymerase epsilon (POLEmut) mutated: Mutations of POLE, gene involved in DNA replication and repair. Commonly high-grade, LVSI, aggressive features in young/thin patients. Highly favorable (>96% 5-year OS; 7-9% of all ECs)
  - MSI "hypermutated" (MMRd): Dysfunctional mismatch repair proteins. Possible benefit to immune checkpoint inhibition. Intermediate outcomes (26-30%)
  - No specific molecular profile (NSMP): Genomically stable, MMR proficient, moderate mutational load. Mostly low-grade EEC with ER, PR positivity, and high response rates to hormonal therapy. Intermediate to favorable outcomes (45-50%)
  - p53 abnormal (p53abn): High somatic copy number alterations and mutational profiles (serous like). Poor prognosis (13-18% of cases but 50-70% of EC mortality)
- **Imaging:** Typical presentation of early-stage disease is a thickened endometrium.

Anatomy

- 1-2 cm muscular uterine wall composed of inner endometrium (epithelial origin), myometrium (mesenchymal origin), and outer serosa (mesenchymal origin)
- Cranial to caudal: *Fundus* is the dome of the uterus which is superior to the opening of the fallopian tubes; *body* is the central portion of uterus; lower uterine segment extending to the *internal cervical os*, which is the constriction in the middle of the uterus above the cervix
- Determining uterine position and degree of flexion is important when sounding for intracavitary brachytherapy. The uterus can be anteverted or retroverted.
- Lymph node drainage:
  - Endometrium has few lymphatics, but subserosa has rich lymphatics, so depth of invasion (DOI) is related to nodal metastases (GOG 33, *Creasman et al. Cancer* 1987).
  - Fundus can drain directly to para-aortics via lymphatics along gonadal vessels and inguinal nodes via round ligament.
  - Fundus and upper body: Hypogastric route
    - Junctional interiliac nodes → common iliac → para-aortic
  - Middle and lower body, internal os: Lateral route to parametrial LNs, then
    - External iliac → common iliac → para-aortic
    - Obturator and internal iliac → common iliac → para-aortic
    - Presacral → para-aortic

Workup

- **History and physical:** Presentation includes vaginal bleeding (classically post-menopause), pelvic pain, and/or dyspareunia. Conduct complete pelvic examination including bimanual examination and rectovaginal exam.
- **Labs:** CBC, CMP, CA125, and LFTs. Consider pregnancy test.
- **Procedures/biopsy:** Endometrial sampling/biopsy—consider dilation and curettage if unable to obtain adequate tissue with endometrial biopsy. Biopsy includes tissue architecture for histology, grading, and LVSI but cannot assess myometrial invasion.
- **Imaging:** Preoperative CXR only for early-stage, low-grade endometrioid endometrial cancer; CT C/A/P or PET-CT if higher risk including FIGO G3, high-risk histology/sarcoma, or suspect extrauterine disease; MRI pelvis if suspected/gross cervical or vaginal involvement

Surgical Staging

- Total extrafascial hysterectomy with bilateral salpingo-oophorectomy, pelvic washings, omental inspection, and lymph node evaluation is standard for EC. Minimally invasive techniques are often employed.

- Options for evaluation of lymph nodes can include pelvic +/− para-aortic (for high-risk features like deep invasion, high-grade, high-risk histology) lymph node dissection or sentinel lymph node biopsy.

GRADE AND STAGING

Note: FIGO uterine cancer staging relies on evaluation of the surgical pathology.

FIGO Grade	
G1	<5% nonsquamous or nonmorular solid growth pattern
G2	5-50% nonsquamous or nonmorular solid growth pattern
G3	>50% nonsquamous or nonmorular solid growth pattern; serous, clear cell, carcinosarcoma, undifferentiated histologies

Molecular Classification	
Good prognosis	POLEmut
Intermediate prognosis	MMRd, NSMP
Poor prognosis	p53abn

Endometrial Cancer FIGO Staging (2023)[a]	
IA1	Limited to endometrial polyp OR confined to endometrium
IA2	Nonaggressive histotype <1/2 myometrial invasion (MI) with ≤ focal LVSI
IA3	Low-grade endometrioid carcinoma limited to uterus and unilateral ovary
IB	Nonaggressive histotypes with ≥1/2 MI and with ≤ focal LVSI
IIA	Invasion of cervical stroma
IIB	Substantial LVSI[b]
IIC	Aggressive histologic types with MI (eg, high-grade histologies)
IIIA1	Spread to ovary or fallopian tube (except if IA3)
IIIA2	Involvement of uterine subserosa or spread through uterine serosa
IIIB1	Vaginal (direct extension or metastasis) and/or parametrial involvement
IIIB2	Metastasis to pelvic peritoneum
IIIC1i	Micrometastasis[a] to pelvic lymph nodes
IIIC1ii	Macrometastasis[a] to pelvic lymph nodes
IIIC2i	Micrometastasis[a] to para-aortic lymph nodes ± pelvic lymph nodes
IIIC2ii	Macrometastasis[a] to para-aortic lymph nodes ± pelvic lymph nodes
IVA	Invades bladder and/or bowel mucosa
IVB	Abdominal peritoneal mets/intraperitoneal carcinomatosis beyond pelvis
IVC	Distant metastases including inguinal lymph nodes and/or peritoneum

[a]Micrometastases defined as ≤2 mm. Macrometastases defined as >2 mm.
[b]As defined in Who 2021: extensive/substantial, at least 5 vessels involved.

TREATMENT ALGORITHM

Operable Endometrioid (Based on FIGO 2009 Staging)			
	Grade 1	Grade 2	Grade 3
IA	Observe	Observe or VBT[a]	VBT
IB	VBT	VBT ± WPRT[a]	WPRT + VBT ± chemo[a]
II	WPRT + VBT		WPRT ± VBT ± chemo[a]
IIIA	Adjuvant chemotherapy ± WPRT with concurrent chemotherapy ± VBT[a]		
IIIB	WPRT with concurrent chemotherapy ± VBT[b] ± adjuvant chemotherapy		
IIIC1	WPRT with concurrent chemotherapy ± VBT + adjuvant chemotherapy. Consider EBRT alone if dMMR		
IIIC2	EFRT with concurrent chemotherapy ± VBT + adjuvant chemotherapy		

Operable Endometrioid (Based on FIGO 2009 Staging)	
IVA	Chemotherapy ± WPRT/EFRT + concurrent chemotherapy ± VBT boost[a]
Other Clinical Scenarios	
Extensive cervical involvement	Preoperative WPRT/EFRT + intracavitary brachytherapy (ICBT) → surgery vs radical hysterectomy if negative margins can be achieved
Vaginal involvement	Preoperative WPRT/EFRT + ICBT → surgery vs definitive chemoRT. If distal vagina involved, need to include inguinal nodes
Adnexal involvement	Chemotherapy with RT recommended based on relative risk factors for local recurrence
Inoperable	WPRT/EFRT + ICBT (like cervical cancer with HR-CTV including endometrial target) with consideration of chemotherapy; consider ICBT alone or progestin IUD trial if early stage
Uterine sarcoma	Generally simple hysterectomy and BSO, consider ovarian preservation in young patients with early-stage disease; role of chemotherapy and radiation is limited.
Other high-risk histologies	Consider the addition of concurrent chemotherapy and adjuvant chemotherapy if not otherwise planned due to stage.
Fertility-sparing	For very low risk (G1 endometrioid adenocarcinoma, limited to endometrium on MRI) can consider 3-6 mo trial of megestrol/ medroxyprogesterone/ progestin IUD and weight management/ lifestyle modification followed by repeat biopsy. If CR → encourage conception w/ sampling q6 mo → TH/BSO with staging after child-bearing complete. Must counsel patients that this strategy is not standard of care.

[a]Consider high-risk factors including substantial LVSI, especially without nodal assessment. Intermediate-risk factors including age >60 years, focal LVSI, large tumor, lower uterine involvement, cervical glandular involvement; EBRT for inadequate LND or >20% risk on Mayo Clinic nomogram (*Alhilli et al. Gyn Oncol* 2013).
[b]May require interstitial brachytherapy if patient had thick or extensive disease at presentation.
VBT, vaginal brachytherapy; WPRT, whole pelvic radiation therapy; EFRT, extended-field radiation therapy.

Chemotherapy

- **Concurrent:** Cisplatin (50 mg/m^2 once weekly) for 2 cycles. Consider weekly paclitaxel for serous carcinoma (50 mg/m^2 once weekly).
- **Adjuvant:** Carboplatin (AUC 5-6 mg min/mL) and paclitaxel (175 mg/m^2) for 3-4 cycles and consider adding pembrolizumab or dostarlimab.

Radiation Treatment Technique

- **SIM:** Supine, arms on chest holding A-bar (above head holding T-bar for EFRT), lower Vac-Lok (add upper Vac-Lok for EFRT), legs straight. Scan full and empty bladder to identify an ITV, from T12 to midfemur (from T10 for EFRT). Isocenter midline, midplane, ~2 cm superior to femoral heads
- **Dose (Fig. 53.1):**
  - EBRT: 45-50.4 Gy in 25-28 fractions at 1.8 Gy/fx. Boost grossly involved lymph nodes to 60-66 Gy. 40 Gy in 2 Gy/fx for patients receiving EBRT without chemotherapy.
  - HDR VBT for prophylaxis: 6 Gy × 5 fractions prescribed to the vaginal surface ($EQD_{2,\alpha/\beta=10}$ = 40 Gy) for VBT alone, 5 Gy × 2 fractions ($EQD_{2,\alpha/\beta=10}$ = 12.5 Gy) with WPRT/EFRT to 45 Gy

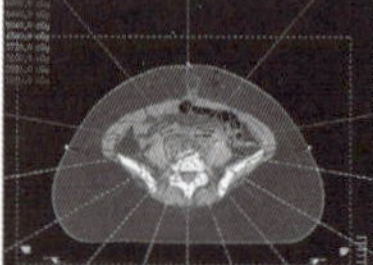
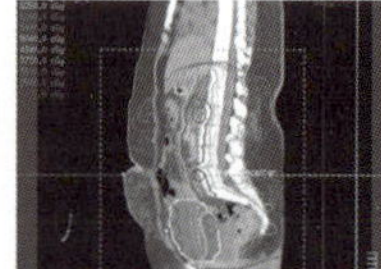
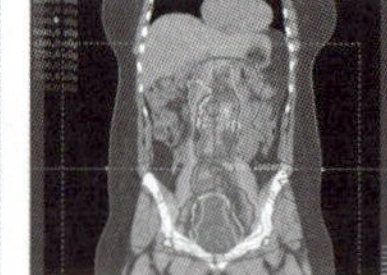

Figure 53.1 Extended-field IMRT (EFRT) plan. *Blue isodose line* representing 50.4 Gy is seen covering nodal CTV and vaginal ITV (*red colorwash*). *Red isodose line* representing 60 Gy is SIB to involved LN. **See color insert.**

- **Targets:**

ITV for Vaginal Cuff	
Include upper 2/3 of vaginal cuff (lower border at the bottom of obturator foramen) and any paravaginal or retracted parametrial tissue. Generate with full and empty bladder.	
CTV for Pelvic Lymph Nodes	
Superior extent at L4/L5. Extend at least 1.5-2 cm or one vertebral body superior to any radiographically involved LNs.	
Include common iliac, external iliac, and internal iliac (hypogastric and obturator).	
Stop external iliac nodes as the external iliac vessels cross the medial portion of the acetabulum or enter the inguinal canal.	
Stop internal iliac nodes as vessels turn laterally before leaving pelvis.	
Stop obturator nodes once vessels leave through obturator foramen.	
Cover presacral space down to S2/S3.	
Special Considerations	
Para-aortic involvement (pathologic or radiographic) or high microscopic risk	Start 1-1.5 cm superior to the left renal vessels (approx. T12) Consider MAG3 renal function scan
Cervical involvement	Cover presacral space to S3/S4
Involvement of distal 1/3 vagina	Add medial inguinal lymph nodes
Posterior involvement to rectovaginal septum, cul-de-sac, or rectum	Add perirectal lymph nodes
Significant rectal gas on sim scan	Extend vaginal ITV to cover rectum
PTV = Vaginal ITV + Pelvic LN CTV + 7 mm	

- **VBT:** Vaginal cuff and proximal ~2 cm of the vagina
  - See **Brachytherapy Chapter** for more details regarding brachytherapy.
- **Technique:** IMRT/VMAT (Fig. 53.1)
- **IGRT:** Weekly CBCT or CT-on-rails, daily kV imaging
- **Dose constraints:**

EBRT	EBRT + Brachy for Intact Uterus
Bladder V45 Gy < 50%	Bladder D2cc < 80 Gy EQD2*
Rectum V45 Gy < 80%	Sigmoid D2cc < 70 Gy EQD2*
Small bowel V40 < 30%	Rectum D2cc < 70 Gy EQD2*
Duodenum V55 < 15 cc, V60 < 2 cc	
Kidney (each) V20 < 33%, V15 < 50%	
Femoral heads V40 < 15%	
Spinal cord <45 Gy	
Bone marrow (V10 Gy < 90%, V40 Gy < 37%)	

*Cumulative EQD_2, including EBRT

Side Effect Management

See Cervical Cancer chapter.

Follow-up

- Physical examination, CT A/P, and CXR q3mo for 2 years, q6mo for 3 years, then annually thereafter
- Vaginal dilators or intercourse 2-3 times per week starting 2-3 weeks after completing radiotherapy to mitigate vaginal stenosis

Notable Trials

Name/Inclusion	Arms	Outcomes*	Notes
		WPRT vs Obs	
PORTEC 1 (*Creutzberg Lancet* 2000; *Creutzberg IJROBP* 2011) 714 stage IB (G2-3) and IC (G1-2) EC s/p TAH-BSO w/o LND	Observation WPRT (46 Gy/23 fx)	Improved 15-y LRR with WPRT (16%) vs Obs (6%); 15-y OS similar with WPRT (52%) vs Obs (60%). Late complications 26% vs 4%	Post hoc high-intermediate risk (HIR) criteria include G3, age >60 y, and MI > 50%
GOG 99 (*Keys et al. Gynecol Oncol* 2004) 392 IB, IC, occult IIA-B EC s/p TAH-BSO HIR = G2-3, LVSI, 2/3 MI	Observation WPRT (50.4 Gy/28 fx)	Recurrence free interval improved with RT (HR 0.42). In HIR subgroup, 2-y LR 6% vs 26%. OS similar	HIR benefit from adjuvant therapy. Most recurrences occur within 18 mo
		VBT vs WPRT	
PORTEC 2 (*Nout Lancet* 2010) 427 stage I-IIA HIR EC s/p TAH-BSO Noninferiority RCT	WPRT (46 Gy/23 fx) VBT to proximal ½ of vagina (HDR 7 Gy × 3 or LDR 30 Gy Rx to 5 mm)	10-y vaginal recurrence similar (3.4% VBT vs 2.4% WPRT). More pelvic recurrence in VBT (6.3%) vs WPRT (0.9%) G1-2 GI toxicity lower in VBT (13%) at end of RT vs WPRT (54%)	Considered to show noninferior to WPRT. Set standard of VBT for HIR patients
GOG 249 (*Randall et al. JCO* 2019) 601 high-risk stages I-II endometrial, serous, or clear cell EC s/p TAH or TLH ± BSO ± LND	WPRT ± VBT VBT + chemotherapy (carboplatin/ paclitaxel × 3)	60-mo RFS with WPRT (0.76) vs VBT/C (0.76). Worse acute toxicity and more nodal recurrences with VBT/C (9% vs 4%)	VBT/C not superior to WPRT and showed worse acute toxicity
		ChemoRT vs RT	
PORTEC 3 (*de Boer et al. Lancet Oncol* 2019) 686 patients with HR IA-IIIC EC s/p TAH or TLH ± BSO ± LND	WPRT/concurrent Cis ×2 ± VBT (48.6 Gy/27 fx) → Carbo/Taxol × 4 WPRT ± VBT (48.6 Gy/27 fx)	Chemo improved OS (81.4% vs 76.1%), FFS (76.5% vs 69.1%), and DM (21% vs 29%) at 5-y. G3+ AE in 60% of chemoRT vs 12% RT alone	On subgroup analysis, benefit seen mainly with stage III, serous, and p53abn disease
NSGO-EC-9501/ EORTC-55991 + MaNGO ILIADE-III (*Hogberg et al. Eur J Cancer* 2010) Pooled analysis of two RCTs of 534 with stages I-III endometrial cancer with high-risk features s/p TAH/BSO ± LND	WPRT (45 Gy/25 fx) → chemo WPRT (45 Gy/25 fx)	Pooled analysis showed improved PFS (69% vs 78%) with chemo/RT and trend toward improved OS	On subgroup analysis, primary benefit seen in serous/ clear cell not endometrioid disease

Name/Inclusion	Arms	Outcomes*	Notes
ChemoRT vs chemo			
GOG 258 (*Matei et al. NEJM* 2019) 736 stage III-IVA or stage I-II clear cell or serous s/p TH-BSO ± LND	WPRT/concurrent Cis (45 Gy/25 fx) ± VBT Carbo/taxol ×4	RFS similar (59% vs 58%), but chemoRT decreased vaginal recurrence (2% vs 7%) and pelvic/PA LN recurrence (11% vs 20%)	ChemoRT had less vaginal and nodal recurrences, but more DM. Chemo alone had higher toxicity
Chemo vs Chemo-IO			
NRG-GY018 (*Eskander et al. NEJM* 2023) 816 stage III with residual disease, IVA, IVB, or recurrent EC Stratified by MMR status	Carbo/taxol + placebo → placebo × 14 Carbo/taxol + pembro → pembro × 14	Pembrolizumab substantially improved PFS at 12 mo in dMMR (38% vs 74%) as well as extended median PFS in pMMR (8.7 vs 13.1 mo)	
RUBY trial (*Mirza et al. NEJM* 2023) 494 advanced stage III, IV, or recurrent EC Stratified by MMR-MSI status, prior EBRT, stage	Carbo/taxol + placebo → placebo × 3 y Carbo/taxol + dostarlimab ×6 → dostarlimab × 3 y	Among dMMR-MSI-H (24% of included patients), dostarlimab dramatically improved PFS (16% vs 61%) at 24 mo Benefit also seen in overall group PFS (36% vs 18%) and OS (56% vs 71%)	
Lymph Node Evaluation			
MRC ASTEC (*ASTEC study group Lancet* 2009) 1408 EC confined to corpus	TH + BSO + peritoneal washings + PA LN palpation Above + LND	LND did not improve RFS or OS	
FIRES (*Rossi et al. Lancet Oncol* 2017) Prospective cohort 385 stage I EC	SLN mapping → pelvic LND ± PA LND	SLNB detected 97% of positive nodes in patients with successful mapping	
WART vs Chemo			
GOG 122 (*Randall et al. JCO* 2006) 396 stage III-IV EC s/p TAH-BSO	WART (30 Gy/10 fx + 15 Gy boost) Doxorubicin/cisplatin × 7 cycles → cisplatin × 1 cycle	Improved 5-y PFS (50% vs 38%) and OS (55% vs 42%) in chemo arm. G3-4 heme toxicity worse with chemo (88% vs 14%)	
RT Modalities			
TIME-C (NRG RTOG 1203; *Yeung et al. JCO* 2022) 289 cervical and endometrial patients receiving postoperative WPRT	3DCRT IMRT	3-y GU toxicity worse with 3DCRT. GI toxicity worse at 1 y with 3DCRT but similar at 3 y	IMRT improves patient-reported GI and GU adverse events compared to 3DCRT

*Primary study end points underlined

VAGINAL CANCER

LAUREN ANDRING • SHANE STECKLEIN • ANUJA JHINGRAN

BACKGROUND

- **Incidence/prevalence:** Least common of all gynecologic cancers (<1500 vaginal cancers diagnosed each year in the United States)
- **Outcomes:** 5-Year survival across all stages is estimated at 50% (SEER data).
- **Risk factors:** Infection with high-risk human papillomavirus (HPV; detected in 75% of vaginal cancers), immunosuppression, early age at coitarche, multiple sexual partners, smoking, increasing age

TUMOR BIOLOGY AND CHARACTERISTICS

- **Pathology:** 80-90% of all vaginal cancers are squamous. Adenocarcinomas classically associated with in utero exposure to diethylstilbestrol (DES), but DES-associated adenocarcinomas are now exceedingly rare. Vaginal adenocarcinoma associated with higher risk of in-field failure and higher risk of distant metastasis. Other rare subtypes include neuroendocrine cancers and melanoma.

ANATOMY

- The average vaginal length is 7-10 cm. Most vaginal cancers arise in the upper vagina.
- Lymph node drainage:
  - Proximal vaginal cancers share the same pattern of spread as cervical cancers:
    - External iliac → common iliac → para-aortic
    - Obturator and internal iliac → common iliac → para-aortic
    - Presacral → para-aortic
  - Distal vaginal cancers may spread through the inguinal lymph nodes similar to vulvar cancers.
  - Invasion of the rectovaginal septum, cul-de-sac, or rectum warrants coverage of the perirectal lymph nodes.

WORKUP

- **History and physical:** Presentation includes postcoital bleeding, irregular or heavy vaginal bleeding, vaginal discharge, pelvic pain, painful/frequent urination.
- **Labs:** CBC, CMP. Consider pregnancy test.
- **Procedures/biopsy:** Lesion biopsy. Examination under anesthesia (EUA) with fiducial placement is critical prior to initiating treatment to delineate extent and location of initial disease to facilitate boost planning.
- **Imaging:** CT abdomen and pelvis and PET-CT (most sensitive) to evaluate for inguinal, pelvic, and para-aortic lymphadenopathy. The vagina is poorly visualized on CT; pelvic MRI with intravaginal gel is the modality of choice for imaging the primary tumor.
- **Referral:** Oncofertility

VAGINAL CANCER STAGING *(FIGO 2012)*

Note: FIGO vaginal cancer staging is based on clinical exam, which does not include many imaging modalities or surgical findings. It allows the following diagnostic tests to determine stage: physical exam, proctoscopy, and cystoscopy. Plain chest radiograph and skeletal radiograph to evaluate for metastases

Clinical Stage	
I	Tumor limited to the vaginal wall
II	Tumor involves the subvaginal tissue but does not extend to the pelvic sidewall
III	Tumor extends to the pelvic sidewall and/or presence of pelvic and/or inguinal lymph node metastasis
IVA	Tumor invades bladder and/or rectal mucosa and/or directly extends beyond the true pelvis
IVB	Spread to distant organs

TREATMENT ALGORITHM

Stage I	Primary surgical resection may be considered but is rarely used
Stage I-IVA	Definitive radiotherapy or chemoradiotherapy
Stage IVB	Chemotherapy or best supportive care. Consider definitive therapy for patients with oligometastatic disease

RADIATION TREATMENT TECHNIQUE

- **SIM:** Supine, frog-leg (if treating inguinal lymph nodes), lower Vac-Lok (add upper Vac-Lok if treating extended fields), arms on chest (above head if treating extended fields). Acquire scans with full and empty bladder. Scan from mid-lumbar spine to mid-femur (extend scan superiorly to T10 if treating extended fields). Place isocenter mid-line, mid-plane, ~2 cm superior to femoral heads.
- **Dose:** If feasible, goal is to treat the tumor with 1- to 2-cm margin to a cumulative dose of 75-90 Gy (EQD_2) using a combination of external beam radiotherapy and interstitial (or intracavitary if original tumor was <7 mm thick) brachytherapy. For some apical lesions where brachytherapy cannot be used, external beam boost to cumulative dose of ~66 Gy may be employed.
- **Targets:** Vagina and paravaginal tissues (ITV), with at least 3-cm distal margin on gross disease, obturator, internal iliac, external iliac, presacral, common iliac, ± inguinal, ± para-aortic lymph nodes
- **Technique:** IMRT/VMAT, to reduce dose to the central pelvis
- **IGRT:** Daily kV imaging with weekly CBCT

CHEMOTHERAPY

- **Concurrent:** Cisplatin (40 mg/m^2 once weekly) for 5-6 cycles; use is extrapolated from cervical cancer data

SIDE EFFECT MANAGEMENT

- Dermatitis: Aquaphor for radiation dermatitis, hydrogel for areas of moist desquamation. Important to encourage hygiene early in treatment course to prevent bacterial and fungal infection; Domeboro Sitz bath 2-3 times daily. If erythema and pain are out of proportion to expected dermatitis, suspect fungal overgrowth and treat empirically with fluconazole.
- Diarrhea: 1st-line Imodium titrating to a max of 8 pills/d; schedule Imodium if refractory on prn dosing → 2nd-line alternating Lomotil 2 pills and Imodium 2 pills every 3 hours → 3rd line tincture of opium
- Cystitis: UA with culture and sensitivity to rule out UTI. Treat if positive. Pyridium for noninfectious radiation cystitis
- Nausea: 1st-line Zofran (8 mg q8h prn) → 2nd-line Compazine (10 mg q6h prn) → 3rd-line Emend (aprepitant) → 4th-line ABH (lorazepam 0.34 mg, diphenhydramine 25 mg, and haloperidol 1.5 mg) 1 capsule q6h

FOLLOW-UP

- Vaginal dilators or intercourse 2-3 times per week after the vagina has healed to mitigate vaginal stenosis
- Interval H&P every 3-6 months for 2 years, then every 6-12 months for 3-5 years, then annually
- Cervical/vaginal cytology as recommended for detection of lower genital tract neoplasia
- Imaging based on symptoms or examination findings suggestive of recurrence

Notable Trials and Papers

Name/Inclusion	Arms	Outcomes	Notes
		Squamous cell carcinoma	
MDACC Experience (*Frank et al. IJROBP 2005*) Retrospective review	193 patients w/ SCC vaginal ca. treated w/ definitive EBRT + BT	5 y DSS 85% (Stg I), 78% (Stg II), 58% (Stg III-IVA) 5-year major complications: 4% (Stg I), 9% (Stg II), 21% (Stg III-IVA)	Patients treated with definitive EBRT + BT have good disease outcomes
		Adenocarcinoma	
MDACC Experience (*Frank et al. Gynecol Oncol 2007*) Retrospective review	26 patients w/ non–DES-related adeno vaginal ca. treated w/ definitive RT	5 y OS 34% (vs 58% SCC) Worse pelvic control and more DM	Adeno histology is associated with worse disease outcomes
		Brachytherapy	
NCDB analysis (*Rajagopalan et al. PRO 2015*)	1530 women with vaginal ca.	BT boost declined from 88% in 2004 to 69% 2011, w/ increased IMRT boost	Showed declining utilization of BT boost for vaginal cancer

Additional guidance: Eifel and Klopp. *Gynecologic Radiation Oncology: A Practical Guide.* Wolters Kluwer; 2016.

VULVAR CANCER

WENDY MCGINNIS • ANUJA JHINGRAN

Background

- **Incidence/prevalence:** Less common gynecologic malignancy with 6470 new cases and 1670 deaths in the United States in 2022 (ACS). Lifetime risk estimated at 0.3%
- **Outcomes:** 5-Year survival 85% localized, 52% regional, all cases 72% (SEER)
- **Demographics:** Average age at diagnosis 68 years
- **Risk factors:** Prior infection with high-risk human papillomavirus (HPV; detected in 50% of vulvar cancers—favorable), immunosuppression, smoking, increasing age, chronic inflammation (eg, lichen sclerosis)

Tumor Biology and Characteristics

- **Pathology:** >75% of all vulvar cancers are squamous cell carcinoma with keratinizing more common (older patients) and warty associated with HPV (younger patients). Adenocarcinoma accounts for most of the remaining epithelial neoplasms. Other rare subtypes include neuroendocrine cancers and melanoma.

Anatomy

- Vulvar cancers can arise from the prepuce, clitoris, labia majora or minora (70% of cases), urethral opening, Bartholin and Skene glands (more likely to be adenocarcinoma), or perineum.
- Lymphatic spread can occur early in disease course. Lymph node drainage:
  - Inguinal → external iliac → common iliac → para-aortic
  - Locally advanced tumors that involve the anus, rectum, or rectovaginal septum may also spread through the internal iliac, presacral, and perirectal lymph nodes.

Workup

- **History and physical:** Presentation includes vulvar lesion/mass or bleeding, pruritus, discharge, dysuria, or pain. Complete pelvic exam including rectovaginal plus inguinal and supraclavicular LN exam. Assess for ability to tolerate treatment and co-occurring HPV-related disease (cervical, vaginal, anal: ~15% of patients). Consider photos.
- **Labs:** CBC, CMP, LFTs, HIV ± β-HCG
- **Procedures/biopsy:** Biopsy of grossly visible lesion(s) and/or radical local excision with HPV testing. Vulvar colposcopy (r/o multifocal disease), cytology, and colposcopy of cervix and vagina (r/o co-primary). Consider EUA with fiducial placement for vaginal involvement, cystoscopy, or proctoscopy as indicated.
- **Imaging:** Pelvic MRI for primary. CT abdomen and pelvis or PET-CT if locoregionally advanced. Consider groin US (most accurate) ± FNA if suspicious nodes.

Vulvar Cancer Staging *(FIGO 2021)*

Note: FIGO vulvar cancer staging is a hybrid of a clinical and surgical staging approach, which includes physical examination, imaging studies, and evaluation of the surgical pathology.

Clinical Stage	
IA	Tumor size ≤2 cm and stromal invasion ≤1 mm[a]
IB	Tumor size >2.0 cm or stromal invasion >1 mm[a]
II	Tumor of any size with extension to adjacent perineal structures (lower 1/3 of urethra, lower 1/3 of vagina, or lower 1/3 of anus)
IIIA	Tumor of any size with extension to upper 2/3 urethra, upper 2/3 vagina, bladder mucosa, rectal mucosa, or regional[b] LN metastases ≤5 mm
IIIB	Regional[b] LN metastases >5 mm
IIIC	Regional[b] LN metastases with ECE
IVA	Disease fixed to pelvic bone, or fixed or ulcerated regional[b] lymph node mets
IVB	Distant metastases

[a]Stromal invasion measures intact basement membrane to deepest point of invasion.
[b]Regional = Inguinal and femoral LN

Treatment Algorithm

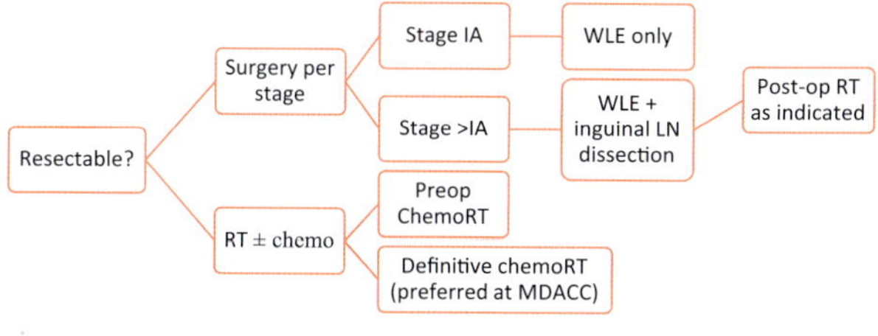

<table>
<tr><td>Stage IA
(≤1 mm invasion)</td><td>Primary: Radical WLE (goal margins 1-2 cm)
• Re-excision preferred for positive margins
Nodes: Can omit groin evaluation for microinvasive disease if no additional risk factors</td></tr>
<tr><td>Stage IB-II
(resectable)</td><td>Primary: Radical WLE (goal margins 1-2 cm)
• Re-excision preferred for positive margins
• Positive margins (additional surgery not feasible) → adjuvant radiotherapy to resection bed and vulva. Add chemo for gross residual, large primary, or LN+
• Consider adjuvant RT for additional risk factors: multifocal disease, dVIN, recurrent disease, LVSI, negative but close margins (≤3-5 mm; controversial), tumor size >4 cm, and >5 mm stromal invasion
Nodes: SLNB (IB) or inguinofemoral lymphadenectomy (II)
• Ipsilateral groin eval for cN0, small (<4 cm), well-lateralized (≥2 cm from vulvar midline) tumors
• If ipsilateral sentinel node does not map → ipsilateral inguinofemoral lymph node dissection
• If ipsilateral SLN macromet → bilateral groin dissection
• If SLN ITC or micromet (<2 mm) → consider adjuvant RT +/− chemo instead of LND (controversial)</td></tr>
<tr><td>LN+
(resectable)</td><td>Primary: See stage IB-II.
Nodes: Bilateral inguinofemoral groin dissection
• Add adjuvant pelvic and inguinal RT for presence of ECE and/or ≥2 involved groin nodes
• Consider observation if only 1 LN+ without risk factors</td></tr>
<tr><td>Unresectable (organ-sparing surgery unlikely to achieve clear margins)</td><td>• Definitive chemoradiation can be employed for patients with unresectable primary or nodal disease
• Treat groin nodes definitively in cases where primary is advanced</td></tr>
</table>

Radiation Treatment Technique

- **SIM:** Supine, frog-leg, lower Vac-Lok (add upper Vac-Lok if treating extended fields), arms on chest (above head if treating extended fields). Radio-opaque markers around lesion, urethra, clitoris, anal verge. Scan with and without bolus. Scan from mid–lumbar spine to mid-femur (extend scan superiorly to T10 if treating extended fields). Place isocenter mid-line, mid-plane, ~2 cm superior to femoral heads.
- **Dose prescribed to volume at risk:**

Adjuvant treatment:

<table>
<tr><td rowspan="4">Vulva</td><td>Margins >5 mm</td><td>45-50 Gy</td></tr>
<tr><td>Margins >1-2 mm but ≤5 mm</td><td>50-54 Gy</td></tr>
<tr><td>Margins <1-2 mm</td><td>54-56 Gy</td></tr>
<tr><td>Positive margins or gross residual disease</td><td>≥60 Gy</td></tr>
<tr><td rowspan="4">Nodes</td><td>Microscopic disease, no ECE</td><td>45-50 Gy</td></tr>
<tr><td>Enlarged nodes, but no ECE</td><td>50-56 Gy</td></tr>
<tr><td>ECE</td><td>60-66 Gy</td></tr>
<tr><td>Gross residual disease</td><td>60-70 Gy</td></tr>
</table>

Definitive treatment:

<table>
<tr><td>Vulva</td><td>Unresectable primary lesion</td><td>60-66 Gy</td></tr>
<tr><td rowspan="4">Nodes</td><td>Suspicious nodes <1 cm</td><td>56-60 Gy</td></tr>
<tr><td>Suspicious nodes 1-2 cm</td><td>60-66 Gy</td></tr>
<tr><td>Suspicious nodes >2 cm</td><td>64-70 Gy</td></tr>
<tr><td>Bulky or fixed nodes</td><td>66-70 Gy</td></tr>
</table>

- Initial external beam treatment: 45 Gy in 25 fractions at 1.8 Gy/fx (consider simultaneous integrated boost to gross disease and/or high-risk clinical target volume(s) to 50-52.5 Gy)

- Boosts: Sequentially boost gross disease and/or high-risk clinical target volume(s) to target dose(s) using external beam treatment at 1.8-2.0 Gy/fx.
- Targets:

CTV primary	
Scenario	**Volume**
Adjuvant (close/positive margin)	Vulva and tumor bed with at least 2 cm margin
Definitive	GTV (delineated based on clinical exam + MRI) + entire vulva + 1 cm margin on any disease outside of vulva Include 3 cm margin on vaginal involvement and 2 cm margin on anorectal, urethral, or bladder involvement
CTV lymph nodes	
N0	Nodal target should extend to bottom of the sacroiliac (SI) joint or the bifurcation of the common iliac
Positive inguinal LN	Raise superior border to the mid-SI joint. Treat bilaterally.
Positive pelvic LN	Raise superior border to the aortic bifurcation
Positive common iliac LN	Consider adding low para-aortic nodes
Positive para-aortic LN	Entire para-aortic nodal CTV should be treated
Proximal ½ vaginal involvement	Add pre-sacral LN (S1-S3)
Anal/anal canal involvement	Add perirectal (including mesorectum) and pre-sacral LN

- **Technique:** IMRT/VMAT, to reduce dose to the central pelvis and mons pubis. Plan with false structure. TLDs at first fraction(s) to ensure adequate dose (Fig. 55.1) – consider evaluation ± bolus.
- **IGRT:** Daily kV imaging
- **Dose constraints (external beam)**
  Bladder V45 Gy < 50%
  Rectum V45 Gy < 80%
  Femoral heads V40 < 15%
  Kidney (each) V20 < 33%, V15 < 50%
  Small bowel V40 < 30%
  Duodenum V55 < 15 cc, V60 < 2 cc
  Spinal cord < 45 Gy max
  Bone marrow V10 Gy < 90%, V40 Gy < 37%

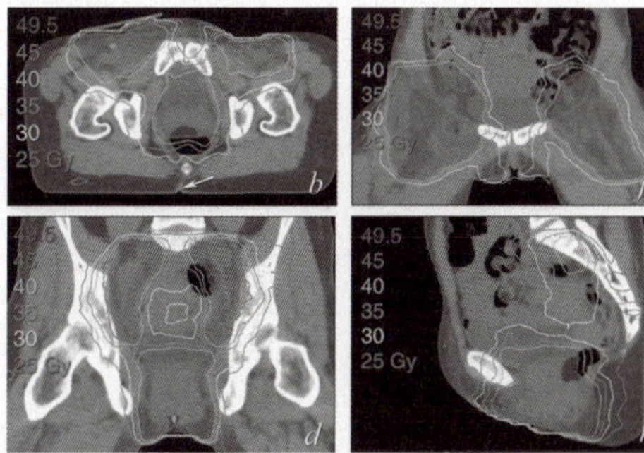

Figure 55.1 Representative treatment plan illustrating coverage of classical CTV (*red colorwash*) and PTV (*purple colorwash*) volumes for a vulvar cancer patient undergoing IMRT. **See color insert**. (Reproduced with permission from Eifel and Klopp, *Gynecologic Radiation Oncology: A Practical Guide*).

Chemotherapy

- **Concurrent:** Cisplatin (40 mg/m² once weekly) for 5-6 cycles, extrapolated from cervical cancer data

Side Effect Management

Interrupting RT significantly worsens outcomes—continue if possible

- Pretreatment: Often severely symptomatic at presentation
  - Address pain control. Consider early palliative care/pain management referral.
  - Treat any preexisting superinfection (*very common;* see below for management).
- Weeks 1-2: Preventative care—keep everything clean and dry
  - Peribottle or handheld shower, hypoallergenic/nonfragrance wipes, sitz baths
  - Gentle soap and water → pat dry (or fan/cool hairdryer). Avoid toilet paper.
- Weeks 3-4: Developing skin erythema/dry desquamation
  - Skin barriers: for example, Mepilex, Aquaphor (any fragrance-free, hypoallergenic ointment)
  - Avoid any skin rubbing (no underwear, loose shorts/skirts, etc.).
  - Sitz baths w/ Domeboro (dilute ½ to ¼ packet)
  - Watch for *candida overgrowth* (brisk erythema disproportionate to RT effect, burning/tingling pain). Manage as complicated yeast infection (3-7 days fluconazole + nystatin powder after cleaning/drying daily prophylactically in thick skin folds)
- Weeks 4-6: Managing moist desquamation and diarrhea
  - Diarrhea: See Cervical Cancer chapter.
  - May need opioids
  - Watch for *bacterial superinfection* (purulent, odorous, dull pain). Treat with antibiotics (staph coverage +/− gram-negative coverage), hibiclens scrub, nonadherent wound dressings, skin protectant (eg, Desitin), BioSeal if bleeding.

Follow-up

- Vaginal dilators or intercourse 2-3 times per week after the vulva has healed to mitigate vaginal stenosis
- Interval H&P every 3-6 months for 2 years, then every 6-12 months for 3-5 years, then annually. Cervical/vaginal cytology as recommended for detection of lower genital tract neoplasia
- Imaging based on symptoms or examination findings suggestive of recurrence

Notable Trials and Papers

Name/Inclusion	Arms	Outcomes	Notes
Adjuvant RT vs Node dissection			
GOG 37 (*Homesley Obstet Gynecol* 1986) 114 Positive groin nodes after vulvectomy + bilateral inguinal lymphadenectomy	RT (45-50 Gy in 5-6.5 weeks) to bilateral pelvic and inguinal nodes Pelvic node resection	6-Year OS 51% for RT group vs 41% for pelvic node resection group	No radiation given to central vulvar area. On subgroup analysis, benefit only if ECE and ≥2 involved nodes
GOG 88 (*Stehman et al. IJROBP* 1992) 58 cN0-1 vulvar SCC	Groin ± pelvic dissection Groin RT (50 Gy/25 fx prescribed to 3 cm depth)	Prematurely closed due to excessive RT groin failures. Groin relapse 18.5% RT vs 0% dissection	Numerous criticisms of this trial including preliminary closure and inadequate depth of prescribed dose
Sentinel lymph node biopsy			
GOG 173 (*Levenback et al. JCO* 2012) 452 vulva SCC cN0 ≥1 mm primary invasion, tumor size 2-6 cm	SLNB → inguinofemoral lymph node dissection	8.3% false-negative nodes, false-negative predictive value 2.0% among tumors <4 cm	

Name/Inclusion	Arms	Outcomes	Notes
GROINSS-V (*Oonk et al. Lancet Oncol* 2010) 403 T1-4 (<4 cm) vulvar SCC	SLNB → inguinofemoral lymph node dissection if SLNB+	Lymphedema 2% vs 25%. Prognosis worse with SLN metastasis >2 mm (69.5% vs 94.4%)	Risk of non-SLN metastasis increased with increasing size of SLN metastasis. All patients with SLN metastasis should have additional groin treatment
GROINSS-VII GOG 270 (*Oonk et al. JCO* 2021) 1535 DOI ≥1 mm, T1-2N0 (<4 cm) s/p SLNB Phase II	SLNB negative → Observation ≤2 mm micromet, no ECE → RT (50 Gy/25-28 fx to ipsi groin and low pelvis) **>2 mm macromet or ECE → completion LND → Adjuvant RT if ≥2 LN+ or ECE	1.6% ipsi groin recurrence with sentinel micromets after RT vs 22% with sentinel macromets. Ipsi groin recurrence 6.9% after IF LND for sentinel macromets	**Protocol amended after excess failures in >2 mm nodal macromet group. Groin RT safe alternative to IF LND for patients with sentinel micromets

Additional guidance: Eifel and Klopp, *Gynecologic Radiation Oncology: A Practical Guide*. Wolters Kluwer; 2016.

OVARIAN CANCER

LAUREN ANDRING • SHANE STECKLEIN • LILIE L. LIN

Background

- **Incidence/prevalence:** 2nd most common gynecologic cancer and 5th most common cause of cancer-related death in women in the United States (19 571 diagnoses, 13 445 deaths in 2019 [CDC]).
- **Outcomes:** 5-Year survival across all stages estimated at 49% (SEER data)
- **Demographics:** Lifetime risk 1 in 77 (1.3%)
- **Risk factors:** Age; family history of breast, ovarian, or colorectal cancers; familial cancer syndromes (hereditary breast and ovarian cancer syndrome, *PTEN* hamartoma syndrome, hereditary nonpolyposis colorectal cancer, Peutz-Jeghers syndrome) obesity; nulliparity; or first pregnancy after age 35

Tumor Biology and Characteristics

- **Pathology:** Epithelial ovarian cancers (EOC) constitute 85-90% of all ovarian cancers and include primary malignancies of the fallopian tube and primary peritoneal cancer. Type I ovarian cancers include low-grade serous, clear cell, endometrioid, and mucinous subtypes and often exhibit mutations in *KRAS*, *BRAF*, or *PTEN* (*Singer et al. JNCI* 2015). Type II ovarian cancers are predominately high-grade serous carcinoma (70% of all ovarian cancers), which are associated with *TP53* mutation (*Ahmed et al. J Pathol* 2010), but also include undifferentiated carcinomas and carcinosarcomas. 10-15% of ovarian tumors are stromal or germ cell tumors.
- **Genetics:** Inherited deleterious mutations in *BRCA1* and *BRCA2* result in ∼40% and 15% lifetime risks of ovarian cancer, respectively. Overall, 18-24% of ovarian cancer patients carry inherited mutations in *BRCA1*, *BRCA2*, *BARD1*, *BRIP1*, *CHEK2*, *MRE11A*, *MSH2*, *MSH6*, *NBN*, *PALB2*, *PMS2*, *RAD50*, *RAD51C*, *RAD51D*, or *TP53* (*Norquist et al. JAMA Oncol* 2016; *Walsh et al. PNAS* 2011). Tumors with mutations in *BRCA* or other homologous recombination pathway genes are hypersensitive to platinum-based chemotherapy and poly(ADP)ribose polymerase (PARP) inhibitors.

Anatomy

- Ovaries lie near the uterine horns at the opening of the fallopian tubes and are connected to the lateral surface of the uterus via the utero-ovarian ligament.
- Lymphatic drainage from the ovaries and fallopian tubes primarily follows the gonadal vessels, and first echelon drainage is the para-aortic and aortocaval nodes. Rarely, ovarian cancers can drain along the round ligament to the inguinal lymph nodes.
- Intraperitoneal dissemination is the primary mechanism of ovarian cancer spread.

Workup

- **History and physical:** Presentation includes bloating, pelvic or abdominal pain, early satiety, urinary frequency, abdominal mass or acites. Abdominal/pelvic exam
- **Labs:** CBC, CMP, LFTs, CA125. Consider pregnancy test.
- **Procedures/biopsy:** Biopsy and/or peritoneal cytology as needed
- **Imaging:** Ultrasound, CT, or MRI abdomen/pelvis, and/or PET. Chest x-ray or CT chest to evaluate lungs
- **Referral:** Genetic risk evaluation for all patients, oncofertility as indicated

Ovarian Cancer Staging (*FIGO* 2017)

FIGO Stage	
IA	Tumor limited to one ovary, with intact capsule, no tumor on surface, negative washings
IB	Tumor involves both ovaries, otherwise like stage IA
IC1	Tumor limited to one or both ovaries with surgical spill
IC2	Tumor limited to one or both ovaries with capsule rupture before surgery or tumor on ovarian surface
IC3	Tumor limited to one or both ovaries with malignant cells in ascites or peritoneal washings
IIA	Extension or implant on the uterus and/or fallopian tubes
IIB	Extension or implant on other pelvic intraperitoneal tissues
IIIA1	Positive retroperitoneal lymph nodes (IIIA1(i) ≤ 10 mm, IIIA1(ii) > 10 mm)
IIIA2	Microscopic extrapelvic (above the brim) peritoneal involvement with or without positive retroperitoneal lymph nodes
IIIB	Macroscopic extrapelvic peritoneal involvement ≤2 cm with or without positive retroperitoneal lymph nodes
IIIC	Like IIIB, but extrapelvic peritoneal involvement is >2 cm; includes extension to capsule of liver and/or spleen
IVA	Pleural effusion with positive cytology
IVB	Hepatic and/or splenic parenchymal metastasis or metastasis to extra-abdominal organs or lymph nodes (including inguinal lymph nodes)

Treatment Algorithm

Stage IA or IB, fertility desired	Unilateral (IA) or bilateral (IB) salpingo-oophorectomy with comprehensive surgical staging
IA-IV, surgically resectable, fertility not desired	Total abdominal hysterectomy, bilateral salpingo-oophorectomy, comprehensive surgical staging, and debulking as needed
Bulky stages III-IV or poor surgical candidate	Consider neoadjuvant chemotherapy with or without interval debulking and total abdominal hysterectomy and bilateral salpingo-oophorectomy

Chemotherapy

- Adjuvant platinum/taxane chemotherapy is employed for all high-grade ovarian cancers. Patients with stage I disease get 3-6 cycles, while 6 cycles are recommended for patients with stages II-IV disease.

- Neoadjuvant chemotherapy may be used in patients with bulky or unresectable disease.
- Intraperitoneal chemotherapy is often recommended for patients with stage II-IV disease who have undergone optimal debulking surgery.
- For patients with BRCA mutation (or BRCA wild-type but <CR), maintenance therapy with PARPi +/− bevacizumab
- At relapse, major determinant of response to additional therapy and outcome is interval between last platinum chemotherapy and disease recurrence.
  - >6 months = Platinum sensitive, consider additional platinum-based chemotherapy, targeted therapy with PARPi +/− bevacizumab, or hormone therapy (tamoxifen, aromatase inhibitors)
  - ≤6 months = Platinum resistant, move to second-line chemotherapy (docetaxel, etoposide, gemcitabine, liposomal doxorubicin [Doxil], topotecan, PARPi ± bevacizumab, HT)

Radiation Treatment Technique

- Radiotherapy is seldom used in the 1st-line treatment of ovarian cancer.
- Prior studies of whole abdominal radiotherapy (WART) showed some efficacy in the curative treatment of ovarian cancer; but due to toxicity, technical challenges, and subsequent improvements in chemotherapy, WART has not been widely adopted.
- The major use of radiotherapy for ovarian cancer is in definitive treatment in select patients with recurrent, persistent, or oligometastatic disease or palliation of bulky disease.
- Radiotherapy may be particularly effective in patients with clear cell (*Hoskins et al. JCO* 2012), mucinous, or endometrioid histology. It is less effective and rarely used for borderline or low-grade serous tumors.
  - GTV should be treated to 60-66 Gy (EQD_2).
  - CTV that includes regions of possible adjacent soft tissue infiltration and adjacent regional lymph nodes should be treated to 45-50 Gy (EQD_2).
  - Can also consider SBRT to 30-50Gy in 3-5 fractions for limited disease
  - 3DCRT, IMRT, or SBRT may be used, depending on location, anatomy, and proximity of critical structures.

Notable Trials and Papers

Name/Inclusion	Arms	Outcomes	Notes
Role of Definitive RT			
Princess Margaret WART vs Pelvic RT (*Dembo et al. Cancer Treat Rep* 1979) Retrospective review 231 patients w/ stage IB-III ovarian ca postoperative	WART Pelvic RT + chlorambucil CHT	RFS improved in WART vs pelvic RT + CHT (64% vs 40%)	WART w/ greatest benefit after R0 resection, independent of stage or histology
British Colombia RT in Clear Cell (*Hoskins et al. JCO* 2012) Retrospective review 241 patients w/ stage I/II clear cell ovarian ca postoperative	Adjuvant CHT: platinum/Taxol Adjuvant CRT: w/ WART	On subset analysis stage IC (excluding rupture only) or II had 20% DFS benefit w/ WART	A subset of patients may have DFS benefit from postoperative WART

Name/Inclusion	Arms	Outcomes	Notes
RT for recurrent, persistent, or oligometastatic disease			
Bae et al. Int J Gynecol Cancer 2023 Retrospective review 79 patients w/ recurrent ovarian ca	Salvage RT w/ conventional fx or SBRT	2 y LC 81%, OS 75% But 2 y PFS only 11% and CHT-free survival 21% Pre-RT platinum resistance and short CA-125 doubling time predictive for 1y CHT-FS (0%, 20%, 54% if both, one, or no risk factors)	RT for salvage of recurrent ovarian ca has good LC, but patients likely to fail elsewhere
MITO RT1 (*Macchia et al. Oncologist* 2020) Retrospective review 261 patients with metastatic, persistent, or recurrent ovarian ca	SBRT to all sites of disease	2 y LC 82%, CR 65%, PR 24% G1/2 toxicity 21%, no G3. 2 y late-tox free survival 95%	Established SBRT is safe and efficacious for recurrent, persistent, or oligomet. Ovarian ca
MITO-RT3/RAD Trial (*Macchia et al. Int J Gynecol Cancer* 2022) Prospective multicenter Ph II trial	SBRT 30-50 Gy in 1, 3, or 5 daily fx to all sites of active disease	Primary end point: clinical CR rate	Estimated accrual: Spring 2023
SMART Trial (*Henke et al. IJROBP* 2022) Ph I trial of 10 patients with recurrent oligometastatic disease	MR-guided SBRT 35 Gy/5 fx	Median PFS 11 mos. Single grade ≥3 toxicity noted	MR-guided SBRT is safe and effective
Systemic therapy			
Review of Ph III PARP-I Trials (*Mirza et al. Annals of Oncol* 2020) SOLO-1, PAOLA-1, PRIMA, and VELIA	PARPi (+/− bevacizumab) as maintenance Placebo	Significant PFS benefit seen in all 4 trials Median PFS benefit ~6 mo for all comers	Established the role for PARPi as maintenance therapy in front line setting of newly diagnosed ovarian ca

SOFT TISSUE SARCOMA

ALISON YODER • ANDREW BISHOP • ASHLEIGH GUADAGNOLO

Background

- **Incidence/prevalence:** Heterogeneous group of solid tumors of mesenchymal cell origin. Rare, ~12 000 cases are diagnosed annually in the United States. Account for 1% of adult cancers.
- **Outcomes:** Disease-specific survival ~60% at 10 years. Prognostic factors for survival: **grade**, size, site, LN involvement, age (older worse). Prognostic factors for local recurrence: **positive margin**, locally recurrent disease, head and neck location, retroperitoneal location, older age
- **Demographics:** Median age at diagnosis is 45-55 years.
- **Risk factors:** Can be associated with genetic syndromes like Li-Fraumeni, tuberous sclerosis, FAP, NF type 1. Prior exposure to ionizing radiation. Majority of cases have no clear predisposing exposure. Injuries have not been associated with an increased risk for developing sarcomas.

Tumor Biology and Characteristics

- **Histologic subtypes:** Over 20 major categories of STS with >60 histologic subtypes. Most common histologies include undifferentiated pleomorphic sarcoma (UPS), liposarcoma, synovial sarcoma, and leiomyosarcoma. Some less common histologic subtypes have distinct clinical characteristics, patterns of spread, and behaviors. Consideration for referral to a sarcoma center should be made with a diagnosis of soft tissue sarcoma.
- **Pathology:** Core biopsy is ideal. Excisional biopsy should be avoided. Important for expert sarcoma pathology review due to rarity and diversity of tumors. Grade is prognostic for LR to an extent, but especially for risk of developing distant metastases and disease-specific survival. Look for signature translocations (ie, synovial sarcoma t(X;18) SS18-SSX1/SSX2, myxoid liposarcoma t(12;16), Ewings sarcoma t(11;22), clear cell sarcoma t(12;22), or alveolar rhabdomyosarcoma t(2;13)). *MDM2* amplification in well-differentiated liposarcoma and dedifferentiated liposarcoma is used to distinguish from benign adipose tumors and poorly differentiated sarcomas (which are negative for amplification). INI1 loss in epithelioid sarcoma is characteristic.
- **Imaging:** Mixed appearances. Generally, on MRI: T1 tumor is isointense, T2 tumor is hyperintense.

Anatomy

- Can occur anywhere, most common location lower extremity ≫ upper extremity = superficial trunk = retroperitoneal > head and neck
- LN involvement in <5% of all cases. More common (15%) in "CARE" tumors: clear cell, (cutaneous) angiosarcoma, rhabdomyosarcoma, and epithelioid sarcoma

Workup

- **History and physical:** Focus on personal/family history of cancer; refer to genetics when appropriate. Ask about functionality of limb for extremity sarcomas, abdominal symptoms for retroperitoneal sarcomas, and pain. Look for open/ulcerating tumors.
- **Procedures/biopsy:** Core needle or incisional biopsy
- **Imaging:** MRI with gadolinium for primary extremity and superficial trunk lesions. CT with contrast for head and neck and retroperitoneal primaries. CT chest for staging. For **retroperitoneal sites**, obtain renal perfusion scan to assess differential renal function prior to RT or surgery. Patients with myxoid liposarcoma should also have CT imaging of the chest, abdomen and pelvis as well as an MRI of the entire spine performed at baseline. MRI brain not recommended except for unique histologies

Treatment Algorithm

Stage I	Surgery alone, WLE (limb sparing if extremity). If R0, can observe if low-grade If recurrent tumor or salvage surgery may be morbid, should consider a combined modality approach
Stages II-III	Favor preoperative RT followed by surgery If upfront surgery is done, recommend post-op RT If upfront unplanned excision with positive margin, should consider preoperative RT followed by re-excision Consider neoadjuvant chemotherapy if high grade and stage T2-T4 In highly select cases, consideration for omitting RT may be reasonable. Factors include small, superficial tumors where widely negative margins can be easily obtained and salvage surgery if the patient were to recur, would not be morbid.
Stage IV	Chemotherapy, immunotherapy (for select histologies), or targeted therapy upfront Supportive care for patients with poor PS Palliative RT Consideration for consolidative local therapy with RT (+/− surgery) in select cases (ie, oligometastatic/oligoprogressive or unresectable, symptomatic primary)

Radiation Treatment Technique

- **SIM:** Depending on anatomic location. Supine position preferred, prone may be needed. For postoperative cases, wire the scar or the entire field to help with target delineation. Do not specifically target drain sites.
  Lower extremity: Vac-Lok for involved extremity. Distal primaries may need CT scan feet first. Frog leg for proximal thigh cases or when needed to create separation with contralateral extremity or decrease inguinal fold. Can elevate noninvolved leg to facilitate better dosimetry and imaging localized on involved leg.
  Upper extremity: Upper Vac-Lok. Arm position depends on location of primary but is usually akimbo. Consider a prone "swimmers" position or abducted arm.
  Distal extremities: Can consider custom cushion +/− aquaplast mask to help with immobilization
  Head and Neck: Prior to SIM, consider dental evaluation/need for stent. Aquaplast mask
  Retroperitoneal: Vac-Lock. Generally arms up (depending on tumor position). For lesions above the iliac crests, the scan should be 4D to account for breathing motion.
- **Dose:**
  Extremity
  Preoperative: 50 Gy in 25 fractions (conventional) is the standard fractionation schedule. If hypofractionation is considered, then preferred regimen is 42.75 Gy in 15 fractions (as per HYPORT-STS).
  Postoperative: 60 Gy at 2 Gy/fx for R0 resection, with field size reduction after 50 Gy. Boost to 64-68 Gy for a positive margin.
  (Despite a higher boost dose, LR is higher for R1/2 resection; in other words, a higher radiation dose does not make up for lack of R0 resection.)
  Considerations: If IMRT preferable for postoperative cases, can also consider a simultaneous-integrated boost technique. (Ex: for R0 resection—CTV2 treated to 59.92 Gy in 28 fractions (2.14 Gy/fx) and CTV1 to 50.4 Gy in 28 fractions (1.8 Gy/fx). See Figure 57.1.
  If there are positive margins postoperatively, can do SIB technique in 30 fractions with doses of 66 Gy, 60 Gy, and 54 Gy to the different CTVs.

Retroperitoneal (RPS)
  50.4 Gy in 28 fractions
- **Target:**
  Preoperative:
  Extremity: GTV + 3-4 cm longitudinally sup/inf along fascial planes and 1.5 cm radially to yield CTV (*Haas et al. IJROBP* 2012; *Salerno et al. PRO* 2021)

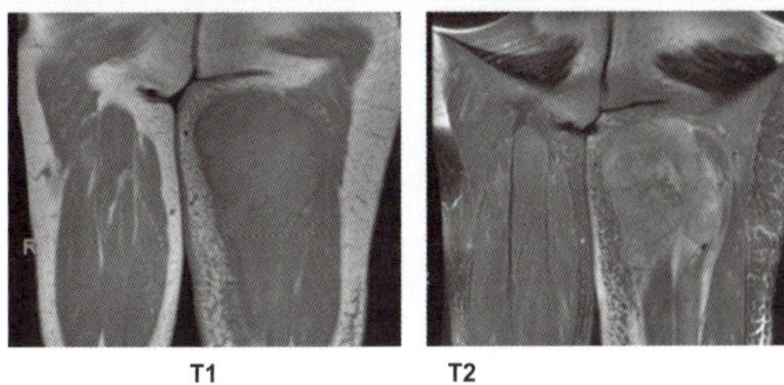

Figure 57.1 Representative coronal images of an MRI of a left lower extremity soft tissue sarcoma located in the upper thigh.

Special case: if subcutaneous tumor: GTV + 3-4 cm circumferential expansion sup/inf and radially, adhering to anatomic barriers

Postoperative:

Virtual GTV = preoperative GTV (if imaging available) or postoperative bed

CTV1 as above (3-4 cm sup/inf, 1.5 cm radially off of vGTV)

Cone down to CTV2 to 60-68 Gy total (vGTV + 2 cm sup/inf, 1.5 cm radially)

*Reference Figure 57.1

RPS: GTV + 1.5 cm symmetric margins to yield CTV (allowing 5 mm into bowel). Trim from liver, bone kidney, etc. as per Baldini guidelines (*Baldini et al.* doi:10.1016/j.ijrobp.2015.02.013)

Note: may need larger CTV if not using 4D sim

Considerations: CTV expansions can be increased in difficult surgical access areas or superficial spreading histologies. CTVs can be trimmed/carved out of bone if not involved. Do not cover elective nodes for any histology other than alveolar rhabdomyosarcoma. PTV expansions typically 0.5-1 cm depending on daily imaging techniques

- **Technique:**

  3DCRT: Consider parallel opposed fields (with nondivergent deep border to spare bone/joint). Other beam arrangements (wedge-pair, obliques, etc.) may be used as well. Asymmetric beam weighting can be used if the tumor is not centrally located.

  IMRT: Unless 3D planning shows a clear benefit in reduced dose to OAR, IMRT/VMAT is routinely done for improved conformality for proximal lower extremities, thoracic, pelvic, retroperitoneal, head and neck sites (Fig. 57.2).

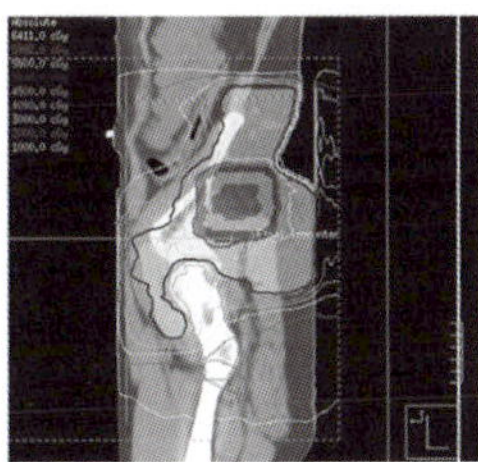

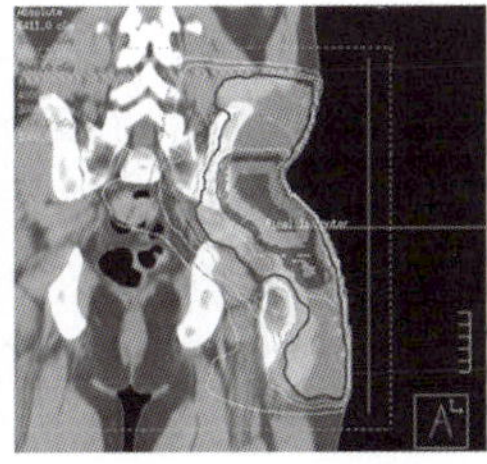

Figure 57.2 Representative sagittal and coronal (L → R) images of an IMRT treatment plan for a 40-year-old male being treated with adjuvant RT following R0 resection of a grade III PNET of the left lower extremity. Using IMRT in this case allowed for reduced dose to the left femoral head/proximal femur. The *red isodose line* represents 59.92 Gy (covering GTV) and *blue* represents 50.40 Gy (covering CTV). **See color insert.**

Adult Extraosseous Ewing Sarcoma: A Different Clinical Entity
Small round blue cell tumor. Very rare. More common in children
Translocation t(11;22) or t(21;22) in 95% of cases
Upfront intensive chemotherapy for everyone
Local tumor treatment is controversial. Consultation at sarcoma specialty center is highly recommended. Often treated with a combined modality approach. However, single modality treatment with surgery or definitive RT can be considered depending on anatomic location and response to chemotherapy
RT Doses • Definitive: 60-66 Gy • Preoperative: 50 Gy • Postoperative: 60 Gy
Adult Rhabdomyosarcoma Sarcoma: A Different Clinical Entity
Adults with RMS do worse than pediatric patients
Alveolar, embryonal, and pleomorphic subtypes
Pediatric RT doses are insufficient. Normally escalate dose closer to standard adult STS doses upward of 60+ Gy in the definitive setting, respecting adjacent normal tissue tolerance
Desmoid Tumors: A Different Clinical Entity
Not technically malignant (does not metastasize) but is a locally aggressive and potentially destructive neoplasm: observed until local progression is painful and/or morbid. The treatment paradigm is complex with improving systemic therapies. Radiation therapy is a local control option. We offer it as an upfront treatment option more commonly in older patients and reserve it as a salvage treatment in younger patients
Definitive treatment schema: 56 Gy in 28 fx
Dermatofibrosarcoma Protuberans: A Different Clinical Entity
Uncommon, low-grade sarcoma of the skin with a characteristic t(17;22) translocation
Primary treatment is surgery, followed by RT for indeterminant/positive margins or if recurrent disease If they have fibrosarcomatous transformation, local treatment is more in line with STS management with both surgery and RT (preoperative preferred)

Note: Cutaneous malignancy may needs bolus

- **IGRT:** Related to modality used and body site.
  Daily kV-aligning to bone typically used. (For 3D planning: consider rotating collimator parallel with long bone for set-up and kV alignment.)
  Weekly CBCT recommended for adequate coverage as tumors can sometimes change on treatment necessitating an adaptive plan (due to either increased or decreased size of tumor while on treatment).
- **Planning directive—Conventional fractionation:**
  Spare at least 1-cm strip of limb circumference/skin
  Avoid treating entire limb circumference >20 Gy when using IMRT
  Avoid treating entire femur circumference to ≥50 Gy
  Spare ½ cross section of weight-bearing bone; V40 < 64%, mean dose < 37 Gy (*Dickie et al. IJROBP* 2009)
  Block part of the joint cavity; V50 < 50%
  Block major tendons: V50 < 50%
- **Planning directive—HYPORT fractionation (15 fractions):**
  Spare 1-cm strip of limb circumference/skin
  Avoid treating entire limb circumference >17 Gy
  Avoid treating entire femur circumference to ≥42.75 Gy
  Spare ½ cross section of weight-bearing bone; V35 < 65%
  Block part of the joint cavity; V42.75 < 50%
- **Planning directive—Retroperitoneal Sarcoma:**
  Bowel Bag: Dmax < 54 Gy, V45 < 195 cc
  Spine: Dmax < 45 Gy
  Liver: Mean < 25 Gy, V30 < 30%
  Kidneys: V20 < 30%, mean < 18 Gy
  Spleen: Mean < 8 Gy
  Bladder: Dmax < 54 Gy, V30 < 50%
  Lungs: V20 < 10%

Surgery

- Mainstay of treatment for soft tissue sarcomas
- Wide local excision with goal of widely negative margin (goal is 2 cm normal tissue around tumor, unless tumor abuts natural barrier to spread like bone or nerve).
- In unirradiated patients with R1 or R2 resection, consider additional surgery or re-excision prior to RT (or preoperative RT to 50 Gy followed by re-excision).

Chemotherapy

- Controversial, as studies have failed to show OS benefit
- We consider neoadjuvant chemotherapy for patients with high-grade, large (>5 cm) tumors. Neoadjuvant chemotherapy is preferred over adjuvant due to a 20-30% response rate to chemotherapy, thus intact measurable disease is important. Typically assess response following 2-4 cycles
- Standard starting chemotherapy regimen involves Adriamycin/ifosfamide for most STS. Other agents commonly used include gemcitabine and docetaxel. Targeted therapy with pazopanib (TKI) and trabectedin (targets FUS-CHOP transcription in myxoid liposarcomas) can be considered as both are FDA approved for advanced STS cases. Can also consider enrolling on trials with other targeted agents (MDM2 inhibitors, immunotherapy).

Side Effect Management

- Skin care: First-line emollients. Topical steroids. Can add Domeboro soaks thereafter. If having further grade 2+ skin toxicity, consider Mepilex. For grade 3 dermatitis, consider Silvadene cream (on weekends or after RT has been completed entirely). Have a low threshold for considering infection/antibiotics in setting of fungating tumors.

Local Recurrences

- In a radiation-naive patient with local recurrence of STS, treat with preoperative radiation (50 Gy) followed by surgery if feasible.
- Generally avoid reirradiation, as complications following reirradiation have been reported to be as high as 80% and reirradiation has not been shown to improve local control for tumors that have been previously irradiated.

Notable Papers

Name/Inclusion	Arms	Outcomes	Notes
Rosenberg et al. *Ann Surg* 1982 43 patients w/ extremity STS. Randomized	LSS +RT: Limb-sparing surgery + postoperative RT to 45-50 Gy to anatomical area + 10-20 Gy tumor bed boost Amputation	Local failure 15% (LSS + RT) vs 0% amputation OS/DFS for LSS + RT 83%/71% vs amputation 88%/78% (*P* = NS)	All patients received postoperative chemo Conclusion: LSS + RT safe for most patients
O'Sullivan et al. *Lancet* 2002 190 patients w/ extremity STS. Randomized	Preoperative RT (50 Gy/25 fx) [postoperative boost if + margins] Postoperative RT (50 Gy/25 fx with boost to 66—70 Gy)	Wound complications (within 90 days of surgery): 35% preoperative vs 17% postoperative (*P* = .01) No difference in LC, DFS, OS	Surgical margin predicts for LF Grade/size predict for DM and OS
Davis et al. *Radiother Oncol* 2005	Analyzed 129 patients from O'Sullivan trial 2 years after treatment	Grade 2+ fibrosis 31% preoperative vs 48% post-operative (*P* = .07) Edema/joint stiffness 18% preoperative vs 23% postoperative (*P* = NS)	Field size predictive for fibrosis and stiffness on MVA ***Conclusion: postoperative RT results in more fibrosis and long-term complications***

Name/Inclusion	Arms	Outcomes	Notes
STRASS, *Bonvalot et al. Lancet Oncol* 2022 266 patients with RPS eligible for RT, previously untreated. Randomized	Surgery alone Preoperative RT (50.4 Gy/28 fx) followed by surgery	Median abdominal recurrence-free survival in RT + surg 4.5 y vs 5.0 y in surg only (*P* = NS)	Preoperative RT not standard for RPS Note: in subgroup analysis outcomes improved for patients with liposarcoma histology
DOREMY, *Lansu et al. JAMA Oncol* 2021 79 patients with myxoid liposarcoma of the extremity or trunk	Single-arm, phase II trial: 36 Gy/18 fx followed by surgical resection	LC 100% at median 25 mos Major wound complication rate: 17%	Extensive pathologic treatment response in 91%
HYPORT *Guadagnolo et al. Lancet Oncol* 2022 120 patients with extremity STS	Single-arm, phase II trial: 42.75 Gy/17 fx followed by surgical resection	Major wound complication rate: 31% 3% of patients had grade >3 late RT toxicity	Conclusion: 42.75 Gy/17 fx comparable to 50 Gy/25 fx in terms of wound complications for preoperative RT in extremity STS. Oncologic outcomes pending

MELANOMA

ALISON YODER • DEVARATI MITRA • ASHLEIGH GUADAGNOLO

Background

- **Incidence/prevalence:** Aggressive skin cancer. Accounts for 1% of all skin cancers in the United States. Incidence is ~97 000 new cases annually, with 8000 deaths annually. Incidence has been increasing over past three decades.
- **Outcomes:** 5-year survival for localized melanomas varies with the degree of spread. Evaluating people diagnosed between 2011 and 2017, regional disease drops 5-year survival from 99% to 68% and again to 30% with metastasis.
- **Demographics:** Median age at diagnosis is 60. White ≫ Hispanic > Black patients. For patients <50 years old, more common in women. For patients >50 years old, more common in men.
- **Risk factors:** Ultraviolet (UV) exposure, family history, history of multiple atypical moles or dysplastic nevi. Increased risk among immunocompromised patients. History of Xeroderma pigmentosum

Tumor Biology and Characteristics

- **Histologic subtypes:** Superficial spreading (70% of cases, arise from pigmented dysplastic nevus), lentigo maligna, nodular, acral lentiginous, and desmoplastic (more likely to be neurotropic, may be amelanotic)
- **Pathology:** Cell of origin is melanocyte. Pathology report should include: Breslow thickness, ulceration, primary tumor mitotic rate, resection margins, microsatellitosis, PNI, LVI, and presence of desmoplasia. If nodal or metastatic involvement, molecular genetic testing should be considered to test for BRAF and NRAS mutational status in patients with cutaneous primaries and KIT mutational status in patients with mucosal primaries.

Anatomy

- Can occur anywhere on skin, predominantly on sun exposed areas. Most common locations in males are the back followed by head/neck. Most common locations in females are the extremities and trunk.

Workup

- **History and physical:** Focused and complete skin examination of the skin and regional lymph nodes with an assessment of melanoma risk factors
- **Procedures/biopsy:** Optimally, an excisional biopsy is preferred for any suspicious, pigmented lesion with 1-3 mm negative margins. Consider full-thickness punch biopsy if in a difficult area (distal digit, face, palms) vs excisional biopsy. Avoid shave biopsies as they give no information on depth.
- **Imaging/labs:** Not recommended for stage 0, IA, IB, and II. Can consider nodal basin ultrasound prior to SLNB in patients with stage I/II disease with equivocal LN physical exam. For stage III-IV or recurrent disease, obtain CT C/A/P w/ contrast or whole-body FDG PET/CT. Obtain MRI brain w/ contrast if clinically indicated or stage IIIB-IV.

Treatment Algorithm

Primary site management	Surgical resection, wide local excision +/– adjuvant RT to primary site (see factors for adjuvant RT to primary site below)
cN0 nodal management	T0 - Stage IB (T1b): Discuss and consider SLNB. (SLNB not required.) Stage IB (T2a) or II: Discuss and offer SLNB Stage IIB/IIC: SLNB. Consider adjuvant systemic agent (*Luke et al. Lancet* 2022)
Clinically occult, pN+, nodal management	Clinically occult/detected nodes by SLNB no longer need CLND per MSTL-2 and DeCOG-SLT. Can consider adjuvant systemic agent
Clinically detected, cN+, nodal management	Consider neoadjuvant + adjuvant systemic agent versus upfront complete therapeutic lymph node dissection (*Patel et al. NEJM* 2023). Consider adjuvant radiotherapy to the nodal basin for patients at high risk of regional relapse (see factors for adjuvant RT to nodal site below)

Radiation Treatment Technique

- **SIM: Primary:** Radiopaque wire to outline scar and/or treatment field. If using electrons, patient positioning is important to allow for en face beam arrangement. Consider lateral penumbra when shaping field to determine PTV.
- **Dose:** Postoperative 30 Gy in 6 Gy/fx, given twice weekly over 2-2.5 weeks (Dmax 30 Gy with goal coverage of D90% [27 Gy]). Alternative TROG regimen: 48 Gy in 2.4 Gy/fx for 20 fractions vs conventional 60 Gy in 30 fx (hypofractionation preferred)
- **Target: Primary:** Primary site/scar + 1.5-2 cm margin = CTV

Factors for Adjuvant RT to Primary Site
Only one factor needed
Pure desmoplastic melanoma (>90% melanoma with desmoplastic features)
Isolated locally recurrent disease
Micro- or macro-satellitosis
Two factors needed
Breslow thickness ≥4 mm
Head and neck location
Ulceration
PNI in head and neck primary or nonhead and neck primary with PNI of large caliber (≥0.1 mm) or named nerves

Factors for Adjuvant RT to Nodal Site: For cN+ Patients	**Lymphedema Risk**
Cervical location (any 1 indication): ECE, ≥2 cm, ≥2 LNs positive	10%
Axillary location (any 1 indication): ECE, ≥3 cm, ≥4 LNs positive	15%
Groin location	30%

Factors for Adjuvant RT to Nodal Site: For cN+ Patients	Lymphedema Risk
BMI <25 kg/m² (any 2 indications): ECE, ≥3 cm, ≥4 LNs positive	
BMI ≥25 kg/m²: Increases threshold to treat. Discuss systemic therapy options, RT complications may outweigh regional control benefits in this anatomic location	
For any site, consider radiation if recurrent disease in a previously dissected nodal basin	

Nodal: Involved nodal region if high-risk features. Do not electively treat LNs.
Head and neck: Involved level plus neighboring levels with additional levels as per risk and degree of nodal evaluation. (High facial/scalp primary include pre/postauricular [superficial] parotid.)
Axilla: Ipsilateral levels I-III. Unless there is a bulky or high disease, we do not electively include supraclavicular field.
Groin: Need 2 or more high-risk factors to consider treating groin, with higher threshold to treat at higher BMIs. Do not electively cover pelvic nodes.

- **Technique:** Generally VMAT/IMRT
  Primary: Bolus needed for primary tumor site treatment. Electrons dosed to D_{max}. Normalize to ≥100% to prevent hot spots >30 Gy. Consider skin collimation when appropriate. May use 3D and VMAT treatment as appropriate
  For head and neck primaries with need for skin collimation and electrons: draw/wire field and cut out field on mask. If near areas of air gap (ie, ear), consider TX-151 bolus (aka "Super Stuff Bolus").
  Nodal:
  Head and Neck: as per standard head and neck setup with VMAT planning, dental clearance, and tongue-lateralizing stent
  Axillary: Ipsilateral arm abducted (preferred) vs akimbo (if patient with limited ROM). Either 3D or VMAT planning (avoid shoulder/AC joint)
  Groin: Frog leg position to decrease skin fold. VMAT planning
- **IGRT:** Daily kV +/− CBCT for hypofractionated schedule. MD verifies IGRT prior to first fraction. If electrons, see set up on table prior to first fraction to verify setup.
- **Planning directive:** For 30 Gy in 5 fractions: evaluate the 24 Gy line on all axial slices. 24 Gy line should be off of any critical structure (brain, eye, brachial plexus, spinal cord, bowel). Evaluate 27 Gy isodose line for target coverage, as opposed to the 30 Gy line (Fig. 58.1). For 48 Gy in 20 fractions regimen: Max dose to brain and spinal cord <40 Gy

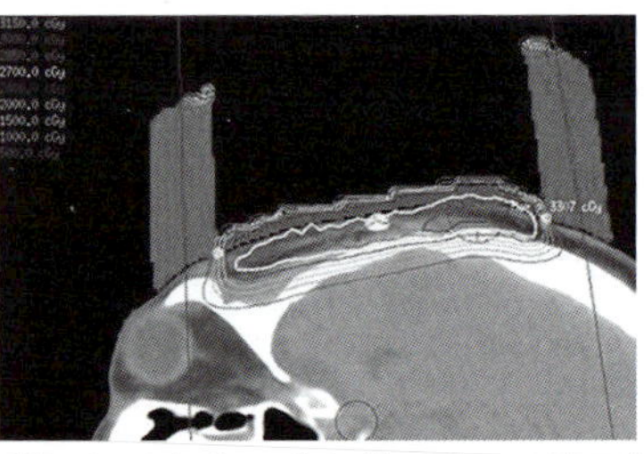

Figure 58.1 Sample RT treatment plan for a patient with a melanoma of the scalp. This patient was treated postoperatively with electrons to the tumor bed to a total dose of 30 Gy in 5 fractions. Note the 27 Gy isodose line in *yellow*, which is used to evaluate target coverage. 30 Gy hotspots are seen in *red*. **See color insert**.

SURGERY

- Primary: Wide local excision with goal of negative margin. Adequate margin is determined by depth of primary.

Primary Tumor Depth	Margin Recommended
In situ	0.5-1 cm
<1.0 mm	1 cm

Primary Tumor Depth	Margin Recommended
1.01-2.0 mm	1-2 cm
>2.0 mm	2 cm

- Nodes:
  - cN0: +/– Sentinel lymph node biopsy. SLNB should be done prior to WLE as to not alter the drainage to the sentinel basin.
  - cN+: Involved/regional nodal basin dissection. For certain head and neck primaries, this will involve superficial parotidectomy. If neoadjuvant systemic therapy is planned, surgeon should place clips in pathologically confirmed nodes prior to starting systemic therapy.

Systemic Therapy

- Stage II: Pembrolizumab for pathologically staged IIB or IIC, with a discussion about benefit versus toxicity.
- Stage III with occult LNs: Anti-PD1 immunotherapy (per Checkmate-248 and Keynote-54) or BRAF/MEK-directed targeted therapy for patients with BRAF V600-activating mutation (per COMBI-AD). Can consider omission for patients with low-risk disease (single SLN+ <1 mm)
- Stage III with gross nodes: Neoadjuvant + adjuvant therapy with anti-PD1 immunotherapy (vs BRAF/MEK-directed targeted therapy for BRAF-activated melanoma)

Side Effect Management

- Side effects may not be present during RT if using 30 Gy in 5 fractions hypofractionated regimen. Advise patients that acute side effects may appear 1-2 weeks after completion of radiotherapy.
- Skin care: First-line emollients. Can add Domeboro soaks. If having further grade 2+ skin toxicity, consider topical steroids (eg, triamcinolone) and Mepilex as needed. Grade 3 dermatitis, consider Silvadene cream. Watch for infection, low threshold antifungal treatment with fluconazole, especially in skin folds.

Follow-up

- Depending on initial stage, complete skin and regional nodal examination every 3-6 months for 2 years. (More frequent follow-ups for higher-stage patients.) Can space to every 3-12 months after.
- For patients with initial stage IIB-III melanoma, consider labs and CT c/a/p or PET/CT to detect asymptomatic recurrence the first 3 years.

Notable Papers

Name/Inclusion	Arms	Outcomes	Notes
Guadagnolo et al. Cancer 2014 Retrospective Review (RR) of 130 patients with desmoplastic melanoma	Surgery alone (45%) Surgery + postoperative RT (55%)	24% of surgery alone patients developed LR at 6 years, dropped to 7% with postoperative RT	Postoperative RT beneficial for desmoplastic melanoma
Strom et al. Cancer 2014 RR of 277 patients with desmoplastic melanoma	Surgery alone (59%) Surgery + postoperative RT (41%)	LR 54% in surgery alone with positive margins vs 14% with postoperative RT	Postoperative RT beneficial for desmoplastic melanoma in most cases Consider omitting postoperative RT if negative margins, depth < 4 mm, no PNI, non-H&N location

Name/Inclusion	Arms	Outcomes	Notes
TROG 02.01, *Burmeister et al. Lancet Oncol* 2012 and *Henderson et al. Lancet Oncol* 2015 250 patients with cN+ s/p LND. Randomized	Lymph node dissection alone Lymph node dissection + adj RT (depending on location/risk factors, see above table)	RT decreased LN recurrence by ~50% No impact on RFS or OS Gr 3-4 toxicities after RT in H&N, axilla, and groin were 8%, 21%, and 29%	Postoperative RT for high-risk LN involvement decreases local recurrence, no impact on OS Trial conducted prior to modern systemic therapy/ immunotherapy
Guadagnolo et al. Lancet Oncol 2009 Review	Review of melanoma patients who received RT	Improved LC with PORT Risk of complications differ with anatomic location	Prior to modern systemic therapy Additional details about fields and planning
MSLT-II, *Faries et al. NEJM* 2017 1934 patients with +SLNB. Randomized	Completion LND Observation	Improved regional control with CLND (3 y 92% vs 77%) No change in melanoma-specific survival (3-y 86% vs 86%)	CLND improves local control but not melanoma-specific survival after positive SLNB
DeCOG-SLT *Leiter et al. Lancet Oncol* 2016 483 patients with +SLNB for micro-metastases. Randomized	Completion LND Observation	DSS 75% with CLND and 77% with observation at 3 years	CLND does not improve DSS for melanoma in patients with micrometastases found on SLNB

NONMELANOMA SKIN CANCER

ALISON YODER • DEVARATI MITRA • ASHLEIGH GUADAGNOLO

BACKGROUND

- **Incidence/prevalence:** Nonmelanoma skin cancers (NMSCs) include basal cell carcinoma and squamous cell carcinoma, which together constitute the most common malignancy worldwide. The highest worldwide incidence is in Australia. Approximately 3.5 million new cases are diagnosed each year in the United States. Incidence rising. Lifetime risk is 1 in 5.
- **Risk factors:** Cumulative exposure to UV light, increasing age, Fitzpatrick skin types 1-4, immunosuppression (HIV and organ transplant), human papillomavirus (HPV), and certain syndromes or genetic disorders (basal cell nevus syndrome [Gorlin syndrome], xeroderma pigmentosum, epidermolysis bullosa, or oculocutaneous albinism).

TUMOR BIOLOGY AND SPECIAL CONSIDERATION

- **Prevention:** Reduction in sun exposure and oral nicotinamide (vitamin B_3) (*Chen et al. N Engl J Med* 2015)
- **Pathology:** BCC (~80%) and SCC (~20%) make up the majority of NMSC. Minority are neuroendocrine, sweat gland, mesenchymal tumors, or lymphomas.
- **Pathologic risk factors** are listed in the Table below.
- **Anatomy:** Predominately occurs on sun-exposed areas. Skin layers are epidermis → papillary dermis → reticular dermis → subcutaneous tissues.

Workup

- **History and physical:** Focused and complete examination of the skin as many may have additional cancers and are at increased risk of developing melanoma.
- **Procedures/biopsy:** Shave/punch/excisional biopsies may be used for diagnosis. Skin biopsy should include the deep reticular dermis if suspicion is high for invasion.
- **Imaging:** The majority of NMSCs can be successfully managed without formal imaging. Consider CT if bony invasion and MRI if orbital involvement or perineural spread depending on presenting symptoms and exam. If there is concern for lymph node spread, it is reasonable to obtain a PET/CT scan.

TABLE 59.1 Risk Factors for Recurrence for Basal Cell Carcinoma (BCC) and Recurrence/Metastasis for Squamous Cell Carcinomas (SCC)

	Low Risk	High Risk
Location/size[a]	L < 20 mm M < 10 mm	L > 20 mm M ≥ 10 mm H > 6 mm
Borders	Well-defined	Poorly defined
Primary vs recurrent	Primary	Recurrent
Immunosuppression	(–)	(+)
Site of prior RT	(–)	(+)
PNI[b] or LVSI	(–)	(+)
Pathology	G1 (SCC) Nodular superficial (BCC)	G2-3 (SCC) Aggressive growth pattern (BCC)
Depth, thickness, or Clark level	<2 mm or I, II, III (SCC)	≥2 mm or IV, V (SCC)

[a]H (mask area), M (cheek, forehead, scalp, neck, pretibial), L (trunk and extremities).
[b]PNI is defined as involvement of large-caliber nerves with a diameter of >0.1 mm.

Treatment Algorithm

Definitive RT is recommended for nonsurgical candidates and clinical instances where skin cancer is located in cosmetically sensitive areas or where surgery might result in a functional deficit—guidelines released by ASTRO (*Porceddu et al. IJROBP* 2020)

T1/T2 operable	Surgical resection (WLE, Mohs, or electrodesiccation for low risk)
T1/T2 inoperable	Definitive RT
cN0 but risk >15% (eg, G3, PNI)	Elective dissection Elective RT (*see ASTRO Guidelines*)
cN+ or pN+	Therapeutic dissection followed by postoperative RT to the nodal bed (unless only 1 LN, <3 cm without ECE)
Postoperative	RT for high risk, SCC T3/T4, recurrent disease, or close/positive margins. May be supplemented by chemotherapy in very select patients
M1	Chemotherapy, clinical trial, or best supportive care

Radiation Treatment Technique

- **SIM:** CT simulation–based treatment planning is recommended for IMRT, history of adjacent RT, or in anticipation of future retreatment. Clinical setup is reasonable for orthovoltage, fixed geometry electronic brachytherapy, and palliation. Wire CTV. Skin collimation for field size <4 cm or for protection of adjacent uninvolved sensitive structures. Bolus to bring dose to the surface.
- **Dose:**
  Definitive RT:
  - For most lesions and optimal cosmesis: 66 Gy/33 fx (2 Gy/fx) or 55 Gy/20 fx (2.75 Gy/fx) delivered daily; 44 Gy/10 fx (4.4 Gy/fx) delivered 4 times a week

- For <2 cm lesions or palliation of large lesions: 50 Gy/15 fx (3.3 Gy/fx); 40 Gy/10 fx (4 Gy/fx), 35 Gy/5 fx (7 Gy/fx) delivered daily
- Skin surface brachytherapy: 40 Gy/8 fx (5 Gy/fx); 44 Gy/10 fx (4.4 Gy/fx) delivered twice or 3 times per week, at least 48 hours apart

Adjuvant RT to primary site:
- 60 Gy/30 fx (2 Gy/fx) or 50 Gy/20 fx (2.5 Gy/fx) delivered daily
- Consider boost to 66 Gy/33 fx if positive margins

Adjuvant RT to regional nodes:
- 66 Gy (2 Gy/fx) for ECE or gross residual adenopathy
- 60 Gy (2 Gy/fx) for no ECE/no residual adenopathy to the involved neck
- 50 Gy (2 Gy/fx) to the undissected neck

- **Target:**

Definitive RT:
- CTV = Primary tumor with 0.5- to 2-cm margin. CTV margin varies based on tumor histology, risk factors, location, and mode of therapy.

Adjuvant RT to primary site:
- CTV = Primary tumor bed with 1- to 2-cm margin +/– ipsilateral parotid and neck nodes, +/– trigeminal or facial nerve pathways
- CTV boost = Primary tumor bed with 0.5- to 1-cm margin

- **Technique:** Electron beam therapy, orthovoltage, brachytherapy, and IMRT in special circumstances (eg, large CTV along scalp convexity, neurotropic spread along CN)
- **Planning directive (for conventional fractionation):** Electron beam doses are prescribed to 90% of D_{max}. Orthovoltage x-ray doses are specified at D_{max} (skin surface). For normal tissue tolerance, refer to Head and Neck section for planning directive tolerances.

SURGERY

- Wide local excision (WLE): Requires the removal of healthy skin; it results in a larger wound.
- Mohs micrographic surgery: Specialized technique for removal of skin cancer. Allows precise microscopic control of the margins by utilizing tangentially cut frozen section histology.
- Curettage and electrodessication (C&E): Commonly performed procedure to remove low-risk BCC and SCC by scraping off the lesion with a curette followed by cauterization. Not recommended for high-risk NMSC.

SYSTEMIC THERAPY

- Vismodegib (Erivedge) and sonidegib (Odomzo) are inhibitors of the sonic hedgehog pathway and FDA approved for adult patients with advanced BCC. Common side effects are GI upset, muscle spasms, fatigue, alopecia, and dysgeusia.
- Topical 5FU (Efudex) is approved for treatment of actinic keratosis (AK) and superficial BCC.
- Concurrent chemoradiation with platinum agents can be considered for patient with high-risk features on a case-to-case basis.
- Neoadjuvant cemiplimab can be considered for stage II-IV SCC (*Gross, NEJM,* 2022).

SIDE EFFECT MANAGEMENT

- Radiation dermatitis: Bland emollient application and sterile nonadherent dressings to keep site clean and moist. Topical steroids (eg, triamcinolone) and Domeboro rinses may be necessary.

FOLLOW-UP

- BCC: H&P, complete skin exam q6-12mo for life
- SCC localized: H&P q3-12mo for 2 years, then q6-12mo for 3 years, and then q1y for life
- SCC regional: H&P q1-3mo for year 1, then q2-4mo for year 2, then q4-6mo for years 3-5, and then q6-12mo for life

Notable Papers

Name/Inclusion	Arms	Outcomes	Notes
Veness et al. *Laryngoscope*, 2005 Retrospective Review (RR) of 167 patients with SCC with nodal involvement	Surgery only (13%) Surgery with adjuvant RT (87%)	Decreased locoregional recurrence w/ PORT (20% vs 43%) Improved 5-y DSS with PORT (73% vs 54%)	Improved LRR and DSS with adjuvant RT for locally advanced SCC
Herman et al. *Eur Arch Otorhinolaryngol* 2016 RR of 107 patients with SCC metastatic to parotid LNs, cN0 cervical nodes	Elective neck dissection + RT (42 patients) RT alone (65 patients)	Local regional control the same between the two arms (1 recurrence in each arm)	PORT (50-60 Gy) to a cN0 neck is a suitable alternative to a neck dissection
TROG 05.01, ***Porceddu et al.*** *JCO* 2018 310 patients with high-risk SCC. Randomized	PORT (60-66 Gy) alone PORT (60-66 Gy) + concurrent carboplatin	LRC was similar for both at 5 years (83% for chemoRT, 87% for RT alone) No difference in OS or DFS	No benefit of adding carboplatin to PORT for high-risk SCC
Van Hezewijk et al. *Radiother Oncol* 2010 RR of 434 nonmelanomatous skin cancers			Electron beam hypofractionation is safe and effective for NMSC

MERKEL CELL CARCINOMA

ALISON YODER • DEVARATI MITRA • ANDREW BISHOP • ASHLEIGH GUADAGNOLO

Background

- **Incidence/prevalence:** Rare aggressive skin cancer with neuroendocrine differentiation. Cell of origin is Merkel cell mechanoreceptor bound to the ends of sensory nerve fibers in the skin. 1500 cases are diagnosed annually in the United States. Incidence has been increasing over the last three decades. Higher incidence rates are reported in Australia and New Zealand.
- **Outcomes:** 5-year survival across all stages is variable. Stage I patients have estimated 5-year OS, 60-80%; stage II, 50-60%; and stage III, 25-45%. High rate of recurrence (local recurrence 25-30%, regional recurrence 50-60%, distant recurrence 30-36%). Worst prognosis of all skin cancers.
- **Demographics:** Median age at diagnosis is 75; majority of patients are older than 50. More common in males (2:1 male to female incidence). 90% of cases occur in white patients.
- **Risk factors:** Immunosuppression (increases risk 10× that of general population). UV exposure. Merkel cell polyomavirus (MCPyV) is detected in over 75% of cases.

Tumor Biology and Characteristics

- **Histologic subtypes:** Small cell, intermediate cell, and trabecular (best prognosis).
- **Pathology:** MCC typically presents as a mass with rare involvement of the epidermis. It is a small, round blue cell tumor. Staining with immunopanel including CK20 (typically positive in paranuclear "dotlike" pattern), CK7, and TTF-1 (both typically negative) is important. Additional IHC staining for neuroendocrine markers should be done (ie, chromogranin, synaptophysin, CD56). MCPyV can be detected via IHC.
- **Genetics:** Associated with mutations in *RB1* and *TP53*, especially in MCPyV-negative tumors.

Anatomy

- Can occur anywhere on skin, predominantly on sun-exposed areas. Most common location is the skin of the head and neck > upper extremities > lower extremities > trunk.

Workup

- **History and physical:** Focused and complete skin examination of the skin and regional lymph nodes
- **Imaging:** PET/CT for staging. Consider CT C/A/P with brain MRI, particularly if PET/CT is unavailable.

Treatment Algorithm

Primary site	Surgical resection, wide local excision, or Mohs +/– adjuvant RT to primary site*
cN0 nodal management	SLNB for staging If SLN positive → clinical trial, multidisciplinary discussion. RT to nodal basin (can consider CLND *Lee, Ann Surg Oncol* 2019; *Perez, Ann Surg Oncol* 2019). Discuss anti-PD1 therapy (*Becker, presented at ESMO* 2022)
cN+ nodal management	Surgical resection consisting of WLE with nodal dissection +/– adjuvant RT to primary site/nodal basin. Discuss anti-PD1 therapy (can consider neoadjuvantly) (*Checkmate 358, Topalian, JCO* 2020)

*Consider observation following WLE if small tumor (<1 cm), without LVSI, and no history of immunosuppression.

Factors for Adjuvant RT to Primary Site
Positive or close margin
LVSI
Consider for tumors >1 cm
Immunocompromised patient

Radiation Treatment Technique

- **SIM:** Depending on anatomic location. Bolus is necessary to ensure that superficial dose is adequate for the skin primary. Wire scar or field
  For head and neck location: Aquaplast mask, wire scar or primary site, draw field, and cut out field on mask if using electrons. Consider skin collimation. If near the ear, consider the use of TX-151 bolus.
- **Dose:**
  Primary:
  Tumor >2 cm, R0 resection → 50-56 Gy at 2 Gy/fx
  R1 resection → 56-60 Gy at 2 Gy/fx
  R2 resection or unresected disease → 60-66 Gy at 2 Gy/fx
  Nodal Basin
  cN0, no nodal evaluation → 46-50 Gy
  cN0, SLNB negative → no RT (unless potential for false-negative SLNB due to anatomic, operator, or histologic failure)
  cN0, SLNB positive, no formal dissection → 50 Gy
  cN+, no dissection → systemic therapy, then consider 50-60 Gy
  cN+, formal dissection with multiple LNs and/or ECE → 50-56 Gy
- **Target:**
  Primary: Primary site/scar + 4-cm margin for CTV; when planning electrons, consider penumbra and need to expand edges of field another 7-10 mm to cover the target.
  Lymph nodes: Involved/sentinel nodal basins
- **Technique:** Consider electrons to get adequate dose to the surface for RT to the primary.
  Consider skin collimation and bolus. Photons may be needed for deep primary tumors and for regional RT.
- **IGRT:** Related to modality used and site of the body. Typically weekly kV for 3D plans
- **Planning directive:** Standard dose constraints for 2 Gy/fx for ROIs nearby

SURGERY

- Primary: Wide local excision with a goal of negative margin when feasible (1- to 2-cm margins). Mohs surgery is an acceptable alternative for smaller lesions. Balance with morbidity of surgery. Avoid complex procedures that would lead to a delay in RT.
- cN0 → sentinel lymph node biopsy. SLNB must be done prior to WLE as to not alter the drainage to the sentinel basin. If SLNB is +, consider completion dissection or RT for cN0.
- cLN+ → Nodal basin dissection

SYSTEMIC THERAPY

- No randomized data with survival benefit, impressive response rates have been seen with immunotherapy (*Nghiem NEJM* 2016; *D'Angelo J Immunother Cancer* 2021; *Kim, Lancet* 2022)
- Immunotherapy considered first line for advanced disease
- Platinum + etoposide can be used—induces response but has poor durability (*Nghiem Future Oncol* 2017).

SIDE EFFECT MANAGEMENT

- Skin care: First-line emollients. Can add topical steroid (eg, triamcinolone), Domeboro soaks thereafter. If having further grade 2+ skin toxicity, consider Mepilex. If grade 3 dermatitis, consider Silvadene cream (on weekends or after RT has been completed entirely).

FOLLOW-UP

- Complete skin and regional nodal examination every 3-6 months for 2 years. (Most recurrences occur within 2 years.) Can space to every 6-12 months thereafter.
- Imaging in LN+ patients on same schedule as above (ie, PET/CT)

NOTABLE PAPERS

Name/Inclusion	Arms	Outcomes	Notes
Strom et al. *Ann Surg Oncol* 2016 RR of 171 patients with merkel cell	All patients treated for merkel cell carcinoma with definitive local therapy who had a surgical lymph node assessment	Improved 3-y LC (91% vs 77%), DFS (57% vs 30%) and OS (73% vs 66%) with PORT DSS improved in node-positive patients (76% vs 48%) but not node negative (90% vs 81%)	Improved disease control and OS with the addition of RT
Bishop et al. *Head Neck* 2015 RR of 106 patients with merkel cell	Most patients were postoperative, 92% with cN0 disease received regional nodal RT to 46 Gy	5-y LRC, DSS, OS were 96%, 76%, and 58%, respectively 5% with long-term grade 3 toxicity	Postoperative RT to primary and nodal basins well-tolerated
Lee et al. *Ann Surg Oncol* 2018 RR of 163 patients with merkel cell with + SLNB	CLND (n = 137) RT (n = 26)	No significant difference in DSS (71% CLND vs 64% RT), NRFS (76% vs 91%) or DFS (52% vs 61%) at 5 years	RT to the nodal basin has similar outcomes to CLND for those with +SLNB

HODGKIN LYMPHOMA

GOHAR MANZAR • JILLIAN GUNTHER

Background

- **Incidence/prevalence:** 10% of all lymphomas in the United States, 8500 new cases per year
- **Demographics:** Predominantly young adults with slight male predominance, bimodal age distribution (peaks at 20 and 65)
- **Risk factors:** Delayed/reduced antigen exposure (single family housing, small family size), immunosuppression, EBV virus exposure, autoimmune disease, radiation exposure especially at young age
- **Outcomes:** Stage I/II: 90-95% OS at 8 years
  Stage III/IV (based on IPS): 0-1, 90%; 2-3, 80%; 4-5, 60% OS at 5 years

IPS, 1 point each: Age ≥ 45, albumin < 4, stage IV, Hgb < 10.5, absolute lymphocyte count < 8%, WBC > 15K, male

Tumor Biology and Characteristics

- **Pathology:**
  - Classical (CD15+/CD30+/CD20–, 95% of cases), nodular sclerosing, mixed cellularity, lymphocyte rich, lymphocyte depleted
  - Nodular lymphocyte predominant Hodgkin lymphoma (NLPHL) (CD15−/CD30−/CD20+/CD45+, 5% of cases) is unlike Classical HL with a unique natural history and is treated differently—located in the groin, axilla, or neck (ie, peripheral locations); usually not mediastinum
- **Imaging:** PET-avid. Typically nodal disease graded utilizing Deauville criteria

Deauville Five-Point Scale for Treatment Response

(*Cheson et al. and Barrington et al. JCO* 2014)

Score	Description	Interpretation
1	No residual uptake	Negative
2	Uptake < mediastinum	Negative
3	Uptake > mediastinum, but ≤ liver	Negative
4	Uptake > liver	Positive
5	Markedly increased uptake and/or any new lesion	Positive
X	New area of uptake unlikely related to lymphoma	Negative

Workup

- **Laboratory studies:** Core needle or excisional biopsy (FNA is not acceptable), CBC w/ diff, LFTs, thyroid function, LDH, ESR, albumin, and pregnancy test; bone marrow biopsy generally not indicated
- **Imaging:** PET scan with contrasted CT component
- **Other studies:** PFT (for bleomycin) and echocardiogram (for doxorubicin)
- **Referrals:** Oncofertility and cardiology

Staging and Risk Stratification

Ann Arbor Staging (Lugano Modification)			
I	Single lymph node region or group of adjacent nodes	**IE**	One extranodal site
II	≥2 node regions on same side of the diaphragm	**IIE**	Stage I/II by nodal extent with limited contiguous extranodal involvement
III	Nodes on both sides of the diaphragm or nodes above diaphragm with splenic involvement		
IV	Noncontiguous extranodal involvement		

Modifiers			
A	No B symptoms	**B**	**B symptoms:** unexplained weight loss >10% over 6 months, drenching night sweats, or fever (>38°C)

The designation X for bulky disease (typically ≥10 cm) is no longer necessary in the AJCC 8th edition; instead, a recording of the largest tumor diameter is required.

Nodal regions ("L/R" are considered to be separate)
Supradiaphragmatic regions: Waldeyer ring, L/R cervical/supraclavicular/occipital/preauricular, infraclavicular nodes, L/R axillary/pectoral, mediastinal, L/R hilar, L/R epitrochoidal/brachial
Infradiaphragmatic regions: Spleen, mesenteric, para-aortic, L/R iliac, L/R inguinal/femoral, L/R popliteal

Unfavorable Risk Factors		
Risk Factor	**GHSG**[a]	**EORTC**
Age		≥50
ESR	>50 if no B symptoms >30 if B symptoms	>50 if A >30 if B
Mediastinal mass	MMR > 0.33	MMR > 0.35
Lymph nodal areas[b]	3 or more	4 or more
Extranodal lesions	Any	
Bulky		

[a]MDACC uses GHSG criteria for risk stratification, ≥1 risk factor = unfavorable risk
[b]Differs between GHSG/EORTC

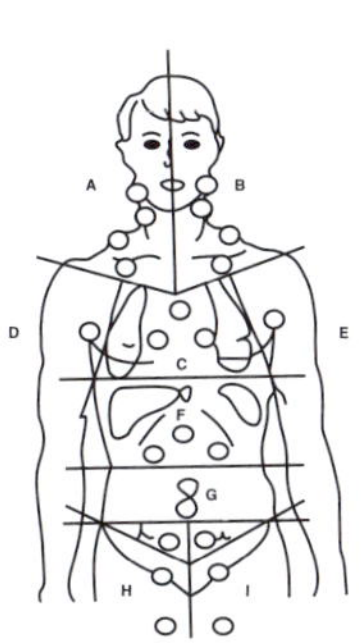

Reproduced with permission from GHSG. https://en.ghsg.org/disease-stages.

Lymph Node Areas (GHSG) for Risk Stratification*	
Right/left	Midline
A/B. Cervical/supraclav/infraclav/subpectoral	**C.** Hilar/mediastinal
D/E. Axilla	**F.** Upper abdomen (spleen, liver, celiac)
H/I. Iliac	**G.** Lower abdomen (spleen, liver, celiac)
K/L. Inguinal/femoral	

*Separate lymph node regions are considered for the purpose of Ann Arbor staging and risk stratification.

Treatment Algorithm

Standard of care treatment regimens exist that involve omission of radiation therapy.

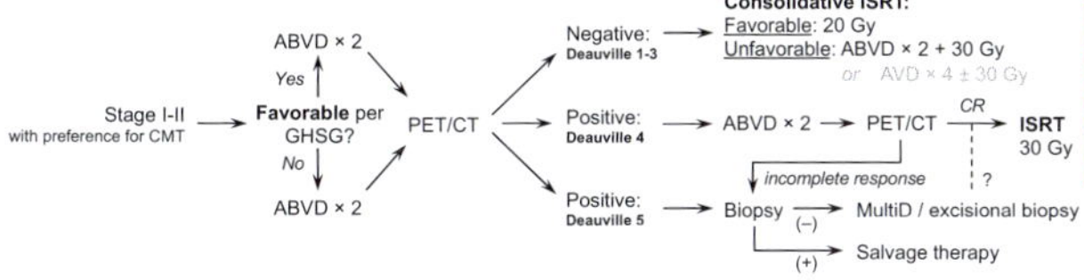

HL 12-2

	Stage/Risk	Systemic therapy	Consolidation RT
Classical Hodgkin	Early favorable: stages I, II nonbulky, and no RF*	2 cycles of ABVD	20 Gy/10 fx, ISRT
	Early unfavorable: stages I, IIA, and ≥1 RF stages IIB and ≥1 RT (no: MMR, ENE, or bulky)	4 cycles of ABVD	30 Gy/15 fx or 30.6 Gy/17 fx, ISRT
	Stage IIB bulky	4-6 cycles of ABVD	30 Gy/15 fx or 30.6 Gy/17 fx, ISRT
	Advanced: stages III, IV	6 cycles of ABVD (with RATHL approach) or AAVD (caution in age >60 or neuropathy)	Consider 30/30.6 Gy for prechemo bulky supradiaphragmatic sites or sites of PR after chemo
NLPHL	Stage IA, contiguous IIA	None	30-30.6 Gy/15-17 fx ISRT** alone
	Stage III, stage IV, or B symptoms	Variable approaches; 3-6 cycles of R-CHOP vs observation vs Rituxan vs ABVD	24-30.6 Gy/12-17 fx ISRT can be considered for sites of bulk or sites of incomplete PET/CT response

*RF, risk factor (as per chart above)

**ISRT, involved site radiation therapy. A slightly more generous involved site is permitted for NLPHL if systemic therapy is not given.

PET/CT imaging should be obtained at minimum after two cycles and at the end of all planned cycles of chemotherapy for early unfavorable and advanced stage cases.

Radiation Treatment Technique

Target Location	Technique	Simulation
Neck	IMRT	Supine, thermoplastic mask
Mediastinum	IMRT with butterfly beam arrangement (AP PA weighted beam angles)	Supine, Vac-Lok indexed with Dabaja/angle board (10-15 degrees), thermoplastic mask, hip stopper, deep inspiratory breath hold
Axilla	IMRT or 3DCRT	Supine, arm slightly akimbo or overhead, Vac-Lok, consider deep inspiratory breath hold for low axilla
Abdomen	IMRT	Supine, arms overhead, Vac-Lok, wing board with T-bar, deep inspiratory breath hold

The goal is to reduce low-dose exposure to adjacent OARs. Depending on patient-specific anatomy and tumor location, other techniques and setups may be more optimal.

- Planning directive

Note that with the prospect of longevity and wanting to avoid RT toxicity, ALARA is the most important guiding principle. Furthermore, exercise caution since many of the below constraints do not apply to 20 Gy treatments.

OAR	Dose Constraint(s)
Heart	Mean < 5 Gy, no higher than 15 Gy
Coronaries	Minimize the maximum dose to individual coronary arteries
Total lung	Mean < 13.5 Gy, V20 < 30%, V5 < 55%
Breasts	Minimize volume >4 Gy (ideally <10%)
Thyroid gland	V25 < 63.5%, minimize V30 Gy

OAR	Dose Constraint(s)
Kidneys	Mean <8 gy;V10 < 30%;V20 < 15% (recommended); < 25% (acceptable)
Ipsilateral parotid glands	Mean < 11 Gy
Submandibular glands	Mean < 11 Gy
Lacrimal glands	V20 < 80%
Spleen	Mean < 10 Gy;V5 ≥ 30;V15 ≤ 20
Liver	Mean < 15;V20 < 30;V30 < 20

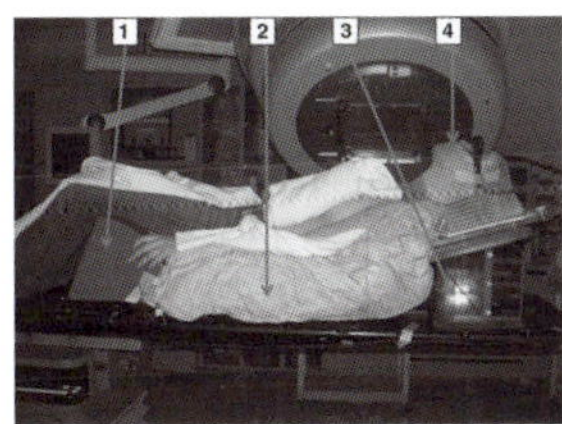

Figure 61.1 Simulation set up for mediastinal HL. (1) Hip stopper, (2) Vac-Lok, (3) Dabaja or incline board at 10-15 degrees, and (4) thermoplastic mask. The patient is wearing goggles that provide real-time visual feedback on the breath cycle.

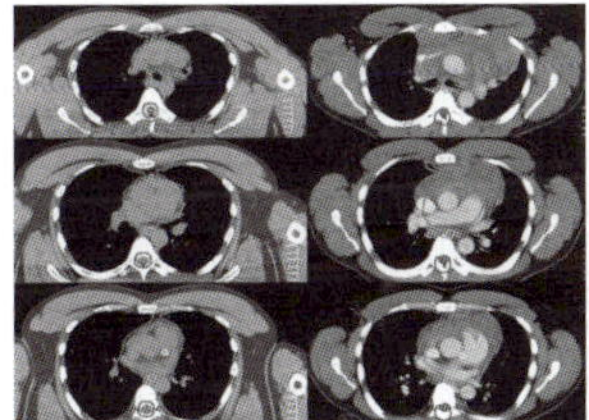

Figure 61.2 Axial view of DIBH (*left* three images) and normal breathing (*right* three images). DIBH can significantly reduce radiation to the coronary arteries, heart, and lungs. Confirm positioning with CT-based IGRT

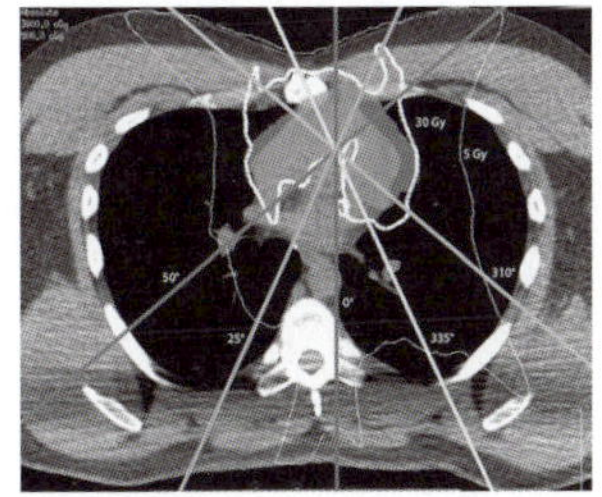

Figure 61.3 Deep inspiratory breath hold with a butterfly technique beam arrangement for anterior mediastinal HL. Anterior beam angles were restricted between 310 and 50 degrees. 30 Gy isodose line is *thick white*; 5 Gy isodose line is *thin white*. AP-PA weighted beam arrangements reduce low-dose spray to breasts and lungs.

Chemotherapy

- ABVD—doxorubicin (Adriamycin), bleomycin, vinblastine, dacarbazine
  Can consider holding bleomycin during latter cycles for early good response on PETCT (eg, RATHL), or if anticipating consolidative RT
- BEACOPP: bleomycin, etoposide, doxorubicin (Adriamycin), cyclophosphamide, vincristine (Oncovin), procarbazine, prednisone
  Not routinely used in the United States due to toxicities (infertility, secondary malignancy)
- AAVD: brentuximab vedotin (Adcetris), doxorubicin (Adriamycin), vinblastine, and dacarbazine
  Preferred upfront therapy for patients with stage III-IV disease

Side Effect Management

- Esophagitis: Xyloxylin (1:1:1 ratio of diphenhydramine, Maalox, viscous lidocaine), 10-15 mL swish/swallow up to 4 times a day
- Pneumonitis (dyspnea or cough): Prednisone 1 mg/kg/d for 2-4 weeks, taper slowly over 2-3 months

Follow-up

- Full-body CT with contrast no more than every 6 months for the first 2 years after treatment; PET/CT **only** if previous Deauville 4-5
- Interim H&P 3 months after completion of therapy then Q6 months for first 3 years, then annually
- Late cardiovascular toxicities: consider echocardiogram/stress and carotid ultrasound if RT to neck Q10 years
- TSH at least annually if RT to neck to evaluate for potential hypothyroidism, supplement with levothyroxine if detected
- Secondary malignancies: Start annual breast screening the earlier of 8-10 years after therapy or age 40 (whatever is sooner) if chest radiation. If RT to chest prior to age 30, screen with mammogram and MRI.

Notable Trials

Study	Design	RFS/PFS/DFS	OS	Conclusion
HD10 *Engert NEJM* 2010 1370 total patients	Stage I or II no risk factors 2 × 2 randomized: 1. ABVD × 2 vs ABVD × 4 2. IFRT 30 vs 20 Gy	**8-y PFS** ABVD × 2 + 20: 87% ABVD × 2 + 30: 85% ABVD × 4 + 20: 90% ABVD × 4 + 30: 88%	**8-y** ABVD × 2 + 20: 95% ABVD × 2 + 30: 94% ABVD × 4 + 20: 95% ABVD × 4 + 30: 94%	Early favorable Hodgkin lymphoma can be treated with ABVD × 2 and 20 Gy
HD11 *Eich JCO* 2010 1395 total patients	Stage IA-IIA and ≥1 risk factors or Stage IIB + ESR ≥30 (no bulky or ENE) 2 × 2 randomized: 1. BEACOPP × 4 vs ABVD × 4 2. IFRT 20 vs 30 Gy	**5-y PFS** ABVD + 30: 87% ABVD + 20: 82% BEACOPP + 30: 88% BEACOPP + 20: 87%	**5-y** ABVD + 30: 94% ABVD + 20: 94% BEACOPP + 30: 95% BEACOPP + 20: 95%	Early unfavorable Hodgkin lymphoma can be treated with AVBD × 4 and 30 Gy

Study	Design	RFS/PFS/DFS	OS	Conclusion
H10 *Andre JCO* 2017 1950 total patients	Favorable or unfavorable, stage I or II with **upfront ABVD × 2 → PET** Favorable patients randomized three ways: 1. ABVD × 1 + 30-36 Gy 2a. PET(−): ABVD × 2 2b. PET(+): BEACOPP + 30-36 Gy Unfavorable patients randomization three ways: 1. ABVD × 2 + 30-36 Gy 2a. PET(−): ABVD × 4 2b. PET(+): BEACOPP × 2 + INRT	**5-y PFS** **PET(+)** ABVD + RT: 77% BEACOPP + RT: 91% **Fav, PET(−)** ABVD × 3 + RT: 99% ABVD × 4: 87% **Unfav, PET(−)** ABVD × 4 + RT: 92% ABVD × 6: 90%	**5-y** **PET(+)** ABVD + RT: 89% BEACOPP + RT: 96% **Fav, PET(−)** ABVD × 3 + RT: 100% ABVD × 4: 100% **Unfav, PET(−)** ABVD × 4 + RT: 98% ABVD × 6: 98%	For interim PET(+) patients, radiation therapy improves PFS For interim PET(+) patients, escalation to BEACOPP + RT improves PFS
HD16 *Fuchs JCO* 2019 1150 total patients	Favorable stage I or II with **upfront ABVD × 2 → PET** Favorable patients randomized three ways: 1. Standard 20 Gy IFRT 2a. PET(−): No further treatment 2b. PET(+): 20 Gy IFRT noninferiority of omitting RT in PET-adapted approach: Δ5-y PFS>10%	**5-y PFS** **Standard combined modality treatment** 1. IFRT: 93.4% **PET-adapted** 2a. No further treatment: 88.4% 2b. IFRT: 93.2%	**5-y OS** **Standard combined modality treatment** 1. IFRT: 98.1% **PET-adapted** 2a. No further treatment: 98.2% 2b. IFRT: 97.9%	For early-stage Hodgkin lymphoma, s/p 2 cycles of ABVD, even for good PET responders, it is not noninferior to omit radiation in terms of PFS
IIB Bulky *Reddy Clin Lymphoma Myeloma Leuk* 2015 149 patients	Retrospective, stage IIB bulky treated with chemotherapy and/or radiation	**8-y** All: 77%	**8-y** ABVD: 89% MOPP: 66% >30.1 Gy: 78% <30.1 Gy: 46%	Excellent outcomes treating IIB bulky patients with chemo and RT
Stage III *Phan JCO* 2011 118 patients	Retrospective, stage III treated with chemotherapy and/or radiation	**15-y DFS** RT: 65%; No RT: 15% Mediastinal RT associated with improved DFS and OS	**15-y** RT: 80% No RT: 29%	Radiation particularly important for disease above the diaphragm. Less effective in abdomen after 6 cycles of ABVD

Study	Design	RFS/PFS/DFS	OS	Conclusion
RATHL *Johnson NEJM* 2016 *Trotman (Abstract)* 2017 1214 total patients	Stage IIB-IV or Stage IIA (bulky or 3+ sites) **Upfront ABVD × 2 → PET1** PET1(−) randomization: 1a. ABVD × 4 1b. ABVD × 2 → AVD × 2 PET1(+) were not randomized and received additional therapy: **BEACOPP-based therapy → PET2** PET2(+) → radiation PET2(−) → BEACOPP-based therapy	**5-y PFS** **PET1(−)** 1a. ABVD × 6: 83% 1b. ABVD × 4 → AVD × 2: 81% **PET1(+):** 66% 11 of 39 patients with stage II bulky with PET1(+) received RT, 1 progression at median follow-up of 52 months	**5-y** **PET1(−)** 1a. ABVD × 6: 95.3% 1b. ABVD ×2 → AVD x2 : 95.0% **PET1(+)**: 85.1%	Dropping last two cycles of bleomycin for good PET responders does not compromise efficacy RT is efficacious for bulky residual disease
RAPID *Radford NEJM* 2015 602 total patients	Stage IA or IIA PET(−) after ABVD × 3 Randomized: 1. IFRT 2. Observation	**3-y** IFRT: 95% Observation: 91% Noninferiority margin of 7% for PFS not met	**3-y** IFRT: 97% Observation: 99%	For early-stage Hodgkin lymphoma, it is not noninferior to omit radiation for good PET responders
ECHELON1 *Ansell NEJM* 2022 664 total patients	Stage III or IV Randomized: 1. Brentuximab vedotin, doxorubicin, vinblastine, and dacarbazine (A+AVD) 2. ABVD	**6-y** A+AVD: 82.3% ABVD: 74.5% HR: 0.68, *P* = 0.04	**6-y** A+AVD: 93.9% ABVD: 89.4% HR: 0.59, *P* = 0.009	For advanced-stage Hodgkin lymphoma, A+AVD has superior frontline efficacy to ABVD with improved PFS and OS

DIFFUSE LARGE B-CELL LYMPHOMA

GOHAR MANZAR • PENNY FANG

Background

- **Incidence/prevalence:** Most common form of high-grade non-Hodgkin lymphoma (NHL); accounts for 30-40% of all NHLs. Approximately 22 000 cases diagnosed in the United States each year
- **Outcomes:** 5-Year survival across all stages estimated at 60% (SEER data)
- **Demographics:** Typically in middle-aged and elderly adults, median age at diagnosis is 64.
- **Risk factors:** Age, HIV infection, immunosuppression, preexisting B-cell lymphoproliferative disorder (eg, follicular lymphoma, chronic lymphocytic leukemia/small lymphocytic lymphoma [CLL/SLL])

Tumor Biology and Characteristics

- **Pathology:** Immunophenotype, CD20+, CD45+, and CD3−. Designated as germinal center B cell (GCB) or nongerminal center B cell/activated B cell (non-GCB/ABC) based on gene expression profiling (GEP) studies *(Alizadeh et al. Nature* 2000)
  - **GCB DLBCL:** Arises from centroblasts in the light zone of the lymph node germinal center and may have chromosomal abnormalities affecting *MYC* [t(8;14), *MYC*;IgH/t(2;8), Igκ; *MYC*/t(8;22), *MYC*;Igλ (observed in 10%)], and *BCL2* [t(14;18), IgH: *BCL2* (observed in 40%)] detected by FISH.
  - **Non-GCB/ABC DLBCL:** Arises from postgerminal center lymphocytes that have committed to plasmablastic differentiation and is characterized by NF-κB activation and blockade of terminal differentiation into plasma cells. In general, GCB DLBCL has a better prognosis than non-GCB/ABC DLBCL.
  - The Hans algorithm *(Hans et al. Blood* 2004) is a widely used immunohistochemical surrogate for gene expression profiling to discriminate GCB and non-GCB/ABC DLBCL.

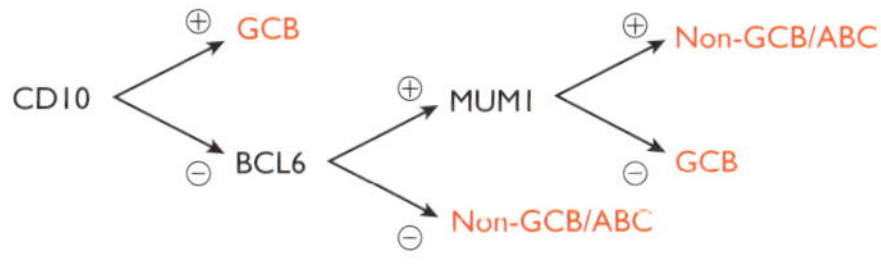

- **Double-hit lymphoma (DHL) and double-protein expression lymphoma:** Aggressive subsets of DLBCL that arise from coexisting genomic rearrangement of *MYC* and *BCL2* or *BCL6* or overexpression of MYC and BCL2 in the absence of simultaneous gene rearrangements (double-protein expression) *(Johnson et al. JCO* 2012). DHL lymphomas are typically GCB DLBCL and have the worst prognosis of all subtypes, while double-protein expression lymphomas are typically non-GCB/ABC DLBCL.
- **Imaging:** ^{18}FDG PET-CT is the most sensitive imaging modality. CT may be used for follow-up. MRI may be useful for imaging the central nervous system (CNS), bulky, or extranodal sites of disease.

Deauville Scale for Treatment Response

(*Cheson et al.* and *Barrington et al. JCO* **2014**)

Score	Description	Interpretation
1	No residual uptake	Negative
2	Uptake < mediastinum	Negative
3	Uptake > mediastinum, but ≤ liver	Negative
4	Uptake > liver	Positive
5	Markedly increased uptake and/or any new lesion	Positive
X	New area of uptake unlikely related to lymphoma	Negative

Workup

- **Laboratory studies:** Core needle or excisional biopsy (FNA is not acceptable, lack tissue architecture), CBC w/diff, ESR, CMP, uric acid, LDH, albumin, bone marrow biopsy (if cytopenic and PET negative)
- **Imaging:** PET/CT, CT with contrast of the neck, chest, abdomen, pelvis
- **Other studies:** Hepatitis B and HIV testing (for rituximab), echocardiogram or MUGA (for doxorubicin). Lumbar puncture is considered for HIV-associated lymphoma, testicular lymphoma, or hit/expression lymphoma.
- **Referrals:** Consider cardiology and infectious diseases.

Ann Arbor Staging System

(*Lugano Modifications, Cheson et al. JCO* **2014**)

See **"Hodgkin Lymphoma"** chapter.

International Prognostic Index

(*Ziepert et al. JCO* **2009**)

One Point per Criterion		**3-Y Overall Survival**	
Age	>60	IPI 0-1	91.4%
ECOG performance status	2, 3, or 4	IPI 2	80.9%
LDH	>Upper limit of normal	IPI 3	65.1%
Extranodal involvement	>1 site	IPI 4-5	59.0%
Ann Arbor stage	III or IV		

Treatment Algorithm for Complete Response to Chemotherapy

Standard-of-care treatment regimens exist that involve omission of radiation therapy. Primary indications for treatment include skeletal, CNS, or testicular involvement of any disease stage, bulky disease of any disease stage, limited-stage and nonbulky disease if only ×3 cycles of R-CHOP, or as palliative/bridging prior to CAR-T cell therapy

Stage I/II*	Nonbulky **and** IPI 0-1	R-CHOP* ×3-4 → 30.6 Gy/17 fx ISRT vs R-CHOP ×4 alone
	Bulky (≥7.5 cm) **or** IPI > 1	R-CHOP* ×6 → 30.6 Gy/17 fx ISRT
Stage III/IV*	Bulky or extranodal (especially osseous) sites of disease	R-CHOP* ×6 → 30.6-36 Gy/17-20 fx ISRT

*For patients with DHL, double-protein expression, or other concerning pathologic features, more aggressive chemotherapy with DA-R-EPOCH can be considered (*Landsburg et al. JCO* 2017).

Treatment Algorithm for Relapsed or Refractory Patients

- The role of radiotherapy for patients with relapsed or refractory DLBCL is individualized and depends on patient- and treatment-related factors, including prior systemic therapy, the extent of disease at diagnosis and relapse, patient performance status, and potential future therapies. Please refer to the International Lymphoma Radiation Oncology Group (ILROG) guidelines for further details and guidance (*Ng et al. IJROBP* 2018).

Radiation Treatment Technique (Not Including Primary CNS or Testicular)

- **Sim:** Highly variable; dependent on area(s) being treated
  - Head and neck: Supine, thermoplastic mask ± bite block, stent as appropriate
  - Axilla: Supine, upper Vac-Lok, arms akimbo
  - Mediastinum: Supine, incline board, upper Vac-Lok, deep inspiration breath hold (DIBH)
  - Abdomen: Supine, upper and/or lower Vac-Lok; consider NPO for 3 hours prior to sim/treatment, may require respiratory motion management
  - Pelvis: Supine, lower Vac-Lok

- **Dose:**

	Response	Dose
Consolidation after chemotherapy	Deauville 1-3	30.6 Gy
	Any Deauville 4-5 residual disease after frontline chemotherapy	Salvage chemotherapy and transplant -or- *30.6-36 Gy to original sites of disease, integrate boost to 45-50 Gy to Deauville 4-5 areas
Relapsed or refractory	Deauville 1-3 after multiple chemotherapy regimens or peritransplant	30.6-36 Gy to original sites of disease with consideration of integrated boost to 40 Gy to previous sites of persistent disease
	Deauville 4-5 after multiple chemotherapy regimens, including SCT	45-50 Gy to sites of gross disease for salvage (curative intent); consider hypofractionated course (eg, 20 Gy in 5 fractions, 30 Gy in 10 fractions, or 37.5 Gy in 15 fractions) for palliation

*For patients with low-volume residual Deauville 4-5 disease, radiation therapy alone can be attempted (in lieu of salvage chemotherapy and autologous stem cell rescue).

- **Targets:**
  - Involved site radiation therapy (ISRT)
    - Prechemotherapy site(s) of disease
    - CTV considers changes in size/extent of the tumor, position of nearby normal tissues and organs, and disease pattern and areas of potential subclinical involvement.
- **Technique:** IMRT/VMAT, though 3DCRT may be appropriate for certain geometries. "Butterfly" technique commonly used for mediastinal lymphoma to minimize dose to the heart, lungs, breasts, and spinal cord (*Voong et al. Radiat Oncol* 2014).
- **IGRT:** Dependent on technique and targets; daily kV, CBCT, or CT on rails
- **Dose constraints:**

Organ/Structure	Dose Constraint(s)
Heart*	Mean < 5 Gy, no higher than 15 Gy
Coronaries and left ventricle*	Max < 5 Gy
Total lung	Mean < 13.5 Gy, V20 < 30%, V5 < 55%
Breasts	Mean < 4 Gy
Thyroid gland	V25 < 63.5%
Kidneys	V5 < 30%, V20 < 33%
Parotid glands	Mean < 5 Gy or ALARA
Submandibular glands	Mean < 11 Gy
Spleen	Mean < 9 Gy
Liver	Max < 10 Gy

*Goal is to keep 5 Gy isodose line off as many critical structures as possible.

Chemotherapy

- **R-CHOP-21: R**ituximab (375 mg/m^2 IV on d1), **c**yclophosphamide (750 mg/m^2 IV on d1), **h**ydroxydaunorubicin (doxorubicin; 50 mg/m^2 IV on d1), **O**ncovin (vincristine; 1.4 mg/m^2 [max dose 2 mg] on d1), and **p**rednisone (40 mg/m^2 po on d1-5) every 21 days.
- **DA-R-EPOCH: R**ituximab (375 mg/m^2 IV on d1), **e**toposide (50 mg/m^2/d IV on d1-4), **p**rednisone (60 mg/m^2 po bid on d1-5), **O**ncovin (vincristine; 0.4 mg/m^2/d IV on d1-4), **c**yclophosphamide (750 mg/m^2 IV on d5), and **h**ydroxydaunorubicin (doxorubicin; 10 mg/m^2/d on d1-4) every 21 days. Subcutaneous Neupogen (filgrastim) is given once daily starting on d6 and continued until WBC count normalizes (can substitute for Neulasta [pegfilgrastim]). Dose-adjusted (DA) protocol increases (etoposide, doxorubicin, cyclophosphamide) or decreases (cyclophosphamide) doses for subsequent cycles based on neutrophil and/or platelet nadirs.

Special Subtypes of DLBCL

- **Primary central nervous system lymphoma (PCNSL)**
  - Classically seen in individuals with primary or acquired immunodeficiency
  - Workup: Slit lamp examination, lumbar puncture, spine MRI (if symptomatic or CSF is positive), HIV test, testicular examination, and testicular ultrasound (especially for men >60 years old)
  - If possible, delay initiation of steroids until biopsy is performed.
  - Treatment:
    - R-MPV (rituximab, high-dose methotrexate, procarbazine, vincristine, ± intrathecal chemotherapy)
    - Complete response: High-dose chemotherapy with autologous stem cell transplant or low-dose whole brain radiotherapy (23.4 Gy in 13 fractions at 1.8 Gy/fx; *Morris et al. JCO* 2013)
    - Residual disease: Whole-brain radiotherapy (30.6-36 Gy, boost gross disease to 45 Gy) or high-dose chemotherapy with autologous stem cell transplant
    - Consider omission of radiation in patients with poor functional status or age >60.
- **Primary testicular lymphoma**
  - Generally seen in men >60 years of age
  - Workup: Lumbar puncture and bilateral testicular ultrasound
  - R-CHOP or DA-R-EPOCH given per standard DLBCL protocol; intrathecal or high-dose methotrexate for CNS prophylaxis
  - High risk of contralateral testicular failure after chemotherapy (*Ho et al. Leuk and Lymphoma* 2017). All patients should receive testicle/scrotal/spermatic cord irradiation to 30.6 Gy in 17 fractions (1.8 Gy/fx) after completing chemotherapy (*Vitolo et al. JCO* 2011).
- **Primary mediastinal B-cell lymphoma**
  - Commonly presents in adolescents and young adults (esp. women)
  - Putatively arises from thymic B cells and has significant molecular overlap with nodular sclerosing Hodgkin lymphoma (NSHL). PMBCL cells are typically weakly positive for CD30 and negative for CD15, which helps discriminate PMBCL from NSHL.
  - DA-R-EPOCH x6 without consolidation radiotherapy for patients with Deauville ≤3 metabolic response on ^{18}FDG PET-CT offers excellent cure rates (*Dunleavy et al. NEJM* 2013).
    - Residual FDG avidity after DA-R-EPOCH should be interpreted cautiously, as not all postchemotherapy metabolic activity denotes active or residual lymphoma and necessitates radiotherapy.
  - For patients with low burden residual PET-CT–avid lymphoma after DA-R-EPOCH, salvage radiotherapy to a dose of 45-50 Gy may be considered. Alternate approaches include salvage chemotherapy followed by autologous stem cell transplant with posttransplant consolidative radiotherapy.
  - For patients with significant disease progression after DA-R-EPOCH, radiation therapy alone is not desirable (*Filippi et al. IJROBP* 2016).
  - Consolidation radiotherapy to 30.0-36.0 Gy is indicated for patients who receive R-CHOP chemotherapy in lieu of DA-R-EPOCH.

Follow-up

- No PET-CT for a minimum of 8 weeks after radiotherapy due to chance of false positives
- H&P and laboratory studies every 3-6 months for 5 years. For stages I and II, repeat imaging only as clinically indicated, and for stages III and IV, CT scan no more often than every 6 months for 2 years and then yearly afterward. TSH at least annually if RT to the neck.
- Secondary malignancies: Start annual breast screening the earlier of 8-10 years after therapy or age 40 if chest radiation

Notable Trials and Papers

Role of consolidation radiotherapy for early and advanced stage

Study	Design	Result	Comment
DSHNHL-2004-3/ UNFOLDER 21/14 (Ongoing; Interim results Held *ICML RT Workshop* 2013)	Phase III trial, 2×2 randomization Early-stage DLBCL IPI = 0-1 with bulky (≥7.5 cm) disease **Arms:** 1A. R-CHOP-21 ×6 1B. R-CHOP-21 ×6 → involved field radiotherapy (IFRT) 2A. R-CHOP-14 ×6 2B. R-CHOP-14 ×6 → involved field radiotherapy	Interim analysis closed arms without RT No RT arms had inferior 3-y EFS (81% vs 65%, *P* = .004)	Supports RT for bulky DLBCL (≥7.5 cm)
SWOG 8736 (*Miller et al. NEJM* 1998; *Stephens et al. JCO* 2016) 308 total patients enrolled on SWOG8736 compared to 56-patient subset treated on S0014	Stage I-IE and nonbulky II-IIE DLBCL 1. CHOP ×8 2. CHOP ×3 + IFRT to 40 Gy (with boost to 50 Gy for residual disease)	On **initial analysis**, CHOP ×3 + IFRT increased: **PFS** (5 y: 77% vs 64%, *P* = .03) **OS** (5 y: 82% vs 72%, *P* = .02) But on **long-term analysis** (median f/u 17.7 y), the curves overlapped: no significant difference in **PFS** (median: 12 vs 11.1 y, *P* = .73) or **OS** (13 vs 13.7 y, *P* = .38) 7 patients died from heart failure in CHOP ×8 arm compared to 1 patient in CHOP ×3 + IFRT arm	An abbreviated course of chemotherapy is comparable to a long course when RT is added No significant difference in cumulative incidence of secondary malignancy
RT in the setting of R-CHOP *Phan et al. JCO* 2010	Retrospective analysis of MDACC patients 469 patients with stage I-IV DLBCL who received R-CHOP ~30% received consolidation IFRT to 30-39.6 Gy	For stage I-II and all stages, RT improved **OS** (HR = 0.52 and 0.29, respectively) and **PFS** (HR = 0.45 and 0.24, respectively), compared to no RT	Consolidation RT improved PFS and OS for all patients

Consolidation radiotherapy for bulky and extralymphatic disease, and bone

Study	Design	Result	Comment
RICOVER-noRTh (*Held et al. JCO* 2014) Post hoc subgroup of 164 patients >60 y with aggressive DLBCL: bulky (≥7.5 cm) and/ or extralymphatic sites of disease	Post hoc subgroup analysis of RICOVER-60 **Comparison:** 1. R-CHOP-14+2R + 36 Gy IFRT 2. Same chemo but no RT after an amendment of RICOVER-60 (RICOVER-*noRTh*)	RT omission in patients with bulky or extralymphatic lymphoma was associated with lower EFS (HR = 2.1, $P = .005$) with trends toward lower PFS (HR = 1.8, $P = .058$) and OS (HR = 1.6, $P = .13$)	Corroborates UNFOLDER trial, supporting RT for bulky DLBCL (≥7.5 cm)
DLBCL involving bone: German High-Grade NHL Study Group (*Held et al. JCO* 2013) 3,840 total patients	Post hoc retrospective subgroup analysis of patients with skeletal involvement from nine consecutive studies	**Improved 3-y EFS** with RT (75% vs 36%; $P < .001$); trend showing improved OS (86% vs 71%; $P = .064$) MVA after adjusting for age, stage, LDH, PS, and IPI: RT reduced risk of an event by 70% ($P < .001$)	**In patients with skeletal involvement:** 1. Rituximab failed to improve EFS or OS 2. Consolidation RT significantly improved EFS
MDACC experience with primary bone DLBCL (*Tao et al. IJROBP* 2015) 102 total patients with primary bone DLBCL	RT administered in 66% of patients 72% of patients received rituximab	Receipt of consolidation RT **improves PFS** (5 y: 88% vs 63%, $P = .007$) **and OS** (5 y: 91% vs 68%, $P = .006$)	Supports consolidation RT for primary bone DLBCL

Omission of RT in low-risk, early-stage DLBCL

Study	Design	Result	Comment
LYSA (*Lamy et al. Blood* 2018) 334 patients stage I-II nonbulky (<7 cm) DLBCL	Phase III randomized trial 1. R-CHOP ×4-6 2. R-CHOP ×4-6 + RT (40 Gy IFRT)	5 y EFS 89% vs 92% (not SS) 5 y OS 92% vs 96% (not SS) PR after 4 cycles of chemotherapy underwent RT regardless of randomization—achieved favorable outcome similar to those with PET CR	R-CHOP ×4-6 = R-CHOP ×4-6 + RT for early-stage, nonbulky DLBCL Predefined study disposition guidelines suggest a role for RT in patients who achieve only a PR to chemo

Study	Design	Result	Comment
FLYER (*Poeschel et al. Lancet* 2019) 592 patients ≤60 y of age, with stage I/II, nonbulky (<7 cm) DLBCL, nl LDH, and ECOG 0-1	Phase III randomized noninferiority trial 1. R-CHOP ×4 + R ×2 2. R-CHOP ×6 Note lack of RT in both arms	No PFS difference at 3 y (96% R ×6-CHOP ×4 vs 94% R-CHOP ×4) Justification for R ×6-CHOP ×4 for low-risk, limited stage, nonbulky DLBCL with RT omission (compared to historical R-CHOP ×3 + RT)	Noninferiority study that did NOT ask an RT question but has influenced chemotherapy recommendations

Bridging RT (bRT) prior to CAR-T cell therapy

The role for RT to bridge CAR-T cell therapy (such as Tisagenlecleucel/Kymriah) in select patients is a rapidly evolving space. General considerations include **1) timing** of bRT (before apheresis with 14 day washout post-RT ≫ after apheresis), **2) dose** (local control vs "bridging" low dose), **3) volume** (treatment of all sites ≫ focal/limited field RT), and **4) technique** (simple vs advanced).

- MDACC experience (*Pinnix et al. Blood Adv. 2020*). 124 patients received Axicel, of which 50% received bridging therapy consisting of only systemic therapy (ST) (n = 45), only bRT (n = 11), or bridging CMT (n = 6). Bridged patients have higher risk disease with increased LDH, disease bulk, and IPI. Median RT dose was 35.2 Gy (range: 10-45 Gy). No SS difference in 1-year PFS and OS for bRT patients vs non-bRT among patients that ultimately got CAR-T. 1-year PFS was lower for ST-bridged patients than non-bRT patients (P = .01). RT bridging had improved PFS compared to ST-bridging (8.9 vs 4.7 months, P = .05). Comprehensive RT encompassing all sites showed a trend toward better PFS than focal RT field size (P = .12), confirmed in subsequent abstracts. No difference in toxicity. Despite the poor prognosis associated with requiring bRT, RT can be an effective bridging strategy.
- Moffitt experience (*Sims et al. IJROBP 2019*). 11 patients with bRT given median 20 Gy (range: 6-36.5 Gy). At 30 days, ORR was 81.8%, CR in 27%. At last follow-up, best ORR was 81.8% and CR in 45%.
- Penn experience (*Wright et al. IJROBP* 2020). 5 patients with bRT, 26 patients without RT or remote RT (>30 days). Median dose 37.5 Gy (range: 20-45 Gy). ORR = 80% for bRT and 64% for no bRT at 30 days. No increased toxicities with bRT

INDOLENT B-CELL LYMPHOMAS

GOHAR MANZAR • SUSAN WU

Follicular Lymphoma

Background and presentation

- **Incidence/prevalence:** Most common indolent non-Hodgkin lymphoma subtype (70% of indolent lymphomas). Commonly presents as asymptomatic lymphadenopathy, rarely with B symptoms. Bone marrow involvement in >70% of patients
- **Outcomes:** Indolent clinical course with possibility of late relapse; median OS > 10 years
- **Demographics:** Median age at diagnosis is 60 years.
- **Risk factors:** Age; common association with a history of autoimmune disease, hepatitis, or chronic immunosuppression, exposure to pesticides or chemical plants. Potential for transformation to more aggressive lymphoma can be high (up to 70% in long-time survivors).

Tumor biology and characteristics

- Arises from the germinal center B cells
  - 85% have t(14;18), which results in Bcl2 overexpression
  - Morphology shows closely packed follicular nodules.

- Immunophenotype: CD10+, Bcl2+, Bcl6+ variable
- Ki-67 significantly lower than DLBCL
- **WHO** 5th **edition reassigned grade as follows:**
  - **Classic follicular lymphoma**, formerly grade 1-3A
  - **Follicular large B-cell lymphoma (FLBCL)**, formerly grade 3B
- IRF4/MUM1 rearrangement, often children/young adult, can present with Waldeyer ring involvement
  - **Follicular lymphoma with uncommon features (uFL)**
- FL with predominantly diffuse growth pattern: typically CD23+, CD10+/−, no IGH:Bcl2 rearrangement, 1p36 del/STAT6 mutations are common with favorable prognosis
- FL with unusual cytologic features: increased large centrocytes, usually high Ki67
- *Formerly*, grade was defined by the number of centroblasts (large cells) per HPF. Grade 1: 0-5 centroblasts/HPF; grade 2: 6-15 centroblasts/HPF; grade 3: >15 centroblasts/HPF; 3A: >15 centroblasts/HPF, but centrocytes are still present; 3B: >15 centroblasts/HPF, centroblasts form solid sheets with no residual centrocytes

Workup

- **History and physical:** Physical examination of all node-bearing areas, assess Waldeyer ring and palpate abdomen for hepatosplenomegaly. Assessment of performance status and B symptoms (night sweats, weight loss, and fevers)
- **Labs:** CBC, CMP, LDH, ESR, uric acid, β2-microglobulin, hep B/C, HIV, and pregnancy test
- **Procedures/biopsy:** Excisional biopsy is preferred. Bone marrow biopsy (bilateral is encouraged but not mandatory). When chemotherapy is planned, consider MUGA/echo and fertility/sperm banking
- **Imaging:** CT neck/C/A/P with contrast and/or PET/CT

Staging *(Lugano modification of Ann Arbor Staging System)*

See "Hodgkin Lymphoma" chapter.

Prognosis

- **FLIPI score** (*Solal-Celigny et al. Blood* 2004)
  - Age > 60
  - Stages III-IV
  - Hemoglobin level < 12 g/dL
  - Number of nodal areas > 4
  - LDH level > ULN

Risk Group (Score)	5-Y OS (%)	10-Y OS (%)
Low (0-1)	90.6	70.7
Intermediate (2)	77.6	50.9
High (≥3)	52.5	35.5

- **FLIPI 2 score** (*Federeico et al. JCO* 2009)
  - Age > 60
  - Hemoglobin level < 12 g/dL
  - Bone marrow involvement
  - β2-microglobulin > upper limit normal
  - Largest diameter of largest involved lymph node > 6 cm

Risk Group (Score)	5-Y OS (%)
Low (0-1)	90.6
Intermediate (2)	77.6
High (≥3)	52.5

Treatment algorithm

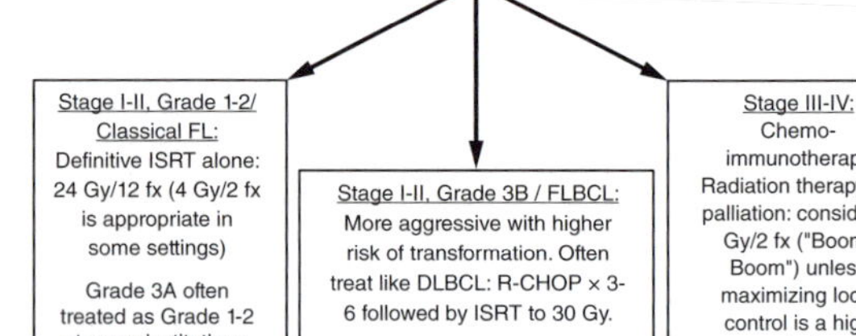

Can consider **observation** if no **GELF criteria are met** for advanced stage FL. If ≥1 GELF criteria are met, this is considered "high" tumor burden, and immediate therapy may be indicated.

Groupe d'Etude des Lymphoes Folliculaires (GELF) criteria:

1. Nodal or extranodal tumor mass >7 cm
2. Systemic or B symptoms
3. Involvement of ≥3 sites each >3 cm
4. Splenomegaly beyond umbilicus
5. Organ compression symptoms
6. Pleural effusion or peritoneal ascites
7. Leukemic with >5 million/L circulating malignant cells
8. Cytopenia (Plt < 100 K/L and/or leukocytes <1 × 10^9/L)

Notable trials

Study	Design	Result	Comment
***Lowry et al.* 2011** Any histologic subtype of non-Hodgkin lymphoma	Noninferiority, phase III RCT Randomized to: 1. Indolent lymphomas (n = 361): 40-45 Gy/20-23 fx vs 24 Gy/12 fx 2. Aggressive lymphomas (n = 640): 40-45 Gy/20-23 fx vs 30 Gy/15 fx	**1-Month overall response** Indolent/40-45 Gy: 93% Indolent/24 Gy: 92% Aggressive/40-45 Gy: 91% Aggressive/30 Gy: 91% No OS or PFS difference, trend for reduced toxicity with lower dose	Established 24 Gy for indolent lymphomas Indolent disease—69% received RT with definitive intent Aggressive disease: 80% received consolidative RT
FORT (*Hoskin et al.* 2014) **FORT update (*Hoskin et al.* 2021)** 548 patients follicular or marginal zone lymphoma treated to 614 sites	Noninferiority, phase III RCT Randomized to: 1. 24 Gy/12 fx 2. 4 Gy/2 fx	**12-wk overall response** 24 Gy/12 fx: 91% 4 Gy/2 fx: 81% **12-wk complete response** 24 Gy/12 fx: 68% 4 Gy/2 fx: 49% Time to progression **not noninferior** for 4 Gy (12.3 vs 19.3 mos **5-y local PFS** in 2021 update: 90% (24 Gy) vs 70% (4 Gy) No OS difference **5-y local PFS s/p 4 Gy:** 88% for MZL vs 68% with FL, which may reflect differing radiosensitivity of these histologies	4 Gy inferior for local progression and time to progression. However, this regimen is pragmatic and well-tolerated, so it is a good option when durable local control is not critical Higher toxicity in 24 Gy (3% vs 1%)

Marginal Zone Lymphoma

Background

- **Incidence/prevalence:** 5-10% non-Hodgkin lymphoma
- **Outcomes:** Indolent disease. Death due to disease is extremely rare. Gastric site has longer time to progression vs nongastric MALT (8.9 vs 4.9 years). 50% gastric, other sites include orbit, lung, skin, thyroid, salivary gland, etc.
- **Demographics:** Variable age groups depending on the subtype
- **Risk factors:** Associated with chronic inflammation: autoimmune disease (Sjögren disease), infections (*Helicobacter pylori*, *Chlamydia psittaci*, *Borrelia burgdorferi*, *Campylobacter jejuni*)

Tumor biology and characteristics

- Neoplasm of mature B cells
- Arise from postgerminal center marginal zone B cells
- B-cell markers: CD19, CD20, CD22+ (CD5/10/23−)
- Characterized by proliferation of cells within a lymphoid area where clonal expansion of B cells occurs. Subtypes include:
  - Splenic marginal zone lymphoma
  - Nodal marginal zone lymphoma
  - Extranodal/Peyer patch marginal zone lymphoma
    - Primary cutaneous marginal zone lymphoma
    - Mucosa-associated lymphoid tissue (MALT) lymphoma

Gastric MALT

Presentation

- Majority present with localized stage I/II extranodal disease
- Most commonly present with abdominal pain and peptic ulcer disease
- B symptoms are uncommon.
- Outcomes: 5-year OS of 90-95% and DFS of 75-80%

Workup

- **History and physical:** Physical examination of all node-bearing areas including Waldeyer ring and for hepatosplenomegaly. Assessment of performance status and B symptoms (uncommon for gastric malt)
- **Labs:** CBC, CMP, LDH, ESR, uric acid, β2-microglobulin, hep B/C, HIV, and pregnancy test. Bone marrow biopsy is not routinely done.
- **Procedures/biopsy:** Endoscopic biopsy with *H pylori* testing by histopathology:
  - If negative → noninvasive testing: Stool antigen test, urea breath test, and blood antibody test
  - PCR or FISH for t(11;18). Translocation associated with lack of response to combination antibiotic therapy
- **Imaging:** CT neck/C/A/P with contrast and/or PET/CT

Staging (*Lugano Staging for Gastrointestinal Lymphomas; Rohatiner et al. Ann Oncol* 1994)

Stage	Involvement	
Stage I	Tumor confined to GI tract. Single primary or multiple noncontiguous lesions	
Stage II	Tumor extends into the abdomen	
	Stage II1	Local node involvement
	Stage II2	Distant node involvement
	Stage IIE	Tumor penetrates the serosa to invade adjacent organs or tissue
Stage III	No stage III in current system	
Stage IV	Disseminated extranodal involvement or concomitant supradiaphragmatic nodal involvement	

Treatment algorithm

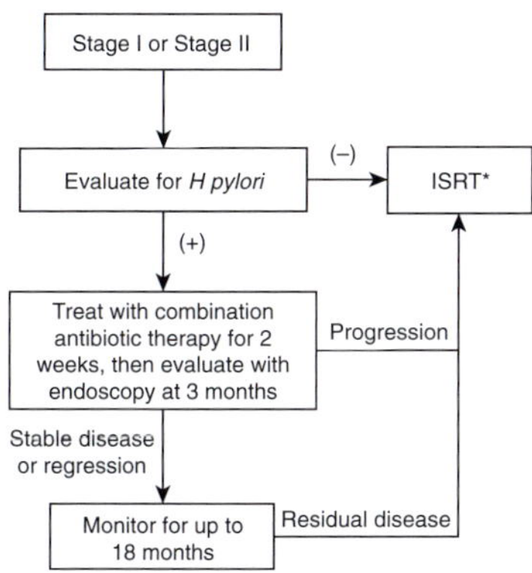

*Can consider ISRT sooner for progression, symptoms or presence of t(11;18).

Radiation treatment technique

Simulation	Supine, upper Vac-Lok cradle, knee wedge, NPO × 4 hours, deep inspiratory breath hold
Target	Entire stomach with a 0.7- to 1.5-cm isometric margin. Cover suspicious perigastric nodes
Dose	24 Gy in 12 fractions or 30 Gy in 15 fractions
Technique	IMRT with daily volumetric imaging. Avoid lateral beams

- Combination antibiotic therapy includes a proton pump inhibitor and antibiotics (eg, clarithromycin, amoxicillin, and omeprazole).
- Consider chemoimmunotherapy for advanced or relapsed disease.

Orbital MALT

Presentation

- Most common nongastric MALT
- Can affect the conjunctiva, eyelid, lacrimal gland, and retrobulbar area
- Associated with *C psittaci*

Treatment approach

- Doxycycline (complete response 65%)
- Consider ISRT if antibiotic therapy failure

Radiation treatment technique

- 4 Gy in 2 fractions can achieve CR in 90% (*Pinnix et al. ASTRO Plenary Session* 2022); for those who do not achieve CR, consider an additional 20 Gy in 10 fractions.

Simulation	Supine. Thermoplastic mask. Skin collimation if indicated
Target	Whole orbit (particularly for retrobulbar or deep conjunctival involvement) or partial orbit
Dose	MDA practice is 4 Gy/2 fx, if no CR → additional 20 Gy/10 fx
Technique	Wedge pair with photons for whole orbit or electrons for conjunctiva only. Consider IMRT if using 20-24 Gy

Primary Cutaneous B-Cell Lymphomas

Background

- Associated with *B burgdorferi* infection, preexisting acrodermatitis chronica atrophicans, and vaccination sites
- 20% of all primary cutaneous lymphomas and divided into five subtypes
  - Primary cutaneous marginal zone B-cell lymphoma (PCMZL)
  - Primary cutaneous follicle center lymphoma (PCFCL)
  - Primary cutaneous diffuse large B-cell lymphoma, leg-type (PCLBCL, LT)
  - Primary cutaneous diffuse large B-cell lymphoma, other (PCLBCL, O)
  - Intravascular large B-cell lymphoma (IVLBCL)

Primary Cutaneous Marginal Zone B-cell Lymphoma (PCMZL)

Tumor biology and characteristics

- Pathology shows nodular to diffuse infiltrates of small to medium lymphocytes, with sparing of the epidermis. A reactive germinal center is frequently seen.
- Marginal zone B cells express CD20, CD79, and bcl-2 and are typically negative for CD5, CD10, and bcl 6; translocation t(18;21) is rare.

Presentation

- Multiple painless, nonulcerative, red to violaceous papules, plaques, or nodules occurring mainly on the trunk or the extremities
- Indolent clinical presentation and spontaneous resolution have been reported.

Treatment approach

- Lesions respond to different treatments (resection, systemic therapy, and radiation). General approach is to treat with least toxic option: ISRT 4 Gy in 2 fractions.
- A noticeable clinical response might not be seen before 4-8 weeks, as effect of radiation may be mostly on the microenvironment rather than on the actual malignant cells.

Outcomes

- The lymphoma-specific survival is close to 100%, while the relapse-free survival for solitary lesions is 77% vs 39% for multifocal lesions.

Primary Cutaneous Follicle Center Lymphoma (PCFCL)

Tumor biology and characteristics

- Pathology demonstrates a monotonous population of large, cleaved follicle center cells, with nodular or diffuse infiltrates sparing the epidermis.
- Cells that are CD20+, CD79a+, and Bcl6+, in a network of CD21+ or CCD35+ follicular dendritic cells
- Rarely express t(14;18) or Bcl2

Presentation

- Difficult to differentiate from PCMZL, as lesions present as nonulcerative plaques or nodules, most commonly on the scalp, forehead, or trunk

Treatment approach

- ISRT 4 Gy in 2 fractions

Outcomes

- Complete remission rates up to 100% and a relapse-free survival of 73-89%; the majority of patients can be salvaged with local radiation.

MISCELLANEOUS HEMATOLOGIC MALIGNANCIES

GOHAR MANZAR • SUSAN WU

Primary Cutaneous T-cell Lymphomas

Mycosis Fungoides (MF)

Background

- Represents 2/3 of cutaneous T-cell lymphoma cases
- Indolent disease may take several years and repeat biopsies for diagnosis
- Incurable disease unless autologous or allogeneic transplant is being considered.

Tumor biology and characteristics

- Pathology shows a clonal T-cell population clustered at the basement membrane of the epidermis.
- Characterized by loss of CD7, CD5, and CD2; dim CD3+; and mature clonal CD4+ and CD45RO+
- Rarely express t(14;18) or bcl2

Presentation

- Presents with patches, but eventually plaques and tumors with or without erythroderma may develop. Concomitant skin infections are frequent.

Workup

- Inspection and determination of the total body surface area involved
- Flow cytometry to determine CD4+/CD8+; if above 4.5, indicates a high level of circulating T-cell lymphoma cells in the blood
- Imaging and bone marrow biopsy in appropriate cases
- When limited to the skin, T1 and T2 are patches or plaques involving more than 10% of the skin; T3 is tumor, and T4 is erythroderma.

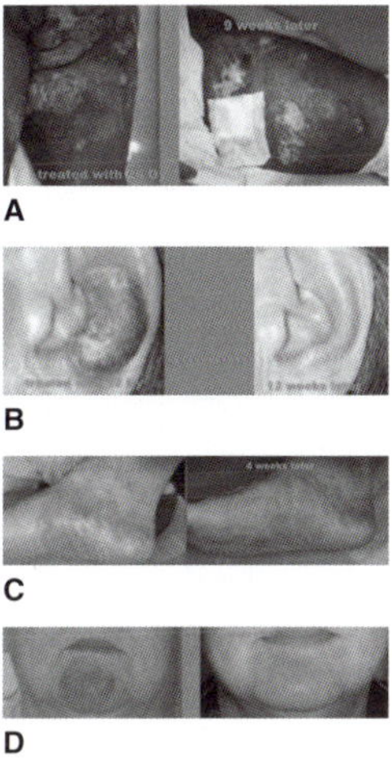

A

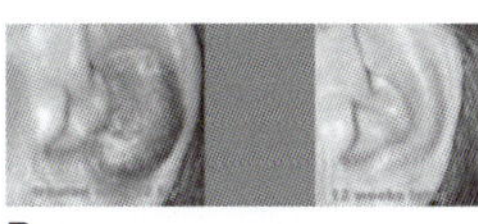

B

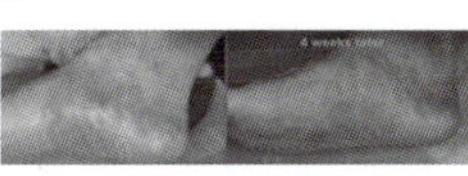

C

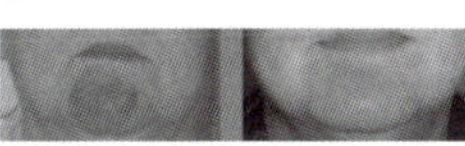

D

Figure 64.1 A–D. Pre- and posttreatment examples of local radiation (4-12 Gy) for the treatment of mycosis fungoides.

Treatment approach

- Initial topical therapies: steroids, chemotherapy, bexarotene gel, phototherapy
- Systemic therapies: retinoids, histone deacetylase inhibitors, denileukin diftitox, monoclonal antibodies, interferon alpha, cytotoxic chemotherapy
- Total skin or local radiation therapy with the goal of avoiding excess skin toxicity
  - TSEBT reserved for substantial body surface area involvement and may take up to 8-12 weeks for maximal response
    - Given in 2 Gy fractions twice per week with boosts/supplemental fields for axilla, shoulders, inframammary folds, groins, perineum, perianal area, soles, and other skinfolds
    - 10-12 Gy overall response rate of 88% with mild toxicity
    - 30-36 Gy for high disease burden or prior to transplant
- Local radiation
  - 4-12 Gy to focal lesions with 1- to 2-cm margin to minimize RT to nonsymptomatic areas. Can retreat with radiation if needed
  - Electron beam RT in most cases starting at 9 MeV with bolus for patch/plaque disease, can consider higher energy for tumors to ensure full skin dose
  - Use simulation CT scan if adjacent to sensitive normal tissue (consider skin collimation also) or unknown tumor depth.

Primary Cutaneous Anaplastic Large Cell Lymphoma (PALCL)

Background

- Second most common type of cutaneous T-cell lymphoma
- Can present along with MF
- May take weeks/months for a response to radiation and wound healing
- Breast implant-associated primary anaplastic large cell lymphoma has the clinical behavior of cutaneous ALCL but is generally less aggressive with higher survival.

Presentation

- Deeper skin involvement than MF and often ulcerative lesions

Treatment approach

- Local radiation
- Responds to doses as low as 6 Gy

Plasma Cell Dyscrasias/Solitary Plasmacytomas

Solitary Plasmacytoma

Background

- **Incidence/prevalence:** 10% of plasma cell neoplasms
- **Outcomes:** Localized disease with no evidence of additional lesions or clinical/laboratory findings consistent with MM (see below for criteria). Excellent locoregional control with radiation (up to 95%)
  - 80% solitary plasmacytoma of bone (SPB): 55-80% progress to multiple myeloma
  - 20% extramedullary plasmacytoma (SEP): 35-50% progress to multiple myeloma
- **Demographics:** Male predominance (2/3 cases); younger median age (55-65) than multiple myeloma
- **Risk factors:** Family prevalence, older age, and male gender

Work-up

- **H&P**, **bone marrow biopsy**, **imaging** (skeletal survey, PET/CT, MRI helpful for long bones or H&N), and **labs** (CBC, CMP including Ca^{2+} and Cr, albumin, LDH, B2M, serum immunoglobulins, free light chains, 24-hour urine and serum electrophoresis with immunofixation)
- **Solitary plasmacytoma** = biopsy-proven solitary lesion of bone or extraosseous tissue AND normal bone marrow AND no myeloma defining events (MDEs, see below) or end-organ damage (no CRAB, ie, no hypercalcemia >11 mg/dL, no renal dysfunction, and no anemia defined as Hgb <10 g/dL)

Treatment approach

- Use CT, PET, and MRI (check marrow signal) for target delineation. PTV expansion depends on tumor location. Neither elective vertebral body (superior/inferior) nor elective nodal coverage is necessary if using PET and MRI.
- Typically ISRT to 40-50 Gy
  - If <5 cm, can consider lower doses on the order of 35 Gy (*Tsang et al. IJROBP* 2001)

Multiple Myeloma

- ***Work-up** same as above, to distinguish solitary plasmacytoma using the revised IMWG criteria:*
  - **Clonal bone marrow plasma cells ≥10%**
  - **OR** biopsy-proven bony or extramedullary **plasmacytoma plus one or more** of the following:
    - ≥1 of the following **CRAB features**:
      - Hyper**C**alcemia (Ca^{2+} >11 mg/dL)
      - **R**enal insufficiency (Cr >2 mg/dL)
      - **A**nemia (Hgb <10 g/dL or > 2 g/dL below normal)
      - **B**one lesions: ≥1 osteolytic lesion on skeletal radiography, CT, or PET/CT; >1 required if marrow <10% clonal plasma cells
  - ≥1 myeloma-defining event (**MDEs**):
    - ≥60% clonal plasma cells in bone marrow
    - >1 lesion on MRI measuring ≥5 mm
    - Serum involved/uninvolved free light chain ratio of ≥100 (provided the involved light chain is ≥100 mg/L

- **Outcomes:** 5-year OS: ~50%
- Polyneuropathy, organomegaly, endocrinopathy, M-protein, skin changes **(POEMS) syndrome**: rare paraneoplastic syndrome due to underlying plasma cell neoplasm

Treatment approach

- Multiple myeloma is considered treatable but generally incurable.
- Typically, for patients ≤65 and with good functional status, initial treatment is a triplet regimen (eg, VRd: Velcade = bortezomib, Revlimid = lenalidomide, and dexamethasone). This is followed by autologous stem cell transplant (ASCT) in appropriate candidates and maintenance therapy.
- RT can be used to palliate lesions or in cases with neurological compromise, for example, cord compression or cranial nerve involvement. Use CT, PET, and MRI (check marrow signal) for target delineation. PTV expansion depending on tumor location. Neither elective vertebral body (superior/inferior) nor elective nodal coverage is necessary.
- Typically ISRT to 20 Gy in 8 fractions to the smallest field possible to avoid jeopardizing stem cell collection in patients who may proceed to ASCT; consider 24 Gy if >5 cm.

Mantle Cell Lymphoma (MCL)

Background

- Usually presents with advanced stage, following an aggressive course
- Male predominance (78%), median age at diagnosis 63 years
- Majority (75%) present in the head and neck
- Age (>60), bulky disease (>5 cm), and stage II → increased treatment failure risk
- Characterized by overexpression of cyclin D and t(11;14)

Prognosis

MCL International Prognostic Index (MIPI) (*Lim et al. Oncol Lett* **2010**)

Points	Age	ECOG PS	LDH (ULN)	WBC (109/L)
0	<50	0-1	<0.67	<6.7
1	50-59	—	0.67-0.99	6.7-9.99
2	60-69	2-4	1.0-1.49	10.0-14.99
3	≥70	—	≥1.5	≥1.5

Risk Group	Median Survival
Low: 0-3 points (44% of patients)	Not reached
Intermediate: 4-5 points (35% of patients)	51 mo
High: 6-11 points (21% of patients)	29 mo

Overall prognosis

- 5-Year freedom from progression, 65% and OS, 76%
- 10-Year freedom from progression, 42% and OS, 64%

Treatment approach

Stage I-II MCL

- Excellent and similar outcomes for chemotherapy, chemoradiation, or radiation alone
- Goal to deintensify therapy to limit treatment-related toxicity
- Stage I/II disease is rare, can consider 24 Gy in 12 fractions as well as 4 Gy in 2 fractions.

Advanced-stage MCL

- RT to palliate bulky nodal or extranodal masses, often after being heavily pretreated
- 4 Gy in 2 fractions is associated with high response rates, although may take up to 4 weeks to respond.
- Consider additional 24-30 Gy if no response after 4 weeks.

BRAIN METASTASES

ALEX SHERRY • AMOL GHIA • THOMAS BECKHAM

BACKGROUND

- **Incidence/prevalence:** Most common adult malignant intracranial tumor. 20-40% of all cancer patients will develop intracranial metastases. ~200-300k diagnosed annually. Incidence is increasing due to the widespread adoption of MRI, where small lesion detection has improved, and increasing long-term survival of metastatic cancer patients.
- **Outcomes:** Widely variable based on presentation, histology, and molecular subtype. Historical median survival for observation 1 month, steroids 2 months, and WBRT 4-6 months. Advances in radiation techniques and systemic therapy have resulted in significantly improved CNS and long-term survival outcomes.

TUMOR BIOLOGY AND ANATOMY

- **Pathology**
  - Most common: lung, breast, melanoma, renal cell, colorectal
  - Commonly hemorrhagic: melanoma, renal cell, choriocarcinoma, thyroid
- **Imaging**: MRI brain with and without contrast. Restaging CT chest/abdomen/pelvis or PET-CT to evaluate systemic disease burden
  - Hematogenous spread to gray-white matter junction (watershed areas) is common, where narrow caliber vessels trap tumor emboli.
  - 80% cerebral hemispheres, 15% cerebellum, 5% brainstem
  - Typical appearance: spherical, solid, or ring-enhancing lesions with surrounding vasogenic edema. Larger lesions may have central necrosis. Tumor is iso- or hypointense on T1 and hyperintense on T2 (occasionally hyperintense on T1 if hemorrhagic). Vasogenic edema is hypointense on T1, hyperintense on T2, best evaluated on FLAIR.
  - Evaluate the proximity of tumor to critical normal tissues (optic apparatus, brainstem, spinal cord, perirolandics/eloquent cortex).

WORK-UP

- **History and physical:** Common presenting symptoms include headache, nausea, vomiting, seizures, focal neurologic deficits, altered mental status, ataxia, and vision changes. Assess neuro exam and performance status. Evaluate the extent and control of intracranial/extracranial disease and the pace of intracranial progression.
- **Labs:** CBC, CMP (tumor markers to r/o CNS primaries vs brain metastases)
- **Imaging/procedures/biopsy:** CT head without contrast to evaluate for hemorrhagic stroke. MRI brain with and without contrast. Differential includes infectious processes (eg, abscess or parasitic infection), infarct, demyelinating disease, vascular abnormalities, or primary CNS malignancy. Biopsy or resection can be considered for a symptomatic lesion if there is no known extracranial primary cancer or long latency from the last known malignancy; for asymptomatic lesions, systemic work-up to establish diagnosis. If leptomeningeal disease is suspected (see Radiation Emergencies section), obtain MRI of the cervical/thoracic/lumbar spine ± contrast, neurology consultation, and CSF cytology.
- **Initial management:** For symptomatic patients, corticosteroids (dexamethasone) 4-16 mg/d in divided doses depending on symptom severity with proton pump inhibitor for gastroprotection. 10 mg IV bolus can be considered. Antiepileptics for seizure (prophylaxis not recommended). Neurosurgery and radiation oncology consults
- **Prognostic factors:** Age, performance status, severity of symptoms, histology, status of primary disease and extracranial metastatic disease, number/size/volume/location of brain metastases, systemic therapy options.
  - **Scoring** (*Sperduto et al. JCO* 2012): histology-specific GPAs are available (https://www.brainmetgpa.com/). Most incorporate performance status, age, extracranial metastasis, and number of brain metastases. Some (lung/melanoma/breast) incorporate histologic subtype and driver mutations.

Management Principles

Brain metastasis treatment paradigms are rapidly evolving. Multidisciplinary evaluation is critical for appropriate treatment selection.

Surgery

- Achieves tissue retrieval for diagnosis/molecular profiling and rapid reduction of mass effect, bleeding, edema, impending herniation, and/or hydrocephalus for patients with large (ie, >3 cm) and/or symptomatic brain metastases.
- Improved OS with surgery + WBRT for single brain metastases compared to WBRT alone.
- Surgery alone results in unacceptable local control rates, and postoperative radiation therapy (typically SRS) is the standard of care.

SRS/SRT

- Preferred treatment for small lesions (typically <2 cm), lesions that are not surgically accessible, and patients who are not surgical candidates.
- SRS preferred over WBRT for limited metastases including postoperative cavities due to improved neurocognitive preservation and no compromise of survival.
- Generally accepted for up to 10 lesions with more limited data for up to 15 lesions.
- Total brain metastases volume, the pace of seeding, histology, and systemic therapy may be more important for treatment selection than the number of metastases.
- Focal therapy is particularly considered for elderly patients who may be more impacted by neurocognitive effects of WBRT.

HA-WBRT

- An alternative option for patients who are not candidates for SRS. Preferred over WBRT if all lesions >5 mm from the hippocampi and no leptomeningeal disease. Use with memantine.

WBRT

- Reserved for patients where SRS or HA-WBRT are contraindicated such as leptomeningeal disease or need for urgent treatment. Use with memantine. For patients with very limited prognosis, best supportive care/hospice should also be considered based on multidisciplinary consensus.

CNS-Active Systemic Therapy

- Rapidly changing paradigms. Reserved for highly selected, small, asymptomatic brain metastases. Lesion location is critical as progression in the brainstem, near optics, or in eloquent cortex may compromise function and salvageability. Multidisciplinary evaluation and patient-centered decision-making is key. Evaluate the likelihood of response to systemic therapy, access to close surveillance, and availability of salvage therapies in decision-making.
  - Melanoma: ipilimumab/nivolumab or dabrafenib/trametinib for *BRAF V600*-mutant
  - Nonsmall cell lung cancer: osimertinib for *EGFR*-mu, alectinib/brigatinib for *ALK*-mu
  - Breast cancer: tucatinib, trastuzumab deruxtecan for *HER2-mu*
  - See Radiation Oncology Principles for further details.
- Close surveillance and early local intervention at time of clinical/radiologic progression is critical.

Recurrence

- Evaluate if local recurrence vs new distant brain metastasis, prior radiation, and surgical history.
- Prior surgery: consider surgery, SRS, systemic therapy, and/or (HA)-WBRT.
- Prior WBRT: consider surgery, SRS, and/or systemic therapy. Repeat WBRT is uncommonly recommended.
- Prior SRS: consider surgery (Cs-131 brachytherapy or postoperative repeat SRS considered in select cases), (HA)-WBRT, systemic therapy.

Radiation Treatment Technique

SRS: stereotactic radiosurgery, single fraction
SRT: stereotactic radiotherapy, 2-5 fx
HA-WBRT: hippocampal avoidance whole brain radiation therapy
WBRT: Whole brain radiation therapy

- **SIM**
  - Supine, head in neutral position, thermoplastic mask, bite block for SRS/SRT
  - Gamma Knife SRS: frame versus frameless (see Special Radiation Techniques).
- **Dose**
  - **SRS** (prescribed to 50-80% isodose line for Gamma Knife and ~80% for LINAC)
    - <4.2 cc — 20-24 Gy (MDACC typically 20 Gy)
    - 4.2-8 cc (or up to 14 cc) — 18 Gy
    - ≥8.0-14 cc, up to 4 cm diameter — 15 Gy
    - Brainstem lesion — *14-18 Gy

      *At MDACC, we typically subtract 2 Gy from recommended dose based on size or fractionate or select the highest dose between 14 and 18 Gy that meets V12 < 1 cc constraint).
  - **SRT:** considered for tumors >2 cm in diameter and based on location/surrounding structure tolerance
    - 3 fx: 27 Gy. May decrease CTV/PTV coverage to 24 Gy if needed
    - 5 fx: 30 Gy. May decrease CTV/PTV coverage to 25 Gy if needed
  - **(HA)-WBRT**: 30 Gy/10 fx
- **Target**
  - **Gamma Knife SRS:** (see Special Radiation Techniques)
  - **SRT or LINAC-based SRS:** GTV (tumor or postoperative cavity) + 2 mm PTV margin (per institutional setup uncertainty and IGRT). CTV may be used on a case-by-case basis (eg, dural margin) and occasionally SIB.
  - **WBRT:**
    - Superior/posterior: Flash skin at cranium by 2 cm. Skin-sparing WBRT may be considered in the absence of dural/calvarial disease.
    - Inferior: C2/C3 inferior border for posterior cranial fossa disease/LMD, otherwise C1/C2
    - Anterior: block lens/anterior orbits. Verify coverage of cribriform plate and middle cranial fossa on cross-sectional imaging
    - Multiple techniques can be utilized to avoid optic lenses (eg, rotate gantry 5 degrees and treat with RAO/LAO technique). Field-in-field dosimetric technique can reduce heterogeneity.
  - **HA-WBRT**: use IMRT/VMAT with planning directive details below.
- **IGRT:**
  - **Gamma Knife SRS:** (see Special Radiation Techniques)
    - **SRT and LINAC-based SRS:** Daily kV, ExacTrac (mounted real-time orthogonal x-ray imaging system)
    - **WBRT:** Weekly mV or daily kV (recommended for HA-WBRT)
- **Planning directive**

SRS	1 Fraction Goal	1 Fraction Hard Constraint
Brainstem	V12 < 1 cc	
Optic chiasm	D_{max} < 8 Gy	D_{max} < 10 Gy
Optic nerve	D_{max} < 8 Gy	D_{max} < 10 Gy
Brain	V12 < 5-10 cc	

SRT	3 Fractions	5 Fractions
Brainstem	V21 < 0.01 cc	V23 < 0.5 cc, V25 < 0.01 cc
Optic chiasm	V17 < 0.01 cc, D_{max} < 18 Gy	V20 < 0.2 cc, D_{max} < 22.5 Gy
Optic nerve	V17 < 0.01 cc, D_{max} < 18 Gy	V20 < 0.2 cc, D_{max} < 22.5 Gy
Spinal cord	V18 < 0.01 cc	V22.5 < 0.25 cc, D_{max} < 25 Gy

Special Scenarios		5 Fractions
Target against brainstem	Brainstem	V25 < 0.5 cc, D_{max} < 30 Gy
Target in brainstem	Brainstem-GTV	V30 < 1 cc, D_{max} < 31 Gy
Target within 3 mm of optics	Optic chiasm	V23 < 0.2 cc, D_{max} < 25 Gy
Target within 3 mm of optics	Optic nerve	V23 < 0.2 cc, D_{max} < 25 Gy
Target against cord	Spinal cord	D_{max} < 26.5 Gy

	10 Fractions HA-WBRT
Brainstem	D_{max} < 34 Gy
Hippocampus	D100% < 9 Gy, D_{max} < 16 Gy
Lens	D_{max} < 5 Gy
Optic chiasm	D_{max} < 33 Gy
Optic nerve	D_{max} < 33 Gy

Side Effect Management

- **WBRT**
  - **Acute:** Fatigue, alopecia, and ototoxicity. Nausea/vomiting/headaches/ vision changes from increased ICP: dexamethasone + PPI, ondansetron, or prochlorperazine.
  - **Long-term:** Neurocognitive impairment. Hippocampal avoidance when achievable. Memantine for all WBRT patients starting day 1 of radiation: 10 mg qd × 1 week then 10 mg bid thereafter for at least 6 months. Consider indefinitely.
- **SRT/SRS**
  - **Acute:** Fatigue, headache, nausea, vomiting. More rarely, based upon size/location of lesion: seizures, focal neurologic deficits, hemorrhage. Consider prophylactic dexamethasone taper for large, edematous, and/or symptomatic lesions. For framed Gamma Knife, pain at pin sites (OTC analgesic/anti-inflammatory meds), periorbital swelling, and infection.
  - **Long-term:** Symptomatic radionecrosis: 5-10% risk, higher with larger volume of treated lesions (>8 cm^3 tumor volume); consider SRT to reduce risk of radionecrosis in these cases vs single-fraction SRS. Diagnosis on conventional MRI can be challenging. Consider MR spectroscopy and perfusion imaging to differentiate recurrence versus radionecrosis: tumor with increased choline (membranes destroyed) and decreased *N*-acetylaspartate (neurons lost) versus radionecrosis with increased lipids and lactate. Asymptomatic: observe with serial imaging. Symptomatic: dexamethasone and slow taper (~1 month) with PPI. If refractory, bevacizumab, vitamin-E/pentoxifylline, hyperbaric oxygen therapy, or surgery

Follow-up

- H&P and MRI brain in 6-12 weeks → repeat every 2-3 months for 1-2 years followed by every 4-6 months indefinitely

Notable Trials

Surgery

Name/Purpose	Arms	Outcomes	Notes
Patchell I (*Patchell et al. NEJM* **1990**) 48 patients with brain metastases with known extracranial tumors	25 patients underwent surgical resection of metastasis + WBRT 23 patients underwent biopsy + WBRT	Recurrence at the site of original metastasis less frequent in surgery group (20% vs 52%; $P < .02$) Median OS improved in surgery arm (40 wk vs 15 wk; $P < .01$)	Patients with surgery + RT live longer, with reduced local recurrence vs RT alone after biopsy **11% of patients* excluded from study as they were found to have second primary tumors or infections following surgery/biopsy

Name/Purpose	Arms	Outcomes	Notes
Patchell II (***Patchell et al. JAMA*** **1998)** 95 patients with single metastases to the brain that were treated with complete surgical resections	WBRT 50.4 Gy/28 fx No adjuvant RT	WBRT reduced local recurrence 46% → 10% ($P < .001$), distant intracranial recurrence 70% → 18% ($P < .01$), and neurologic death 44% → 14% ($P = .003$)	Patients with cancer and single brain metastases have fewer recurrences and are less likely to die of neurologic causes when treated with WBRT after surgical resection
MD Anderson **(*Mahajan et al. Lancet Oncol* 2017)** 132 patients with complete resection of 1-3 brain metastases (maximum diameter ≤4 cm)	Postoperative SRS (12-16 Gy) in a single fraction Observation	1-year freedom from local recurrence improved in the SRS arm 42% → 72% ($P = .015$)	Postoperative SRS of the surgical cavity significantly lowers local recurrence compared with observation alone
N107C/CEC•3 **(*Brown et al. Lancet Oncol* 2017)** 194 patients with single resected brain metastasis with cavity ≤ 5	Postoperative SRS (12-20 Gy) WBRT (30 Gy/10 fx or 37.5 Gy/15 fx)	Median cognitive-deterioration–free survival was improved in the SRS arm 3.0 months → 3.7 months ($P < .00031$) Median OS similar at 12.2 months vs 11.6 months	Decline in cognitive function is more frequent with postoperative WRBT vs SRS, with no OS difference between the groups

SRS for multiple brain metastases

Name/Purpose	Arms	Outcomes	Notes
JLGK0901 **(*Yamamoto et al. Lancet Oncol* 2014)** Prospective nonrandomized observational study of patients with 2-4 vs 5-10 brain mets treated with SRS alone (20-22 Gy)	2-4 brain metastases 5-10 brain metastases	OS was similar between 2-4 vs 5-10 brain metastases groups (median 10.8 months for both; noninferiority $< P$ .0001) Adverse events were similar between cohorts	Suggests that in patients treated with SRS without WBRT with 5 to 10 brain metastases is noninferior to that in patients with two to four brain metastases
MDACC (*Li et al. ASTRO* 2020) Patients with 4-15 untreated brain metastases	SRS (15-24 Gy) WBRT (30 Gy/10 fx with memantine)	LC at 4 months similar (95% vs 87%, $P = .79$) as was OS (35 vs 34 months, $P = .59$) Improved cognitive function at 1 and 6 months ($P = .012$) per HVLT_R_TR score	Neurocognitive deterioration reduced with SRS vs WBRT. No difference in local control/OS

Neurocognitive function

Name/Purpose	Arms	Outcomes	Notes
MD Anderson (***Chang et al. Lancet Oncol*** **2009)** 58 patients with 1-3 brain metastases	SRS + WBRT (30 Gy in 12 fx) SRS alone (15-24 Gy)	Deterioration in learning/memory function was significantly reduced with SRS alone 52% → 24% SRS&WBRT improved distant recurrence (27% vs 73%; *P* = .0003) at 1 y	Patients with limited brain metastases treated with SRS plus WBRT have a greater risk of a significant decline in learning and memory compared to SRS alone
RTOG 0614 (*Brown et al. Neuro-Onc* 2013) 554 patients with brain metastases receiving WBRT But only 149 analyzable patients	Memantine + WBRT Placebo + WBRT	Primary end point was preserved delayed recall at 24 weeks, which trended toward improvement in the memantine arm but not statistically significant (*P* = .059), limited by reduced statistical power due to 34% death rate prior to 24-week assessment	Memantine is well tolerated with a favorable toxicity profile and should be used concurrently with WBRT in patients with reasonable life expectancy
Alliance N0574 **(*Brown et al. JAMA* 2016)** 213 patients with 1-3 brain metastases	SRS alone (18-22 Gy) SRS + WBRT (30 Gy in 12 fx)	Cognitive decline more frequent with WBRT (92% vs 64% SRS alone) WBRT improved 12 month local control (90% vs 73%) and distant control (92% vs 70%) there is no survival compromise with SRS alone	SRS alone should be standard of care in patients with 1-3 brain metastases
CC001 (*Brown et al. JCO* 2020) 518 patients with brain metastases receiving WBRT + memantine	HA-WBRT + memantine WBRT+ memantine	6-month cognitive failure reduced with HA-WBRT (HR 0.74; *P* = .02) OS, PFS, toxicity profiles all similar between both arms	HA-WBRT + memantine better preserves cognitive function and patient-reported symptoms. Should be standard of care in patients with good PS and reasonable life expectancy

SPINE METASTASES

JULIANNA BRONK • AMOL GHIA

BACKGROUND

- **Incidence/prevalence:** Osseous disease third most common site of metastases. The spine most common site of bone metastases. 70% involve thoracic spine, 20% lumbar, and 10% cervical. Breast, lung, and prostate account for 50-60% of cases.
- **Radiosensitive histologies:** Breast, prostate, ovarian, and neuroendocrine carcinoma. Patients achieve symptomatic relief and effective local control rates with conventional external beam radiotherapy (cEBRT).
- **Radioresistant histologies:** Sarcoma, melanoma, chordoma, hepatobiliary, and renal cell carcinoma. Do not have good local control rates with conventional radiation. Radiosurgery should be considered.
- **Intermediate resistance histologies:** Lung, colon, and thyroid. Treatment typically dependent on institutional classification and experience

WORKUP

- **History and physical:** Characterize pain: Mechanical pain worse with movement and neurologic pain worse when supine. Pain is the most common initial presenting symptom and usually precedes neurologic deficits. Mechanical pain indicates possible need for stabilization. Inquire about neurologic deficits that indicate possible acute cord compression. Does patient have known cancer diagnoses? Ask about prior surgery, prior radiation therapy, concurrent chemotherapy. Assess performance status and ability to tolerate simulation/treatment. Perform complete neurologic examination.
- **Imaging:** MRI T1 with/without contrast of entire spine to delineate disease and identify other sites of involvement. Axial T2 to localize spinal cord. CT myelogram is useful in postoperative SRS above the conus where instrumentation causes increased T2 artifact signal making cord visualization difficult.
- **Surgery consult:** Patient should be evaluated by neurosurgery or spine surgery to determine the need for emergent decompression or spine stabilization prior to radiation therapy.

GENERAL TREATMENT OVERVIEW

- **Disease touching the cord (MESCC grade IC or greater)?** If the patient is a surgical candidate, we prefer surgery followed by radiation therapy. If not a surgical candidate but otherwise meets clinical indications for SSRS as outlined below, proceed with SSRS respecting spinal cord dose tolerance. Otherwise, cEBRT (see Radiation Emergencies)
- **Assess the need for surgical stabilization:** Refer patient to neurosurgery or spine surgery for assessment of spine stability and need for stabilization prior to RT based on SINS score (spine instability neoplastic score; *Fisher Radiat Oncol* 2014). **Score 0-6, stable; 7-12, indeterminate; and 13-18, unstable**.
- **Spine radiosurgery:**
  Indications: Reirradiation, radiation-resistant histology, oligometastatic, oligoprogressive
  Contraindications: >3 spinal level involvement, poor PFS, unable to tolerate SRS simulation or treatment (eg, lay flat for an extended period of time)

Component	Score
Location	
Junctional (O-C2; C7-T2; T11-L1; L5-S1)	3
Mobile spine (C3-6; L2-4)	2
Semirigid (T3-10)	1
Rigid (S2-5)	0
Mechanical pain	
Yes	3
No	2
Pain-free lesion	1

Component	Score
Bone lesion	
Lytic	2
Mixed (lytic/blastic)	1
Blastic	0
Radiographic spinal alignment	
Subluxation/translation present	4
Deformity (kyphosis/scoliosis)	2
Normal	0
Vertebral body collapse	
>50% collapse	3
<50% collapse	2
No collapse with >50% body involved	2
None of the above	0
Posterolateral involvement	
Bilateral	3
Unilateral	1
None of the above	0

RADIATION TREATMENT TECHNIQUE

Conventional radiotherapy (cEBRT)

- **SIM:** Varies by site and technique. Consider patient pain tolerance.
- **Dose:** Typically 30 Gy in 10 fractions or 20 Gy in 5 fractions; 20 Gy in 8 fractions for lymphoma/multiple myeloma
- **Target:** One vertebral body above and below the site of disease + soft tissue extension + 1-2 cm laterally from the vertebral body
- **Technique:** Depends on level. In general:
  - Cervical (C1-C7): Opposed lateral
  - Thoracic (T1-T12): AP:PA or PA
  - Lumbar (L1-L5): AP:PA or PA
  - Sacrum: Laterals, AP:PA, or 3 field (PA: laterals)

Spine stereotactic surgery

- **SIM:** MRsim preferred, patient supine, Klarity SBRT system, head/neck/shoulder Aquaplastic mask for c-spine (Fig. 66.1).

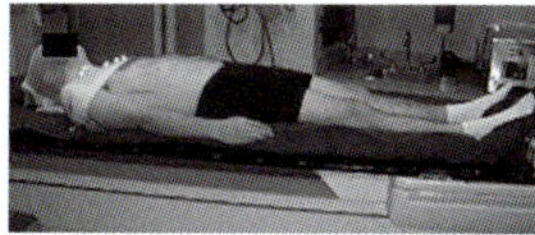
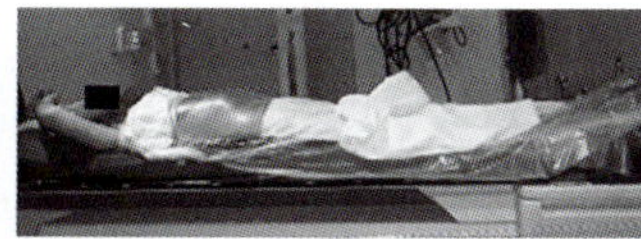

Figure 66.1 Typical set-up for cEBRT (left picture) and SSRS (right picture). Note the use of a highly indexable and adjustable Klarity SBRT system, which typically includes a wingboard with customized vacuum bag, respiratory belt, knee bridge and cushion, and angled foot positioner for immobilization.

- **Dose: *Dosing and target dependent on IGRT availability and physics support.** MDACC SSRS simultaneous integrated boost (SIB) technique:

	Radioresistant (GTV/CTV/fx)	Radiosensitive (GTV/CTV/fx)
No prior RT	24 Gy/16 Gy/1 fx	18 Gy/16 Gy/1 fx
Prior cEBRT	27 Gy/24 Gy/3 fx	27 Gy/21 Gy/3 fx

- **Image fusion:** Axial T1 and/or T1+C for GTV. Identify true cord on axial T2 MRI for intact. CT myelogram preferred for postoperative cases as hardware causes T2 artifact

- **Target (based on SSRS consensus guidelines;** ***Cox et al. IJROBP*** **2012):**
  Intact tumor
  GTV: Visible tumor on CT or MRI
  CTV: Contiguous at-risk bone as per guidelines (1 echelon beyond; see below) + 5 mm expansion around paraspinal/soft tissue extension of disease
  PTV: Depends on institutional setup uncertainty. No expansion at MDACC
  Postoperative:
  GTV: Preoperative disease + residual disease in postoperative imaging
  CTV: Same as intact, if bone resected, contour virtual CTV referring to postoperative consensus guidelines (*Redmond et al. IJROBP* 2017)
  PTV: Same as intact

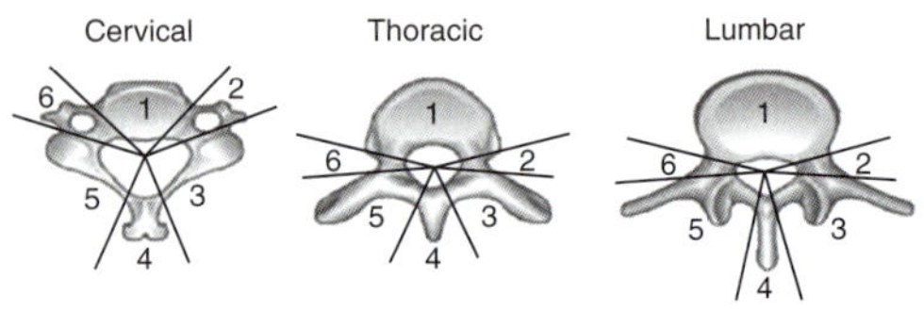

Figure 66.2 Anatomic classification system for consensus target volumes for spine SRS adapted from the international SRS consortium consensus guidelines. *1*, Vertebral body; 2, left pedicle; 3, left transverse process and lamina; *4*, spinous process; *5*, right transverse process and lamina; and *6*, right pedicle. (Adapted from Cox BW, Spratt DE, Lovelock M, et al. International Spine Radiosurgery Consortium consensus guidelines for target volume definition in spinal stereotactic radiosurgery. *Int J Radiat Oncol Biol Phys*. 2012;83(5):e597-605. Copyright © 2012 Elsevier. With permission.)

- **Planning directive constraints:** *PRV expansion based on institutional setup uncertainty. *No PRV expansion used at MDACC*
  Spinal cord:
  Single fraction: V8-10 Gy ≤ 1 cc, $D_{0.01cc}$ < 10-12 Gy
  Three fraction (prior cEBRT): 9 Gy ≤ 1 cc, $D_{0.01cc}$ ≤ 10 Gy
  Cauda equina:
  Single fraction: V12-14 Gy ≤ 1 cc, $D_{0.01cc}$ < 16 Gy
  Three fraction (prior cEBRT): 12 Gy ≤ 1 cc, $D_{0.01cc}$ ≤ 18 Gy
  Esophagus:
  Single fraction: V12 Gy ≤ 1 cc, $D_{0.01cc}$ < 17 Gy
  Three fraction (prior cEBRT): 12 Gy ≤ 1 cc, $D_{0.01cc}$ ≤ 21 Gy
- **Treatment planning:** VMAT. Goal GTV D_{min} > 14 Gy/1 fx or > 21 Gy/3 fx (*Bishop IJROBP* 2015). GTV coverage typically 80-90%
- **IGRT:** Daily ExacTrac, CBCT, and orthogonal ports prior to treatment and ExacTrac "snapshot" between each beam

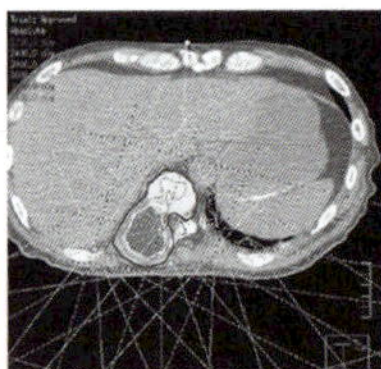 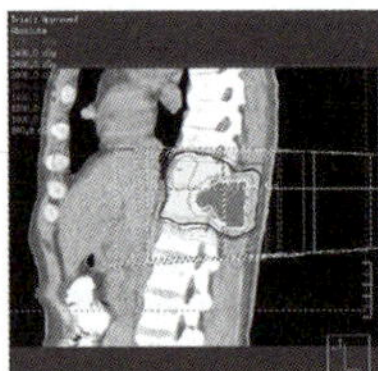 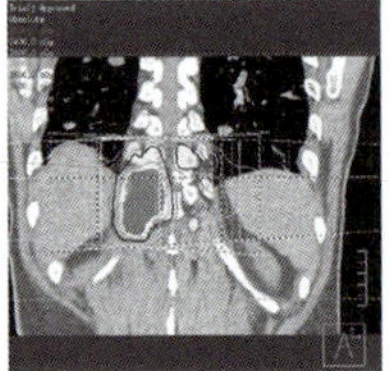

Figure 66.3 Representative treatment plan of a patient undergoing SSRS in axial, sagittal, and coronal (L → R) cross-sectional views. The CTV is highlighted in *yellow color* wash and GTV in *red*. The *blue isodose line* represents 16 Gy and *white isodose line* 24 Gy. This patient was treated with a single fraction. **See color insert.**

Side Effect Management

Acute

- **Pain flare:** Incidence 20-63%. Typically self-limiting and salvageable by treating with dexamethasone 4 mg bid over 5-7 days
- **Esophagitis:** Dietary modifications (pureed/bland/soft food, frequent small meals), topical anesthetics (magic mouthwash, etc.), analgesics (acetaminophen, narcotics)

Late

- **Vertebral body fracture:** Rates range from 10% to 40%, although a significant portion is asymptomatic. Risk correlated to dose/fraction, SINS, and preexisting fracture
- **Myelopathy:** <1%
- **Radiculopathy:** ~10% sensory radiculopathy risk and 3% motor radiculopathy risk. Risk greatest if disease involves the foramen
- **Esophageal stricture or perforation:** <1%

Follow-up

- Every 3 months with MRI of the entire spine w/contrast for 1-2 years and then every 6 months.
- Local control expected to be >90% at 1 year in radiation-naive patients regardless of histology and >75% in those receiving reirradiation.

Notable Trials

Name/Purpose	Study	Outcomes	Notes
MDACC prospective phase I/II trial (*Garg Cancer 2012*) 61 patients with 63 spinal tumors	Received 18-24 Gy in a single fraction	• 1- and 2-year LC rates were 91% and 88%, respectively • No significant differences in outcomes with respect to tumor histology • 87% of patients with complete or partial pain relief	Two patients experienced grade 3 and grade 4 neurologic toxicities
MDACC prospective phase I/II trial (*Wang Lancet Oncol* 2012) 149 patients with 166 metastatic spine tumors	Received a total dose of 27-30 Gy, typically in 3 fractions	• 1- and 2-year LC rates of 80.5% and 72.4%, respectively • 92.9% of patients reported some degree of pain relief with a significant reduction in opioid use from baseline to 3 (P = .021) and 6 months (P = .011) post SSRS	Rare instances of nonneurologic grade 3 toxicities were reported with no grade 4 toxicities noted
Phase II RTOG 0631 trial (*Ryu PRO* 2014) 44 patients with metastatic spine tumors	Received 16 Gy SSRS in a single fraction 65 institutions successfully credentialed	Adopted spinal cord constraints in the study have been reported to be safe with a D_{max} of 10 Gy, ≤0. cc or ≤10% of partial spinal cord	Phase III component comparing single-dose 16 Gy SSRS to single-dose 8 Gy cEBRT for pain control and QoL unpublished
Phase II/III CCTG SC.24/TROG 17.06 trial (*Sahgal Lancet Oncol* 2021) 229 patients with metastatic spine tumors among 18 institutions	24 Gy in 2 fractions SSRS 20 Gy in 5 fractions conventional EBRT	At 3 months, 35% of patients who received SSRS and 14% cEBRT had a complete response for pain (P = .0002), which was durable at 6 months post SSRS	SSRS at 24 Gy in 2 fx superior to cEBRT in improving the complete response rate for pain

NONSPINE BONE METASTASES

ALEX SHERRY • QUYNH-NHU NGUYEN

BACKGROUND

- **Incidence/prevalence:** Approximately 350 000 patients die each year with bone metastases. Pain is the most common presenting symptom, and bone metastases are most common cause of cancer-related pain.
- **Demographics:** Third most common site of metastatic disease (1st lung, 2nd liver). Axial skeleton more commonly involved (spine > pelvis > ribs > femur > skull)
- **Outcomes:** Highly variable, dependent on histology and extent of disease. In general, 90% of patients with at least partial relief, 60% of patients with significant relief, and 30% of patients pain-free off medication.
- Radiation for bone metastases constitutes ~40% of radiation treatments in the United States.

BIOLOGY AND PATHOLOGY

- **Pathology:** Most to least common: Breast > prostate > thyroid > kidney > lung. Bone metastases can occur either by direct extension or via hematogenous spread. Alters normal bone remodeling process mediated by osteoblasts and osteoclasts and can present as either lytic (classically kidney, myeloma, melanoma, non–small cell lung), blastic (classically prostate and small cell lung), or mixed (breast cancer, gastrointestinal, squamous) lesions

WORKUP AND EVALUATION

- **History and physical:** Identify the source of pain, severity, weight-bearing ability, neurologic deficits, pain medication use, performance status, and systemic disease burden.
- **Imaging:** Bone scan (technetium-99) for asymptomatic blastic bone mets. Uptake in bone scan more indicative of osteoblastic activity and may not be as reliable for lytic lesions. Plain films generally insensitive for detecting early medullary lesions. For focal assessment of symptomatic lesions, plain films to assess fracture risk, CT, or PET/CT, MRI, PSMA scan. For myeloma, get skeletal survey.
- **Biopsy:** Consider if no prior hx of cancer, site of 1st relapse, or multiple primary cancers.
- **Fracture risk:** Consult orthopedics if surgical stabilization is needed prior to RT. Use Mirels criteria, a weight-based scoring system to assess fracture risk (*Mirels et al. Clin Orthop Res* 1989) and the need for orthopedic evaluation prior to radiation (table below).
- Predictors of pathologic fracture of the femur: >30-mm axial cortical involvement or circumferential cortical involvement >50%, based on analysis of Dutch Bone Metastases Study (*Van der Linden et al. J Bone Joint Surg Br* 2004)

Mirels Score			
Score	1	2	3
Site	Upper extr	Lower extr	Peritrochanteric
Pain	Mild	Mod	Severe/Mechanical
X-ray	Blastic	Mixed	Lytic
% of shaft	0-33%	33-66%	67-100%

Score	Fracture Risk
0-6	**0%**
7	**5%**
8	**33%**
9	**57%**
10-12	**100%**

TREATMENT PRINCIPLES

- If significant fracture risk (Mirels score ≥ 8, >30 mm femoral cortical involved, >50% cortical involvement) and operative candidate (medically fit, life expectancy > 3 months, proximal/distal bone of sufficient quality to support fixation device) → prophylactic surgical fixation followed by radiation therapy
- Consider prophylactic radiation to asymptomatic nonspine bone metastases involving the hip, sacroiliac joint, or long bones with >33-66% cortical thickness or for tumors ≥ 2 cm (*Gillespie et al. ASTRO* 2022)
- Numerous dose and fractionation regimens are available based on the goals of treatment and patient evaluation.

- Palliative intent:
  - 8 Gy in 1 fraction (limited life expectancy < 3 months, PS ≥ 2)
  - 20 Gy in 5 fractions or 30 Gy in 10 fractions
  - Palliative reirradiation is safe and feasible. Achieves ~50% overall response rate (*Chow et al. Lancet Oncol* 2013)
  - Evaluate the potential for marrow suppression when considering large treatment fields or multiple sites, particularly for patients with upcoming chemotherapy
- Local control + palliative intent:
  - Regimens vary and include 12-24 Gy in 1 fraction, 27-36 Gy in 3 fractions, and 25-40 Gy in 5 fractions.
  - Greater and more durable pain relief with SBRT (12/16 Gy in 1 fraction) compared to 30 Gy in 10 fractions (*Nguyen JAMA Oncology* 2019)
  - To select a regimen, consider (among other factors) prognosis, performance status, mental status, acuity, hospitalization status, histology, radioresistance, response to systemic therapy, disease burden (oligometastatic vs polymetastatic), pace of progression, and anticipated need for and utility of durable local control; ability to achieve organ-at-risk constraints; prior radiation; tumor size and location; and salvage potential and morbidity of in-field recurrence.

Radiation Treatment Technique

- **SIM:** Varies by site and technique. Consider patient pain tolerance.
- **Target:** Contour GTV. Ensure soft tissue components encompassed using aid of diagnostic CT or MR as applicable. PTV = GTV + 0.5-2 cm (depending on setup reliability, patient's ability to stay still, and use of daily IGRT). Add 0.5-2 cm to block edge for dose buildup when using 3DCRT. Anticipate future radiation fields for marginal progression when designing beams and blocks. Postoperative: Cover the entire rod (both myeloma and nonmyeloma tumors); split joint space. Leave untreated strip of the skin.
- **Technique:** Depends on location. 2D or 3DCRT with palliative intent, beam arrangement varies by site. IMRT/VMAT or radiosurgery for dose escalation.
- **Planning directive:**
  - Palliative regimens: avoid significant hotspots in organs at risk
  - Dose-escalation general constraints below; others site-specific. Generally prioritize constraints over target coverage.

	1 Fraction	3 Fractions	5 Fractions
Brachial plexus/ peripheral nerves	D_{max} < 17.5 Gy	D_{max} < 24 Gy	D_{max} < 30.5 Gy
Skin	D_{max} < 26 Gy	D_{max} < 33 Gy	D_{max} < 39.5 Gy
Bowel	D_{max} < 12.4 Gy	D_{max} < 22.2 Gy	D_{max} < 35 Gy
Trachea	D_{max} < 20.2 Gy	D_{max} < 30 Gy	D_{max} < 40 Gy
Esophagus	D_{max} < 15.4 Gy	D_{max} < 25.2 Gy	D_{max} < 35 Gy

Surgery

- Done to prevent and/or treat pathologic fractures. For pelvic lesions, orthopedic surgeons typically opt for total hip arthroplasty if the lesion involves the neck and if the patient is able to tolerate. Other options include proximal hip endoprosthesis, intramedullary rods (if lesion in the midbone), or compression hip screw and side plate.

Systemic Therapy

- RANK-L inhibitors (denosumab): Monoclonal antibody that inhibits the RANK/RANK-L pathway (involved in osteoclast maturation and activity). Has been shown to decrease skeletal-related events in patients with bony mets from advanced cancers when compared to zoledronic acid (*Lipon Eur J Cancer* 2012). Approved for use in metastatic solid tumors. Typically given subcutaneously 120 mg q4wk and continued indefinitely
- Bisphosphonates (zoledronic acid, pamidronate): Inhibit osteoclast activity, preventing bone resorption. Used in castrate-resistant prostate cancer and breast cancer. Typically given IV q3-4wk (dose adjusted for creatinine clearance). Can also be given q3mo

- Systemic radionuclides (radium-223 and others): selective absorption into bone metastases. Consider for patients with diffuse osteoblastic osseous involvement without visceral disease as adjuvant to EBRT or first-line therapy in asymptomatic patients without high-risk lesions (impending fracture, mechanical instability, high-risk location)

Notable Trials

Name/Purpose	Study	Outcomes	Notes
RTOG 97-14 (*Hartsell et al. JNCI* 2005) 898 breast and prostate patients With 1-3 painful bone metastases	8 Gy in 1 fraction 30 Gy in 10 fx	Complete and partial response rates were 15% and 50% in the 8 Gy arm vs 18% and 48% in the 30 Gy arm. Retreatment was higher in 8 Gy arm vs 30 Gy arm (18% vs 9%), with less acute toxicity in the 8 Gy arm (10% vs 17%)	SFRT may be appropriate (8 Gy in 1 fx) for palliation in select cases in breast and prostate cancer patients with painful bony metastases
Chow et al. Meta-analysis (*Chow et al. JCO* 2007) 16 published randomized trials from 1986 onward	Evaluating 8 Gy in 1 fx regimen vs 30 Gy in 10 fx	SF and MF were found to be equivalent in palliation of pain with CR rates of 23% vs 24% for SF and MF, respectively, and OR rates of 58% and 59%. Retreatment rate 2.5× higher with SF (95% CI, 1.76-3.56, $P < .00001$). No difference in pathologic fracture risk	There is a significantly higher retreatment rate with SF palliative RT
MD Anderson (*Nguyen et al. JAMA Onc* 2019) 160 patients with mostly nonspine bone lesions	12-16 Gy SBRT 30 Gy in 10 fx	Statistically significant improved pain response improved with SBRT at 2 weeks (62% vs 36%), 3 months (73% vs 49%) and 9 months (77% vs 46%)	Pain response rates improved with single-fraction SBRT and should be considered for patients with bone metastases and long life expectancy

RADIATION EMERGENCIES

ALEX SHERRY • CHENYANG WANG • MARY MCALEER

Cord Compression

- **Definition:** Acute potentially life-threatening or morbid event caused by cancer for which radiation therapy may be therapeutic and/or offer palliation
- **Incidence/prevalence:** Breast, lung, and prostate account for 50-60% of cases. 70% involve thoracic spine, 20% lumbar, 10% cervical.
- **Pathophysiology:** Most commonly due to external compression caused by tumor eroding through the vertebral body from hematogenous seeding (95% of cases).

Rarely caused by intramedullary tumor. Obstructed epidural venous plexus drainage leads to vasogenic edema with nerve injury and progression to spinal cord infarction.

- **Outcomes:** Median OS ~3 months. Pretreatment ambulatory status biggest predictor of functional outcome. If ambulatory, median OS ~7 months; if nonambulatory, OS ~1.5 months

Workup

- **History:** Patient must be seen and assessed immediately. Inquire about pain and its features (radicular/mechanical/positional), motor/sensory/bowel/bladder deficits, and duration of symptoms. *Back pain is the most common initial presenting symptom and precedes neurologic deficits and is typically worse when lying down. Establish whether patient has known cancer diagnosis with pathology or elevated cancer biomarker (PSA, AFP, CEA, etc.). Assess performance status. Inquire about prior radiation treatment and last chemotherapy.
- **Examination:** Complete neurologic examination with clinical localization. Evaluate motor, sensory, and reflex function. Check for saddle anesthesia, rectal tone, spasticity, atrophy, and flaccidity.
- **Imaging:** Must image the entire spine as patients may have epidural disease outside primary symptomatic site. MRI with at least T1 and T2 sequences, preferable with and without contrast. Enhancing mass usually best visualized on T1 + C and cord impingement on T2 as CSF is bright (Fig. 68.1). Characterize the degree of compression using the Bilsky system (***Bilsky et al. J Neurosurg Spine* 2010**), and describe spinal stability with the SINS system (see Spine Metastases chapter). Consider CT myelogram if contraindication to MRI.

Bilsky Grade	Definition
0	Disease confined to bone
1a	Epidural impingement without indentation of the thecal sac
1b	Indentation of the thecal sac but not touching the cord
1c	Cord abutment without compression
2	Cord compression with cerebrospinal fluid visible
3	Cord compression without visible cerebrospinal fluid

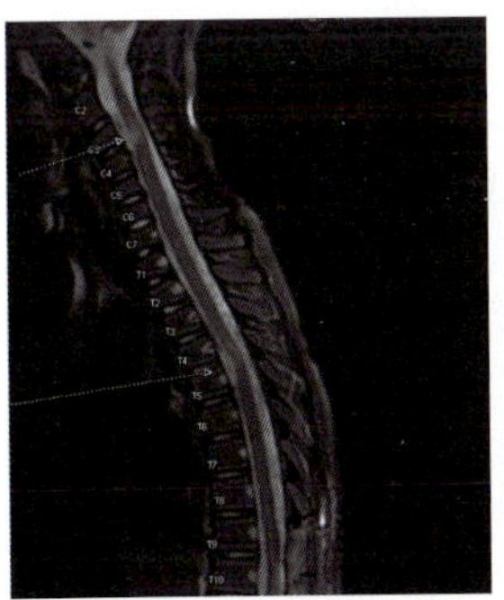

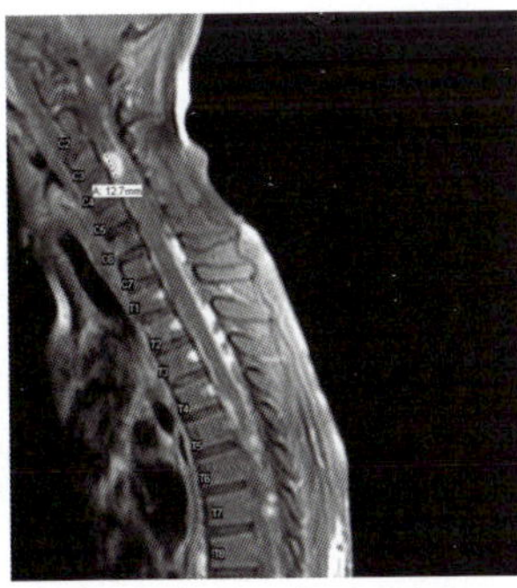

Figure 68.1 MRI T2-FLAIR **(left)** and T1 + C **(right)** sequences showing cord compression at C3-C4 and T4-T5 presenting in a 7-year-old male with a new diagnosis of a primitive neuroectodermal tumor. T2 sequence clearly shows the cord impingement with loss of bright CSF signal in areas where tumor has invaded the spinal canal (*arrows*).

Treatment principles

- Must establish a cancer diagnosis before radiation therapy, either with tissue, or in emergent scenarios with multidisciplinary discussion, elevated biomarker(s).
- Begin steroids: Dexamethasone 10 mg IV loading dose → 4 mg IV every 6 hours. Start proton pump inhibitor for GI prophylaxis and monitor blood sugar in patients with diabetes. For patients on immunotherapy/targeted therapy, consider discussion with medical oncologist, as feasible, on steroid use.

- Neurosurgery consult to evaluate for decompression and/or stabilization. For non-hematologic malignancies, level I evidence supporting superior functional outcomes for surgical decompression → radiation vs radiation alone. Surgery is especially considered for patients with radioresistant tumors, in-field recurrence within previously radiated sites, or mechanical instability. Postoperative radiation typically starts 2-4 weeks after surgery.
- If surgery is not recommended, patients with high-grade (Bilsky grade 3) cord compression and focal neurologic deficits should initiate radiation emergently (same day as consultation).

Radiation treatment technique

- **SIM:** Varies by site and technique. Consider patient pain tolerance and give PRN pain medications prior to simulation and treatment. An incline board at 10-15 degrees may be used for patients who are unable to tolerate lying fully spine due to severe refractory pain. In emergent cases where CT-based simulation may not be available (evening, weekends), clinical setup should be used (refer to Clinical Setup chapter for further details).
- **Dose:** Most common: 30 Gy in 10 fractions, 20 Gy in 5 fractions, or 8 Gy in 1 fractions; 20 Gy in 8 fractions for lymphoma/multiple myeloma. Consider radiosurgery postoperatively after decompression for oligometastatic or radioresistant histology (see Spine Metastases chapter for more detail).
- **Target:** Place field borders one vertebral body above and below site of disease + soft tissue extension + 1-2 cm laterally from the vertebral body.
- **Technique:** Depends on level. In general:
  - Cervical (C1-C7): Opposed lateral beams
  - Thoracic (T1-T12): AP:PA or PA
  - Lumbar (L1-L5): AP:PA or PA
  - Sacrum: Opposed laterals, AP:PA, or 3 field (PA:laterals)

Side effect management

- Pain management: NSAIDs, acetaminophen, narcotics. Initiate bowel regimen if narcotics are prescribed.
- Esophagitis: Dietary modification (pureed/bland/soft food, frequent small meals), topical anesthetics (magic mouthwash, glutamine), analgesics (acetaminophen, narcotics)
- Nausea: Antiemetics prior to treatment and PRN. First-line Zofran, add second line if needed
- Diarrhea: First-line Imodium titrating to a max of 8 pills/day → second-line alternating Lomotil and Imodium
- Cystitis: Rule out UTI, analgesics, cranberry juice, phenazopyridine.

Reirradiation

- If cord compression is identified in a previously irradiated field and the patient is not a candidate for surgery, SSRS, or spine simultaneous integrated boost (SSIB) (*Farooqi et al. Pract Radiat Oncol* 2019), conventional reirradiation may be offered to select patients.
- Consider life expectancy and extent of neurologic deficit since likelihood of restoring neurologic function is low, but reirradiation may limit progression and offer palliation.
- Based on analysis by *Nieder et al. IJROBP* 2006, risk of myelopathy is <3% if the following conditions are met:
  - Interval between radiation courses ≥6 months
  - Cumulative spinal cord BED ≤ 135 Gy assuming α/β value of 2 for cervical/thoracic cord and 4 for lumbar cord
  - ≤98 Gy BED delivered in any single course

Leptomeningeal Disease

Background

- **Definition:** Tumor involvement of the CSF or leptomeninges (pia mater and arachnoid). Note: Involvement of the dura mater does not constitute LMD as CSF is between pia and arachnoid meningeal layers.
- **Incidence/prevalence:** Diagnosed in ~5% of all cancer patients, most commonly in the breast, lung, and melanoma. Risk factors for LMD include piecemeal brain metastasis resection, resection of metastasis with dural involvement, and multiple brain metastases, particularly those in the posterior fossa.
- **Outcomes:** Prognosis is poor with median survival of 4 months or less with conventional WBRT; however, use of proton craniospinal irradiation (pCSI) may

significantly improve overall survival in select patients based on a phase II randomized study (*Yang et al. JCO* 2022).

Workup

- Patients often present with multifocal neurologic symptoms, as disease can involve the entire neuroaxis: For example, combination of cranial neuropathy and extremity weakness. Headache, cerebellar dysfunction, altered mental status, seizure, and cauda equina syndrome are also possible presenting symptoms.
- Patients suspected of having LMD should have MRI of the complete neuroaxis (brain and cervical, thoracic, lumbar spine) as well as lumbar puncture for CSF cytology analysis if no gross seeding identified on spine imaging. Note: (1) LP should be performed ***after*** spine imaging is completed to prevent false-positive sampling and/or unnecessary procedure if gross evidence of LMD seeding along the spinal cord/cauda nerve roots and (2) sensitivity of CSF cytology ~50%, thus repeating LP to increase sensitivity to 85-95% is warranted in patients with high clinical suspicion or radiographic findings concerning for LMD.

Treatment principles

- Symptomatic patients should receive dexamethasone as outlined in the section on "Cord Compression" above, with medical oncology consultation as needed regarding steroid use in patients on immune/targeted therapies.
- Selected patients may be treated comprehensively with pCSI. Consider for KPS 60 or greater, cytologic or radiographic diagnosis of LMD, and ability to meet organ at risk constraints after accounting for prior radiation. Obtain weekly CBC during pCSI. Hold systemic therapy during pCSI and at least 1-2 weeks before and after depending on the agent (longer washout for targeted therapy/selected chemotherapy vs immunotherapy). Consider emergent focal photon treatment to areas of gross areas of disease or patients with rapidly declining neurologic status or performance status rather than pCSI.
- For patients who are not candidates for pCSI, focal palliation may be offered including WBRT or spine radiation. Note that symptomatic sites may not have radiographic correlate. Localized treatment to suspected site of disease in these patients is reasonable (eg, RT to lumbosacral spine in patient with cauda equina syndrome).
- Patients treated with either pCSI or WBRT should be offered memantine.
- Referral to neuro-oncology for intrathecal therapy evaluation

Proton CSI treatment technique

- **SIM:** Supine, arms at side, Aquaplast mask over head, full-body Vac-Lok. Scan from the vertex of the skull through coccyx.
- **Dose:** 30 Gy in 10 fractions, junction every 3-4 fractions
- **Target:** Whole neuroaxis including brain (contour and cover cribriform plate) and spinal canal (contour thecal sac and place field border ~1 cm or one vertebral body inferior to the thecal sac for dosimetric margin). Do not cover the vertebral body (preserve marrow for systemic therapy) unless also treating selected symptomatic vertebral body metastases.
- **Technique:** Passive scatter proton therapy. Use RPO/LPO for the brain and three PA spine fields covering down to the thecal sac inferiorly. Feather the junctions after 3-4 fractions to avoid junctional hotspots in the cord.

SVC Syndrome

- **Definition:** Obstruction of blood flow through the superior vena cava
- **Incidence/prevalence:** 60-80% caused by malignancy of which 50% NSCLC, 25% SCLC, 10% NHL. Note 20-40% caused by benign processes (thrombosis from intravascular devices such as catheters or pacemakers, infection). 60% of patients present without prior cancer diagnosis.
- **Outcomes:** If SVC syndrome is appropriately managed, survival is comparable to patients with the same tumor type/stage without SVC syndrome.

Workup and treatment

- **History and physical:** Assess respiratory status, signs of airway compromise (stridor, oropharyngeal swelling), and ability of patients to lie down supine. Presenting symptoms include dyspnea, swelling of the face/arm/chest, laryngeal edema causing hoarseness/stridor, cough. Symptoms may be worsened with bending forward or lying down. Most cases will have associated pleural effusion. Evaluate for swelling/discoloration of the neck, face, and upper extremities. Focused neurologic assessment.
- **Imaging:** Chest x-ray, CT of the chest with contrast. Consider US if with concern for thrombus. CT of the head if concern for cerebral edema.

Treatment principles

- Supportive measures can be considered such as elevating head of bed, supplemental oxygen, steroids, diuretics.
- As majority of patients present with undiagnosed cancer, must establish tissue diagnosis prior to initiating radiation unless severe SVC causing airway compromise or, rarely, coma secondary to cerebral edema.
- Consider minimally invasive techniques for rapid diagnoses (sputum/pleural fluid cytology, biopsy of superficial nodes, BM biopsy for lymphoma, cancer biomarkers such as AFP or β-HCG). Alternatively, obtain tissue with CT or bronchoscopic-guided needle techniques.
- For patients with severe symptoms, rapid relief can be achieved with intraluminal stenting to allow time for establishment of a pathologic diagnosis and prior to treatment with chemotherapy/radiation therapy.
- For chemosensitive histologies (SCLC, lymphoma, germ cell tumors), can treat with chemotherapy alone.
- Expected time to relief ~3-14 days dependents upon histology.

Radiation treatment technique

- **SIM:** Generally upper Vac-Lok, arms above head, incline board if unable to lie flat
- **Dose:** If clinically stable, treat to appropriate dose for the primary histology (eg, 66 Gy in 33 fractions for NSCLC). For palliative intent, 30 Gy in 10 fractions or 20 Gy in 5 fractions. Can consider 3-4 Gy for the first few fractions and then convert to definitive dosing.
- **Target:** Contour GTV. CTV = GTV + 0.5- to 2-cm margin (depending on histology). PTV = CTV + 0.3-1 cm depending on setup and patient's ability to lay still.
- **Technique:** For definitive, consider IMRT. For palliative or rapid initiation of treatment, 3DCRT or 2D (AP/PA, obliques)

Side effect management

- Esophagitis: Dietary modifications (pureed/bland/soft food, frequent small meals), topical anesthetics (magic mouthwash, glutamine), analgesics (acetaminophen, narcotics)
- Cough: Tessalon Perles, Tussin (dextromethorphan)

Airway Compromise

- **Incidence/prevalence:** Approximately 80 000 cases of malignant airway obstruction occur annually.
- Can lead to cough, dyspnea, and pneumonia and cause significant morbidity and/or mortality

Treatment principles

- Nonradiation treatment options include therapeutic bronchoscopy with resection or stenting and surgery. These treatment options may provide rapid relief and tissue for diagnostic workup if needed.
- For candidates for definitive radiation therapy, bronchoscopy is preferred to allow for treatment planning and appropriate fractionation.

Radiation treatment technique

- Palliative radiation therapy can be offered, typically external beam for emergent cases.
- 45 Gy in 15 fractions, 30 Gy in 10 fractions (ASTRO guidelines preference), or 20 Gy in 5 fractions. If plan is to convert to definitive therapeutic intent, give 3-4 Gy for the first few fractions and then switch to a definitive dosing regimen.

Uncontrolled Bleeding

- **Incidence/prevalence:** Occurs in 6-10% of cancer patients most typically in the form of hemoptysis, upper/lower GI bleed, epistaxis, hematuria, or vaginal bleeding

Workup

- Assess the patient to confirm hemodynamic stability and rule out platelet abnormality, coagulopathy, or iatrogenic (anticoagulants) cause of bleeding.

Treatment principles

- **Nonradiation treatment options**
  - Packing, if accessible, is the least invasive approach and may achieve rapid hemostasis, or cauterization as appropriate.
  - Endoscopy (EGD, colonoscopy, bronchoscopy, cystoscopy) can achieve rapid hemostasis and provide tissue for diagnostic workup.

- IR embolization can achieve rapid hemostasis but requires the identification of feeder artery that will not result in significant normal tissue ischemia if embolized.
- Surgery is appropriate for some patients with localized disease (eg, hysterectomy).

- **Radiation therapy:** Typically takes days to weeks to achieve hemostasis. If patient is a candidate for definitive treatment, preferable to achieve rapid hemostasis with nonradiation treatment to allow for definitive planning and fractionation.

Radiation treatment technique

- Dosing varies by site, prognosis, severity of bleeding, and desire to convert to definitive treatment.
- Consider 30 Gy in 10 fractions, 20 Gy in 5 fractions, 8-10 Gy in 1 fraction, "Quad-shot" for HN cancer (*Corry et al. Radiother Oncol* 2005): 14.8 Gy in 4 fractions bid with >6-hour interfractional interval. If possibly converting to definitive intent, give 3-4 Gy for the first few fractions and then convert to definitive dosing.

Notable Trials

Name/Purpose	Study	Outcomes	Notes
***Patchell et al. Lancet* 2005** 101 patients with MRI evidence of cord compression with at least 1 symptom (including pain) and expected survival of > 3 mo	Surgery + RT (30 Gy in 10 fx) RT alone (30 Gy in 10 fx)	Primary end point of ambulation at 3 mo improved (84% vs 57%) with surgery Among patients unable to ambulate at the time of treatment, surgery improved return to ambulation (62% vs 19%)	Surgery + PORT offers superior outcomes compared to RT alone in patients with spinal cord compression
***Yang et al. JCO* 2022** 63 patients with LMD from breast cancer or non–small cell lung cancer randomized 2:1 to pCSI or phase II	Proton CSI Photon-based involved-field radiotherapy (WBRT or focal spine)	CNS PFS improved with pCSI (2 vs 8 mo; $P < .001$) and OS improved from 6 to 10 mo ($P = .04$) No difference in grade 3/4 toxicity rates	pCSI vs photon-based IFRT may improve PFS and OS in patients with select histologies and reasonable KPS (>60)

BENIGN DISEASE: NONNEURAL

JULIANNA BRONK • SHALIN SHAH

Heterotopic Ossification

- Heterotopic ossification (HO) is the formation of extraskeletal bone in muscle and soft tissues. It typically appears in the periarticular soft tissues following tissue injury from trauma or surgery. While the estimated frequency varies widely between 10% and 80% of cases, ~10% result in extensive HO, resulting in pain and impairment in the elbow, thigh, pelvis, and shoulder.
- Highest risk of HO is in patients with previous history of HO, either on the ipsilateral or contralateral side (following second surgery, the risk may be as high as 100%).
- Pain and immobility are the clinical hallmarks of this diagnosis. Typically, radiodense "eggshell calcifications" may be initially seen on plain radiographs of the joint. Management of HO generally involves surgery and prophylactic radiotherapy but may also include medical management.
- Surgery: Remove clinically meaningful ossifications resulting in discomfort.
- Medical management: NSAIDs (indomethacin) and COX-2 inhibitors have shown promising results in reducing the risk of HO development in the perioperative setting.

- Radiation: Typically completed 8 hours prior to or within 72 hours after surgery
- Low-dose radiation has been an effective technique in reducing the risk of HO formation. Both preoperative (8 hours prior to surgery) and postoperative (within 72 hours after surgery) regimens demonstrate efficacy in reducing the risk of HO. Single-fraction doses of 7 Gy in the preoperative setting and postoperative setting demonstrate excellent efficacy with low toxicity, including no worsening of wound healing (*Seegenschmiedt IJROBP* 2001). An example field for a patient with heterotopic ossification treated in the postoperative setting is demonstrated in Figure 69.1.

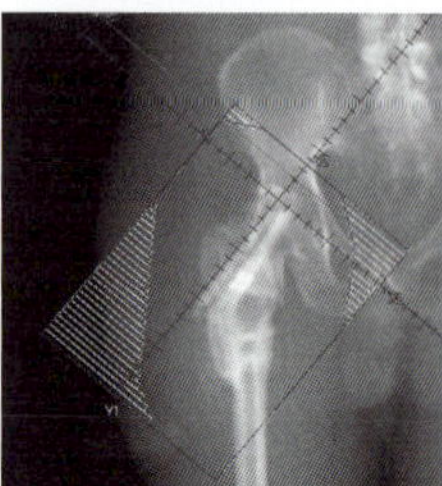

Figure 69.1 Standard AP field for heterotopic ossification.

Keloid

- Keloids are defined as areas of irregular fibrous tissue formed at the site of a scar or injury. Unlike hypertrophic scars, keloids do not regress over time and can slowly progress beyond initial wound edges. They may result in local pain and inflammation as a consequence of their infiltrating character.
- They occur more frequently in areas of high skin tension and are often seen in the upper body, around the joints, and in the earlobes.
- While the exact cause of keloids remains unknown, a genetic/racial predisposition, particularly in individuals of African descent, has been identified.
- Surgical resection of keloids is the initial treatment, with >50% recurrence rates seen in most series.
- Nonradiation options following surgery include pressure silicone dressings, intralesional injections of steroids/5FU/interferon/bleomycin or topical treatment with imiquimod, mitomycin C. Postop Laser therapy is an ongoing area of investigation.
- Radiation helps to reduce the rate of keloid formation after surgery to 20-25%. Detailed coordination following surgery is required to optimally reduce the rate of keloid formation, with radiation typically initiated within 24 hours of operation.
- Typical radiation dose-fractionation schemes vary from single-fraction 7.5-10 Gy to 12-25 Gy in 3 or 4 Gy fractions. Electrons are utilized to optimize dose to the scar with a 1-cm margin, with bolus applied to ensure generous coverage to the postoperative field.
- Depth of coverage is generally not specified as long as the postoperative field is well treated.

Gynecomastia

- Gynecomastia, a benign proliferation of breast tissue, is the most common breast condition in older men (24-65% prevalence), attributed to increased adiposity/obesity seen with aging.
- Gynecomastia incidence can be exacerbated by the use of androgen deprivation therapy in men with prostate cancer, particularly in those receiving older generation antiandrogen monotherapy (eg, bicalutamide 150 mg).
- This breast enlargement is frequently painful (mastodynia) and is a significant toxicity for many men receiving androgen deprivation therapy.
- Radiation given prophylactically (at time of bicalutamide initiation) may reduce the incidence of both gynecomastia and breast pain. Radiation is slightly less effective when given after gynecomastia and breast pain have already started (*Perdona Lancet Oncol* 2005).
- Classically, radiation has been delivered to a dose of 12-15 Gy in 3 Gy fractions, but single-dose treatment of 9-12 Gy has also been investigated.
- Tamoxifen (usually 20 mg daily) appears to be more effective than radiation therapy for gynecomastia and breast pain when given prophylactically, as well as after gynecomastia/breast pain has already started. However, tamoxifen requires a longer treatment course (6-12 months) and has a slightly higher toxicity profile compared to radiation therapy.
- Prophylactic tamoxifen or radiotherapy should be considered for men treated with long-term antiandrogen therapy.

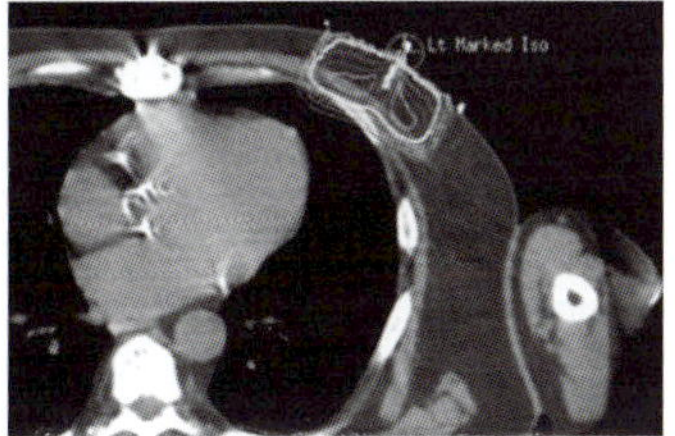

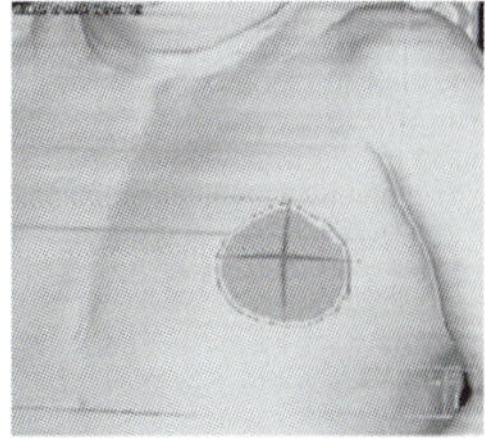

Figure 69.2 Standard electron field for gynecomastia. Field is a 5-6 cm diameter circle centered on each nipple. Depth measured on CT simulation.

Dupuytren Contracture

- Dupuytren disease (palmar fibromatosis) and Ledderhose disease (plantar fibromatosis) are benign but progressive proliferation of fibroblasts and myofibroblasts. This disorder begins with subcutaneous nodules that can progress to "cording" of tendons and connective tissue hardening.
- Eventually, the disorder results in severe flexion contractures of the metacarpophalangeal or proximal interphalangeal joints, limiting the use of the hands or causing impaired ambulation. The most commonly affected joints are the 4th/5th fingers of the hand and 1st/2nd toes of the foot.
- In more than half of patients, disease progression will occur 5 years after diagnosis. Steroids may be used for small, painful nodules, though the disease will likely progress. Collagenase is effective in patients with limited contractures but with short-term efficacy. If a patient is functionally limited as a consequence of the disorder, surgical intervention is recommended.
- Radiation is typically implemented in the early stages of the disease to limit progression, particularly in patients with asymptomatic lesions or minimal contracture. A dose of 30 Gy in 10 fractions (split course with a 12-week break) is preferred at MDACC. Targeted disease includes palpable cords and nodules with 1- to 2-cm proximal/distal and 1-cm lateral margins, respecting anatomical constraints. Orthovoltage (120 kV) or electrons with bolus are used to ensure adequate surface/superficial dose coverage.
- Radiation was able to reduce the risk of progression in a significant number (>70%) of patients with early-stage lesions but rarely results in the complete regression of hallmark nodules and cords. Long-term data demonstrates the most utility for radiation when utilized early in the disease course.

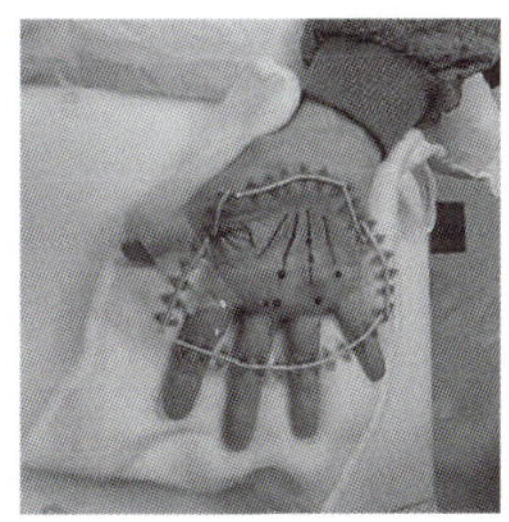

Figure 69.3 Standard field and setup for Dupuytren contracture. Palpated nodules and cords are marked at the time of simulation. Treatment borders are wired with care to spare the thenar muscles and nail beds if feasible. Note the use of a customized Klarity cushion for hand immobilization and setup reproducibility.

Osteoarthritis

- Osteoarthritis (OA), the most common joint disease in adults globally, affects 1 in 7 Americans and incidence is expected to increase with increasing life expectancy. OA can affect both large and small joints, most commonly the hand, knee, or hip.
- Etiology is thought to be multifactorial; however, pathogenesis is related to continuous degeneration of cartilage between bones in the joint driven by proinflammatory mechanisms that lead to degradation of the extracellular matrix.
- Clinical diagnosis of peripheral OA if following present: persistent use-related joint pain, age $\geq$ 45 years, morning stiffness lasting $\leq$ 30 min.
- Risk factors: older age (90% are over the age of 45 years), female sex, higher BMI, family history of OA, joint alignment and shape, or previous joint injury
- Management of OA is focused on palliation of symptoms, improving joint function, slowing disease progression and preventing disability—conservative management including lifestyle modification, weight loss, education, and exercise is often first line.
- Topical pain relievers and systemic analgesics including NSAIDs and acetaminophen can be used but are associated with increased risk of cardiovascular events, GI bleeding, and kidney toxicity if used long term. Intra-articular glucocorticoids and surgery (ie, total joint arthroplasty or arthrodesis) are reserved for severe OA.
- Low-dose radiation therapy (LDRT) to joints affected by OA has been shown to improve mobility and lead to moderate to long term pain relief due to anti-inflammatory effects.
- Dose: 6 Gy (1 Gy/fraction, 2-3 fractions per week) or 3 Gy (0.5 Gy/fraction, 2-3 fractions per week)—multiple studies indicate 60-70% of patients will have significant pain relief. A second course of LDRT (same dose and fraction) can be considered at 6-8 weeks if needed for persistent pain (30-40% of patients).

Small joints:

- Target: entire affected joint and cartilage, surrounding bursa, muscular insertion sites and surrounding soft tissue structures; consider shielding nail beds to prevent growth defects
- Technique: orthovoltage or 6 MV photon beam prescribed to joint midpoint (parallel opposed or PA with bolus). Consider immobilization devices (thermoplastic masks for the extremity or vac lock bags) for treatment reproducibility.

Large joints (knee or hip):

- Target: entire affected joint and cartilage, surrounding bursa, muscular insertion sites, and surrounding soft tissue structures; consider gonadal shielding
- Technique: knee: AP or lateral opposed photon beam prescribed to joint midpoint; hip: AP parallel opposed beams using higher energies (10 MV or greater). Similar immobilization devices can be used as with oncologic therapy.
- Treatment is very well tolerated with minimal acute side effects reported.

CLINICAL SETUP

JULIANNA BRONK • JARED OHRT • PETER BALTER

STATEMENTS OF CALIBRATION

- For each beam, there will be a reference point/geometry for which 1 MU will deliver 1 cGy of dose.
- The most commonly used reference geometries for linear accelerators are source surface distance (SSD) and source axial distance (SAD) (Fig. 70.1):

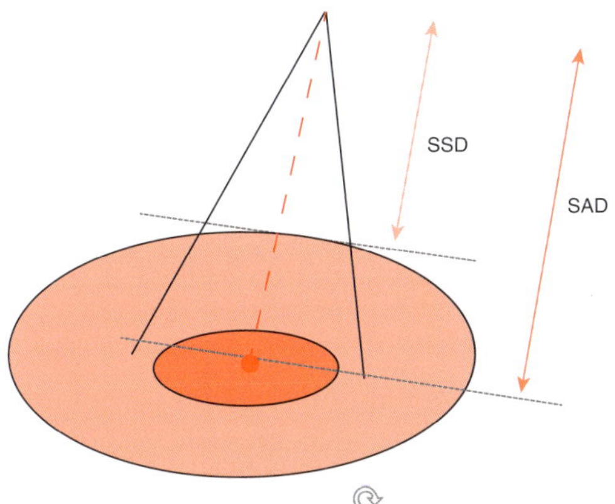

Figure 70.1 Illustration highlighting the difference between SAD and SSD techniques for referencing geometries. Note how the SSD technique maintains constant distance between the source and skin of the patient, whereas the SAD references the isocenter (*maroon spot*).

- For this section, we will assume that the isocenter distance will be 100 cm as this is most common on modern linear accelerators that would be used for these types of setup. For machines with other SAD distances, please consult your physics staff.
- SSD calibration: 100 cm to the surface, D_{max} depth for a 10 × 10 cm field 1 MU = 1 cGy (water). Uses constant distance between source and surface/skin. The **patient** is moved for each field.
- SAD calibration: 100 cm to the calculation point, D_{max} depth for a 10 × 10 cm field 1 MU = 1 cGy (water). Uses constant distance between source and the isocenter (100 cm for the modern linear accelerator). The **gantry** is moved for each field.
- Please check with your physics staff to understand how your machine is calibrated, different machines in the same department may be calibrated differently.

Photons:

- To perform calculations, you will need a depth correction factor (PDD and/or TMR tables) and Scatter factors (Sc: collimator scatter, Sp: phantom scatter, these may be combined as an output factor [OF] for cases with no blocking where OF = Sc × Sp).

$$MU = \frac{\text{Prescribed Dose per Field}}{\text{Calibration in } \frac{cGy}{MU} \times \text{Inverse Square Factor} \times \text{Depth Factor} \times Sc \times Sp \times \text{Other}}$$

	Inverse Square Factor (ISF)				
	SAD Calibrated Machines	**SSD Calibrated Machines**	**Depth Correction Table**	**Sc**	**Sp**
SAD Setup	1.000	$\left(\frac{100\,\text{cm}}{100\,\text{cm} + D_{max}[\text{cm}]}\right)^2$ *Typical values* *1.032 for 6X* *1.059 15X*	TMR	Field size per collimator display	Blocked field size at 100 cm when taking blocking or missing tissue into account
SSD Setup	$\left(\frac{100\,\text{cm} + D_{max}[\text{cm}]}{100\,\text{cm}}\right)^2$ *Typical values* *0.969 for 6X* *0.944 for 15X*	1.000	PDD		
Extended SSD	$\left(\frac{\textit{Distance from source to calc point}}{100\,\text{cm} + D_{max}[\text{cm}]}\right)^2$	$\left(\frac{100\,\text{cm} + D_{max}[\text{cm}]}{\textit{Distance to calc point}}\right)^2$	TMR *use the field size at the plane of measurements*		Blocked field size scaled from 100 cm to the distance to calc point*

$$^*\textit{Scaled Field size} = (\textit{field size}\,@100\,\text{cm})\,x\,\frac{\textit{distance to calculation point}[\text{cm}]}{100\,\text{cm}}$$

Other: Off-axis factors and beam attenuation factors such as wedge factors, tray factors, and other attenuations. *These factors are usually found in machine-specific tables but any case that requires the use of these should be avoided for clinical setups so this factor should be 1.000 for these cases.*

Electrons:

- To perform calculations, you will need depth correction (PDD) tables and cone factors. If you will be treating at nonstandard SSD you will need to know how your institution corrects for distances for electrons.

$$\text{MU} = \frac{\text{Prescribed Dose per Field}}{\text{Calibration in } \frac{cGy}{\text{MU}} \times \text{Distance Factor} \times \text{Normalization} \times \text{Cone Factor}}$$

- Distance Factor: Depending on your institution, this may be inverse square with an energy-dependent effective source distance, or this could be an air gap factor, if you are not treating at the nominal calibration distance (100 SSD), please contact your physicist.
- Normalization: The isodose lines used for target coverage, chosen from the electron PDD curve for the energy and the cone being used, this is generally between 80% and 90% and would be expressed as a decimal value, that is, percent/100 so 90% = 0.90, etc.
- Cone factor: Corrects from the calibration cone for that machine/energy to the one used for treatment.
- Note: Field size corrections for blocking were not included as it is not recommended to have performed clinical setups with significant blocking that would change the PDD and/or cone factor

General Landmarks

- T1: Most prominent posterior process
- T3: Suprasternal notch, root of spine of scapula
- T4: Sternal angle and 2nd rib
- T5: Carina
- T7: Bottom of scapula
- T9: Xiphoid process
- L4: Top of iliac crest
- S2: Posterior superior iliac spine

General Rules

- SAD setup is generally used for photon-based plans to treat deep lesions.
- SSD setup is generally used for electron or orthovoltage-based plans to treat superficial lesions or for single-field treatment.
- Dose falloff: 6 MV ~3.5% per cm; 18 MV ~2.0% per cm, deeper than D_{max}
- Calculated MUs are ~110% of field prescription (eg, prescribe 150 cGy anticipate ~170 MU).
- Agreement between independent calculations must be ±3% (or within 1 MU, whichever is larger).
- If separation <20 cm, consider 6 MV photons.

General Field Setup

First: Decide on setup (SAD vs SSD)
Second: Beam arrangement
Third: Beam energy
Fourth: Treatment depth
Fifth: Field size (X,Y)

- Whole brain: 20 × 20 cm opposed lateral fields covering the entire head, rotate collimator to block face, typical separation 15 ± 2 cm. Expected MUs/field = 166 ± 5 for 300 cGy, 6 MV based on machine calibrated at 100 SSD + D_{max} depth
- Spine: Center field at site of epidural disease or compression, cover 1 vertebral body above and below target vertebral body, expand to cover soft tissue extension, laterally cover 1-2 cm from edge of vertebral body. Review patient records for possible overlap of previous treatment.

General Treatment Plans

	Field(s) Setup	General Doses
Whole brain radiation	L lateral 50%/R lateral 50% prescribed to midplane	30 Gy in 10 fractions
Superior vena cava syndrome	AP 50%/PA 50%	30 Gy in 10 fractions
Painful bone metastasis	AP 50%/PA 50%	30 Gy in 10 fractions or 8 Gy in 1 fraction
Cervical spine	L lateral 50%/R lateral 50%	30 Gy in 10 fractions PA 100% L lateral 50%/R lateral 50% ~50% PA/L lateral ~25%/R lateral ~25%
Thoracic spine	AP ~33%/PA ~67% **OR** PA 100%	
Sacral spine	L lateral 50%/R lateral 50% **OR** AP ~33%/PA ~67% **OR** ~50% PA/L lateral ~25%/R lateral ~25%	
Palpable surface	Electrons	Variable

ABBREVIATIONS

^{18}F	fluorine 18
^{18}F PSMA	prostate-specific membrane antigen
^{18}FDG-PET	fluorodeoxyglucose-positron emission tomography
2DCRT	2-D conformal radiation therapy
3DCRT	3-D conformal radiation therapy
4DCRT	4-D conformal radiation therapy
4DCT	4-D computed tomography
5-FU	fluorouracil
^{68}Ga	gallium
6-MP	mercaptopurine
β-hCG	beta-human chorionic gonadotropin
A1AT	alpha-1 antitrypsin
ABH	lorazepam, diphenhydr-amine, haloperidol
ABMT	autologous bone marrow transplant
ABS	American Brachytherapy Society
ABVD	Adriamycin, bleomycin, vinblastine, dacarbazine
AC	Adriamycin cyclophosphamide
ACh	acetylcholine
AChE	acetylcholine esterase
AChR	acetylcholine receptor
ACS	American Cancer Society
ACTH	adrenocorticotropic hormone
ADC	apparent diffusion coefficient
ADH	antidiuretic hormone
ADT	androgen deprivation therapy
AE	adverse event
AF	applicator factor
AFP	alpha-fetoprotein
AJCC	American Joint Committee on Cancer
ALARA	as low as reasonably achievable
ALK	anaplastic lymphoma kinase
ALL	acute lymphoblastic leukemia
ALN	axillary lymph node
ALND	axillary lymph node dissection
ALT	alanine transaminase
AML	acute myelogenous leukemia
AP	anterior-posterior
APBI	accelerated partial breast irradiation
APCs	antigen-presenting cells
APR	abdominoperineal resection
ARR	absolute risk reduction
AS	active surveillance
AST	aspartate aminotransferase
ASTRO	American Society for Radiation Oncology
AT/RT	atypical teratoid/rhabdoid tumor
ATC	anaplastic thyroid cancer
ATM	ataxia-telangiectasia mutated
AUA	American Urological Association
AUC	area under curve
AV	anal verge
AVM	arteriovenous malformation
AZO	phenazopyridine
BBB	blood-brain barrier
BCC	basal cell carcinoma
BCF	biochemical failure
BCG	bacille Calmette-Guerin
BCL	B-cell lymphoma
BCM	breast cancer mortality
BCNU	carmustine
BCS	breast-conserving surgery
BCSM	breast cancer–specific mortality
BEACOPP	bleomycin, etoposide, doxorubicin (Adriamycin), cyclophosphamide, vincristine (Oncovin), procarbazine, prednisone
BED	biologically effective dose
BEP	bleomycin, etoposide, cisplatin
BID	two times a day
BI-RADS	breast imaging-reporting and data system
BM	bone marrow
BMBx	bone marrow biopsy
BMI	body mass index
BMT	bone marrow transplant
BOT	base of tongue
BP	blood pressure
bPFS	biochemical progression-free survival
BPH	benign prostatic hyperplasia
BSO	bilateral salpingo-oophorectomy
BT	brachytherapy
BUN	blood urea nitrogen

C&E	curettage and electrodessication	**CSF**	cerebrospinal fluid
CAPOX	capecitabine/oxaliplatin	**CSI**	craniospinal irradiation
CAR-T	chimeric antigen receptor-T cells	**CSS**	cancer-specific survival
CBC	complete blood count	**CT**	computed tomography
CBCT	cone beam CT	**CTCAE**	common terminology criteria for adverse events
CCNU	lomustine	**CTCL**	cutaneous T-cell lymphoma
CCRT	concurrent chemoradiation therapy	**CTV**	clinical target volume
CCSK	clear cell sarcoma of the kidney	**CV**	cardiovascular
CCSS	Childhood Cancer Survivor Study	**CW**	chest wall
CDC	Centers for Disease Control and Prevention	**CXR**	chest x-ray
CEA	carcinoembryonic antigen	**DA**	dose-adjusted
cEBRT	conventional external beam radiation therapy	**DAHANCA**	Danish Head and Neck Cancer Study Group
CF	conventional fractionation	**DAMPs**	damage-associated molecular patterns
CFS	colostomy-free survival	**DBCG**	Danish Breast Cancer Group
CF-WBI	conventionally fractionated whole-breast irradiation	**DCIS**	ductal carcinoma in situ
cGE	cobalt gray equivalent	**DD**	death dose
ChemoRT	chemoradiotherapy	**DD4A**	vincristine/dactinomycin/doxorubicin
CHF	congestive heart failure	**ddAC**	dose-dense AC
CHT	chemotherapy	**ddMVAC**	dose-dense methotrexate, vinblastine, adriamycin, cisplatin
CI	conformity index	**DE-EBRT**	dose-escalated external beam radiation therapy
CIMP	CpG island methylator phenotype	**DE-RT**	dose-escalated radiation therapy
CIN	chromosomal instability	**DES**	diethylstilbestrol
CKD	chronic kidney disease	**DEXA**	dual-energy x-ray absorptiometry
CLL	chronic lymphocytic leukemia	**DF**	distant failure
cLN	clinically palpable lymph node	**DFS**	disease-free survival
CLND	completion lymph node dissection	**DHL**	double-hit lymphoma
CMF	cyclophosphamide, methotrexate, and fluorouracil	**DI**	diagnostic imaging
CML	chronic myelogenous leukemia	**DIBH**	deep inspiration breath hold
CMP	comprehensive metabolic panel	**DIPG**	diffuse intrinsic pontine gliomas
CMT	combined modality treatment	**DLBCL**	diffuse large B-cell lymphoma
CN	cranial nerve	**DLI**	dermal lymphatic invasion
CNS	central nervous system	**DLT**	dose-limiting toxicity
COG	Children's Oncology Group	**DM**	distant metastasis
COX-2	cyclooxygenase-2	**DMFS**	distant metastasis-free survival
CP	chest pain	**dMMR**	deficient mismatch repair
CR	clinical response	**dMMR-MSI-H**	deficient mismatch repair, microsatellite instability-high
Cr	creatinine	**DMSO**	dimethyl sulfoxide
CRC	colorectal cancer	**DNA**	deoxyribonucleic acid
CREON	pancrelipase	**DNA-PKcs**	DNA-dependent protein kinases
CRM	continual reassessment method	**DOI**	depth of invasion
CRPC	castrate-resistant prostate cancer	**DPFS**	distant progression-free survival
CRT	chemoradiation therapy	**DR**	disease recurrence

DRE	digital rectal exam
DRR	digitally reconstructed radiography
DSB	double-strand break
DS-GPA	diagnosis-specific graded prognostic assessment
DSS	disease-specific survival
DTPA	diethylenetriaminepentaacetate
DVH	dose-volume histogram
dVIN	differentiated vulvar intraepithelial neoplasm
DWI	diffusion-weighted imaging
DX	diagnosis
EBCTCG	Early Breast Cancer Trialists' Collaborative Group
EBRT	external beam radiation therapy
EBUS	endobronchial ultrasound
EBV	Epstein-Barr virus
ECC	epirubicin, cisplatin, capecitabine
ECE	extracapsular extension
ECF	epirubicin, cisplatin, 5-fluorouracil
ECG	electrocardiogram
ECOG	Eastern Cooperative Oncology Group
ECX	epirubicin, cisplatin, capecitabine
EDRT	escalated dose radiotherapy
EFRT	extended field radiation therapy
EFS	event-free survival
EFT	Ewing family of tumors
EGD	esophagogastroduodenoscopy
EGFR	epidermal growth factor receptor
EGFR-MAPK	EGFR-mitogen-activated protein kinase
EI-CESS	European Intergroup Cooperative Ewing Sarcoma Studies
EMVI	extramural vascular invasion
ENE	extranodal extension
ENI	elective nodal irradiation
EOC	epirubicin, oxaliplatin, capecitabine
EORTC	European Organisation for Research and Treatment of Cancer
EP	etoposide, cisplatin
EPIC	Expanded Prostate Cancer Index Composite
EPID	electronic portal imaging device
EPP	extrapleural pneumonectomy
EQD2	equivalent dose at 2 Gy
ER	estrogen receptor
ERCP	endoscopic retrograde cholangiopancreatography
ESBC	early-stage breast cancer
ESMO	European Society of Medical Oncology
ESR	erythrocyte sedimentation rate
ES-SCLC	extensive stage small cell lung cancer
ESTRO	European Society of Therapeutic Radiation Oncology
ETE	extrathyroid extension
EtOH	ethanol
ETV	evaluation target volume
EUA	examination under anesthesia
EUS	endoscopic ultrasound
EWS	Ewing sarcoma
FA	focal anaplasia
FAC	fluorouracil, Adriamycin, and cyclophosphamide
FAP	familial adenomatous polyposis
FAS-L	Fas ligand
FB	free breathing
FDA	Food and Drug Administration
FDG	fludeoxyglucose
FEV1	forced expiratory volume (1 second)
FFDM	freedom from distant metastasis
FFDP	freedom from distant progression
FFLF	freedom from local failure
FFLR	freedom from local recurrence
FFS	failure-free survival
FGFR	fibroblast growth factor receptor
FH	favorable histology
FIGO	International Federation of Gynecology and Obstetrics
FISH	fluorescence in situ hybridization
FLAIR	fluid-attenuation inversion recovery
FLIPI	Follicular Lymphoma International Prognostic Index
FLOT	fluorouracil/leucovorin/oxaliplatin/docetaxel
FNA	fine needle aspiration
FOLFIRINOX	folinic acid, fluorouracil, irinotecan, oxaliplatin

FOLFOX folinic acid, fluorouracil, oxaliplatin
FOM floor of mouth
FOV field-of-view
FS fat-suppressed
FSH follicle-stimulating hormone
FSRS fractionated stereotactic radiosurgery
GBC gallbladder cancer
GBM glioblastoma multiforme
GCB germinal center B cell
G-CSF granulocyte colony-stimulating factor
GCT germ cell tumor
GEJ gastroesophageal junction
GEP gene expression profiling
GERD gastroesophageal reflux disease
GFAP glial fibrillary acidic protein
GFR glomeruli filtration rate
GH growth hormone
GHSG German Hodgkin Study Group
GI gastrointestinal
GIST gastrointestinal stromal tumor
GM-CSF granulocyte-macrophage colony-stimulating factor
GnRH gonadotropin-releasing hormone
GOG Gynecologic Oncology Group
GP glossopharyngeal
GPAs graded prognostic assessments
GS genomically stable
GTR gross total resection
GTV gross tumor value
GU genitourinary
GVHD graft versus host disease
H&N head and neck
H&P history and physical examination
HA hinge angle
HAV hepatitis A virus
HB hepatitis B
HBsAg hepatitis B surface antigen
HBV hepatitis B virus
HCC hepatocellular carcinoma
HCG human chorionic gonadotropin
HD high dose
HDAC histone deacetylase
HDR high-dose rate
HER-2 human epidermal growth factor receptor 2
HF hypofractionated
HF-WBI hypofractionated whole-breast irradiation
HGG high-grade glioma
HIV human immunodeficiency virus
HL Hodgkin lymphoma
HLA human leukocyte antigen
HN head and neck
HNC head and neck cancer
HNPCC hereditary nonpolyposis colorectal cancer
HNSCC head and neck squamous cell carcinoma
HO heterotopic ossification
HPF high-powered field
HPV human papillomavirus
HPV16 human papillomavirus 16
HR hazard ratio
HR-CTV high-risk clinical target volume
HSCT hematopoietic stem cell transplantation
HSV-1 herpes simplex virus type 1
HT hormone therapy
HTN hypertension
HVA homovanillic acid
HVL half-value layer
HVLT-R Hopkins Verbal Learning Test-Revised
HYPORT-STS hypofractionated radiotherapy for soft tissue sarcoma study
IAC internal auditory canal
IBC inflammatory breast cancer
IBD inflammatory bowel disease
IBTR ipsilateral breast tumor recurrence
IC induction chemotherapy
ICBT intracavitary brachytherapy
ICP intracranial pressure
ICRP International Commission on Radiological Protection
ICRT intracavitary radiation therapy
ICRU International Commission on Radiation Units and Measurements
iCTV internal clinical target volume
ICV infraclavicular
IDH isocitrate dehydrogenase
IDL isodose line
IFNγ interferon-gamma

IFRT	involved-field radiotherapy
IGBT	image-guided brachytherapy
IGF-1	insulin growth factor 1
IGRT	image-guided radiation therapy
iGTV	internal gross tumor volume
IHC	immunohistochemistry
IJROBP	*International Journal of Radiation Oncology, Biology, Physics*
IJV	internal jugular vein
IL	interleukin
IL-2	interleukin-2
ILROG	International Lymphoma Radiation Oncology Group
IM	internal mammary/internal margin
IMA	internal mammary artery
IMC	internal mammary chain
iMLD	ipsilateral mean lung dose
IMN	internal mammary nodes
IMPT	intensity-modulated proton therapy
IMRT	intensity-modulated radiation therapy
INR	international normalized ratio
INRT	involved nodal radiation therapy
INSS	International Neuroblastoma Staging System
IO	immune oncology
IPI	International Prognostic Index
IPS	International Prognostic Score
IPSS	International Prostate Symptom Score
IQ	intelligence quotient
IR	interventional radiology
IRB	Institutional Review Board
IRS	intergroup rhabdomyosarcoma
ISRT	involved site radiation therapy
ISUP	International Society of Urologic Pathologist
ITC	isolated tumor cell
ITMIG	International Thymic Malignancy Interest Group
ITV	internal target volume
iTVI	internal tumor-vessel interface
IUD	intrauterine device
IUGR	intrauterine growth restriction
IV	intravenous/irradiated volume
IVC	inferior vena cava
IVF	in vitro fertilization
IVLBCL	intravascular large B-cell lymphoma
IVP	intravenous
JPA	juvenile pilocytic astrocytoma
KPS	Karnofsky Performance Status
KUB	kidney, ureter, and bladder
KV	kilovoltage
LABC	locally advanced breast cancer
LAO	left anterior oblique
LAR	low anterior resection
LC	local control
LC-CRT	long-course chemoradiation
LDCSI	low-dose craniospinal irradiation
LDH	lactate dehydrogenase
LDR	low-dose rate
LDR-PB	low-dose rate prostate brachytherapy
LET	linear energy transfer
LF	local failure
LFTs	liver function tests
LGG	low-grade glioma
LH	luteinizing hormone
LHRH	luteinizing hormone–releasing hormone
LINAC	linear accelerator
LL	left lateral
LLO	left lateral oblique
LMD	leptomeningeal disease
LN	lymph node
LND	lymph node dissection
LOET	late onset efftox model
LOH	loss of heterozygosity
LP	lumbar puncture
LPFS	local progression failure-free survival
LPO	left posterior oblique
LR	local recurrence
LRC	locoregional control
LRF	locoregional failure
LRFS	locoregional failure survival
LRR	local recurrence rate
LRRFS	locoregional recurrence–free survival
LSS	limb-sparing surgery
LS-SCLC	limited-stage small cell lung cancer
LUL	left upper lobe
LUTS	lower urinary tract symptoms
LV	left ventricle
LVI	lymphovascular invasion

LVSI	lymphovascular stromal invasion
MAC	meta-analysis of chemotherapy
MALT	mucosa-associated lymphoid tissue
MB	medulloblastoma
MCC	Merkel cell carcinoma
MCL	mantle cell lymphoma
MCPyV	Merkel cell polyomavirus
mCRC	metastatic colorectal cancer
mCRPC	metastatic castrate-resistant prostate cancer
MD	medical doctor
MDA	MD Anderson
MDACC	MD Anderson Cancer Center
MDP	methylene diphosphonate
MDR	medium-dose rate
MDS	myelodysplastic syndrome
MDSC	myeloid-derived suppressor cells
MEC	mucoepidermoid carcinoma
MEN1	multiple endocrine neoplasia type 1
MEN2	multiple endocrine neoplasia type 2
MESCC	metastatic epidural spinal cord compression
MF	mycosis fungoides
MFO	multifield optimization
MFS	metastasis-free survival
MGMT	O^6-alkylguanine-DNA alkyltransferase
MHC	major histocompatibility complex
MIBG	meta-iodobenzylguanidine
MIP	maximum intensity projection
MIPI	MCL International Prognostic Index
MLB	multilumen balloon
MLD	metachromatic leukodystrophy
MM	multiple myeloma
MMC	mitomycin C
MMG	mammogram
MMMT	malignant mixed müllerian tumor
MMR	mediastinal mass ratio
MMT	mixed malignant tumor
MOPP	mechlorethamine, vincristine, procarbazine, prednisone
MR	magnetic resonance
MRA	magnetic resonance angiogram
MRC	Medical Research Council
MRCP	magnetic resonance cholangiopancreatography
MRI	magnetic resonance imaging
MRM	modified radical mastectomy
mRNA	messenger RNA
MS	multiple sclerosis
MSI	microsatellite instability
MSK	musculoskeletal
MSKCC	Memorial Sloan Kettering Cancer Center
MSSA	methicillin-susceptible *Staphylococcus aureus*
MTC	medullary thyroid cancer
MTD	maximal tolerated dose
MTV	mucosal target volume
MTX	methotrexate
MUGA	multigated acquisition scan
MV	megavolt
MVA	multivariable analysis
MVAC	methotrexate, vinblastine, Adriamycin, and cisplatin
MyoD1	myogenic differentiation 1
MZL	mantle zone lymphoma
NAC	neoadjuvant chemotherapy
NASH	nonalcoholic steatohepatitis
NB	neuroblastoma
NCCN	National Comprehensive Cancer Network
NCCTG	North Central Cancer Treatment Group
NCDB	National Cancer Database
NCIC	National Cancer Information Center
NED	no evidence of disease
NEJM	*New England Journal of Medicine*
NF	neurofibromatosis
NF1	neurofibromatosis type 1
NFT	no further treatment
NGGCT	nongerminomatous GCT
NHEJ	nonhomologous end-joining
NHL	non-Hodgkin lymphoma
NK	natural killer
NLPHL	nodular lymphocyte predominant Hodgkin lymphoma
NMSC	nonmelanoma skin cancer

NNT number needed to treat
NovoTTF Novocure tumor treating fields
NPC nasopharyngeal carcinoma
NPO nothing by mouth
NPV negative predictive value
NPX nasopharynx
NRFS nodal recurrence-free survival
NS not significant
NSABP National Surgical Adjuvant Breast and Bowel Project
NSAIDs nonsteroidal anti-inflammatory drugs
NSCLC non–small cell lung cancer
NSHL nodular sclerosing Hodgkin lymphoma
NTCP normal tissue complication probability
NTR near-total resection
NWTS National Wilms' Tumor Society
OAR organs at risk
OC oral cavity
ODI optical distance indicator
OER oxygen enhancement ratio
OF output factor
OPC oropharyngeal cancer
OPX oropharynx
OR odds ratio
ORR objective response rate
OS overall survival
OTC over-the-counter
PA posterior-anterior
PAI pubic arch interference
PALCL primary anaplastic large cell lymphoma
PAMPs pathogen-associated molecular patterns
PARP poly(ADP-ribose) polymerase
PARPi poly(ADP-ribose) polymerase inhibitor
PBI partial breast irradiation
PBRT prostate bed radiation therapy
PC posterior commissure
PCA prostate cancer
PCFCL primary cutaneous follicle center lymphoma
PCI prophylactic cranial irradiation
PCLBCL primary cutaneous diffuse large B-cell lymphoma
PCMZL primary cutaneous marginal zone B-cell lymphoma
PCNSL primary central nervous system lymphoma
PCOS polycystic ovarian syndrome
PCP primary care physician
pCR pathologic complete response
PCR polymerase chain reaction
PCSM prostate cancer–specific mortality
PCSS prostate cancer–specific survival
PCV procarbazine, lomustine, vincristine
PD progressive disease
PD-1 programmed cell death protein 1
PDAC pancreatic ductal adenocarcinoma
PDD percent depth dose
PDE phosphodiesterase
PDE5 phosphodiesterase type 5
PDGF platelet-derived growth factor
PDGFR platelet-derived growth factor receptor
PD-L1 programmed death-ligand 1
PDR pulsed dose rate
PE photoelectric effect
PEG percutaneous endoscopic gastrostomy
PeIN penile intraepithelial neoplasia
PET positron emission tomography
PFS progression-free survival
PFT pulmonary function test
PGI prompt gamma imaging
pGS pathologic Gleason score
PLAP placental alkaline phosphatase
pLN pathologic lymph node
PLND pelvic lymph node dissection
PLT platelet
PM parametria
PMBCL primary mediastinal B-cell lymphoma
PMH past medical history
PMN polymorphonuclear cell
PMRT postmastectomy radiation therapy
PNA pneumonia
PNET primitive neuroectodermal tumor
PNI perineural invasion
PNS peripheral nervous system
PO by mouth

PORT	postoperative radiation therapy
PP	pair production
PPI	proton pump inhibitor
PPV	positive predictive value
PR	partial response
PR/SD	partial response/stable disease
PRL	prolactin
PRN	as needed
PRT	pharyngeal-targeted radiation therapy
PRV	planning risk volume
PS	performance status
PSA	prostate-specific antigen
PSMA	prostate-specific membrane antigen
PSMA-PET	prostate-specific membrane antigen positron emission tomography
PSPT	passive scattering proton therapy
PSRT	pharyngeal-sparing radiation therapy
pSV	pathologic seminal vesicle specimen
PTC	percutaneous transhepatic cholangiography
PTV	planning target volume
PY	pack years
QA	quality assurance
QD	every day
QOD	every other day
QOL	quality of life
QUANTEC	quantitative analyses of normal tissue effects in the clinic
RAI	radioactive iodine
RAO	right anterior oblique
RB	retinoblastoma
RBC	red blood cell
RBE	relative biological effectiveness
RC	regional control
RCC	renal cell carcinoma
R-CHOP	rituximab-cyclophosphamide, doxorubicin, vincristine, prednisone
RCT	randomized controlled trial
RDL	recommended dose level
RF	radiofrequency
RFA	radiofrequency ablation
RFS	recurrence/relapse-free survival
RHDVRT	reduced high-dose volume radiation therapy
RILD	radiation-induced liver disease
R-MPV	rituximab, methotrexate, procarbazine, and vincristine
RMS	rhabdomyosarcoma
RMT	retromolar trigone
RNA	ribonucleic acid
RNI	regional nodal irradiation
ROI	region of interest
ROM	range of motion
RP	retroperitoneal
RPA	recursive partitioning analysis
RPLND	retroperitoneal lymph node dissection
RPO	right posterior oblique
RPS	retroperitoneal sarcoma
RR	risk ratio or relative risk
RT	radiation therapy
RTK	rhabdoid tumor of the kidney
RTOG	Radiation Therapy Oncology Group
RT-PCR	real-time PCR
SABR	stereotactic ablative radiotherapy
SAD	source axial distance
SBC	secondary breast cancer
SBO	small bowel obstruction
SBRT	stereotactic body radiation therapy
SC	short course
SCC	squamous cell carcinoma
SCD	source to calibration distance
SCLC	small cell lung cancer
SCM	sternocleidomastoid
SCRT	sequential chemoradiation therapy
SCT	stem cell transplantation
SCV	supraclavicular
SD	stable disease
SDCSI	standard-dose craniospinal irradiation
SEER	surveillance, epidemiology, and end results
SEP	solitary extramedullary plasmacytoma
SERD	selective estrogen receptor degrader
SERM	selective estrogen receptor modulator
SF	single fraction
SFO	single-field optimization
SFRT	single-fraction radiotherapy
SHH	sonic hedgehog
SHIM	sexual health inventory for men
SI	sacroiliac
SIADH	syndrome of inappropriate antidiuretic hormone secretion

SIB	simultaneous integrated boost
SIM	simulation
SINS	spine instability neoplastic score
SIOP	International Society of Paediatric Oncology
SIR	score index for radiosurgery
SLL	small lymphocytic lymphoma
SLN	sentinel lymph node
SLNB	sentinel lymph node biopsy
SLND	sentinel lymph node dissection
SM	setup margin/surgical margin
SMA	superior mesenteric artery
SMN	second malignancy
SMV	superior mesenteric vein
SND	selective neck dissection
SNEC	small cell neuroendocrine carcinoma
SNL	sentinel lymph node
SNUC	sinonasal undifferentiated carcinoma
SOB	shortness of breath
SOBP	spread-out Bragg peak
SOC	standard of care
SOD	superoxide dismutase
SPB	solitary plasmacytoma of bone
SPD	source to point distance
SRS	stereotactic radiosurgery
SRT	stereotactic radiotherapy
SS	statistically significant
SSBs	single-strand breaks
SSD	source surface distance
SSRS	spine stereotactic radiosurgery
STD	sexually transmitted disease
STIR	short T1 inversion recovery
STR	subtotal resection
STS	soft tissue sarcoma
STV	scanning target volume
SUV	standardized uptake value
SV	seminal vesicle
SVC	superior vena cava
SVI	seminal vesicle involvement
TACE	transcatheter arterial chemoembolization
TAD	targeted axillary dissection
TAE	transanal excision
TAH	total abdominal hysterectomy
TAM	tamoxifen
TBI	tolerance by inhibiting
TCGA	The Cancer Genome Atlas
TCHP	paclitaxel, carboplatin, Herceptin, pertuzumab
TCR	T-cell receptor
TFE	turbo field echo
TG	tamoxifen, Genox
THP	paclitaxel, Herceptin, pertuzumab
TID	three times a day
TIL	tumor-infiltrating lymphocyte
TKI	tyrosine kinase inhibitor
TLD	thermoluminescent dosimetry
TLH	total laparoscopic hysterectomy
TLM	transoral laser microsurgery
TME	total mesorectal excision
TMR	tissue maximum ratio
TMZ	temozolomide
TNBC	triple-negative breast cancer
TNF	tumor necrosis factor
TNM	tumor, nodes, metastasis classification system
TNT	total neoadjuvant therapy
ToGA	trastuzumab for gastric cancer
TORS	transoral robotic surgery
TPF	docetaxel, cisplatin, fluorouracil
TROG	Trans-Tasman Radiation Oncology Group
TRUS	transrectal ultrasound
TS	tumor size
TSE	turbo spin echo
TSEBT	total skin electron beam therapy
TSH	thyroid-stimulating hormone
TTF	tumor-treating fields
TTF1	thyroid transcription factor-1
TTP	time to progression
TURBT	transurethral resection of bladder tumor
TURP	transurethral resection of the prostate
TV	treated volume
TVC	true vocal cord
TVI	tumor-vessel interface
TVL	tenth-value layer
UA	urinalysis
UCSF	University of California San Francisco

Ucx urine culture
UH unfavorable histology
ULN upper limit of normal
UPS undifferentiated pleomorphic sarcoma
URI upper respiratory infection
US ultrasound
USPSTF United States Preventive Services Task Force
UTI urinary tract infection
UV ultraviolet
VA Veterans Administration
VAA vincristine/actinomycin D/Adriamycin
VAC vincristine/dactinomycin/cyclophosphamide
VATS video-assisted thoracic surgery
VB vertebral body
VBT vaginal brachytherapy
VCE vincristine/carboplatin/etoposide
VDC vincristine/doxorubicin/cyclophosphamide
VDC/IE vincristine/doxorubicin/cyclophosphamide (VDC) alternating w/ ifosfamide/etoposide (IE)
VEGF vascular endothelial growth factor
vGTV virtual gross tumor volume
VIP VP-16/ifosfamide/cisplatin
VMA vanillylmandelic acid
VMAT volumetric-modulated arc therapy
VOD veno-occlusive disease
VTE venous thromboembolism
WA wedge angle
WAGR WT, aniridia, GU malformations, retardation
WAI whole-abdomen irradiation
WART whole pelvic radiation therapy
WBC white blood cell count
WBI whole-breast irradiation
WBRT whole-brain radiation therapy
WF weighting factor
WHO World Health Organization
WLE wide local excision
WLI whole-lung irradiation
WPRT whole-pelvis RT
WT Wilms tumor
WV-PTV whole ventricular planning target volume
WVRT whole ventricle RT
XRT radiation therapy

Page numbers followed by "f" denote figures; those followed by "t" denote tables

D

F

J

K

M

O

P

T

BT 2-3

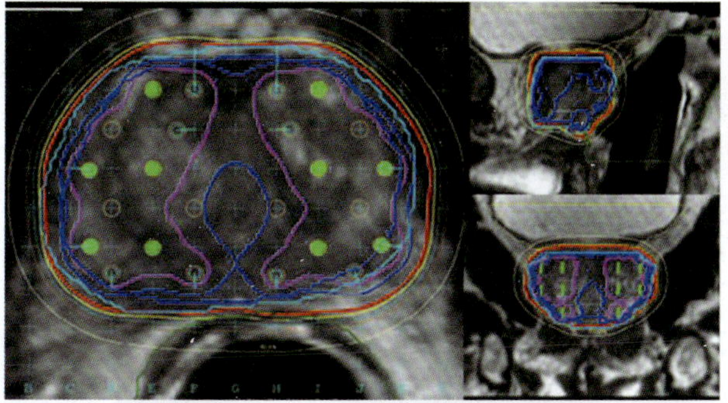

A

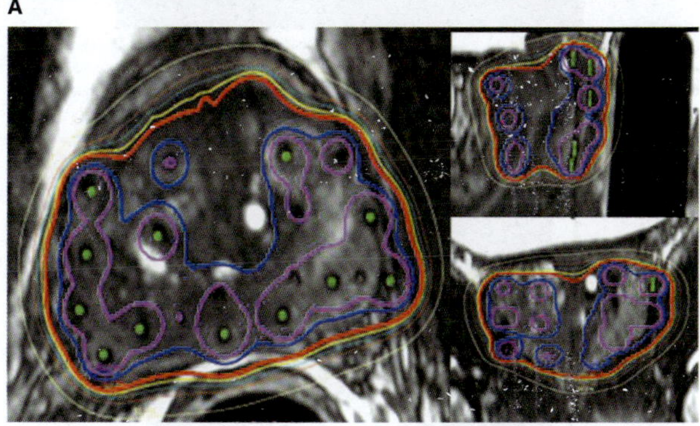

B

Figure 6.1 Example MRI LDR preplan **(A)** and D0 **(B)** plan for 144 Gy I-125 brachytherapy monotherapy implant to treat intermediate-risk prostate cancer. Showing the 100%, 150%, and 200% isodose lines.

PT 2-9

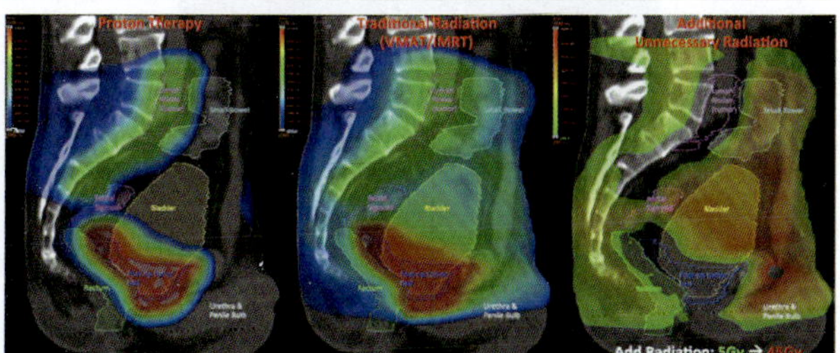

Figure 7.2 Comparative plan showing intensity-modulated proton therapy (*left*) vs a VMAT/IMRT plan (*middle*). Excess radiation dose (*right*) is calculated by subtracting the proton therapy plan from the VMAT/IMRT plan.

HGG 3-7

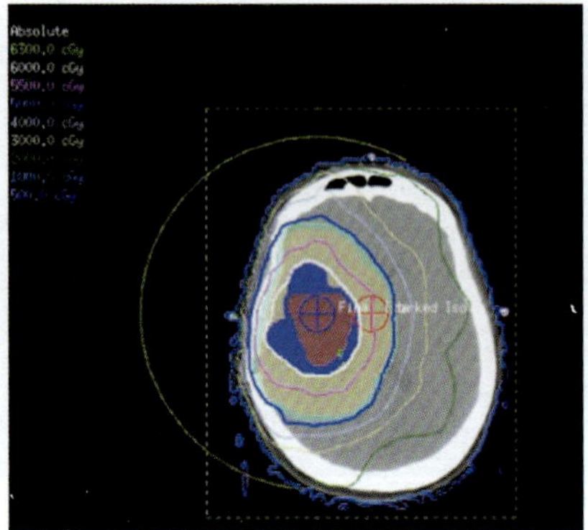

Figure 10.2 Representative plan for a patient with a grade 4 glioblastoma. The 60-Gy isodose line (*white*) can be seen surrounding the red GTV/resection cavity (*red color wash*). The 50-Gy isodose line (*blue*) covers GTV + 2 cm (*tan color wash*), which is expanded to include hyperintense signal on T2-FLAIR sequence.

OC 5-3

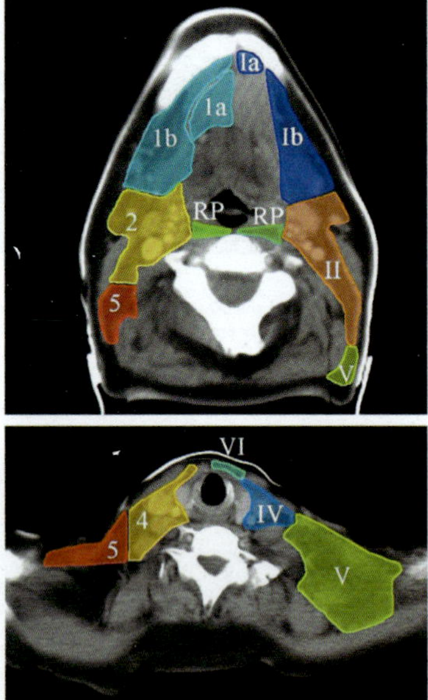

Figure 23.2 Axial CT images showing LN levels at the lower edge of the mandible (*upper panel*) and low neck (*lower panel*). (Reprinted from Grégoire V, Levendag P, Ang KK, et al. CT-based delineation of lymph node levels and related CTVs in the node-negative neck: DAHANCA, EORTC, GORTEC, NCIC, RTOG consensus guidelines. Radiother Oncol. 2003;69(3):227-236. Copyright © 2003 Elsevier Ireland Ltd. With permission.)

OC 5-4

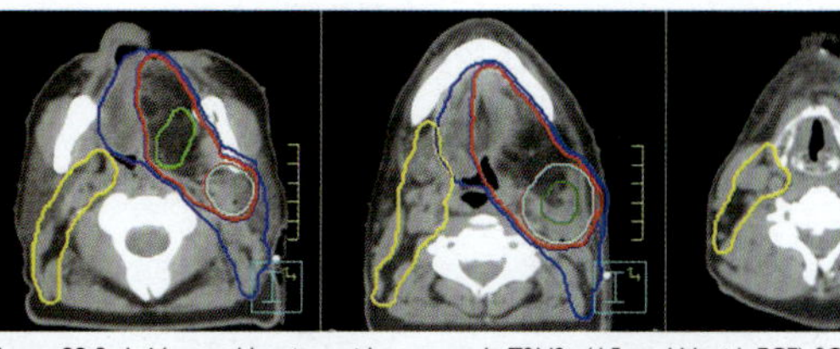

Figure 23.3 A 64-year-old patient with a resected pT2N2a (4.5 cm LN with ECE) SCC of the oral tongue reconstructed with a pectoralis flap treated with chemoRT. GTV (*green*), GTV-N (*forest green*), CTV63 (*aqua*), CTV60 (*red*), CTV57 (*blue*), and CTV54 (*yellow*) in 30 fractions.

TC 5-30

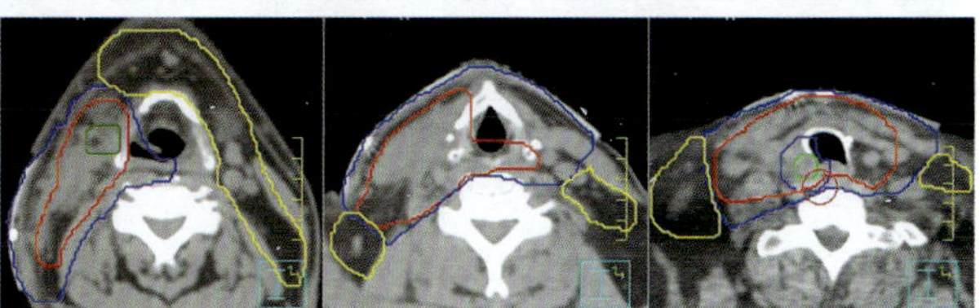

Figure 28.1 A 74-year-old patient with four previous resections for papillary thyroid cancer. Following surgery, he was found to have a 3-cm right level II node with ECE, 2/10 level right level III nodes up to 2 cm, as well as a right tracheal sidewall mass resected with SM+. Contours shown are GTV-LN (*green*), CTV63 (*purple*), CTV60 (*red*), CTV57 (*blue*), and CTV54 (*yellow*). Treatment was delivered utilizing simultaneous integrated boost in 30 fractions.

UHNP 5-34

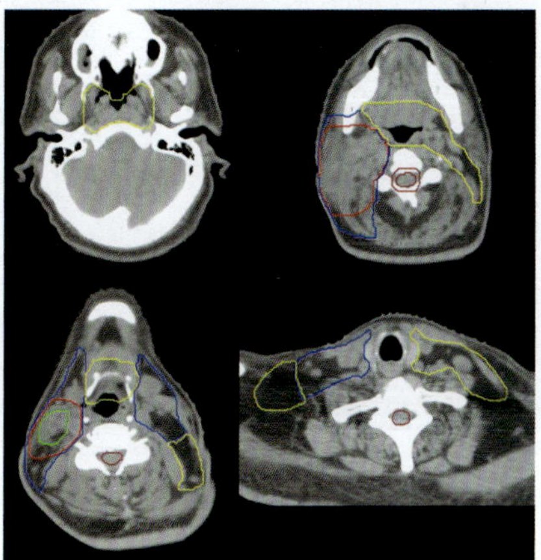

Figure 29.1 Target volumes for CUP with metastasis to right LN levels II-III, showing CTVHD (*red*), CTV_{ID} (*blue*), and CTV_{ED} (*yellow*).

SCLC 6-13

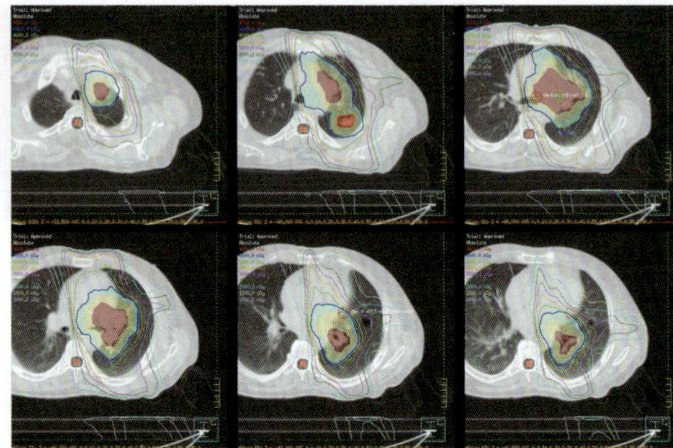

Figure 32.3 Limited stage SCLC IMRT plan. 45 Gy isodose line showed in blue surrounding PTV (*sky blue color wash*), CTV (*tan*), and GTV (*red*). Note sparing of contralateral lung.

ESOPHAGEAL 6-25

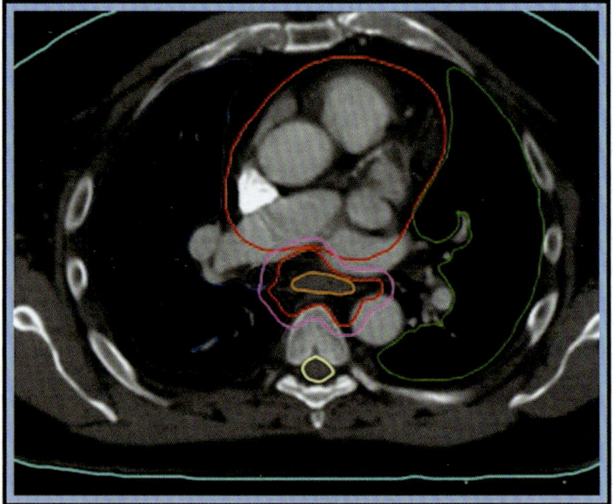

Figure 35.2 Representative cross-sectional image illustrating typical contours for an esophageal adenocarcinoma patient. GTV, CTV, and PTV contours showed in *orange*, *red*, and *pink*, respectively.

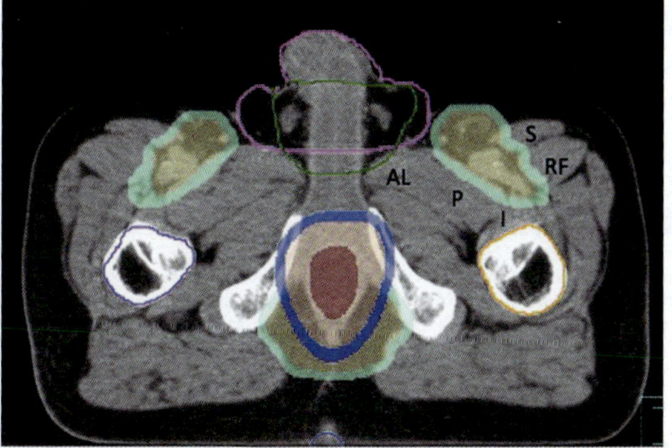

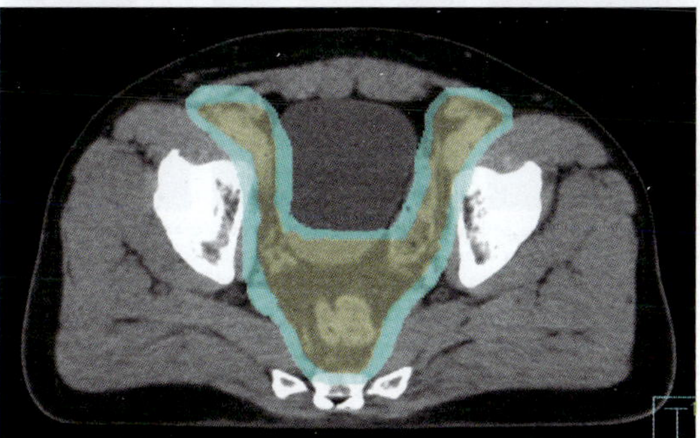

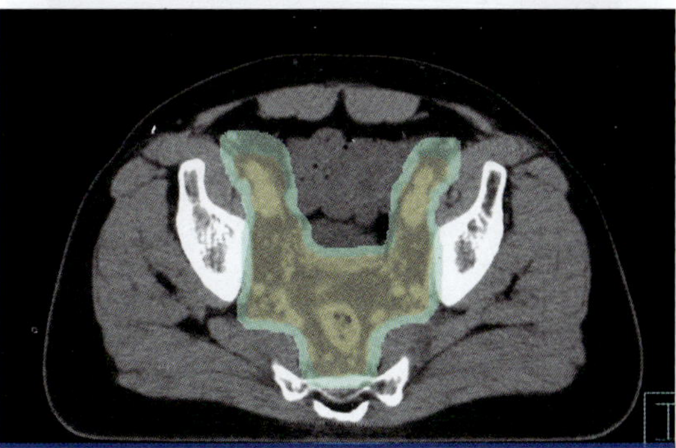

Figure 37.1 RTOG Atlas (used for RTOG 0529): https://www.rtog.org/CoreLab/ContouringAtlases/Anorectal.aspx. (Australasian GI Trials Group Atlas: *Ng et al. Int J Radiat Oncol Biol Phys* 2012; Inguinal Nodal Atlas: *Kim et al. Pract Radiat Oncol* 2012.)

PC 7-13

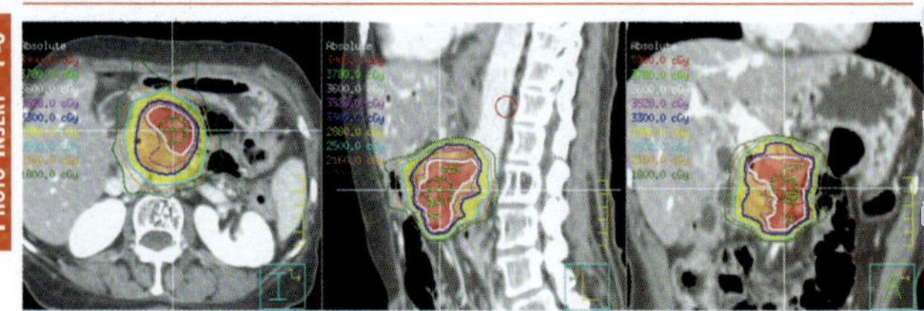

Figure 38.1 Representative cross-sectional axial, sagittal, and coronal images (L→R) from a SBRT treatment plan for locally advanced pancreatic cancer. The *white* isodose line represents 36 Gy encompassing the *red color* wash, which delineates PTV3 (tumor-vessel interface minus PRV). The *sky-blue* isodose line represents 25 Gy, which is encompassing the *yellow contour* that represents PTV1 (gross tumor + TVI + 3 mm). This patient had fiducials placed, which was used daily for image guidance along with CBCT.

GC 7-17

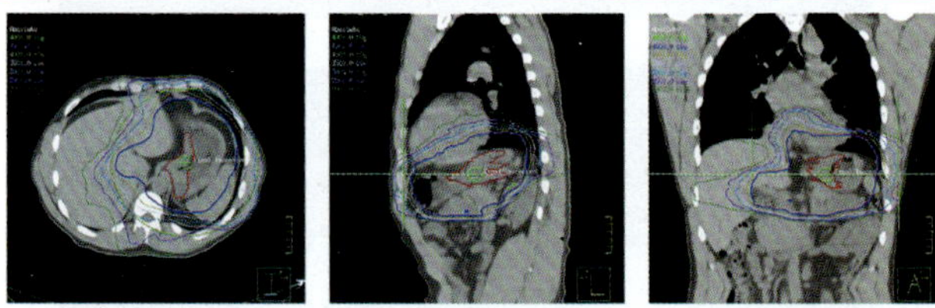

Figure 39.2 Representative axial, sagittal, and coronal cross-sectional images (L → R) illustrating a typical IMRT treatment plan for preoperative radiation for gastric adenocarcinoma. The 45-Gy isodose line is shown in *blue*, which encompasses the MTV (*red line*), involved and elective nodes, with a 1-cm expansion. This patient's primary tumor was located at the GEJ extending 4 cm into the cardia.

LABC 8-17

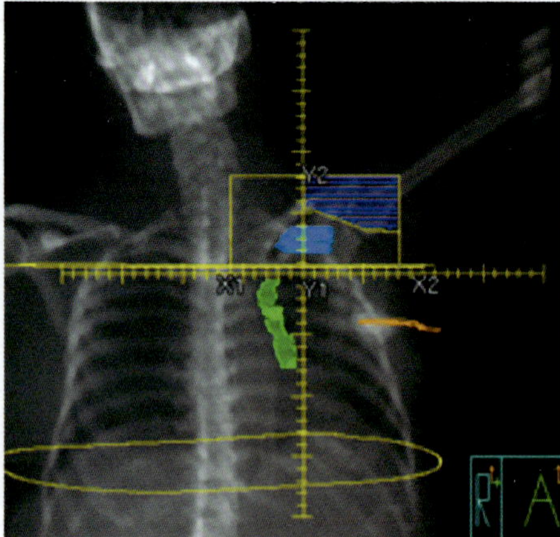

Figure 44.1 Supraclavicular/infraclavicular field design: DRR matched to nondivergent tangent fields. Contours: blue, level III axilla on DRR; green, IM nodes in 1st 3 interspaces; orange, mastectomy scar. Lines: yellow, superior and inferior borders of tangent fields. Blocks: purple, humeral head block.

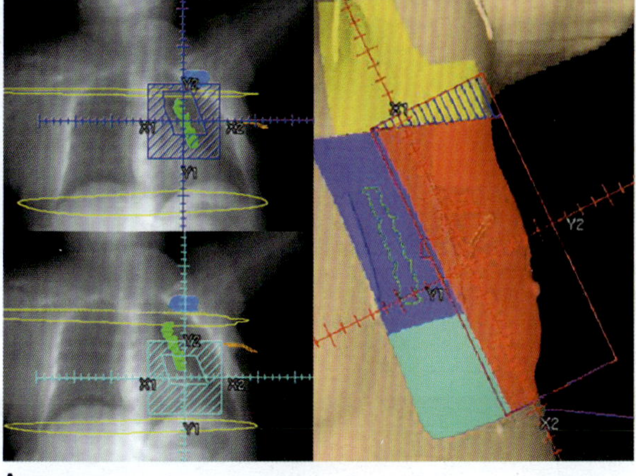

A

Figure 44.2 A. IMC Field Design: DRRs and skin rendering matched to nondivergent tangent fields and SCV field. Contours: Blue, Level III axilla on DRR; Green, IM nodes in 1st 3 interspaces; Orange, Mastectomy scar. Lines: Yellow, Superior and inferior borders of tangent fields. Fields: Yellow, AP oblique SCV field; Purple/Aqua, appositional upper and lower IMC fields; Red, Medial tangent field.

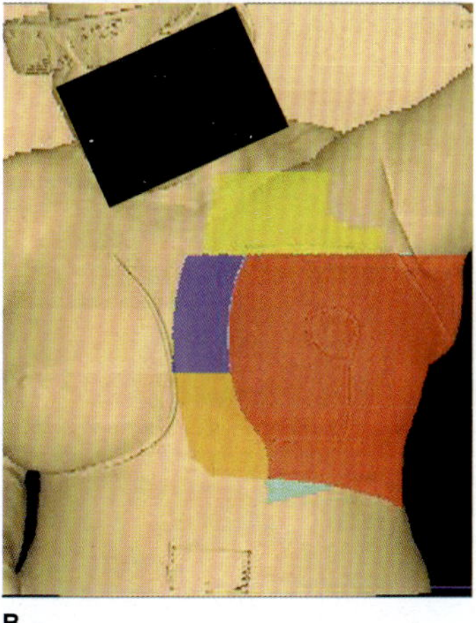

B

Figure 44.2 B. Composite Skin Rendering of Comprehensive Treatment Fields (w/o Boost). Fields: Yellow, AP oblique SCV field; Purple/Orange, appositional upper and lower IMC fields; Red/Aqua, Medial and lateral tangent fields.

PC 9-9

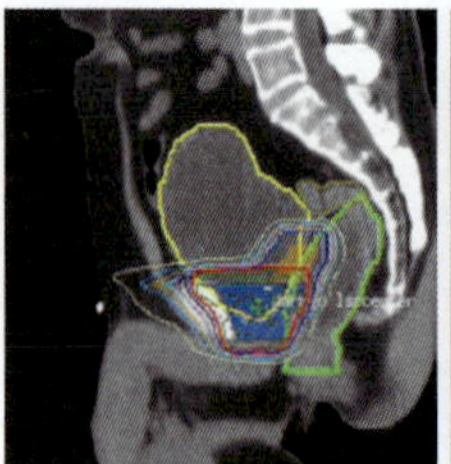

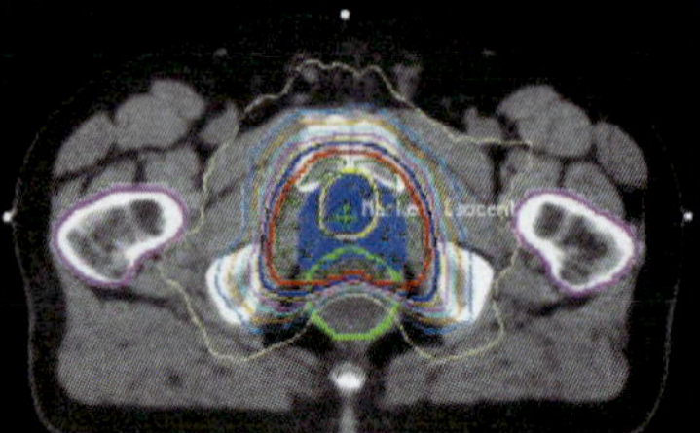

Figure 47.1 Sagittal and axial views showing an RT plan treating the prostate fossa to 70 Gy (*blue color wash*) and SV fossa (*yellow color wash*) to 63 Gy.

BC 9-13

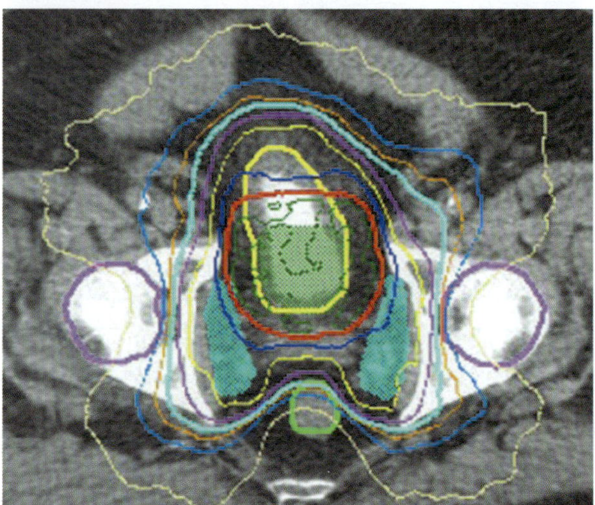

Figure 48.2 IMRT bladder conservation radiation plan treating to 45 Gy (*blue isodose line*) in 25 fractions to LNs and whole bladder followed by a sequential boost to the bladder resection cavity to 64.8 Gy (*red isodose line*) in 36 fractions.

CC 10-3

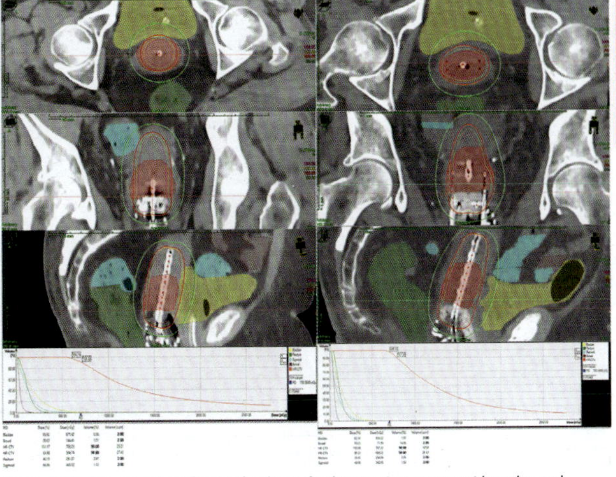

Figure 52.2 Plan comparison: fraction 1 utilizes a fixed intracavitary system with tandem and ovoids, fraction 2 utilizes a hybrid applicator with interstitial needles.

EC 10-9

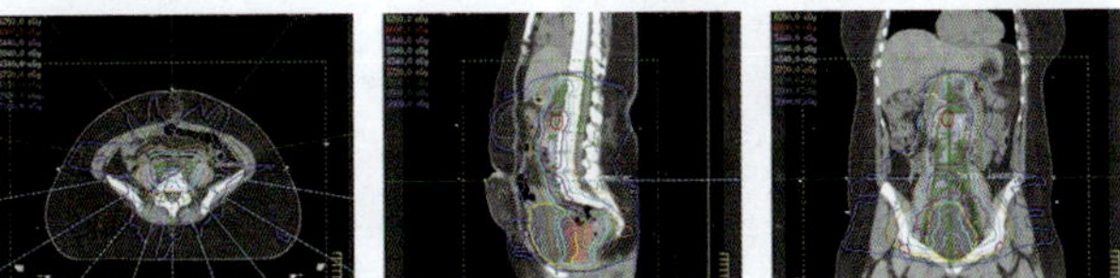

Figure 53.1 Extended-field IMRT (EFRT) plan. *Blue isodose line* representing 50.4 Gy is seen covering nodal CTV and vaginal ITV (*red colorwash*). *Red isodose line* representing 60 Gy is SIB to involved LN.

VC 10-18

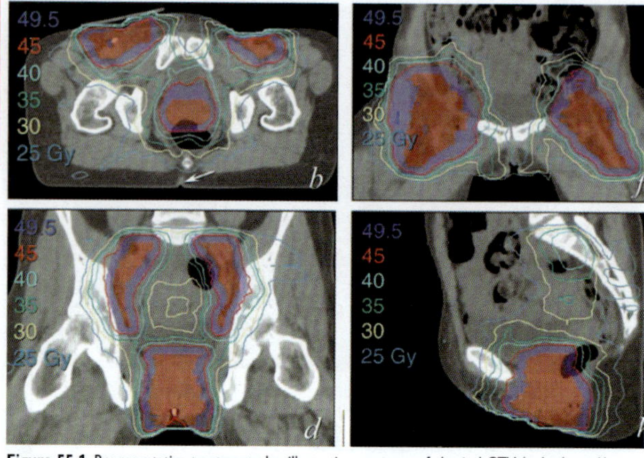

Figure 55.1 Representative treatment plan illustrating coverage of classical CTV (*red colorwash*) and PTV (*purple colorwash*) volumes for a vulvar cancer patient undergoing IMRT. (Reproduced with permission from Eifel and Klopp, *Gynecologic Radiation Oncology: A Practical Guide*).

STS 11-3

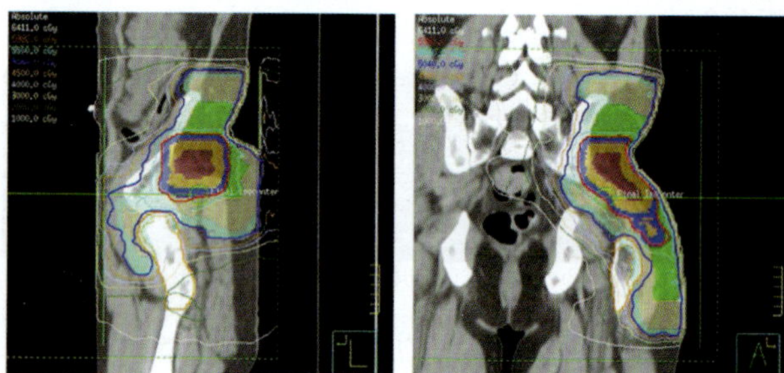

Figure 57.2 Representative sagittal and coronal (L → R) images of an IMRT treatment plan for a 40-year-old male being treated with adjuvant RT following R0 resection of a grade III PNET of the left lower extremity. Using IMRT in this case allowed for reduced dose to the left femoral head/ proximal femur. The *red isodose line* represents 59.92 Gy (covering GTV) and *blue* represents 50.40 Gy (covering CTV).

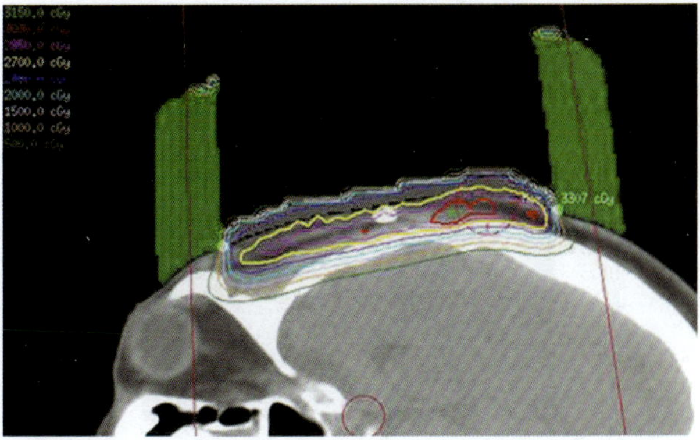

Figure 58.1 Sample RT treatment plan for a patient with a melanoma of the scalp. This patient was treated postoperatively with electrons to the tumor bed to a total dose of 30 Gy in 5 fractions. Note the 27 Gy isodose line in *yellow*, which is used to evaluate target coverage. 30 Gy hotspots are seen in *red*.

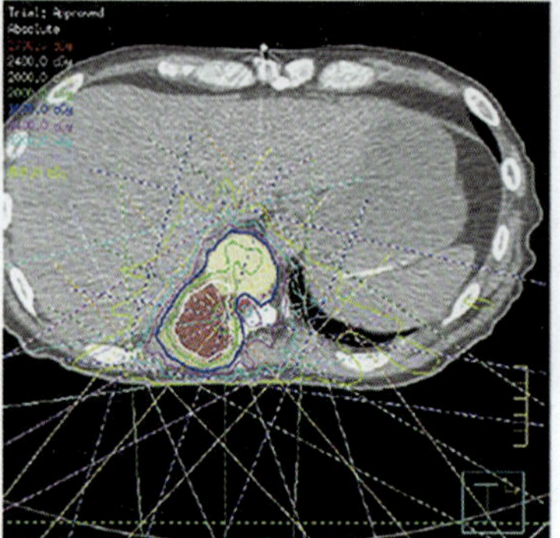

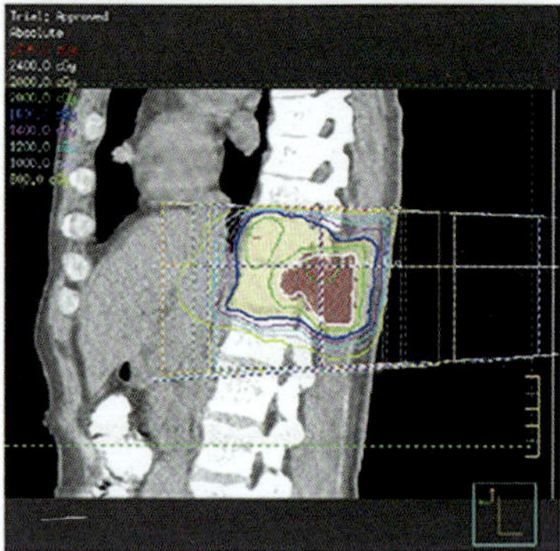

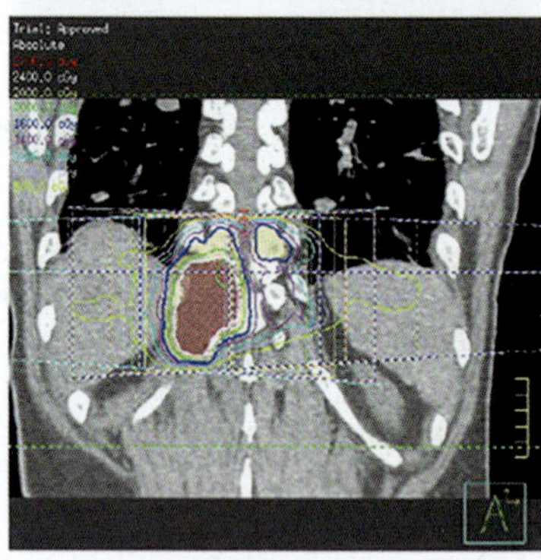

Figure 66.3 Representative treatment plan of a patient undergoing SSRS in axial, sagittal, and coronal (L → R) cross-sectional views. The CTV is highlighted in *yellow color* wash and GTV in *red*. The *blue isodose line* represents 16 Gy and *white isodose line* 24 Gy. This patient was treated with a single fraction.